Medicinal Plants: Anti-diabetic and Hypoglycaemic Activities

A.B. RAY
Professor (Retd.)
Department of Medicinal Chemistry, I.M.S.
Banaras Hindu University
C-38, Ashokpuram, Dafi, B.H.U.
Varanasi 221005 (U.P.)

J.P.N. CHANSOURIA
Senior Research Officer (Retd.),
Institute of Medical Sciences
Banaras Hindu University
24 Gandhinagar, Naria,
Varanasi 221005 (U.P.)

S. HEMALATHA
Reader
Department of Pharmaceutics, I.T.
Banaras Hindu University
Varanasi 221005 (U.P.)

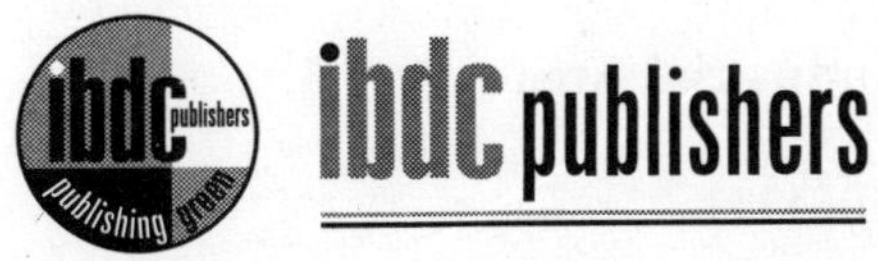

Published by

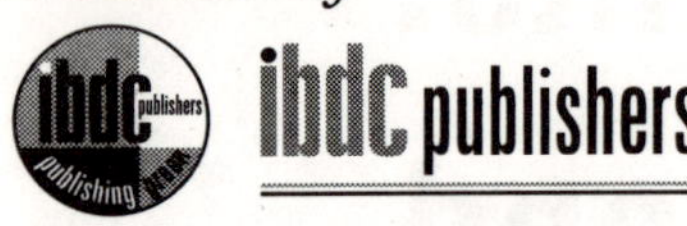

Khushnuma Complex Basement
7, Meerabai Marg (Behind Jawahar Bhawan)
Lucknow 226 001 U.P. (INDIA)
Tel. : 91-522-2209542, 2209543, 2209544, 2209545
Fax : 0522-4045308
E-Mail : ibdco@airtelmail.in

First Edition 2010

ISBN 978-81-8189-537-0

Composed & Designed at :

Panacea Computers
3rd Floor, Agarwal Sabha Bhawan, Subhash Mohal
Sadar Cantt. Lucknow-226 002
Phone : 0522-2483312, 9335927082
E-mail : prasgupt@rediffmail.com

Printed at:

Salasar Imaging Systems
C-7/5, Lawrence Road Industrial Area
Delhi - 110 035
Tel. : 011-27185653, 9810064311

Biswapati Mukherjee
M.Sc., Ph.D.
Former Professor and Executive Director
S.N. Pradhan Centre for Neurosciences
University of Calcutta
Kolkata-700020, India
Board Member
Asian Network of Research on Antidiabetic Plants (ANRAP)
BIRDEM, Dhaka, Bangladesh

AF 144/P 35 Saha Institute Co-operative
Kolkata-700101
Mobile : 91-9831187834
Fax : 91-33-22233260
e-mail : mukherjee.biswapati@gmail.com

Foreword

There are around 170 million people worldwide suffering from diabetes, almost five times more than the estimates ten years ago. This number may probably double by the year 2030. WHO has already forecast that in India alone the number of people with diabetes is likely to exceed 79 million by the year 2030. Diabetes with its complications is becoming a pandemic disease and if not properly controlled, the affected nations, will have to divert a lion's share of their health budget for its management.

Though there are several hypoglycaemic drugs available and newer agents and technologies are coming up but none is adequate for diabetic care. There is thus need for alternative strategies for combating this dreadful disease. Here lies the importance of the plant drugs which are being used in different forms from time immemorial for the treatment of diabetes in the Ayurveda and other traditional systems of medicine. Attention of the modern scientists has now been turned towards plants for development of ideal antidiabetic drugs. Tremendous work has been carried out so far on chemical and pharmacological aspects on huge number of plants in search of hypoglycaemic agents, but we are yet to receive the ideal drug for diabetes. This research on plant medicine is to be continued with further zeal and motivation to reach our goal for complete win over diabetes. In this endeavour a good compendium, describing the research work so far done on plants having antidiabetic/hypoglycaemic activity is necessary for future guidance to the scientific workers.

This book entitled, **"Medicinal Plants : Antidiabetic and Hypoglycaemic Activities"** written by Professor A.B. Ray, Dr. J.P.N. Chansouria and Dr. S. Hemlata will meet that demand. The authors are well known in their respective fields of research. They have collected carefully informations on the hypoglycaemic and antidiabetic activities of the plants on which work has been done during last thirty five years. These have been arranged alphabetically with concise description of the work supported by up-to-date references. In the Appendix of the book, very useful chapters on ***Antidiabetic herbal formulations, Dietary fibres in the management of diabetes, Hypoglycaemic glycans, Hypoglycaemic plant lectins and list of hypoglycaemic phytochemicals have been added.***

The readers may have a glimpse into the informations on about 600 plants before using any one of these as antidiabetic drug or initiating further research. I believe this book will find place by the side of the working desks of the students and researchers of modern science, pharmacy and ayurveda, interested in the eradication of diabetes and in the libraries of all biomedical institutions throughout the world.

I congratulate the authors for preparing such an authentic and useful document about plant medicine of diabetes.

B. Mukherjee

(Biswapati Mukherjee)

Preface

Drug potential of plants is well documented. The usefulness of medicinal plants as drugs, food supplements and also as adjuvant therapy in the management of diabetes mellitus, a metabolic disorder, has also been amply demonstrated by numerous research publications. Several review articles on the role of medicinal plants in the management of diabetes mellitus have appeared but what a researcher in this area needs is not merely a review but the total work done in the area, the findings of different workers on a particular plant as well of the plants that have been investigated and the present book fulfils that requirement. It is a compilation of brief summary of the publications in the area during the last 35 years in a systematic manner. In the book the plants, investigated for their anti-diabetic activity, have been arranged in alphabetical order and the research findings on the anti-hyperglycaemic, hypoglycaemic and antioxidant activity of each plant are presented in an orderly fashion;— the findings of similar nature are grouped together though the references are in chronological order. A brief description of each plant has been provided mainly on the basis of the information furnished by Wikipedia, the free encyclopedia. The common names of the plants and their Hindi (H.) and Sanskrit (S.) names have been shown, wherever possible. The essential sources of abstracts of research publications are Medicinal and Aromatic Plant Abstracts (MAPA) and online database of Pub Med., a service of the US National Library of Medicine. Besides the main text, the book provides an Appendix which covers the topics like Anti-diabetic herbal formulations, Dietary fibres in the management of diabetes, Phytochemicals with anti-diabetic potential etc. The structures of the plant-derived chemicals together with their sources and appropriate references are shown in a tabular form. We are thankful to Dr. Biswapati Mukherjee, Former Professor and Executive Director, S. N. Pradhan Centre for Neurosciences, Kolkata and Board Member, Asian Network of Research on Anti - diabetic Plants, Dhaka, for writing the Foreword of the book. We hope that the book will be helpful to researchers in the area and to all those who are interested to know the useful contribution of plants in controlling this rather dreadful disease.

A B Ray
J. P. N. Chansouria
S. Hemalatha

INTRODUCTION

Diabetes mellitus is known to mankind since antiquity. The disease has been mentioned in the **Vedas**, which is considered to be the first documented knowledge about it. Even in Ayurvedic classics, aetiological factors, symptomatology and management of diabetes mellitus have been described in great detail.

Diabetes mellitus, a group of metabolic disorders, is characterized by an excess of sugar in the blood and urine, hunger, thirst and gradual loss of body weight. It is caused either by inadequate secretion or action of insulin or both. Prolonged hyperglycaemia adversely affects almost all tissues and organs of the body, particularly eyes, nerves, kidneys and blood vessels.

Diabetes mellitus has emerged as a major global health problem. Epidemiological profile and future trends indicate that there may be 354 million patients suffering from this crippling disease world wide by the year 2030. Rapid economic development and urbanization of Asian countries, particularly India, has immensely contributed to a sharp increase in the incidence of the disease in this part of the globe. The incidence of diabetes mellitus in India is increasing at an alarming rate and it is predicted that India may have the maximum number of diabetic patients in the world by the end of the year 2030. .

The major predisposing factors of the disease include sedentary habits, changes in the life style and food habits which are usually linked with affluence. .The complications associated with this disease further worsen the situation and adversely affect all the systems of the body. Diabetic patients become more vulnerable to a number of degenerative complications and associated angiopathies etc.

It is known that hypertriglyceridaemia leading to atherosclerosis is more common in diabetic patients than in non-diabetics. Further, an increased incidence of stroke, coronary heart disease and peripheral vascular disorders in diabetic patients indicate that lipid metabolism is also deranged in this disease. In general, diabetes and its complications cut down the life expectancy and quality of life.

The treatment of diabetes mellitus primarily aims at achieving effective control of the elevated blood sugar levels. Proper and effective management of the disease help in correcting the metabolic disturbances and decreasing the incidence of its complications. Insulin and other oral anti-diabetic agents like biguanides, sulfonylureas and thiozolidinediones are known to help in effectively controlling hyperglycaemia but none of them are free from side effects. Chronic administration of insulin may lead to the development of insulin resistance, auto insulin antibodies, accidental hypoglycaemia and sensitivity reaction etc. Similarly, oral anti-diabetic agents may cause lactic acidosis, prolonged hypoglycaemia, hepatic toxicity and gastrointestinal disturbances etc. Apart from this, these anti-diabetic agents do not effectively address the diabetic complications. Therefore, search for an effective anti-diabetic agent with minimal side effects is warranted and this can be accomplished probably from plants, a vast store house of diverse chemical entities.

Potent hypoglycaemic activity, elicited by numerous plant extracts and the phytochemicals (alkaloids, saponins, flavonoids, polysaccharides, peptides, amino acids etc.) present in the extracts may provide important leads to the development of newer and effective anti-diabetic agents with minimum side effects. Numerous plants have also shown promising antioxidant activity, which may be useful in preventing some of the diabetic complications and protecting pancreas, kidney and liver of diabetic animals.

All the above mentioned properties of hypoglycaemic plants make them suitable candidates for ameliorating diabetes mellitus and its complications. Since diabetes is a multi-factorial disorder with several complications, it would be most desirable to use multiple therapeutic approaches. As the hypoglycaemic activity of several herbal extracts and pure phytochemicals has been confirmed in experimental and clinical studies, the WHO expert committee has recommended that the traditional medicinal herbs should be further investigated.

The use of plants with proven hypoglycaemic activity as adjuvant to known anti-diabetic drugs has been reported to reduce the doses and frequency of intake of chemical drugs. This may also help in minimizing the undesirable side effects of commercially available anti-diabetic drugs.

In this volume, the authors present a brief account of the work done on anti diabetic plants and published during the last 35 years or so. It is hoped that the information furnished in this book would familiarize the researchers in this area of investigation with the work already done in this field and help them planning future work for the development of more effective anti-diabetic drugs of plant origin.

APPENDIX

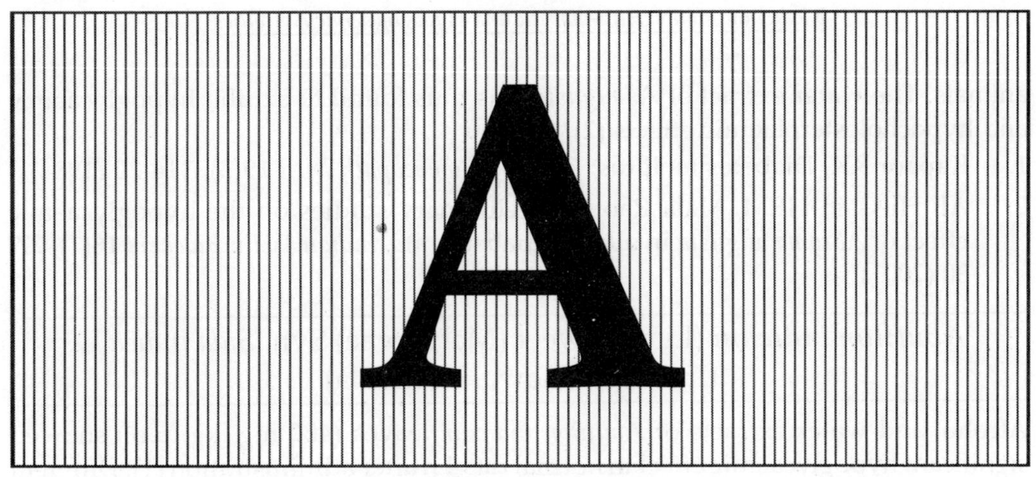

Abelmoschus moschatus Medik (Malvaceae) Syn. *Hibiscus abelmoschus* (Muskmallow)

Abelmoschus moschatus is an aromatic and medicinal plant, which is native to India. The seeds have a sweet, flowery fragrance similar to that of musk. Different parts of the plant have uses in traditional and complimentary medicine.

Intravenous injection of myricetin, a constituent of *Abelmoschus moschatus*, decreased the plasma glucose concentrations in a dose-dependent manner in streptozotocin-induced diabetic rats. Myricetin, at the effective dose (1.0 mg/kg), significantly attenuated the increase of plasma glucose, induced by an intravenous glucose challenge test in normal rats. This was obviously due to increase of glucose utilization by myricetin, which was substantiated from the observed enhancement of glycogen synthesis in isolated hepatocytes of streptozotocin-diabetic rats. These results suggested that myricetin has an ability to enhance glucose utilization to lower plasma glucose in diabetic rats lacking insulin.

Liu IM, SS Liou, TW Lan, FL Hsu JT Cheng; Myricetin as the active principle of *Abelmoschus moschatus* to lower plasma glucose in streptozotocin-induced diabetic rats, *Planta Med* **71**(7), 617-21 (2005)

Abroma augusta Linn. (Sterculiaceae) (Devils cotton)

Abroma augusta is one of the two species of the genus *Abroma* and it is regarded as the Asian species. *A. augusta* is reported as an effective plant drug for the treatment of diabetes mellitus. It is claimed to be a deep acting drug (1). Treatment of diabetic rats with the aqueous extract (4 ml) of the plant for 16 weeks resulted in a gradual but significant fall in fasting blood glucose level and improvement of glucose tolerance. The extract also showed improvements in the levels of serum total cholesterol, LDL-cholesterol and triacylglycerol, which are elevated in diabetic animals. The water extract of *A. augusta* was thus found to exhibit hypoglycaemic and hypocholesterolaemic effects (2).

1. Kapoor KK, Diabetes mellitus; *Indian J Homoeopath Med* **19**(3), 114-20 (1984)
2. Ali Hussain HEM, Mala Rao JK; Preliminary studies on the hypoglycaemic effect of *Abroma augusta* in alloxan diabetic rats, *Indian J Clin Biochem* **16**(1), 77-80 (2001)

Abutilon indicum (Linn.) Sweet (Malvaceae) Syn. *Sida indica* L. (Indian mallow, H. Atibala)

Alcohol and water extracts of *Abutilon indicum* leaves (400 mg/kg, p.o.) showed significant hypoglycaemic effect in normal rats 4 h after administration (1). Different extracts of A. indicum leaves showed significant hypoglycaemic activity at a dose of 400 mg/kg but the aqueous extract was most potent in reducing the blood glucose level. The presence of steroids, sapogenins and flavonoids were detected in the leaves of the plant (2).

1. Seetharam YN, G Chalageri, SR Setty, Bheemachar; Hypoglycaemic activity of *Abutilon indicum* leaf extracts in rats, *Fitoterapia* **73**(2), 156-59 (2002)
2. Lakshmayya, NR Nelluri, Pramod Kumar, NK Agarwal, TS Gouda, SR Setty; Phytochemical and pharmacological evaluation of leaves of *Abutilon indicum, Indian J Trad Knowledge* **2**(1), 79-83 (2003)

Acacia arabica Lam. (Fabaceae Leguminosae) (H. Babul)

Acacia arabica is the gum-Arabic tree of India but it yields a gum inferior to the true gum-Arabic, a product of *Acacia senegal*, abundant in dry tropical West Africa.

Administration of powdered seeds of *Acacia arabica* in doses of 2, 3 and 4 g/kg body weight to normal rabbits exerted a significant hypoglycaemic effect. The hypoglycaemic effect was not significant in alloxan diabetic rabbits. From this study it was concluded that the powdered seeds of *A. arabica* act by initiating the release of insulin from pancreatic *beta* cells of normal rabbits.

Wadood A, N Wadood, SA Shah; Effects of *Acacia arabica* and *Caralluma edulis* on blood glucose levels of normal and alloxan diabetic rabbits, *J Pak Med Assoc* **39**(8), 208-12 (1989)

Acacia catechu (L.) Willd., Oliv. (Fabaceae Leguminosae) (Catechu, H. Katha)

Acacia catechu is a deciduous, thorny tree, found in China, India and the Indian Ocean area. Hypoglycaemic activity of *A. catechu* seed diet was studied in normal albino rats.

Singh KN, RK Mittal, KC Barthwal; Hypoglycaemic activity of *Acacia catechu*, *Acacia suma*, and *Albizzia odoratissima* seed diets in normal albino rats, *Indian J Med Res* **64**(5), 754-57 (1976)

Acacia coriacea DC (Fabaceae Leguminosae) (Dogwood)

Acacia coriacea occurs throughout northern Australia and its seeds contain slowly digesting carbohydrate. It was observed that incorporation of the flour made from the seeds of *A. coriacea* into wheat bread (18 g/82 g wheat flour) significantly reduced the initial rise in plasma glucose levels and the area under the plasma glucose curve in six healthy subjects. Thus, *Acacia* flour when used to dilute wheat flour in the manufacture of breads, produces a very palatable food, which could be useful in the diets of diabetic individuals.

Thorburn AW, JC Brand, V Cherikoff, AS Truswell; Lower postprandial plasma glucose and insulin after addition of *Acacia coriacea* flour to wheat bread, *Aust N Z J Med* **17**(1), 24-26 (1987)

Acacia suma (Roxb.) Voigt (Fabaceae Leguminosae) Syn. *Acacia polyacantha* Willd

The hypoglycaemic activity of *Acacia suma* seed diet was assessed in normal albino rats.

Singh KN, RK Mittal, KC Barthwal; Hypoglycaemic activity of *Acacia catechu*, *Acacia suma*, and *Albizzia odoratissima* seed diets in normal albino rats, *Indian J Med Res* **64**(5), 754-57 (1976)

Acalypha ciliata Forsk (Euphorbiaceae)

Extract of the roots of *Acalypha ciliata*, a medicinal plant of Garhwal, India, exhibited hypoglycaemic activity.

Uniyal SK, S Bahuguna, OP Sati; Biological screening of extracts of some medicinal plants from Garhwal, *Herba Hungarica* **29**(1-2), 37-41 (1990)

Acanthopanax senticosus (Rupr. et Maxin) Harms (Araliaceae) Syn. *Eleutherococcus senticosus* (Siberian ginseng, Devils root)

Eleuthero is the new name for Siberian ginseng in the United States. It is different from both American ginseng and *Panax ginseng*. Eleuthero is used widely in eastern Asia as a tonic to enhance overall well-being. The saponin, isolated from the leaves of *Acanthopanax senticosus,* was tested for its hypoglycaemic effect. The saponin (100, 200 mg/kg, ip) was found to decrease blood sugar levels in various cases of experimental hyperglycaemia, induced by injection of adrenaline, glucose and alloxan, without affecting the levels of blood sugar in normal mice (1).

Oral administration (three times daily for 3 days) of an aqueous extract of the root of *A. senticosus* to rats that had received fructose-rich chow for 4 weeks reversed the elevated value of the glucose-insulin index (the product from areas under the curve of glucose and insulin during the intra-peritoneal glucose tolerance test), indicating that this herb has the ability to improve insulin sensitivity. Experiments also showed that this extract delayed the development of insulin resistance in rats. It may thus be used as an adjuvant therapy for patients with insulin resistance (2).

An ethanol (50%) extract of *A. senticosus* stem bark was found to reduce body weight and insulin resistance in high fat diet-induced hyperglycaemic and hyperlipidemic ICR mice. Treatment of insulin-resistant ob/ob mice with fatty livers for a period of 8 weeks reversed the hepatomegaly and specifically lowered circulating glucose and lipids, and enhanced insulin action in the liver. These changes culminated in inhibition of triglyceride synthesis in non-adipose tissues including liver and skeletal muscle. The ethanol extract of *A. senticosus* stem bark was thus proved to be an effective treatment for insulin resistance and hepatic steatosis in ob/ob mice by decreasing hepatic lipid synthesis (3).

1. Sui DY, ZZ Lu, SH Li, Y Cai; Hypoglycaemic effect of saponin isolated from leaves of *Acanthopanax senticosus* (Rupr. et Maxin.) Harms, *Zhongguo Zhong Yao Za Zhi* **19**(11), 683-85 (1994) [Article in Chinese]
2. Liu TP, CS Lee, SS Liou, IM Liu, JT Cheng; Improvement of insulin resistance by *Acanthopanax senticosus* root in fructose-rich chow-fed rats, *Clin Exp Pharmacol Physiol* **32**(8), 649-54 (2005)
3. Park SH, SG Lee, SK Kang, SH Chung; *Acanthopanax senticosus* reverses fatty liver disease and hyperglycaemia in ob/ob mice, *Arch Pharm Res* **29**(9), 768-76 (2006)

Acanthophyllum squarrosum Boiss (Caryophyllaceae)

The enhancing potential of saponins, isolated from *A. squarrosum,* on intranasal insulin absorption was studied and compared with that of Quillaja total saponin and sodium cholate. *A. squarrosum* saponin showed considerable insulin absorption enhancing effect and can possibly be used to increase insulin bioavailability *via* nasal route. However, the potential toxic effects of this saponin on nasal mucosa need evaluation.

Sajadi Tabassi SA, H Hosseinzadeh, M Ramezani, E Moghimipour, SA Mohajeri; Isolation, characterization and study of enhancing effects on nasal absorption of insulin in rat of the total saponin from *Acanthophyllum squarrosum, Curr Drug Deliv* **3**(4), 399-404 (2006); *Indian Journal of Pharmacology* **39**(5), 226-230 (2007)

Achillea ligustica All. (Asteraceae/Compositae) (Ligurian yarrow)

Achillea is a genus of flowering plants, commonly referred to as yarrow and are found in Europe and temperate areas of Asia. These plants typically have frilly, hairy, aromatic leaves. The antioxidant activities of the methanol extract of *A. ligustica* and of its fractions were carried out using two different *in vitro* assays (2,2-diphenyl-1-picrylhydrazyl test and lipid peroxidation of liposomes assay) and two different sets of result were obtained. Methanol extract showed higher radical scavenging activity on DPPH (IC_{50} of 50 μg/ml) than by lipid peroxidation of liposomes (IC_{50} of 416 μg/ml). The activity probably resides in the phenolic fraction of the extract as it showed an IC_{50} value of 22 mg /ml on DPPH test. The *alpha*-amylase inhibition assay was applied to evaluate anti-diabetic activity of the extracts. The methanol extract showed weak activity while its n-hexane-soluble fraction was quite active.

Conforti F, MR Loizzo, GA Statti, F Menichini; Comparative radical scavenging and anti-diabetic activities of methanolic extract and fractions from *Achillea ligustica* ALL, *Biol Pharm Bull* **28**(9), 1791-94 (2005)

Achyranthes aspera Linn. (Amaranthaceae/Chenopodiaceae) (H. Chirchidi, S. Apamarga)

Oral administration of powdered whole plant of *A. aspera* (2, 3 and 4 g/kg) produced a significant dose-related hypoglycaemic effect in normal as well as in diabetic rabbits. Similar effect was also observed with aqueous and methanol extracts of the plant. A 7-day acute toxicity study in rabbits (8 g/kg p.o.) did not reveal any adverse or side effects of this folk medicine.

Akhtar MS., J Iqbal; Evaluation of the hypoglycaemic effect of *Achyranthes aspera* in normal and alloxan-diabetic rabbits, *J Ethnopharmacol* **31**(1), 49-57 (1991).

Achyrocline satureioides (Lam) DC (Asteraceae)

Oral administration (20 mg/kg q.d) of achyrofuran, a prenylated dibenzofuran isolated from an extract of *Achyrocline satureioides*, significantly lowered blood glucose levels in db/db mouse model for type-2 diabetes.

Carney JR, JM Crenisky, RT Williamson, J Luo; Achyrofuran, a new anti-hyperglycaemic dibenzofuran from the South American medicinal plant *Achyrocline satureioides*, *J Nat Prod* **65**(2), 203-05 (2002).

Aconitum carmichaeli Debeaux (Ranunculaceae) (Chinese aconite)

The plant is native to China and bears extraordinary flowers on a sturdy plant. The whole plant is highly toxic.

See Glycans in Addendum for aconitans A, B, C and D (1, 2).

Oral administration of Hei-Shug-Pian, the fire-processed product of the root of *A. carmichaeli* (12.5-50 mg/kg), to strptozotocin-induced diabetic rats decreased plasma glucose level in a dose-dependent manner after 120 min. Under treatment conditions, the uptake of glucose into soleus muscle was increased and the incorporation of glucose into glycogen of hepatocytes was enhanced. The plasma glucose-lowering effect of Hei-Shug-Pian was eliminated by blockade of opioid μ-receptors. The findings led to infer that the drug lowers the plasma glucose concentrations of streptozotocin-induced diabetic rats through activation of mu (μ) opioid receptors (MOR) of peripheral tissues, resulting in enhanced glucose utilization (3).

1. Konno C, M Murayama, K Sugiyama, M Arai, M Murakami, M Takahashi, H Hikino; Isolation and hypoglycaemic activity of aconitans A, B, C and D, glycans of *Aconitum carmichaeli* roots, *Planta Med* **(2)**, 160-61 (1985)
2. Hikino H, M Kobayashi, Y Suzuki, C Konno; Mechanisms of hypoglycaemic activity of aconitan A, a glycan from *Aconitum carmichaeli* roots, *J Ethnopharmacol* **25**(3), 295-304 (1989).
3. Liou SS, IM Liu, MC Lai; The plasma glucose lowering action of Hei-Shug-Pian, the fire-processed product of the root of Aconitum (*Aconitum carmichaeli*), in streptozotocin-induced diabetic rats, *J Ethnopharmacol* **106**(2), 256-62 (2006)

.*Acosmium panamense* Benth. Yakolev (Fabaceae)

Oral administration of water extract of *A. panamense* bark, at doses of 20 and 200 mg/kg, significantly lowered the plasma glucose levels in streptozotocin-induced diabetic rats within 3 h. Butanol extract of the plant bark, at doses of 20 and 100 mg/kg, showed similar effect. Glibenclamide, used as reference, showed hypoglycaemic effect very much like the extracts.

Andrade-Cetto A, H Wiedenfeld; Hypoglycaemic effect of *Acosmium panamense* bark on streptozotocin diabetic rats, *J Ethnopharmacol* **90**(2-3), 217-20 (2004)

Acrocomia mexicana Karw.ex Mast. (Arecaceae) (Feather palm)

Methanol extract of *A. mexicana* showed a significant blood sugar lowering effect in normal and alloxan-diabetic mice, when administered at 2.5 to 40 mg/kg i.p.

doses, and it exhibited a dose-dependent response in the mice models. Coyolosa, a new tetrahydropyran compound and assumed to be an unusual disaccharide, was isolated from this extract and it also showed hypoglycaemic activity.

Perez S, RM Perez, C Perez, MA Zavala, R Vargas; Coyolosa, a new hypoglycaemic from *Acrocomia mexicana, Pharm Acta Helv* **72**(2), 105-11 (1997)

Adhatoda vasica (L) Nees (Acanthaceae)
(S. Simha Mukhi, H. Vasa)

The plant is found throughout India and particularly in the Himalayan mountain area up to 1.000 meters above sea level. In Sanskrit, the plant is called "Simha mukhi" because the shape of its flowers resembles a lion's head. In addition to respiratory stimulant activity, the alcoholic extract of the leaves of the plant exhibits hypoglycaemic activity.

Rao VSN, KS Krishnaiah; Pharmacological investigations on *Adhatoda vasica* Nees (Vasaka), *Ind Vet J* **58**(2), 107-11 (1981)

Adiantum capillus-veneris Linn. (Adiantaceae)
(Black Maidenhair Fern)

Adiantum capillus-veneris is a species of fern, native to western and southern Europe, Africa, North and Central America. Aqueous extract of the fern was prepared by boiling dried plant material with water. An improvement in glucose tolerance was observed in Swiss mice that were loaded with glucose after the extract had been given by oral gavage. Similar result was observed with an alcoholic extract, prepared by macerating dried plant material with 80% ethanol.

Neef H, P Deelereq, G Lackeman; Hypoglycaemic activity of selected European plants, *Phytother Res* **9**(1), 45-48 (1995)

Aegle marmelos Correa (Rutaceae)
(S. Bilwa, H. Bael)

Aegle marmelos is a fruit-bearing tree, which is cultivated throughout India, Sri Lanka, Java and in the Philippines. It is widely used in Indian Ayurvedic medicine for the treatment of diabetes mellitus. Different parts of the plant, particularly the leaves and fruits of the plant, are most commonly used for the purpose but use of root bark and seeds are also on record.

The aqueous extract of *A. marmelos* leaves and alcoholic extract of its fruits were found to significantly lower the blood sugar levels of normal rabbits but were virtually ineffective in diabetic animals (1). Aqueous and alcoholic extracts of *A. marmelos* leaves, at a dose of 500 mg/kg, produced hypoglycaemia in normal fasting rats (3).The aqueous extract of root bark of *A. marmelos*, used in Sri Lanka for the treatment of diabetes, showed significant hypoglycaemic activity in rats (2).

The potential anti-diabetic effect of *A. marmelos* leaf extract was studied in alloxan-induced animal model. Oral administration of *A. marmelos* leaf extract to diabetic animals brought down the blood glucose level near control levels. An increased glucose tolerance was also observed in animals, given the leaf extract prior to the experiment. A significant decrease in liver glycogen, observed in diabetic rats, was brought to almost the normal level by treatment with leaf extract. The leaf extract treatment also decreased the blood urea and serum cholesterol levels. The extract produced an effect similar to that observed in animals treated with insulin injection (4). Similar anti-diabetic effect was also observed with the alkaloid fraction of the leaf extract (5). The leaf extract also exhibited anti-hyperglycaemic effect in alloxanised rabbits (6). The leaf extract is also reported to exhibit hypoglycaemic effect in normoglycaemic rats and anti-hyperglycaemic activity by increasing the plasma insulin levels in streptozotocin-induced diabetic rats (8). The effects of *A. marmelos* leaf extract on histological and ultra structural changes in tissues of streptozotocin-induced diabetic rats were studied by light and electron microscopic examination. The changes in the liver and kidney tissues and the altered functions of pancreatic *beta*-cells and the acinar cells of rats, rendered diabetic with streptozotocin (45 mg/kg b.w.), were almost normalised by treatment with the leaf extract (7). Malate dehydrogenase (MDH) is an important enzyme in glucose metabolism and its variation contributes to the pathological status of diabetes. The kinetic parameters of MDH were studied in the liver of streptozotocin-induced diabetic rats and also the potential of the leaf extract of *A. marmelos* as an anti-diabetic agent was investigated. The K_m value (Michaelis-Menten constant) of the liver enzyme (MDH) increased significantly, in both crude and purified preparations in the diabetic state when compared to the respective controls. Insulin as well as leaf-extract treatment of the diabetic rats brought about a reversal of K_m'values to near normal. The fact that leaf extract of *A. marmelos* was found to be as effective as insulin in restoration of blood glucose and body weight to normal levels suggested , the use of *A. marmelos* as a potential hypoglycaemic agent (9). Biochemical studies in streptozotocin-induced diabetic rats confirmed the potent hypoglycaemic activity of an aqueous extract *A. marmelos* leaves and suggested it to be an oral substitute for insulin (10).

Administration of a methanol (70%) extract of *A. marmelos* to alloxan-induced diabetic rats showed that the treatment lowered alloxan-induced lipid peroxidation and altered superoxide dismutase and catalase enzymes to reduce oxidative stress (11). The anti-diabetic and antioxidant activities of methanol extract of the plant were superior to those of other commonly used herbal drugs (16). The effect of alcoholic extract of *A. marmelos* leaves on glucose tolerance in glucose induced hyperglycaemic rats (Charles foster) was studied. Oral administration of the extract of *A. marmelos* (250 mg/kg) to the animals for seven consecutive days, showed significant improvements in their ability to utilize the external glucose load. Average blood glucose lowering caused by *A. marmelos* was found to be 67% and it was speculated that increased utilization of glucose, either by direct stimulation of glucose uptake or by the mediation of enhanced insulin secretion was the probable mechanism of action (12). Oxidative stress induced by alloxan has been shown to damage pancreatic *beta*-cells and produce hyperglycaemia in rats. Oxidative stress, produced by alloxan, was significantly lowered by the administration of methanol extract of *Aegle marmelos* leaves. This was evident from a significant decrease in lipid peroxidation, conjugated diene and hydroperoxide levels in serum as well as in liver. *Aegle marmelos* extract effectively reduced the oxidative stress and produced a reduction in blood sugar (18). Estimation of glucose, urea and glutathione-S-transferase (GST) in plasma, glutathione (GSH) and malondialdehyde (MDA) levels in erythrocytes in control, diabetic as well as in diabetic albino rats receiving aqueous extract of *A. marmelos* leaves revealed a decrease in blood glucose level at the end of four weeks in diabetic rats receiving the *A. marmelos* leaf extract compared to the diabetic rats. Leaf extract treated group also showed an increase in erythrocyte GSH and a decrease in MDA in comparison to untreated diabetic animals. Owing to hypoglycaemic and antioxidant properties, *A. marmelos* leaf extract was considered to be useful in the long-term management of diabetes (20). A suspension of *A. marmelos* leaf powder was formulated and the prepared suspension reduced blood glucose level in alloxan-induced diabetic rabbits (22). Albino rats were treated with ethanol extract of two varieties (sweet and bitter) of *A. marmelos* leaves and their blood glucose lowering effect was studied using glucose oxidase assay method. Both the varieties exhibited hypoglycaemic activity in a dose dependent manner. Sweet variety (250 and 500 mg/kg) produced maximum blood glucose reduction at 6h, while the bitter variety at the same dose levels showed maximum reduction at 8h and this continued upto 24h (13).

Kamalakkanan and his group studied the hypoglycaemic activity of aqueous extract of *A. marmelos* fruit and published four papers. Administration of an aqueous extract of *Aegle marmelos* fruits (250 mg/kg) twice daily for 1 month to streptozotocin-induced diabetic rats and determination of blood glucose, plasma insulin, glycosylated hemoglobin, liver glycogen, and change in body weight led to the conclusion that treatment with the fruit extract reversed the effects of diabetes on these biochemical parameters to near-normal levels (14), Oral administration of the water extract (125 and 250mg/kg) of *A. marmelos* fruits twice a day for 4 weeks resulted in significant reductions in blood glucose, plasma thiobarbituric acid reactive substances, hydroperoxides, ceruloplasmin and *alpha*-tocopherol in streptozotocin-induced diabetic Wistar rats. A significant elevation in reduced glutathione and vitamin C was also noted in diabetic rats. The extract at a dose of 250mg/kg was more effective than glibenclamide (15). The fruit extract was also found to exhibit anti-oxidative activity in streptozotocin-induced diabetic rats. The depressed activities of superoxide dismutase, catalase and glutathione peroxidase and lowered glutathione content in the heart and pancreas of diabetic rats were found to increase on treatment with *A. marmelos* fruit extract. The activity of the antioxidant enzymes was found to be increased in the hepatic and renal tissues of diabetic animals treated with the fruit extract (17, 19). The protective effect of an aqueous extract of *A. marmelos* fruits on the histopathology of the pancreas in streptozotocin-induced diabetic rats was studied. Oral administration of *A. marmelos* fruit extract (125 and 250 mg/kg twice daily) to diabetic rats for a period of 30 days resulted in a significant increase in the weight of the pancreas and insulin levels associated with a significant decrease in fasting blood glucose levels. The fruit extract treated groups showed improved functional state of the pancreatic *beta*-cells and partially reversed the damage caused by streptozotocin to the pancreatic islets. The extract was thus found to exhibit protective effects on the pancreas (21).

Oral administration of aqueous extract of *A. marmelos* seeds (250 mg/kg) was found to decrease blood glucose level by 35.1% in normal healthy rats 6h after administration, by 41.2% in subnormal and by 33.2% in mild diabetic rats in glucose tolerance test after 2 h. Treatment of severely diabetic rats for 14 days with a dose of 250 mg/kg reduced the fasting blood glucose level by 60.84%. It also brought about a fall in the level of total cholesterol with an increase in HDL-cholesterol and a decrease in LDL-cholesterol and triglycerides. Aqueous extract of *A. marmelos* seeds was thus proved to possess anti-diabetic and hypolipidaemic effects in diabetic rats (23).

1. Vyas DS, VN Sharma, HK Sharma, NK Khanna; Preliminary study on anti-diabetic properties of *Aegle marmelos* and *Enicostemma littorale*, *J Res Indian Med Yoga Homoeopath* **14**(3-4),63-66 (1979)

2. Karunanayake EH, J Welihinda, SR Sirimanne, G Sinna dorai; Oral hypoglycaemic activity of some medicinal plants of Sri Lanka, *J Ethnopharmacol* **11**(2), 223-31 (1984).

3. Hema CG, K Lalithakumari; Screening of pharmacological actions of *Aegle marmelos*, *Indian J Pharmacol* **20**(2-4), 80-85 (1988)

4. Ponnachan PT, CS Paulose, KR Panikkar, Effect of leaf extract of *Aegle marmelose* in diabetic rats, *Indian J Exp Biol* **31**(4), 345-47 (1993)

5. Ponnachan PT, CS Paulos, KR Panikar; Hypoglycaemic effect of alkaloids of preparation from leaves of *Aegle marmelos*, *Amala Res Bull* **13**(Aug), 37-39 (1993)

6. Rao VV, SK Dwivedi, D Swarup,; SR Sharma; Hypoglycaemic and anti-hyperglycaemic effects of *Aegle marmelos* leaves in rabbits; *Curr Sci* **69**(11), 932-33 (1995)

7. Das AV, PS Padayatti, CS Paulose, Effect of leaf extract of *Aegle marmelose* (L.) Correa ex Roxb. on histological and ultra-structural changes in tissues of streptozotocin induced diabetic rats, *Indian J Exp Biol* **34**(4), 341-45 (1996}

8. Sharma SR, SK Dwivedi, VP Varshney, D Swarup; Anti-hyperglycaemic and insulin release effects of *Aegle marmelose* leaves in streptozotocin-diabetic rats,

Phytother Res **10**(5), 426-28 (1996)

9. Seema PV, B Sudha, PS Padayatti, A Abraham, KG Raghu, CS Paulose, Kinetic studies of purified malate dehydrogenase in liver of streptozotocin-diabetic rats and the effect of leaf extract of *Aegle marmelose* (L.) Correa ex Roxb, *Indian J Exp Biol* **34**(6), 600-02 (1996}
10. Bhavapriya V, S Govindasamy; Biochemical studies on the hypoglycaemic effect of *Aegle marmelos* (Linn) Correa ex Roxb in streptozotocin induced diabetic rats, *Indian Drugs* **37**(10), 474-477 (2000)
11. Sabu MC, R Kuttan; Inhibitory effect of *Aegle marmelos* on lipid peroxidation and anti-oxidant enzymes in blood and tissue in diabetic rats, *Amala Res Bull* **21**, 21-27 (2001)
12. Sachdewa A, D Raina, AK Srivastava, LD Khemani, Effect of *Aegle marmelos* and *Hibiscus rosa sinensis* leaf extract on glucose tolerance in glucose induced hyperglycaemic rats (Charles foster), *J Environ Biol* **22**(1), 53-57 (2001)
13. Rao PR, MD Babu, RVK Rao, S Nimmi; Comparative study of sweet and bitter varieties of *Aegle marmelos* (L) Correa in hypoglycaemic activity in rabbits, *J Nat Remedies* **2**(1), 88-91 (2002)
14. Kamalakkanan N, M Rajadurai, PS Prince, Effect of *Aegle marmelos* fruits on normal and streptozotocin-diabetic Wistar rats, *J Med Food* **6**(2), 93-98 (2003)
15. Kamalakkanan N, PS Prince; Hypoglycaemic effect of water extracts of *Aegle marmelos* fruits in streptozotocin diabetic rats, *J Ethnopharmacol* **87**(2-3), 207-10 (2003)
16. Sabu MC, R Kuttan; Antioxidant activity of Indian herbal drugs in rats with alloxan-induced diabetes, *Pharmaceut Biol* **41**(7), 500-05 (2003)
17. Kamalakkanan N, PSM Prince; Effect of *Aegle marmelos* Correa. (Bael) fruit extract on tissue antioxidants in streptozotocin diabetic rats, *Indian J Exp Biol* **41**(11), 1285-88 (2003)
18. Sabu MC, R Kuttan, Anti-diabetic activity of *Aegle marmelos* and its relationship with its antioxidant properties, *Indian J Physiol Pharmacol* **48**(1), 81-88 (2004)
19. Kamalakkannan N, PS Mainzen Prince; Anti-diabetic and antioxidant activity of *Aegle marmelos* extract in streptozotocin-induced diabetic rats, *Pharmaceut Biol* **42**(2), 125-30 (2004)
20. Upadhya S, KK Shanbhag, G Suneetha, M Balachandra Naidu, S Upadhya; A study of hypoglycaemic and antioxidant activity of *Aegle marmelos* in alloxan induced diabetic rats, *Indian J Physiol Pharmacol* **48**(4), 476-80 (2004)
21. Kamalakkanan N, PS Prince; The effect of *Aegle marmelos* fruit extract in streptozotocin diabetes: a histopathological study, *J Herb Pharmacother* **5**(3), 87-96 (2005)
22. Kalaiselvan V, V Ravichandran, A Dharamsi; Formulation and standardisation of *Aegle marmelos* suspension, *Hamdard Medicus* **18**(3), 55-58 (2005)

23. Kesari AN, RK Gupta, SK Singh, S Diwakar, G Watal; Hypoglycaemic and anti-hyperglycaemic activity of *Aegle marmelos* seed extract in normal and diabetic rats, *J Ethnopharmacol* **107**(3), 374-79 (2006)

Aerva lanata (L.) Juss. ex Schultes (Amaranthaceae) (S. Bhadram)

The effect of an alcoholic extract of *A. lanata* on blood glucose and other biochemical parameters was studied in alloxan-induced diabetic rats. The plant extract was found to reduce the increase of blood sugar in alloxan-induced diabetic rats. Chronic administration of *A. lanata* extract significantly reduced the blood sugar of alloxan-induced diabetic rats. From the results of the investigation, the plant extract was suggested to have anti-diabetic activity with the ability to ameliorate biochemical damages in alloxan-induced diabetic rats.

Vetrichelvan T, M Jegadeesan; Anti-diabetic activity of alcoholic extract of *Aerva lanata* (L.) Juss. ex Schultes in rats, *J Ethnopharmacol* **80**(2-3), 103-07 (2002).

Aesculus assamica Griff. (Sapindaceae)

Aesculus assamica is a widespread species in the tropical and subtropical monsoon forest zone from Northeast India eastward to South China and North Vietnam. Assamicin I and II, the two novel triterpenoid saponins, isolated from the roots of *Aesculus assamica*, were found to enhance glucose uptake into 3T3-L1 adipocytes and exhibit insulin-like activity.

Sakurai T, T Nishimura, N Otake, Y Xinsheng, K Abe, M Zeida, H Nagasawa, S Sakuda; Assamicin I and II, novel triterpenoid saponins with insulin-like activity from *Aesculus assamica* Griff, *Bioorg Med Chem Lett* **12**(5), 807-10 (2002).

Aesculus hippocastanum Linn. (Sapindaceae Hippocastanaceae) (Horse chestnut)

It is a large deciduous tree, commonly known as Horse-chestnut that is native to a small area in the mountains of Southeast Europe. It is widely cultivated throughout the temperate world. Its fruits are green, spiky capsules containing one or more nut-like seeds called horse-chestnuts. Escins-Ia, Ib, IIa, and IIb, the triterpene oligoglycosides isolated from the seeds of horse chestnut tree (*A. hippocastanum*), were found to exhibit hypoglycaemic activity in the oral glucose tolerance test in rats. Escins-IIa and IIb were more active than the other triterpene glycosides. The chemical structures of the all the compounds were fully determined on the basis of chemical and physicochemical evidence (1, 2).

1. Yoshikawa M, E Harada, T Murakami, H Matsuda, N Wariishi, J Yamahara, N Murakami, I Kitagawa; Escins-Ia, Ib, IIa, IIb, and IIIa, bioactive triterpene oligoglycosides from the seeds of *Aesculus hippocastanum* L.: their inhibitory effects

on ethanol absorption and hypoglycaemic activity on glucose tolerance test, *Chem Pharm Bull* (Tokyo) **42**(6), 1357-59 (1994).

2. Yoshikawa M, T Murakami, H Matsuda, J Yamahara, N Murakami, I Kitagawa; Bioactive saponins and glycosides. III. Horse chestnut. (1): The structures, inhibitory effects on ethanol absorption, and hypoglycaemic activity of escins Ia, Ib, IIa, IIb, and IIIa from the seeds of *Aesculus hippocastanum* L, *Chem Pharm Bull* (Tokyo) **44**(8), 1454-64 (1996).

Agarista mexicana (Hemsl.) Judd. (Ericaeae)

It is a shrub or tree, distributed in the mountainous areas of Mexico and Central America, Oral administration of a chloroform extract (100 , 150 mg/kg) of the plant produced a significant hypoglycaemic effect in normal as well as in diabetic mice and rats (1). The triterpenes (12-ursene and a novel triterpene based on stigmastane skeleton), isolated from the chloroform extract of the dried stem of *A. mexicana* by bioactivity-directed fractionation, were tested for hypoglycaemic activity in normal and alloxan-induced diabetic CD-1 mice. Intra-peritoneal administration of the triterpenes (50 mg/kg b.w.) produced a significant hypoglycaemic effect (comparable to tolbutamide) in normal as well as in diabetic mice (2).

1. Perez GRM, GS Perez, MA Zavala, GSC Perez; Effect of *Agarista mexicana* and *Verbesina persicifolia* on blood glucose level of normoglycaemic and alloxan-diabetic mice and rats, *Phytother Res* **10**(4), 351-53 (1996)
2. Perez GRM, SR Vargas; Triterpenes from *Agarista mexicana* as potential anti-diabetic agents, *Phytother Res* **16**(1), 55-58 (2002)

Agrimony eupatoria Linn. (Rosaceae) (Agrimony)

The plant is found abundantly throughout England, on hedge-banks and on all waste places. It is also quite common in Scotland. Incorporation of agrimony into the diet (62.5 g/kg) and drinking water (2.5 g/l) countered the weight loss, polydipsia, hyperphagia and hyperglycaemia of streptozotocin-induced diabetic mice. Aqueous extract of agrimony (1 mg/ml) stimulated the transport of 2-deoxy-glucose, oxidation of glucose and incorporation of glucose into glycogen in mouse abdominal muscle. The activity is comparable with 0.1 μM insulin. In acute 20 min tests, 0.25-1 mg/ml aqueous extract of agrimony evoked a stepwise stimulation of insulin secretion from the BRIN-BD11 pancreatic *beta*-cell line. The effect of extract was glucose-independent and was not evident in BRIN-BD11 cells exposed to a depolarizing concentration of KCl. The ability of agrimony extract to enhance insulin secretion was dependent on use of heat during extract preparation. The presence of anti-hyperglycaemic, insulin-releasing and insulin-like activity in *A. eupatoria* was thus demonstrated.

Gray AM, PR Flatt; Actions of the traditional anti-diabetic plant, *Agrimony eupatoria* (agrimony): effects on hyperglycaemia, cellular glucose metabolism and insulin secretion, *Brit J Nutr* **80**(1), 109-114 (1998).

Ajuga iva (L.) Schreiber (Lamiaceae / Labiatae) (Herb ivy)

Ajuga or Carpet bugle is a genus of annual and perennial herbaceous flowering plants in the mint family Lamiaceae. El-Hilaly and co-workers studied the hypoglycaemic effect of the lyophilised aqueous extract of *Ajuga iva,* a plant used in the treatment of diabetes in Moroccan folk medicine, in normal and streptozotocin-induced diabetic rats. Single and repeated oral administration of the extract at a dose of 10 mg/kg produced a slight but significant decrease in plasma glucose levels in normal rats 6 h after administration and after 3 weeks of treatment. Plasma glucose levels of streptozotocin-induced diabetic rats were also significantly reduced 6 h after oral administration of the extract. Repeated oral administration of the extract to these diabetic rats significantly decreased their plasma glucose levels, which became normal after 1 week of treatment. From the results of the investigation, aqueous extract of the whole plant of *A. iva* was proved to possess a strong hypoglycaemic effect in diabetic rats (1). In addition to its hypoglycaemic effect in normoglycaemic and diabetic rats, aqueous extract of *Ajuga iva* whole plant (10 mg/kg) produced a small but significant decrease in plasma cholesterol levels and caused a significant decrease in plasma triglycerides on sub-chronic dosing for up to 21 days in normal rats. In streptozotocin-induced diabetic rats, a single dose as well as a treatment for 3 weeks with the extract produced a significant decrease in plasma cholesterol and triglyceride levels. A lyophilised aqueous extract of *Ajuga iva* whole plant was thus found to exhibit hypolipidaemic activity, in addition to its hypoglycaemic effect in normoglycaemic and diabetic rats (3). The lyophilised aqueous extract of *A. iva* was found to be fairly non-toxic as no adverse effect was observed in mice after a single oral dose as high as 14 g/kg of this extract. However, single intra-peritoneal injection of the extract (1500-5500 mg/kg b.w.) produced a dose-dependent increase in adverse effects in the general behaviour and the mortality rate (LD_{50} of acute intra-peritoneal dose was 3.6 g/kg). Histopathological examination of the brain, liver and the kidneys at the end of a three-month study showed normal architecture suggesting no morphological disturbances. In view of the hypoglycaemic and hypolipidaemic activity, and its relatively non-toxic nature, *Ajuga iva* may be a candidate for development as an anti-diabetic agent in humans (2).

1. El-Hilaly J, B Lyoussi; Hypoglycaemic effect of the lyophilised aqueous extract of *Ajuga iva* in normal and streptozotocin diabetic rats, *J Ethnopharmacol* **80**(2-3), 109-13 (2002).
2. El-Hilaly J, ZH Israili, B Lyoussi; Acute and chronic toxicological studies of *Ajuga iva* in experimental animals, *J Ethnopharmacol* **91**(1), 43-50 (2004).

3. El-Hilaly J, A Tahraoui, ZH Israili, B Lyoussi; Hypolipidaemic effects of acute and sub-chronic administration of an aqueous extract of *Ajuga iva* L. whole plant in normal and diabetic rats, *J Ethnopharmacol* **105**(3), 441-48 (2006)

Albizzia lebbeck (Linn.) Benth (Fabaceae Leguminosae) (H. Siris)

It is a large spreading tree having large leaves and clusters of greenish-yellow flowers and long seed pods that clatter in the wind. The antioxidant potential of an aqueous extract of *A. lebbeck* was studied in diabetic rats. Oxidative damage in the liver and kidneys of alloxan-induced diabetic rats was evidenced by a marked increment in the levels of thiobarbituric acid reactive substances and conjugated dienes, and also by a distinct lowering in reduced glutathione content. All these parameters showed a tendency to retrieve towards normalcy on administration of *A. lebbeck* extract. The antioxidant enzymes, that registered a decline in activity in diabetic rats due to alloxan exposure, returned to normalcy on administration of the plant extract indicating the antioxidant efficacy of the drug in resisting oxidative insult. The findings provide a rationale for further studies on isolation of active principles from the plant and their pharmacological evaluation.

Resmi CR, MR Venukumar, MS Latha; Antioxidant activity of *Albizzia lebbeck* (Linn.) Benth. in alloxan diabetic rats, *Indian J Physiol Pharmacol* **50**(3), 297-302 (2006).

Albizzia odoratissima Benth. (Fabaceae Leguminosae) (Ceylone Rosewood,, S. Bhusiris, H. Kala Siris)

Albizzia odoratissima is identified by its dark green foliage, grey bark with irregular cracks and darker patches. It yields pale yellowish white fragrant flowers, which appear from April to June. *Albizzia odoratissima* seed diet exhibited hypoglycaemic activity.

Singh KN, RK Mittal, KC Barthwal; Hypoglycaemic activity of *Acacia catechu*, *Acacia suma*, and *Albizzia odoratissima* seed diets in normal albino rats, *Indian J Med Res* **64**(5), 754-57 (1976)

Allium cepa Linn. (Alliaceae) (Onion, S. Palandu, H. Piyaj)

Allium cepa is known only in cultivation, but related wild species are known to occur in Central Asia. Archaeological and literary evidence suggests that onion cultivation probably took place around 3000 BC in ancient Egypt. The bulbs from the onion family have been used as a food source for millennia.

1n 1965, Galal and Gawad reported the anti-diabetic activity of Egyptian onion (1). Thereafter, Augusti and co-workers published a series of papers (2-6) describing the effects of a hypoglycaemic principle of onion (2), the effect of allicin (diallyl disulphide-oxide) on alloxan diabetes (3), the effect of long-term feeding of this principle on alloxan-induced diabetic rats (4), isolation of hypo- and hyper-glycaemic agents from *Allium cepa* (5) and the effect of allyl propyl disulphide obtained from onion on alloxan diabetes (6).

Jain and Vyas reported the hypoglycaemic action of onion on rabbits (7) and Augusti and co-workers studied the effect of allyl propyl disulphide, isolated from onion, on glucose tolerance of alloxan-induced diabetic rabbits (8). The administration of allyl propyl disulphide to normal volunteers after a 12-hour fast caused a significant fall in the levels of blood glucose, a significant rise in serum insulin during the subsequent 4 hours and prevented the expected rise of serum free fatty acid levels (9). An active hypoglycaemic fraction of onion was claimed to be half as active as phenformin in lowering the fasting blood sugar of alloxan-induced diabetic rabbits. It also improved their glucose tolerance. The supplementation of food of diabetic patients with the residue, left after expression of juice from onion, controlled their hyperglycaemia (10). Gas chromatographic analysis of the hypoglycaemic fractions of onion was also conducted (11). Gupta and co-workers studied the anti-hyperglycaemic effect of onion and its various fractions (12, 13).

Diphenylamine, isolated from mature onion bulbs, was identified as one of the active anti-hyperglycaemic agents of onion. Cooking was found to decrease the diphenylamine content. A correlation between the diphenylamine content of the ether extracts of onions and their hypoglycaemic activity was observed. A simple and rapid UV spectrophotometric method for the determination of diphenylamine in Polish and Arabic onions has been described (14, 15).

Oral administration of S-methyl cysteine sulphoxide, a sulphur containing amino acid isolated from onion, daily (200 mg/kg b.w.) for a period of 45 days to alloxan-induced diabetic rats, controlled significantly their blood glucose and lipids in serum and tissues and altered the activities of liver hexokinase, glucose 6-phosphatase and HMG CoA reductase towards normal levels. These effects were comparable to those of glibenclamide and insulin (16, 17). Oral administration of S-methylcysteine sulfoxide and S-allylcysteine sulfoxide to alloxan-induced diabetic rats for a month is reported to ameliorate their diabetic conditions, being characterized by glucose intolerance, weight loss, depletion of liver glycogen, etc. (18). S-methyl cysteine sulphoxide like other S-alkyl cysteine sulfoxides decompose into a variety of thiosulfinates and polysulfides by the action of an enzyme allinase, present in onion. These volatile degradation products, present in the oils of onion, possess anti-diabetic, antibiotic, hypocholesterolaemic, fibrinolytic and various other biological actions (19). In addition to control of blood sugar levels in rats, S-methyl cysteine sulfoxide ameliorated the diabetic conditions significantly, viz. maintenance of body weight and lowering the levels of malondialdehyde, hydroperoxide and conjugated dienes in tissues exhibiting antioxidant effect on lipid peroxidation in experimental diabetes. As an antioxidant, S-methyl cysteine sulfoxide proved to be better than glibenclamide and insulin (22). Onion increased the fasting serum high-density lipoprotein levels, and demonstrated alleviation of hyperglycaemia in streptozotocin-induced diabetic rats. The hypoglycaemic and hypolipidaemic actions of *A. cepa* were associated with antioxidant activity, since onion decreased superoxide dismutase activities (23).

The effect of feeding diet containing freeze-dried onion powder (3%) was examined in albino rats, rendered diabetic with streptozotocin. Dietary onion partially reversed the abnormalities in plasma albumin, urea, creatinine and inorganic phosphorus and produced a significant reduction in hyperglycaemic status of diabetic animals. Hepatic cholesterol, triglycerides and phospholipids, which were elevated under diabetic condition, were countered significantly by dietary onion. Diabetic rats fed onion diet also exhibited lowered lipid peroxides in circulation and in urine when compared to diabetic control group (20). Callus cultures of onion in comparison to natural bulbs of onion indicated much higher anti-diabetic activity (21).

The effects of onion juice on biochemical parameters, enzyme activities and lipid peroxidation were studied in alloxan-induced diabetic rats. The increased levels of glucose, urea, creatinine and bilirubin, the increased activities of aspartate aminotransferase, alanine aminotransferase, lactate dehydrogenase, and alkaline and acid phosphatases and the increased concentration of thiobarbituric acid reactive substances and the activity of glutathione S-transferase in plasma, liver, testes, brain, and kidney in alloxan-diabetic rats were restored to their normal levels by treatment of the diabetic rats with repeated doses of onion juices (24).

1. Galal EE, MA Gawad; Anti-diabetic activity of Egyptian onion "*Allium cepa*" extract, *J Egypt Med Assoc*;**48**(Suppl),14-45 (1965)
2. Augusti KT; Studies on the effects of a hypoglycaemic principle from *Allium Cepa* Linn, *Indian J Med Res* **61**(7), 1066-71 (1973)
3. Mathew PT, KT Augusti; Studies on the effect of allicin (diallyl disulphide-oxide) on alloxan diabetes. I. Hypoglycaemic action and enhancement of serum insulin effect and glycogen synthesis, *Indian J Biochem Biophys* **10**(3), 209-12 (1973)
4. Augusti KT; Effect of long term feeding of hypoglycaemic principles from plants on alloxan diabetes, *Indian J Exp Biol* **11**(5), 445-47 (1973)
5. Mathew PT, KT Augusti; Isolation of hypo- and hyperglycaemic agents from *Allium cepa* Linn, *Indian J Exp Biol* **11**(6), 573-75 (1973)
6. Augusti KT; Effect of alloxan diabetes of allyl propyl disulphide obtained from onion, *Naturwissenschaften* **61**(4), 172-73 (1974).
7. Jain RC, CR Vyas; Letter: Hypoglycaemic action of onion on rabbits, *Br Med J* **2**(921), 730 (1974)
8. Augusti KT, VC Roy, M Sempler; Effect of allyl propyl disulphide isolated

from onion (*Allium cepa* L.) on glucose tolerance of alloxan diabetic rabbits, *Experientia* **30**(10), 1119-20 (1974)

9. Augusti KT, ME Benaim; Effect of essential oil of onion (allyl propyl disulphide) on blood glucose, free fatty acid and insulin levels of normal subjects, *Clin Chim Acta* **60**(1), 121-23 (1975)
10. Mathew PT, KT Augusti; Hypoglycaemic effects of onion, *Allium cepa* Linn. on diabetes mellitus - a preliminary report, *Indian J Physiol Pharmacol* **19**(4), 213-17 (1975)
11. Augusti KT; Gas chromatographic analyses of onion principles and a study on their hypoglycaemic action, *Indian J Exp Biol* **14**(2), 110-12 (1976).
12. Sharma KK, RK Gupta, S Gupta, KC Samuel; Anti-hyperglycaemic effect of onion: effect on fasting blood sugar and induced hyperglycemia in man, *Indian J Med Res* **65**(3), 422-29 (1977).
13. Gupta RK, S Gupta, KC Samuel; Blood sugar lowering effect of various fractions of onion, *Indian J Exp Biol* **15**(4), :313-14 (1977).
14. Karawya MS, SM Abdel-Wahab, MM El-Olemy, NM Farrag; Diphenylamine, an anti-hyperglycaemic agent from onion and tea, *J Nat Prod* **47**(5), 775-80 (1984).
15. Smoczkiewiczowa A, B Ostrowska, J Jasiczak, M Olszak, H Rychlinska; Method of estimation of diphenylamine as hyperglycaemic agent in onion (*Allium cepa* L.) *Herba Pol* **36**(3), 97-109 (1990).
16. Kumari K, KT Augusti; Anti-diabetic effects of S-methylcysteine sulphoxide on alloxan diabetes, *Planta Med* **61**(1), 72-74 (1995).
17. Kumari K, BC Mathew, KT Augusti; Anti-diabetic and hypolipidaemic effects of S-methyl cysteine sulfoxide isolated from *Allium cepa* Linn, *Indian J Biochem Biophys* **32**(2), 49-54 (1995)
18. Sheela CG, K Kumud, KT Augusti; Anti-diabetic effects of onion and garlic sulfoxide amino acids in rats, *Planta Med* **61**(4), 56-57 (1995).
19. Augusti KT; Therapeutic values of onion (*Allium cepa* L.) and garlic (*Allium sativum* L.), *Indian J Exp Biol* **34**(7), 634-40 (1996)
20. Babu PS, K Srinivasan; Influence of dietary capsaicin and onion on the metabolic abnormalities associated with streptozotocin-induced diabetes mellitus, *Mol Cell Biochem* **175**(1-2), 49-57 (1997)
21. Kelkar SM, GS Kaklij, VA Bapat; Determination of anti-diabetic activity in *Allium cepa* (onion) tissue cultures, *Indian J Biochem Biophys* **38**(4), 277-79 (2001).
22. Kumari K, KT Augusti; Anti-diabetic and antioxidant effects of S-methyl cysteine sulfoxide isolated from onions (*Allium cepa* Linn) as compared to standard drugs in alloxan diabetic rats, *Indian J Exp Biol* **40**(9), 1005-09 (2002).
23. Campos KE, YS Diniz, AC Cataneo, LA Faine, MJ Alves, EL Novelli; Hypoglycaemic and antioxidant effects of onion, *Allium cepa*: dietary onion addition,

antioxidant activity and hypoglycaemic effects on diabetic rats, *Int J Food Sci Nutr* **54**(3), 241-46 (2003).

24. El-Demerdash FM, MI Yousef, NI El-Naga; Biochemical study on the hypoglycaemic effects of onion and garlic in alloxan-induced diabetic rats, *Food Chem Toxicol* **43**(1), 57-63 (2005).

Allium sativum Linn (Alliaceae) (Garlic, H. Lehsun.)

Allium sativum, commonly known as garlic, is a close relative of onion. It has a characteristic pungent, spicy flavour that mellows and sweetens considerably with cooking. Garlic finds an important place in the alternative system of medicine for the treatment various human ailments including diabetes mellitus. Augusti and co-workers reported some early work on the effect of long-term feeding of the aqueous extract of garlic on normal rats (1), the effect of allicin, a garlic constituent, on alloxan diabetes (2) and the hypoglycaemic effects of garlic in sucrose-fed rabbits (4). Jain and Vyas (3) reported the effect of garlic in alloxan-induced diabetic rabbits, while Chang and Jhonson (5) reported the anti-diabetic activities of garlic and its effect on carbohydrate metabolism and lipid synthesis in rats. The effect of garlic oil on the pancreas of experimental diabetes in guinea pigs was also studied (6). Thai workers (8) published a report of phase II clinical trial of garlic in the treatment diabetes mellitus. A fraction derived from garlic was also reported to exhibit hypolipidaemic and hypoglycaemic activity in albino rats, house rats and gerbils. The blood sugar lowering effect was attributed to increased insulin response (7).

Administration of S-allyl cysteine sulphoxide, a sulphur containing amino acid of garlic, to alloxan-induced diabetic rats at a dose of 200 mg/kg b.w, significantly decreased the concentration of serum lipids, blood glucose and activities of enzymes like alkaline phosphatase, acid phosphatase and lactate dehydrogenase and liver glucose-6-phosphatase. Intestinal and liver HMG CoA reductase and liver hexokinase activities also increased (9). Oral administration of garlic constituents, S-methylcysteine sulphoxide and S-allylcysteine sulphoxide, to alloxan-diabetic rats for a month ameliorated their diabetic conditions like glucose intolerance, weight loss and depletion of liver glycogen. In this respect garlic sulphoxides were comparable to glibenclamide and insulin but S-allyl cysteine sulphoxide controlled lipid peroxidation better than the other two drugs. It also significantly stimulated *in vitro* insulin secretion from *beta* cells, isolated from normal rats. The beneficial effects of S-allyl cysteine sulphoxide could, therefore, be due to both its antioxidant and its secretagogue actions (10, 11). S-allyl cysteine sulphoxide was found to combat the nicotine-induced peroxidative damage in rats to some extent. It decreased the concentrations of thiobarbituric acid reactive substances (TBARS), hydroperoxides, and conjugated dienes in liver, lungs and heart and increased the activities of catalase and superoxide dismutase and the levels of antioxidants like vitamins A,

C, and E in the liver. The effects were compared with the standard antioxidant vitamin E. (15). Both garlic oil and diallyl trisulfide have been reported to improve glycaemic control in streptozotocin-induced diabetic rats through increased insulin secretion and increased insulin sensitivity (18).

Administration of an extract of garlic bulb (500 mg/kg/day) in hyperthyroid animals decreased the serum glucose concentration as well as the serum thyroid hormones. The reductions in serum glucose and thyroid hormone concentrations in the garlic extract-treated group were comparable to that in propyl thiouracil-treated animals. The findings indicate that garlic bulb extract may prove to be effective in the treatment of thyroxine-induced hyperglycaemia (14). The effects of garlic juice on biochemical parameters, enzyme activities and lipid peroxidation were studied in alloxan-induced diabetic rats. Garlic juice was found to exert antioxidant and anti-hyperglycaemic effects and consequently alleviate liver and renal damage caused by alloxan-induced diabetes (16). Effect of garlic on blood glucose and histopathology of pancreas of alloxan-induced diabetic rats was studied. Garlic was able to reduce blood glucose significantly compared with the control group. However, no significant change in morphometric factors (volume density of *beta* cells, volume density of islets, percent of *beta* cells, number of islets per square millimeter, average area of islets and average volume density of *beta* cell in whole pancreas) between treated and untreated diabetics was observed (17).

Anti-diabetic effects of ajoene, derived from garlic, were investigated in genetically diabetic KK-A(y) mice. The levels of plasma glucose in four-week-old male KK-A(y) mice, kept on a laboratory diet containing 0.05% of ajoene for 8 weeks, were significantly suppressed compared with the control group. The results of detailed investigation suggest that hyperglycaemia and hypertriglyceridemia are suppressed by ajoene treatment (19).

The antioxidant properties of garlic compounds representing the four main chemical classes, alliin, allyl cysteine, allyl disulfide, and allicin, were studied. Alliin scavenged superoxide, while allicin suppressed the formation of superoxide by the xanthine/xanthine oxidase system, Alliin, allyl cysteine, and allyl disulfide all scavenged hydroxyl radicals. Allyl disulfide was also a lipid peroxidation terminator. All these compounds exhibited different patterns of antioxidant activities as protective compounds against free radical damage (20).

Oral administrations of an ethanol (95%) extract of garlic (45 mg/kg b.w./day for 4 weeks) to alloxan-induced diabetic mice significantly lowered their serum glucose levels and nociceptive responses. The therapeutic potential of ethanol extract of garlic for anti-hyperglycaemic and anti-nociceptive effects in diabetes was suggested (12). The effects of oral administration of an ethanol extract of garlic (0.1, 0.25 and 0.5 g/kg body wt.) for 14 days on the level of serum glucose, total cholesterol, triglycerides, urea, uric acid, creatinine, aspartate amino transferase (AST) and alanine amino transferase (ALT) in normal and streptozotocin-induced diabetic rats were evaluated. The extract significantly decreased serum glucose, total cholesterol, triglycerides, urea, uric acid, creatinine, AST and ALT levels in normal and streptozotocin-induced diabetic rats. It increased serum insulin in diabetic rats but not in normal rats. The anti-diabetic effect of the extract was more effective than that observed with glibenclamide (21).

Dasture and coworkers (13) reviewed different therapeutic uses of garlic including its anti-diabetic activity.

1. Augusti KT, PT Mathew; Effect of long-term feeding of the aqueous extracts of onion (*Allium cepa* Linn.) and garlic (*Allium sativum* Linn.) on normal rats. *Indian J Exp Biol* **11**(3), 239-41 (1973)
2. Mathew PT, KT Augusti; Studies on the effect of allicin (diallyl disulphide-oxide) on alloxan diabetes I. Hypoglycaemic action and enhancement of serum insulin effect and glycogen synthesis, *Indian J Biochem Biophys* **10**(3), 209-12 (1973)
3. Jain RC, CR Vyas; Garlic in alloxan-induced diabetic rabbits, *Am J Clin Nutr* **28**(7), 684-85 (1975)
4. Zacharias NT, KL Sebastian, B Philip, KT Augusti; Hypoglycaemic and hypolipidaemic effects of garlic in sucrose fed rabbits, *Indian J Physiol Pharmacol* **24**(2), 151-54 (1980)
5. Chang ML, MA Johnson, Effect of garlic on carbohydrate metabolism and lipid synthesis in rats, *J Nutr* **110**(5), 931-36 (1980)
6. Begum H, MA Bari; Effect of garlic oil on the pancreas of experimental diabetes in guineapigs, *Bangladesh Med Res Counc Bull* **11**(2), 64-68 (1985).
7. Dixit VP, R Sinha; Hypolipidaemic effect of a fraction derived from garlic (*Allium sativum*) in albino rats, house rats and gerbils, *Indian Zoologist* **9**(182), 147-49 (1985)
8. Sitprija S, C Plengvidhya, V Kangkaya, S Bhuvapanich, M Tunkayoon; Garlic and diabetes mellitus phase II clinical trial, *J Med Assoc Thai* **70**(Suppl. 2), 223-27 (1987)
9. Sheela CG, KT Augusti, Anti-diabetic effects of S-allyl cysteine sulphoxide isolated from garlic *Allium sativum* Linn, *Indian J Exp Biol* **30**(6), 523-26 (1992).
10. Sheela CG, K Kumud, KT Augusti, Anti-diabetic effects of onion and garlic sulfoxide amino acids in rats, *Planta Med* **61**(4), 356-57 (1995).
11. Augusti KT, CG Sheela; Anti-peroxide effect of S-allyl cysteine sulfoxide, an insulin secretagogue, in diabetic rats, *Experientia* **52**(2), 115-20 (1996).
12. Rajendra Kumar G, KP Reddy; Reduced nociceptive responses in mice with alloxan-induced hyperglycaemia after garlic (*Allium sativum* Linn.) treatment, *Indian J Exp Biol* **37**(7), 662-66 (1999)
13. Dasture AV, PH Kulkarni; Therapeutic excellence of garlic (*Allium sativum* Linn.), *Deerghayu International* **15**(57), 28-32 (1999)

14. Tahiliani P, A Kar; Mitigation of thyroxine-induced hyperglycaemia by two plant extracts, *Phytother Res* **17**(3), 294-96 (2003).

15. Helen A, K Krishnakumar, PL Vijayammal, KT Augusti; A comparative study of antioxidants S-allyl cysteine sulfoxide and vitamin E on the damages induced by nicotine in rats, *Pharmacology* **67**(3), 113-17 (2003)

16. El-Demerdash FM, MI Yousef, MI El-Naga; Biochemical study on the hypoglycaemic effects of onion and garlic in alloxan-induced diabetic rats, *Food Chem Toxicol* **43**(1), 57-63 (2005).

17. Jelodar GA, M Maleki, MH Motadayen, S Sirus; Effect of fenugreek, onion and garlic on blood glucose and histopathology of pancreas of alloxan-induced diabetic rats, *Indian J Med Sci* **59**(2), 64-69 (2005)

18. Liu CT, H Hse, CK Lii, PS Chen, LY Sheen; Effects of garlic oil and diallyl trisulfide on glycaemic control in diabetic rats, *Eur J Pharmacol* **516**(2), 165-73 (2005).

19. Hattori A, N Yamada, T Nishikawa, H Fukuda, T Fujino; Anti-diabetic effects of ajoene in genetically diabetic KK-A(y) mice, *J Nutr Sci Vitaminol* **51**(5), 382-84 (2005).

20. Chung LY; The antioxidant properties of garlic compounds: allyl cysteine, alliin, allicin, and allyl disulfide, *J Med Food* **9**(2), 205-13 (2006)

21. Eidi A, M Eidi, E Esmaeili; Anti-diabetic effect of garlic (*Allium sativum* L.) in normal and streptozotocin-induced diabetic rats, *Phytomedicine* **13**(9-10), 624-29 (2006)

Allophyllus cominia (L.) Swartz (Sapindaceae) (Christmas Berry)

Phytochemical screening of an extract of *A. cominia* detected the presence of free amines, free phenolics, tannins, leucoanthocyanidines, saponins, triterpenes, and steroids. In view of the reported hypoglycaemic activity of these groups of compounds, it would be interesting to study their pharmacological activity.

Rodriguez TV, JV Gonzales, LM Sanchez, MN Perez, EM Faz; Detection and determination of chemical groups in an extract of *Allophylus cominia* (L.), *J Herb Pharmacother* 5(4), 31-38 (2005)

Aloe arborescens Mill. var. ***natalensis*** Berger (Asphodelaceae) (Candelabra aloe, Kidachi aloe)

Aloe arborescens occurs naturally in areas of South Africa, Mozambique and Zimbabwe. The glycans, arborans A and B, isolated from the leaves of the plant, showed hypoglycaemic activity (1, See Hypoglycaemic Glycans in Appendix.). Low-dose streptozotocin-induced diabetic ICR mice were fed basal diet supplemented with 2% kidachi aloe from 31 days before to 73 days after induction of diabetes by streptozotocin injection. The diet supplemented with kidachi aloe suppressed the elevation of blood sugar level and significantly decreased the incidence of insulitis. A 10 KDa fraction, derived from kidachi aloe also showed similar activity. It has been suggested that this fraction protects islets of Langerhans from the destruction caused by the methyl radical from streptozotocin (2).[

1. Hikino H, M Takahashi, M Murakami, C Konno, Y Mirin, M Karikura; Isolation and hypoglycaemic activity of arborans A and B, glycans of *Aloe arborescens* var. *natalensis* leaves, *Int J Crude Drug Res* **24**(4), 183-186 (1986)
2. Beppu H, K Shimpo, T Chihara, T Kaneko, I Tamai, S Yamaji, S Ozaki, H, Kuzuya, S Sonoda; Anti-diabetic effects of dietary administration of *Aloe arborescens* Miller components on multiple low-dose streptozotocin-induced diabetes in mice; Investigation of hypoglycaemic action and systemic absorption dynamics of aloe components, *J Ethnopharmacol* **103**(3), 468-77 (2006)

Aloe barbadensis Miller (Asphodelaceae)
Syn. *Aloe vera* (L.) Burm.
(S. Ghrita kumari, H. Gwarpatha)

The genus Aloe is a group of plants including *Aloe vera* that are empirically known to have various medicinal properties. *Aloe vera* is native to North Africa and also cultivated in Turkey. It is classified as a succulent, which means that it stores water in its leaves for possible periods of drought. Its thick leaf structure makes it prone to be grouped with cacti, but the rosette formation of its leaves is indicative of its relationship with lily family. The dried sap of the aloe plant (aloes) is one of several traditional remedies used for diabetes in the Arabian Peninsula. The anti-diabetic activity of aloes was studied in 5 patients with non-insulin-dependent diabetes and in alloxan-induced Swiss albino mice. Daily ingestion of half a teaspoonful of aloes for 4-14 weeks significantly lowered the fasting serum glucose level in every patient with no change in body weight. In normal mice, administration of aloes (500 mg/kg twice daily) induced hypoglycaemia after 5 days while in diabetic mice, the fasting plasma glucose level was significantly reduced by aloes after 3 days. The hypoglycaemic activity of aloes was compared with glibenclamide (1).

The effects of the exudate of *Aloe barbadensis* leaves (aloes) and its bitter principle were studied on plasma glucose levels of alloxan-diabetic mice. The hypoglycaemic effect of a single oral dose of aloes (500 mg/kg) on serum glucose level was insignificant whereas intra-peritoneal administration of its bitter principle (5 mg/kg) was highly significant and extended over a period of 24 h. In chronic studies, aloes was administered twice daily and the bitter principle was administered once a day for 4 days. The maximum reduction in plasma glucose level was observed at the 5th day in both cases. It is considered that the hypoglycaemic effect of aloes and its bitter principle is mediated through stimulating synthesis and/or release of insulin from the *beta* cells of Langerhans (2).

The clinical effectiveness of *Aloe vera*, a popular herbal remedy, was reviewed. Even though oral administration of *Aloe vera* might be a useful adjunct for lowering blood glucose in diabetic patients as well as for reducing blood lipid levels in patients with hyperlipidaemia, the reviewers are of the opinion that clinical effectiveness of oral or topical *Aloe vera* is not sufficiently defined at present (4). The controversial reports on the hypoglycaemic activity of *Aloe vera* are probably due to differences in the parts of the plant used or due to the model of diabetes chosen. The results of investigation revealed that *A. vera* leaf pulp, which was ineffective in lowering the blood sugar level of non-diabetic rats, showed hypoglycaemic activity in type-1 (IDDM) and type-2 (NIDDM) diabetic rats. Surprisingly, *A. vera* leaf gel extract showed hyperglycaemic activity in NIDDM rats. It was, therefore, concluded that the pulps of *Aloe vera* leaves devoid of the gel could be useful in the treatment of non-insulin dependent diabetes mellitus (5).

Effects of oral administration of an alcoholic extract of *A. vera* gel were studied on normal fasted rats, oral glucose-loaded rats and also on streptozotocin-induced diabetic rats. The extract, at a concentration of 200 and 300 mg/kg of body weight, was found to maintain the glucose homeostasis by controlling the carbohydrate metabolizing enzymes. Oral administration of the extract, at a concentration of 300 mg/kg body weight for 21 days, resulted in a significant reduction in fasting blood glucose, thiobarbituric acid reactive substances, hydroperoxides, superoxide dismutase, catalase and glutathione peroxidase and significant improvement in reduced glutathione in the pancreas of streptozotocin-induced diabetic rats, when compared with untreated diabetic rats. The ethanol extract appeared to be more effective than glibenclamide in controlling oxidative stress (6-7). The potential anti-hyperlipidaemic efficacy of the ethanol extract of *Aloe vera* leaf gel was studied in streptozotocin induced diabetic rats. Oral administration of *Aloe vera* gel extract (300 mg/kg b.w. daily) to streptozotocin-induced diabetic rats for a period of 21 days resulted in a significant reduction in fasting blood glucose, hepatic transaminases, plasma and tissue cholesterol, triglycerides, free fatty acids and phospholipids and a significant improvement in plasma insulin. The results of the detailed study provided a scientific rationale for the use of *Aloe vera* as an anti-diabetic agent (9). Five phytosterols (lophenol, 24-methyl-lophenol, 24-ethyl-lophenol, cycloartanol, and 24-methylene-cycloartanol) were isolated from anti-hyperglycaemic *Aloe vera* gel. After administration of the five phytosterols for 28 days fasting blood glucose levels decreased to different degrees. The phytosterols derived from *Aloe vera* gel have a long-term blood glucose controlling effect and would be useful for the treatment of type-2 diabetes mellitus (10).

The role of some inorganic elements like vanadium, zinc, sodium, potassium, calcium, copper, manganese, and traces of chromium in the improvement of impaired glucose tolerance and their indirect role in the management of diabetes mellitus are being increasingly recognized. The fact that treatment with the ash of *Aloe vera* leaf gel also resulted in hypoglycaemic action supported the presence of various inorganic trace elements in the gel. (8).

The positive influence of *Aloe vera* on the healing of full-thickness wounds in diabetic rats is reported. It has been conjectured that *Aloe vera* treatment of wounds in diabetic rats enhance the process of wound healing by influencing phases such as inflammation, fibroplasia, collagen synthesis and maturation, and wound contraction. These effects may be due to the reported hypoglycaemic effects of the aloe gel (3).

1. Ghannam N, M Kingston, IA Al-Meshaal, M Tariq, NS Parman, N Woodhouse; The anti-diabetic activity of aloes: preliminary clinical and experimental observations, *Horm Res* **24**(4), 288-94 (1986)
2. Ajabnoor MA; Effect of aloes on blood glucose levels in normal and alloxan diabetic mice, *J Ethnopharmacol* **28**(2), 215-20 (1990)
3. Chithra P, GB Sajithlal, G Chandrakasan, Influence of *Aloe vera* on the healing of dermal wounds in diabetic rats, *J Ethnopharmacol* **59**(3), 195-201 (1998)
4. Vogler BK, E Ernst; *Aloe vera*: a systematic review of its clinical effectiveness, *Brit J Gen Pract* **49**(447), 823-28 (1999)
5. Okyar A, A Can, N Akev, G Baktir, N Sutlupinar; Effect of *Aloe vera* leaves on blood glucose level in type I and type II diabetic rat models, *Phytother Res* **15**(2), 157-61 (2001)
6. Rajasekaran S, K Sivagnanam, K Ravi, S Subramanian; Hypoglycaemic effect of *Aloe vera* gel on streptozotocin-induced diabetes in experimental rats, *J Med Food* 7(1), 61-66 (2004).
7. Rajasekaran S, K Sivagnanam, S Subramanian; Modulatory effects of *Aloe vera* leaf gel extract on oxidative stress in rats treated with streptozotocin, *J Pharm Pharmacol* **57**(2), 241-46 (2005).
8. Rajasekaran S, K Sivagnanam, S Subramanian; Mineral contents of *Aloe vera* leaf gel and their role on streptozotocin-induced diabetic rats, *Biol Trace Elem Res* **108**(1-3), 185-95 (2005).
9. Rajasekaran S, K Ravi, K Sivagnanam, S Subramanian; Beneficial effects of *Aloe vera* leaf gel extract on lipid profile status in rats with streptozotocin diabetes, *Clin Exp Pharmacol Physiol* **33**(3), 232-37 (2006)
10. Tanaka M, E Misawa, Y Ito, N Habara, K Nomaguchi, M Yamada, T Toida, H Hayasawa, M Takase, M Inagaki, R Higuchi; Identification of five phytosterols from *Aloe vera* gel as anti-diabetic compounds, *Biol Pharm Bull* **29**(7), 1418-22 (2006)

Alpinia galanga (L) Willd. (Zingiberaceae) (Thai ginger)

Alpinia galanga is a plant in the ginger family. It is used in cooking, especially in Indonesian and Thai cuisine. The plant, which is native to South Asia and Indonesia, grows from rhizomes. *A. galanga* rhizomes, which are sweet and aromatic, are a common ingredient in Thai soups and curries.

The effects of *Alpinia galanga* rhizome on blood glucose levels were studied. While powdered rhizome of *A. galanga* and its methanol and aqueous extracts significantly lowered the blood glucose in normal rabbits, no significant reduction in blood glucose was observed in alloxan-induced diabetic rabbits. The hypoglycaemic effect of *A. galanga* in normal rabbits was comparable to gliclazide.

Akhtar MS, MA Khan, MT Malik; Hypoglycaemic activity of *Alpinia galanga* rhizome and its extracts in rabbits, *Fititerapia* **73**(7-8), 623-28 (2002)

Amaranthus caudatus Linn (Amaranthaceae) (Velvet flower, Red Cockscomb)

Amaranthus caudatus is a species of annual flowering plant. Leaves and seeds of the plant are edible, and are frequently used as a source of food in India and South America. *A. caudatus* can grow anywhere and grows best in full sun. It can handle a variety of conditions, both humid and arid. The red colour of the inflorescences of *A. caudatus* is due to a high content of betacyanin.

The antioxidant and anti-diabetic activities of the seeds of two varieties of *Amaranthus caudatus* (Oscar blanco and Victor red) were studied. Oil, squalene and phenolic contents of the two varieties were determined. The two varieties contained different levels of squalene but their antioxidant activity did not differ significantly from each other. However, significant differences were noticed in relation to their anti-diabetic activity (inhibition of *alpha*-amylase activity). *A. caudatus* var. Oscar blanco was superior to the other variety.

Comforti F, G Statti, MR Loizzo, G Sacchetti, F Poli, F Menichini; *In vitro* antioxidant effect and inhibition of *alpha*-amylase of two varieties of *Amaranthus caudatus* seeds, *Biol Pharm Bull* **28**(6), 1098-102 (2005)

Amaranthus esculentus Bess (Amaranthaceae) (Amaranth grain)

Glycaemic index of grain amaranth, wheat and rice preparations was studied in NIDDM subjects. Diets containing 50 g carbohydrate equivalent were given and post-prandial blood glucose levels estimated at different intervals. Glycaemic index calculated for different experimental diets showed that 25:75 combination of amaranth and wheat can be considered as low glycaemic index food (1)

Anti-oxidative and anti-diabetic effects of amaranth grain and its oil were studied in streptozotocin-induced diabetic rats (2). Supplementation of diet of diabetic rats with amaranth grain (500 g/kg diet) significantly decreased the level of serum glucose and increased the level of serum insulin. Serum concentration of the enzymes, GOT and GPT were also normalised. It also significantly increased the activities of superoxide dismutase and glutathione-reductase and decreased catalase, peroxidase and glutathione-peroxidase activities in diabetic rats. Similar results were obtained by supplementation with Amaranth oil (100 g/kg diet).

1. Chaturvedi G, G Sarojini, N Nirmala, Nirmalamma, D Satyanarayana; Glycaemic index of grain amaranth, wheat and rice in NIDDM subjects, *Plant Foods Hum Nutr* **50**(2), 171-78 (1997)
2. Kim HK, MJ Kim, HY Cho, EK Kim, DH Shin; Antioxidative and anti-diabetic effects of amaranth (*Amaranthus esculantus*) in streptozotocin-induced diabetic rats, *Cell Biochem Funct* **24**(3), 195-99 (2006)

Ambrosia maritima L. (Asteraceae/Compositae). (Ragweeds)

Ambrosia maritima is a herb that grows wildly in Egypt. The effects of different solvent extracts of this herb on blood glucose levels of rats were studied. The one and half hour post-prandial blood glucose was reduced significantly after administration of the water, aqueous alcohol (50%) or petroleum ether extracts, while two hour post-prandial blood glucose level was reduced significantly after the administration of ethyl ether or the petroleum ether extract. The fasting blood glucose was reduced only by total water or the alcoholic extract. No significant change of insulin level 2 hours and 1.5 hours after glucose ingestion was observed either by petroleum ether or aqueous alcoholic extract,

Ammar NM, SY Al-Okbi, IH Badawy; The hypoglycaemic effect of different extracts of *Ambrosia maritima* L. Compositae, *J Islamic Acad Sci* **6**(4), 298-301 (1993)

Amomum xanthioides Wall. ex Baker (Zingiberaceae)

An aqueous ethanol extract of *A. xanthioides* at a concentration of 0.5 mg/ml stimulated glucose uptake in 3T3-L1 adipocytes. The extract significantly potentiated insulin-stimulated glucose uptake in a dose dependent manner at a concentration range of 0.02 to 0.5 mg/ml. It is surmised that the anti-diabetic activity of the plant extract is mediated through the stimulation of glucose uptake and potentiation of insulin action (1).

In a preliminary study, methanol extract of *A. xanthioides* showed strong inhibitory activity against yeast *alpha*-glucosidase *in vitro*. Bioactivity directed fractionation of the extract led to the isolation of an active constituent, which was identified as quercetrin. The inhibitory activity of the isolated quercetrin against yeast *alpha*-glucosidase at the concentration of 0.5 mg/ml was more than that of acarbose, a commercial *alpha* glucosidase inhibitor (2).

1. Kang Y, HY Kim; Glucose uptake stimulatory activity of Amomi Semen in 3T3-L1 adipocytes, *J Ethnopharmacol* **92**(1), 103-105 (2004)
2. Kim Y-M, M-J Kim, JA Zhang, H-J Joo, Ji-Y Hwang, J-I Kim, Y-S Choi; Isolation of an active compound with *alpha*-glucosidase inhibitory activity from *Amomum xanthioides* Wallich, *The FASEB J* **21**, 845.4 (2007)

Amorphophallus konjac K.Kocl. (Araceae) syn. *A. rivieri* (Konjak, Devils tongue, Voodoo lily)

It is a perennial plant, growing from a large corm and having large leaves (1.3 m across), which are divided into numerous leaflets. It is native to warm subtropical to tropical eastern Asia, from Japan and China south to Indonesia. The corm of konjac is often colloquially referred to as a yam, although it bears no marked relation to tubers of the family Diascoreaceae.

The effects of konjac extract on insulin sensitivity in insulin resistant rats, induced by high fat diet, were evaluated. Wistar rats, fed on high fat diet for 4 weeks, developed insulin resistance and treatment with konjac extract (1.5, 3.0 g/kg/d) for 4 weeks decreased their fasting blood glucose, serum total cholesterol, triglycerides and LDL-c levels while increased HDL-c/total cholesterol ratio in comparison to untreated high fat diet fed rats. There was no significant effect on insulin level. Konjac extract could improve insulin sensitivity, elevate glycogen, and decrease triglycerides in liver and skeletal muscle. From the results of the investigation, it was inferred that konjac extract could promote glycogen syntheses and adjust blood lipid metabolism so as to improve insulin resistance in high fat diet fed rats (1).

The roots/yams of *A. konjac*, known to exhibit hypoglycaemic effects on diabetic subjects, yielded three oligosaccharide fractions. Of these, the fraction named as KOS-A, was found to have nitric oxide (NO*) free radical regulation effect. At concentrations less than 1.5 mM, KOS-A positively decreased streptozotocin-induced NO* level of islets, but normal NO* release for non- streptozotocin-treated islets was not affected within the range. At 15 mM, KOS-A played a contrary role and increased NO* level of islets both with and without streptozotocin treatment. Increased insulin secretion appeared parallel to the decrease of NO*, and normal insulin release was not affected by KOS-A at less than 1.5 mM. KOS-A was shown to be a tetrasaccharide with Mw of 666 Daltons. The hypoglycaemic function of *A. konjac* might be related with free radical attenuation and lower risks of islets damage from NO* radical (2).

Glucomannan is the main polysaccharide obtained from the tubers of the *Amorphophallus konjac* plant. This soluble fibre, with an extraordinarily high water-holding capacity, is highly effective in the treatment of obesity, presumably due to the satiety sensation that it produces. It has also been shown to be a hypoglycaemic and hypoinsulinemic agent and this activity is probably due to the fact that it delays gastric emptying and slows down glucose delivery to the intestinal mucosa. Some of the adverse side effects of this fibre are flatulence, abdominal pain and oesophageal obstruction. (3)

1. Mao CP, ML Xie, ZL Gu; Effects of konjac extract on insulin sensitivity in high fat diet rats, *Acta Pharmacol Sin* **23**(9), 855-59 (2002).

2. Lu XJ, XM Chen, DX Fu, W Cong, F Ouyang; Effect of *Amorphophallus konjac* oligosaccharides on STZ-induced diabetes model of isolated islets, *Life Sci* **72**(6), 711-19 (2002).

3. Gonzalez CA, MN Fernandez, AM Sahagun, VJJ Garcia, LMJ Diez, PAP Calle, RLJ Castro, VM Sierra; Glucomannan: properties and therapeutic applications, *Nutr Hosp* **19**(1), 45-50 (2004) [Article in Spanish].

Ampelopsis grosse-dentata W.T.Wang (Vitaceae)
(Snake wine vine)

Snake wine vine grows in warm climates from Yunnan to Hainan. The tender stems and leaves of the snake vine have traditionally been made into a healthy tea for treating common cold and various other diseases. The tea has a mild and rich taste, with a striking sweetness that develops in the mouth some minutes after drinking the tea. The plant is rich in flavonoids.

The hypoglycaemic action of total flavone of *A. grossedentata* was studied on alloxan-induced diabetic mice, on epinephrine and glucose-induced hyperglycaemic mice as well as on normal mice. The flavone had better therapeutic action on alloxan-induced diabetic mice, and could significantly lower the blood glucose levels of epinephrine and glucose- induced hyperglycaemic mice but had no significant effects on blood glucose levels of normal mice. Acute toxicity test of the flavone revealed its toxicity to be very little.

Zhong ZX, JP Qin, GF Zhou, XF Chen; Experimental studies of hypoglycaemic action on total flavone of *Ampelopsis grossedentata* from Guangxi, *Zhongguo Zhong Yao Za Zhi* **27**(9), 687-89 (2002) [Article in Chinese].

***Ammi visnaga* (L)** Lam. (Apiaceae/Umbelliferae)
(Toothpick weed)

The plant grows in fields and sandy places and it is found from Central Europe to West Asia and North Africa. The leaves of the plant are chewed for their pleasant aromatic flavour. Skin contact with the sap has been reported to cause photo-sensitivity and/or dermatitis in some people. The fruiting pedicel is used as a toothpick and is sold as toothpicks in Egyptian markets.

The aqueous extract of *A. visnaga* fruits at a dose of 20 mg/kg significantly reduced blood glucose level of normal rats 6h after a single oral administration and 9 days after repeated oral administration. The hypoglycaemic activity is more pronounced in streptozotocin-induced diabetic rats. The findings justify clinical use of the aqueous extract of the fruits of the plant by the Moroccan people.

Jouad H, M Maghrani, M Eddouks; Hypoglycaemic effect of aqueous extract of *Ammi visnaga* in normal and streptozotocin-induced diabetic rats, *J Herbal Pharmacother* **2**(4), 19-29 (2002).

Anacardium occidentale Linn. (Anacardaceae) (Cashew, H, Kaju)

Cashew is a commercially important plant and different parts of the plant are used for different purposes. The cashew "apple," the enlarged fully ripe, fruit may be eaten raw, or preserved as jam. The juice is made into a beverage (Brazil cajuado) or fermented into a wine. Cashew nut of commerce is generally obtained by roasting the shells and separating the nuts from vesicant shells. Cashew nut shell liquid is vesicant but is a commercially useful starting material for some polymers. Stems exude a clear gum, Cashawa gum, used in pharmaceuticals and as a substitute for gum arabic. Shell oil is used in folk remedies for various ailments.

The protective effect of aqueous extract of *A. occidentale* leaves against steptozotocin-induced diabetes was evaluated in rats. The extract significantly inhibited the hyperglycaemic action of streptozotocin. Diabetic manifestations in pre-treated rats after streptozotocin administration were reduced suggesting that the extract may involve direct inhibition of streptozotocin (1). Anti-diabetic activity of the leaf extract was also evaluated using alloxan (80 mg/kg b.w., i.p.)-induced hyperglycaemic rabbits. The maximum lowering of blood sugar levels in both normal and alloxanised rabbits was found to be at a dose of 400 mg/kg b.w. (2).

The hypoglycaemic effect of extracts of *A. occidentale* stem-bark was studied in normoglycaemic and in streptozotocin-treated diabetic rats. In one set of experiments, graded doses of the aqueous and methanol extracts of *A. occidentale* stem-bark (100-800 mg/kg p.o.) were separately administered to groups of fasted normal and fasted diabetic rats and a dose, which produced maximal hypoglycaemic effects in both fasted normal and diabetic rats, was found to be 800 mg/kg p.o. At this dose, aqueous and methanol extracts of *A. occidentale* stem-bark significantly reduced the mean basal blood glucose concentrations of fasted normal and fasted diabetic rats. The hypoglycaemic effect of the methanol extract of the plant was slightly more pronounced than that of the aqueous extract in both the normal and diabetic rats examined. The authors suggested that hypoglycaemic activity of the plant extracts could possibly be attributed to their terpenoid and/or coumarin contents. However, the mechanism of hypoglycaemic activity of these compounds remains speculative and seems unlikely to be due to the stimulation of pancreatic *beta*-cells and subsequent secretion of insulin (4).

Stigmast-4-en-3-ol and stigmast-4-en-3-one, isolated from the hexane extract of the bark of *Anacardium occidentale,* produced significant hypoglycaemic activity in healthy dogs after intravenous administration at a dose of 1.3 mg/kg body weight. The reported hypoglycaemic activity of extracts of the bark of the cashew plant is probably due to the presence of these compounds (5).

Rats fed on diet, enriched with fructose, showed significant increases in plasma glucose, total cholesterol, triglycerides, total cholesterol/HDL-cholesterol ratio, malonyldialdehyde, total protein, urea and creatinine. Administration of methanol extract of the stem bark of *A. occidentale* to fructose fed rats significantly prevented these changes. From the results of detailed investigation, it was inferred that methanol extract of *A. occidentale* stem bark at a dose of 200 mg/kg body weight might be a safe remedy for hyperglycaemia (6).

Insulin is a rather expensive drug and the availability and affordability of insulin are the major problems for treating diabetes, particularly for type-1 diabetes, in poor countries. Traditional medicines are suitable under such conditions and many plants have been used for this purpose. *Anacardium occidentale* is one of the important plants used for this purpose (3).

1. Kamtehouing P, SD Sokeng, PL Moundipa, P Watcho, HB Jatsa, D Lontsi; Protective role of *Anacardium occidentale* extract against streptozotocin-induced diabetes in rats, *J Ethnopharmacol* **63,** 95-99 (1998)
2. Esimone CO, JM Okonta, CO Ezugwu; Blood sugar lowering effect of *Anacardium occidentale* leaf extract in experimental rabbit model, *J Nat Remedies* **1**(1), 60-63 (2001)
3. Akah PA, CO Okoh, SV Nwafor; Phytotherapy in the management of diabetes mellitus, *J Nat Remedies* **2**(1), 4-10 (2002)
4. Kurihara H, H Fukami, A Kusumoto, Y Toyoda, H Shibata, Y Matsui, S Asami, JA Ojewole; Laboratory evaluation of the hypoglycaemic effect of *Anacardium occidentale* Linn (Anacardiaceae) stem-bark extracts in rats, *Methods Find Exp Clin Pharmacol* **25**(3), 199-204 (2003).
5. Alexander-Lindo RL, EY Morrison, MG Nair; Hypoglycaemic effect of stigmast-4-en-3-one and its corresponding alcohol from the bark of *Anacardium occidentale* (cashew), *Phytother Res* **18**(5), 403-07 (2004).
6. Olatunji LA, JL Okwusidi, AO Soladoye; Anti-diabetic effect of *Anacardium occidentale* stem bark in fructose-fed diabetic rats, *Pharmaceut Biol* **43**(7), 589-93 (2006)

Ananas comosus **Linn. (Bromeliaceae)** ***Syn. Ananas sativus*** **(Pineapple, H. Ananas)**

Anti-diabetic, anti-hyperlipidaemic and anti-oxidative activities of an ethanol extract of *A. comosus* leaves were investigated in diabetic-dyslipidaemic rats induced by alloxan and a high-fat / high-cholesterol diet. The leaf extract, at the dose of 0.40 g/kg, significantly inhibited the increase in blood glucose in diabetic rats in oral glucose tolerance test, but did not cause any hypoglycaemic activity in normal rats. After 15 days of treatment of diabetic dyslipidaemic rats with *A. comosus* leaf extract, significant decrease of blood glucose, triglycerides, total cholesterol and LDL-c levels, significant increase of serum HDL-c levels and significantly lowered lipid peroxidation products of blood, brain, liver and kidneys were observed in comparison with those of untreated diabetic dyslipidemic rats. These data suggested anti-diabetic, anti-dyslipidaemic and anti-oxidative activities of the ethanol extract of *A. comosus* leaves.

Xie W, D Xing, H Sun, W Wang, Y Ding, L Du; The effects of *Ananas comosus* L. leaves on diabetic-dyslipidaemic rats induced by alloxan and a high-fat/high-cholesterol diet, *Am J Chin Med* **33**(1), 95-105 (2005).

Andrographis paniculata **Nees (Acanthaceae) (H. Kalmegh, S. Bhunimba)**

Kalmegh is an annual herb. It is extremely bitter, acrid, cooling and laxative. Kalmegh is found throughout the plains of India and other Asian countries. In Ayurveda the drug has been described as antipyretic and hepatoprotective.

Andrographis paniculata is one of the commonly used herbs by the diabetic patients in Pampanga, Philippines. A significant decrease in blood glucose concentration was demonstrated in rats on glucose tolerance test, when an aqueous extract (2g/kg) was administered orally. However, the extract failed to lower the blood glucose level when it was administered intraperitoneally. From the results of the investigation, it was suggested that the extract inhibits glucose absorption along the intestine (1). The blood glucose lowering effects of aqueous extract of *Andrographis paniculata* was studied in normoglycaemic and streptozotocin-induced hyperglycaemic rats. Significant reduction in blood glucose level (52.90%) was observed when hyperglycaemic rats were treated with aqueous extract of *A. paniculata* (50 mg/kg b.w.). This effect was enhanced when freeze-dried material was used (5). The aqueous decoction of the plant could restore impaired estrous cycle in alloxan-induced diabetic rats (6).

Development of diabetic complications is known to be the result of oxidative stress and an ethanol extract of aerial parts of *A. paniculata* was shown to possess not only an anti-hyperglycaemic property, but also the property of reducing oxidative stress in diabetic rats. Oral administration of the extract (400 mg/kg b.w.), twice a day for 14 days significantly increased body weight and reduced fasting serum glucose in diabetic but not in normal rats. The levels of thiobarbituric acid-reactive substances in liver and kidney were significantly lower and the level of glutathione in liver was significantly higher in the extract-treated diabetic rats in comparison with those of vehicle treated diabetic rats. The extract significantly increased the activity of superoxide dismutase and catalase but no significant effect on glutathione peroxidase activity was observed in diabetic rats. The effect of the extract was comparable to that of metformin (2). Oral administration of the extract at different doses significantly reduced the fasting serum glucose level in streptozotocin-induced diabetic rats compared to the vehicle (distilled water)-treated rats. This effect was dose-dependent. In the glucose tolerance test, an oral administration of the extract at the same doses suppressed the elevated glucose level in normal and diabetic rats. The extract caused significant reduction of fasting serum triglyceride but not cholesterol levels. The anti-diabetic property of the ethanol extract of *A paniculata* may be attributed, at least in part, to increased glucose metabolism. Its hypotriglyceridaemic effect is also beneficial in the diabetic state (3)

Oral administration of andrographolide, an active principle in the leaves of *A. paniculata,* decreased the plasma glucose concentrations of streptozotocin-induced diabetic rats in a dose-dependent manner. Andrographolide, at the effective dose (1.5 mg/kg), significantly attenuated the increase of plasma glucose induced by an intravenous glucose challenge test in normal rats. In the isolated soleus muscle of streptozotocin-induced diabetic rats, andrographolide enhanced the uptake of radioactive glucose in a concentration-dependent manner. The results of detailed investigation suggest that andrographolide can increase the glucose utilization to lower plasma glucose in diabetic rats lacking insulin (4).

1. Ahmad M, M Asmawl; A study of the hypoglycaemic property of *Andrographis paniculata* Nees, *7th Asian Symp Med Plants (ASOMPS VII)*, Manila, February 2-7, (1992).
2. Zhang XF, BK Tan; Anti-hyperglycaemic and anti-oxidant properties of *Andrographis paniculata* in normal and diabetic rats, *Clin Exp Pharmacol Physiol* **27**(5-6), 358-63 (2000).
3. Zhang XF, BK Tan; Anti-diabetic property of ethanolic extract of *Andrographis paniculata* in streptozotocin-diabetic rats, *Acta Pharmacol Sin* **21**(12), 1157-64 (2000)
4. Yu BC, CR Hung, WC Chen, JT Cheng; Anti-hyperglycaemic effect of andrographolide in streptozotocin-induced diabetic rats, *Planta Med* **69**(12), 1075-79 (2003)
5. Huson R, AH Pihie, M Nallappan, Screening for anti-hyperglycaemic activity in several local herbs of Malaysia, *J Ethnopharmacol* **95**(2-3), 205-08 (2004).
6. Reves BA, ND Bautista, NC Tanquilut, RV Anunciado, AB Leung, GC Sanchez,

RL Magtoto, P Castronuevo, H Tsukamura, KL Maeda; Anti-diabetic potentials of *Momordica charantia* and *Andrographis paniculata* and their effects on estrous cyclicity of alloxan-induced diabetic rats, *J Ethnopharmacol* **105**(1-2), 196-200 (2006)

Anemarrhena asphodeloides Bunge (Asphodelaceae/Liliaceae) (Xilingzhimu)

The hypoglycaemic activity of the glycans anemarans A, B, C and D, isolated from the rhizomes of *A. asphodeloides,* were studied (1) [See glycans in Appendix.]

A hot-water extract of the rhizomes of the plant was found to lower the blood glucose level in alloxan-induced diabetic mice. Hypoglycaemic activity-guided fractionation of this extract yielded a new glycoside, pseudoprototimosaponin AIII, which was comparable with the chemically known prototimosaponin AIII. These compounds exhibited hypoglycaemic effects in a dose-dependent manner in streptozotocin-induced diabetic mice but showed no effect on glucose uptake and insulin release. It was on this basis that the mechanism of hypoglycaemic effect was considered to be due to inhibition of hepatic gluconeogenesis and/or glycogenolysis (2).

The water extract of the rhizomes of *A. asphodeloides* (90 mg/kg) reduced blood glucose levels in KK-Ay mice 7 h after oral administration and also tended to reduce their serum insulin levels. Based on these results, the mechanism for the anti-diabetic activity of *A. asphodeloides* aqueous extract was considered to be due to decreased insulin resistance. The xanthone glycosides mangiferin and neomangiferin (7-O-β-D-glucopyranosyl-mangiferin), isolated from the rhizomes of the plant were considered to be active constituents of the plant. Mangiferin lowered the blood glucose level of KK-Ay mice 3 weeks after oral administration. However, no effect on the blood glucose level in normal mice was seen, indicating that mangiferin could be useful in treating type-2 diabetes. It also improved hyperinsulinemia and, on insulin tolerance test, reduced blood glucose levels of KK-Ay mice. From these findings, it was considered to exert its anti-diabetic activity by decreasing insulin resistance (3-5).

With an objective to investigate whether an ethanol extract of *A. asphodeloides* stimulates insulin secretion and if so, to elucidate the mechanism behind this effect, isolated pancreatic islets of normal Wistar rats and spontaneously diabetic Goto-Kakizaki (GK) rats were batch incubated or perifused to study the effect of the extract on insulin release. It was observed that the extract stimulates insulin secretion both at 3.3 and 16.7 mM glucose in islets of normal Wistar and diabetic GK rats. In perifusions of islets, the extract also increased insulin secretion that returned to basal levels when the extract was omitted from the perifusate. Mangiferin showed no effect on insulin secretion of islets. It was inferred that the extract contains an active substance (TH2), which is responsible for this effect (6).

1. Takahashi M, C Konno, H Hikino, Isolation and hypoglycaemic activity of anemarans A, B, C and D, glycans of *Anemarrhena asphodeloides* rhizomes, *Planta Med* No. (2), 100-02 (1985)
2. Nakashima N, I Kimura, M Kimura, H Matsuura, Isolation of pseudoprototimosaponin AIII from rhizomes of *Anemarrhena asphodeloides* and its hypoglycaemic activity in streptozotocin- induced diabetic mice, *J Nat Prod* **56**(3), 345-50 (1993).
3. Hong YF, GY Han, XM Guo, Isolation and structure determination of xanthone glycosides of *Anemarrhena asphodeloides Yao Xue Xue Bao* **32**(6), 473-75 (1997) [Article in Chinese].
4. Miura T, H Ichiki, I Hashimoto, N Iwamoto, M Kato, M Kubo, E Ishihara, Y Komatsu, M Okada, T Ishida, K Tanigawa; Anti-diabetic activity of a xanthone compound, mangiferin, *Phytomedicine* **8**(2), 85-87 (2001).
5. Miura T, H Ichiki, N Iwamoto, M Kato, M Kubo, H Sasaki, M Okada, T Ishida, Y Seino, K Tanigawa; Anti-diabetic activity of the rhizoma of *Anemarrhena asphodeloides* and active components, mangiferin and its glucoside, *Biol Pharm Bull* **24**(9), 1009-11 (2001).
6. Hoa NK, DV Phan, ND Thuan, CG Ostenson, Insulin secretion is stimulated by ethanol extract of *Anemarrhena asphodeloides* in isolated islet of healthy Wistar and diabetic Goto-Kakizaki rats, *Exp Clin Endocrinol Diabetes* **112**(9), 520-25 (2004).

Angelica archangelica Linn. (Apiaceae) (Garden Angelica, Wild Celery)

Angelica archangelica is a biennial plant from the umbelliferous family Apiaceae and it grows wild in Finland, Sweden, Norway, Denkark, Greenland and Iceland. It is cultivated in France in marshy lands.

An organic compound containing equal parts of Antimony and Tin has been extracted from *Angelica archangelica*. The compound was found to inhibit the appearance of interleukin-2 receptors, lymphocyte proliferation and oxidative metabolism.

Claude MJ, MJ Pierre; New organic derivatives of metals with phospholipids, use of these derivatives, process for isolating the derivatives from plants and pharmaceutical compositions containing them, PCT Int Appl. WO 91,13892 (CL C07F9/10, 1991

Angelica dahurica (Hoffm.) Franch. & Sav(Apiaceae/Umbelliferae)

A number of coumarins were isolated from the roots of the plant. The effects of these coumarins on actions of adrenaline, ACTH and insulin were studied.

Kimura Y, H Ohminami, H Arichi, H Okuda, K Baba, M Kozawa, S Arichi; Effects of various coumarins from roots of *Angelica dahurica* on actions of adrenaline, ACTH and insulin in fat cells, *Planta Med* **45**(3), 183-87 (1982)

Angylocalyx pynaertii De Wild. (Fabaceae / Leguminosae)

The bark extract of *Angylocalyx pynaertii* was found to be a potent inhibitor of mammalian α- L-fucosidases. Fifteen polyhydroxylated alkaloids were isolated from this extract. The alkaloids are structurally related to sugars and the minimum structure and stereochemical requirements to be α- L-fucosidase inhibitor have been discussed.

Asano N, K Yasuda, H Kizu, A Kato, J-Q Fan, RJ. Nash, George WJ. Fleet, RJ Molyneux; Novel α-L-fucosidase inhibitors from the bark of *Angylocalyx pynaertii* (Leguminosae), *FEBS J* **268**(1), 35-41(2001)

Annona squamosa Linn. (Annonaceae) (Custard apple, H. Shareefa, Seetaphal)

Annona squamosa is a species native to the tropical America. Its exact native range is unknown due to extensive cultivation, but thought to be in the Caribbeans. Anti-diabetic properties of aqueous and ethanol extracts of the young leaves of the plant as well as of the fruit pulp of *Annona squamosa* were studied.

The anti-diabetic activity of an alcoholic extract of *A. squamosa* leaves was investigated in rats with type-2 diabetes mellitus, induced with standardised doses of streptozotocin and nicotinamide. Graded doses of the extract suspended in gum acacia were administered to normal and experimental diabetic rats for 12 days and their effects on fasting plasma glucose levels, serum insulin levels, serum lipid profiles and changes in body weight were studied. Liver glycogen levels and pancreatic TBARS levels were evaluated additionally for experimental diabetic rats. The findings showed that the alcoholic extract of *A. squamosa* leaves had significant potential in ameliorating the diabetic conditions in diabetic rats. No significant effect was observed in normal rats (1). The effects of oral administration of an ethanol extract of *A. squamosa* leaves at different doses to normal and streptozotocin-induced diabetic rats as well as to alloxan-induced diabetic rabbits were studied. At a dose of 350mg/kg body weight, the extract reduced the fasting blood glucose level within 1 h and the peak blood glucose at 1 h during glucose tolerance test in normal rats. In alloxan-induced diabetic rabbits, the same dose of the extract also reduced fasting blood glucose level and improved glucose tolerance. Similar effect was also observed in streptozotocin-induced diabetic rats. Treatment of severely diabetic rabbits for 15 days with a dose of 350 mg/kg of the extract reduced fasting blood glucose level by 52.7% and urine sugar by 75% (4).

The claims of anti-diabetic activity of aqueous extract of young leaves of *A. squamosa* was verified by administration of leaf extract in drinking water to normal and streptozotocin-nicotinamide-induced diabetic rats for 12 days. The findings of the study supported the anti-diabetic claims of *A. squamosa* and the activity was compared with standard glibenclamide (2). Oral administration of the aqueous extract of *A. squamosa* leaves to diabetic rats for 30 days significantly reduced the levels of blood glucose, lipids and lipid peroxidation, but increased the activities of plasma insulin and antioxidant enzymes, like catalase, superoxide dismutase and glutathione peroxidase. It also reduced the activities of glutathione (6).

Effect of the fruit pulp of the edible fruit of *A. squamosa* was studied on various biochemical parameters. Fruit pulp increased the net protein utilization in normal healthy rabbits as well as in alloxan-induced diabetic animals when compared with the control group of rabbits. It also increased the total haemoglobin content in normal and diabetic rabbits. Fruit pulp improved the liver function, characterised by reduction of serum SGOT, SGPT, ALKP and bilirubin levels, in normal as well as in diabetic rabbits. It also brought down urine sugar levels in diabetic rabbits (3, 5).

1. Shirwaikar A, K Rajendran, C Dinesh Kumar; Oral anti-diabetic activity of *Annona squamosa* leaf alcohol extract in NIDDM rats, *Pharmaceut Biol* **42**(1), 30-35 (2004)
2. Shirwaikar A, K Rajendran, C Dinesh Kumar, R Bodla; Anti-diabetic activity of aqueous leaf extract of *Annona squamosa* in streptozotocin-nicotinamide type-2 diabetic rats, *J Ethnopharmacol* **91**(1), 171-75 (2004).
3. Gupta RK, AN Kesari, G Watal, V Tandon; Nutritional effect of fruit pulp of *Annona squamosa* in normal healthy and alloxan-induced diabetic rabbits, *Chem Biol Interface: Synergistic New Frontiers,* New Delhi, India, P-22-46 November 21-26, 2004
4. Gupta RK, AN Kesari, PS Murthy, R Chandra, V Tandon, G Watal; Hypoglycaemic and anti-diabetic effect of ethanolic extract of leaves of *Annona squamosa* L. in experimental animals, *J Ethnopharmacol* **99**(1), 75-81 (2005).
5. Gupta RK, AN Kesari, G Watal , PS Murthy, R Chandra, V Tandon; Nutritional and hypoglycaemic effect of fruit pulp of *Annona squamosa* in normal healthy and alloxan-induced diabetic rabbits, *Ann Nutr Metab* **49**(6), 407-13 (2005)
6. Kaleem M, M Asif, QU Ahmed, B Bano; Anti-diabetic and antioxidant activity of *Annona squamosa* extract in streptozotocin-induced diabetic rats, *Singapore Med J* **47**(8), 670-75 (2006)

Anoectochilus formosanus Hayata (Orchidaceae) (Jewel orchids)

Orchids of the genus *Anoectochilus* are sometimes called "Jewel orchids" because of their attractive venation. They are found in moist areas with deep shade and from the Himalayas to tropical and subtropical Asia, Australia, Papua New Guinea and the Pacific Islands.

The anti-hyperglycaemic and antioxidant effects of an aqueous extract of *A. formosanus* were studied in streptozotocin-induced diabetic rats. Diabetic rats were randomly divided into two groups and treated orally by gavage either with vehicle (distilled water) or with aqueous extract of the plant (1 and 2 g/kg), once a day for 21 days. At the end of the 21 days, a reduction in the levels of fasting blood glucose, serum fructosamine, triglycerides and total cholesterol was observed in diabetic rats having the plant extract (2 g/kg) compared with vehicle-treated diabetic rats. Renal lipid peroxidation levels were significantly lower and renal reduced glutathione concentrations were significantly higher in the plant extract-treated diabetic rats compared with vehicle-treated diabetic rats. The diabetic kidney in the vehicle-treated group showed a decrease in catalase, but the activity of glutathione peroxidase was increased. Treatment with aqueous extract of *A. formosanus* reversed the activity of catalase, but not of glutathione peroxidase. These results indicate that the plant extract (1 and 2 g/kg) not only possesses an anti-hyperglycaemic effect, but also reduces oxidative stress in diabetic rats.

Shih CC, YW Wu, WC Lin; Anti-hyperglycaemic and anti-oxidant properties of *Anoectochilus formosanus* in diabetic rats, *Clin Exp Pharmacol Physiol* **29**(8), 684-88 (2002).

Anthocleista vogelii Planch (Gentianaceae / Loganiaceae)

Aqueous extract of finely divided roots of the plant (100, 400 and 800 mg/kg) induced significant hypoglycaemic activity in a dose-dependent fashion at 2h after oral administration in mice and rats. In normoglycaemic rabbits, the extract (800 mg/kg, p.o.) similarly reduced blood glucose level in a statistically significant manner. The extract (400 and 800 mg/kg, p.o.) also caused reduction of blood glucose levels in alloxan-induced diabetic animals. *A. vogelii* was thus proved to possess a favourable hypoglycaemic activity both in normal and hyperglycaemic animals comparable to chlorpropamide.

Abuh FY, C Wambebe, PP Rai; Hypoglycaemic activity of *Anthocleista vogelii* (Planch) aqueous extract in rodents, *Phytother Res* **4**(1), 20-24 (1990).

Antidesma madagascariense Lam. (Euphorbiaceae)

The plant is found in Tropical evergreen mountain forest of Mauritus. The effects of *Antidesma madagascariense* leaf extract on the transport of D-glucose, L-tyrosine, fluid and electrolytes (Na^+ and K^+) across rat everted intestinal sacs were studied. The sacs were mounted in an organ bath containing KHB buffer. Incubation with aqueous *A, madagascariense* extracts (>0.375 mg/ml) significantly stimulated the mucosal disappearance and serosal appearance of glucose and fluid. The concentration of glucose accumulated in the intestinal tissues also increased significantly compared to that found in the controls. Incubation with the plant extract (0.75 mg/ml) significantly enhanced Na^+ uptake and transport but not K^+ transport. Aqueous extract of *A. madagascariense* produced stimulatory effects on the transport of glucose, fluid and Na^+ as were found with insulin. It has been hypothesised that bioactive phytochemicals of the plant extract interfere with the Na^+/glucose carrier, and thus enhance the transport of glucose, Na^+ and fluid across rat everted intestinal sacs. It was proposed that *A. madagascariense* leaf extract might represent a possible alternative dietary supplement for the treatment of type-2 diabetes.

Mahomoodally MF, AG Fakim, AH Subratty; Stimulatory effects of *Antidesma madagascariense* on D-glucose, L-tyrosine, fluid and electrolyte transport across rat everted intestine, comparable to insulin action *in vitro*, *Br J Biomed Sci* **63**(1), 12-17 (2006)

Apocynum venetum Linn (Apocynaceae Euphorbiaceae) (Indian Hemp, Dogbane)

The Chinese herbs, *Apocynum venetum, Ginkgo biloba, Morus alba* and *Rhododendron dauricum,* were shown to have strong hydroxyl radical scavenging activities.

Cao Y, Q Chu, J Ye; Determination of hydroxyl radical by capillary electrophoresis and studies on hydroxyl radical scavenging activities of Chinese herbs, *Anal Bioanal Chem* **376**(5), 691-95 (2003)

Aporosa lindleyana (Wight.) Baill. (Phyllanthaceae)

The aqueous and alcoholic extracts of *A. lindleyana* (100 mg/kg) significantly reduced the blood glucose level of normal as well as of alloxan induced diabetic rats 3 h after oral administration of the extracts. The anti-hyperglycaemic activity of *A. lindleyana* was compared with tolbutamide, an oral hypoglycaemic agent.

Jayakar B, B Suresh; Anti-hyperglycaemic and hypoglycaemic effect of *Aporosa lindleyana* in normal and alloxan induced diabetic rats, *J Ethnopharmacol* **84**(2-3), 247-49 (2003).

Arachis hypogaea Linn. (Fabaceae) (Peanut, Groundnut, H. Mungphali)

The aqueous extract of *A. hypogaea* caused a significant decrease of fasting blood glucose level of both normal and alloxan-induced diabetic rats. The extract also caused a significant decrease in serum triglyceride, total cholesterol, HDL-cholesterol and LDL-cholesterol in both normal and alloxan-induced diabetic rats.

Bilbis LS, RA Shehu, MG Abubakar; Hypoglycaemic and hypolipidaemic effects of aqueous extract of *Arachis hypogaea* in normal and alloxan-induced diabetic rats,

Phytomedicine **9**(6), 553-55 (2002).

Aralia cachemirica Decne (Araliaceae) (Himalayan spikenard)

Aralia (Spikenard) is a genus of the plant family Araliaceae. The genus is native to Asia and the Americas, with most species occurring in mountain woodlands. The aqueous and alcoholic extracts of *A. cachemirica* at a dose of 250 mg/kg showed statistically significant hypoglycaemic activity in glucose loaded animals but no effect was observed in normal fasted rats.

Bhat ZA, SH Ansari, HM Mukhtar, T Naved, JI Siddiqui, NA Khan; Effect of *Aralia cachemirica* Decne root extracts on blood glucose level in normal and glucose loaded rats, *Pharmazie* **60**(9), 712-13 (2005).

Aralia dasyphylla Miq. (Araliaceae)

The plant occurs in China, Vietnam, Malaysia, and Indonesia.The total saponins, isolated from the plant, exhibited hypoglycaemic effect on a model of alloxan-induced diabetes in rats.

Yi YH, JQ Gu, K Xiao, ZZ Wang, HW Lin; Studies on triterpenoids and their glycosides from *Aralia dasyphylla* Miq, *Yao Xue Xue Bao* **32**(10), 769-72 (1997) [Article in Chinese].

Aralia elata Seem (Araliaceae) (Japanse angelica tree)

Aralia elata is native to eastern Russia, China, Korea, and Japan. The plant is sometimes cultivated for its exotic appearance. *Aralia elata* is closely related to the American species *Aralia spinosa*, with which it is easily confused. In Japan, the shoots are eaten in the spring. They are picked from the end of the branches and fried.

Oleanolic acid 28-O-β-D-glucopyranoside, isolated from the root bark of *A. elata*, was found to be an active anti-hyperglycaemic compound in a model of alloxan-induced diabetic rats at a dose 100 mg/kg p.o. The contents of the liver glycogen, which were lowered by alloxan injection, were also increased by this compound (1). The hypoglycaemic activities of oleanolic acid and nine oleanolic acid glycosides obtained from the root cortex of *A. elata* were determined by monitoring inhibition effect on the elevation of plasma glucose level by oral sucrose tolerance test in rats, and some structure-activity relationships were found. The structure of elatoside E, the hypoglycaemic component isolated from the root cortex of *A. elata*, was settled as oleanolic acid 3-O-[β-D-xylopyranosyl (1α2)]-[β-D-glucopyranosyl (1α3)]-a-L-arabinopyranoside (2, 4).

Of the five new saponins, isolated from the young shoots of the plant, elatosides G, H and I (glycosides of oleanolic and hydroxy oleanolic acids) were found to exhibit potent hypoglycaemic activity in the oral glucose tolerance test in rats (3)

1. Kim OK, EB Lee, SS Kang; Anti-hyperglycaemic constituent of *Aralia elata* root bark, *Korean J Pharmacogn* **24**(3), 219-22 (1993)
2. Yoshikawa M, H Matsuda, E Harada, T Murakami, N Wariishi, J Yamahara, N Murakami; Elatoside E, a new hypoglycaemic principle from the root cortex of *Aralia elata* Seem.: structure-related hypoglycaemic activity of oleanolic acid glycosides, *Chem Pharm Bull* (Tokyo) **42**(6), 1354-56 (1994).
3. Yoshikawa M, S Yoshizumi, T Ueno, H Matsuda, T Murakami, J Yamahara, N Murakami; Medicinal foodstuffs: I. Hypoglycaemic constituents from a garnish foodstuff "Taranome" the young shoot of *Aralia elata* Seem: Elatosides G, H, I, J and K, *Chem Pharm Bull* (Tokyo) **43**(11), 1878-82 (1995).
4. Yoshikawa M, T Murakami, E Harada, N Murakami, J Yamahara, H Matsuda; Bioactive saponins and glycosides. VII. On the hypoglycaemic principles from the root cortex of *Aralia elata* Seem.: Structure related hypoglycaemic activity of oleanolic acid oligoglycoside, *Chem Pharm Bull* (Tokyo) **44**(10), 1923-27 (1996).

Aralia mandshurica Rupr (Araliaceae) Syn. *A. elata*

Oral administration of the saponins from *A. mandshurica* did not affect plasma lactic acid, glucagon, insulin or liver glycogen levels in exercised rats. Plasma glucose levels in resting rats were decreased by saponin extracts of the plant.

Martinez B, EJ Staba; The physiological effects of *Aralia, Panax* and *Eleutherococcus* on exercised rats, *Jpn J Pharmacol* **35**(2), 79-85 (1984)

Areca catechu Linn. (Arecaceae Palmae) (Betel nut, H. Supari)

Areca catechu, known commonly as Betel nut tree, grows in the tropical Pacific, Asia, and parts of East Africa. *A. catechu* is grown for its economically important seed crop, the Betel nut. Areca palms are grown in India, Malaysia, Taiwan and many other Asian countries for their seeds. Arecoline is the major alkaloid of Betel nut,

Subcutaneous administration of the alkaloid fraction of *A. catechu* at the dose levels of 0.20 and 0.25 mg/kg b.w. showed hypoglycaemic activity. The hypoglycaemia lasted for 4-6 hours.

Chempakam B, Hypoglycaemic activity of arecoline in betel nut *Areca catechu* L., *Indian J Exp Biol* **31**(5), 474-75 (1993).

Aronia melanocarpa (Michx.) Elliott (Rosaceae) (Black chokeberry)

The chokeberries (*Aronia*) are two species of deciduous shrubs, native to eastern North America and most commonly found in wet woods and swamps. Its flowers are white but fruits are black.

Anthocyanins, derived from the plant, exhibited hypoglycaemic activity in alloxan-induced diabetic rabbits and streptozotocin-induced diabetic rats. The sugar concentration in blood serum was substantially decreased by daily administration of the plant-derived anthocyanins in alloxanised rabbits. The pigment also prevented the loss of body weight and generation of oxygen free radicals, as was evident from the lowering of thiobarbituric acid reactive substances (1, 2).

Incorporation of the extract of *A. melanocarpa* leaves into drinking water and its intra-peritoneal administration significantly reduced the blood glucose level of normal and streptozotocin-induced diabetic rats (3).

The low calorie juice of *A. melanocarpa* (sugar free, with artificial sweeteners) might be a valuable adjunct to the complex therapy of patients with diabetes mellitus. No increased blood glucose level was observed 1h after ingestion of 200 ml *Aronia* juice. On the contrary, lower fasting blood glucose concentrations were measured in 16 patients with insulin dependent diabetes and in 25 patients with non-insulin dependent diabetes. The daily intake of 200 ml *Aronia* juice over a period of 3 months was effective in lowering fasting blood glucose levels in 21 patients with non-insulin dependent diabetes. *Aronia* had a beneficial effect on HbA1c, total cholesterol and lipid levels. Accumulated data illustrated the hypoglycaemic potential of *Aronia* juice (4).

1. Jankowski A, J Niedworok, B Jankowska; The influence of *Aronia melanocarpa* Elliot on experimental alloxan-induced diabetes in the rabbits, *Herba Pol* **44**(4), 409-16 (1998).
2. Jankowski A, J Niedworok, B Jankowska; The influence of *Aronia melanocarpa* Elliot on experimental diabetes in the rats, *Herba Pol* **45**(4), 345-53 (1999).
3. Maslov DL, OM Ipatova, Olu Abakunova, TA Tsvetkova, VN Prozorovskii; Hypoglycaemic effect of an extract from *Aronia melanocarpa* leaves, *Vopr Med Khim* **48**(3), 271-77 (2002) [Article in Russian]
4. Simeonov SB, NP Botushanov, EB Karahanian, MB Pavlova, HK Husianitis, DM Troev; Effects of *Aronia melanocarpa* juice as part of the dietary regimen in patients with diabetes mellitus, *Folia Med* (Plovdiv) **44**(3), 20-23 (2002)

Artemisia abyssinica Schultz.bip (Asteraceae) (Artemisia)

An aqueous decoction of *A. abyssinica* significantly decreased the blood glucose level of alloxan-induced diabetic mice over a period of 6 hours. In normal mice, however, an increase in the level of blood glucose was observed 2 and 4 hrs after the drug administration. Phytochemical screening revealed the presence of alkaloids, flavonoids, sterols, terpenes, tannins and volatile oils (1).

The essential oil of *Artemisia abyssinica* was examined for its potential radical scavenging activities. The ability of this volatile oil to act as a non-specific donor for hydrogen atoms or electrons was checked in the diphenylpicrylhydrazyl (DPPH) assay and it showed positive results. However, the oil from *A. abyssinica* exhibited a paradoxical effect, when tested for a hydroxyl radical scavenging agent using deoxyribose degradation assay (2).

1. Mossa JS; Phytochemical and biological studies on *Artemisia abyssinica*, an anti-diabetic herb used in Arabian folk medicine, *Fitoterapia* **56**(5), 311-14 (1985).

2. Burits M, K Asres, F Bucar; The antioxidant activity of the essential oils of *Artemisia afra*, *Artemisia abyssinica* and *Juniperus procera*, *Phytother Res* **15**(2), 103-08 (2001)

Artemisia afra Jacq. ex Willd. (Asteraceae)

Artemisia afra is a common species of the genus *Artemisia* in Africa, with a wide distribution from South Africa, to areas reaching to the North and East. *Artemisia afra* is a well-known medicinal plant in Africa, and is still used effectively by people of many cultures.

The essential oil of *Artemisia afra* was examined for its potential radical scavenging activities. The ability of this volatile oil to act as a non-specific donor of hydrogen atoms or electrons was checked in the diphenylpicrylhydrazyl assay and it showed positive results. The oil of *A. afra* was also found to be an effective hydroxyl radical scavenging agent when assessed in the deoxyribose degradation assay. In the *in vitro* assay for non-enzymatic lipid peroxidation in liposomes, the oil of *A. afra* displayed antioxidant potential.

Burits M, K Asres, F Bucar; The antioxidant activity of the essential oils of *Artemisia afra*, *Artemisia abyssinica* and *Juniperus procera*, *Phytother Res* **15**(2), 103-08 (2001)

Artemisia cannariensis Lee (Asteraceae)

A sesquiterpenic lactone (vulgarin), isolated from an extract of *A. cannariensis*, showed highly significant hypoglycaemic effects when administered orally or intravenously.

Peran S, AM De-Diego, F Arcas, A Mate, M Morell; Effect of a new hypoglycaemic drug on the blood sugar in rats, *Rev Iber Endocrinol* **23**(134), 171-78 (1976) [Article in Spanish]

Artemisia capillaris Thunb (Asteraceae/Compositae)

Artemisia capillaris is a bushy sub-shrub which is grown for its aromatic, finely-divided, gray-green foliage. The effects of *A. capillaris* on blood glucose and lipid in mice were studied and its effective mechanism was explained. The hyperglycaemic effects in alloxan-induced diabetic mice were significantly inhibited by *A. capillaris* but the change of fasting blood glucose in normal and hyperlipidaemic mice was not significant. The results of the study indicated that the hypoglycaemic effect of *A. capillaris* was comparable to that of biguanide-drugs and that the plant drug could be used to protect and treat diabetes mellitus and its chronic complications.

Pan J, G Liu, H Lin, Z Qiu, L Chen; Effects of *Artemisia capillaris* on blood glucose and lipid in mice, *Zhong Yao Cai* **21**(8), 408-11 (1998) [Article in Chinese].

Artemisia dracunculus Linn. (Asteraceae) (Tarralin)

An ethanol extract of *A dracunculus* inhibited aldose reductase (ALR2), a key enzyme involved in diabetic complications. The inhibitory activity was comparable with quercitrin, a known ALR2 inhibitor. Bioactivity guided fractionation of this ethanol extract yielded four bioactive compounds with ALR2 inhibitory activity. These compounds were identified as 4, 5-di-O-caffeoylquinic acid, 6-demethoxycapillarisin, 2',4'-dihydroxy-4-methoxydihydrochalcone and davidigenin (1).

The anti-hyperglycaemic activity of an ethanol extract of *A. dracunculus* (known as Tarralin) was studied in diabetic and non-diabetic animals. Tarralin treatment by gavage (500 mg/kg b.w./day for 7 days) lowered elevated blood glucose levels in genetically diabetic KK-A (*gamma*) mice. The activity was comparable to the known anti-diabetic drugs, troglitazone (30 mg/kg b.w./day) and metformin (300 mg/kg b.w./day). Tarralin also reduced blood insulin concentrations in KK-A(*gamma*) mice like the other two drugs. Similar effects were also observed in streptozotocin-induced diabetic mice. Tarralin significantly decreased phosphoenolpyruvate carboxykinase (PEPCK) mRNA expression in streptozotocin-induced diabetic rats. In non-diabetic animals, treatment with Tarralin did not significantly alter PEPCK expression, blood glucose or insulin concentrations. It was also shown to increase the binding of glucagon-like peptide (GLP-1) to its receptor *in vitro* (2).

1. Logendra S, DM Ribnicky, H Yang, A Poulev, J Ma, EJ Kennelly, I Raskin; Bioassay-guided isolation of aldose reductase inhibitors from *Artemisia dracunculus*, *Phytochemistry* **67**(14), 1539-46 (2006)
2. Ribnicky DM, A Poulev, M Watford, WT Cefalu, I Raskin; Anti-hyperglycaemic activity of Tarralin, an ethanolic extract of *Artemisia dracunculus* L, *Phytomedicine* **13**(8), 550-57(2006)

Artemisia herba alba Asso (Asteraceae/Compositae) (White wormwood)

Artemisia herba alba is an important Iraqi folk medicine for the treatment of diabetes mellitus. Oral administration of an aqueous extract (0.39 g/kg) of the aerial parts of this plant to normoglycaemic and alloxan-induced diabetic rabbits produced significant hypoglycaemic activity, which was consistent and time-dependent. While aqueous extracts of leaves and barks of the plant produced a significant reduction in blood glucose level, the aqueous extract of roots and methanol extract of the aerial parts of the plant were virtually ineffective (1-2). The efficacy and toxicity of *A. herba alba* were assessed. The aqueous extract of the aerial parts of the plant (0.39 g/kg b.w. for 2-4 weeks), fed to diabetic rats and rabbits, significantly reduced their blood glucose level, prevented elevation of glycosylated haemoglobin level and showed a hypoliposis effect, in addition to the protection against body weight loss of diabetic animals (3). The aqueous extract of the plant produced an initial hyperglycaemia which was followed by hypoglycaemia in normoglycaemic and alloxan-treated rabbits and mice. The extract (0.3g/kg) also significantly increased the gastro-intestinal transit time (4)

1. Twaij HA, AA Al-Badr; Hypoglycaemic activity of *Artemisia herba alba, J Ethnopharmacol* **24**(2-3), 123-26 (1988).
2. al-Khazraji SM, LA al-Shamaony, HA Twaij; Hypoglycaemic effect of *Artemisia herba alba.* I. Effect of different parts and influence of the solvent on hypoglycaemic activity, *J Ethnopharmacol* **40**(3), 163-66 (1993)
3. Al-Shamaony L, SM al-Khazraji, HA Twaij; Hypoglycaemic effect of *Artemisia herba alba.* II. Effect of a valuable extract on some blood parameters in diabetic animals, *J Ethnopharmacol* **43**(3), 167-71 (1994).
4. Marrif HL, BH Ali, KM Hassan; Pharmacological studies on *Artemisia herba alba* in rabbits and mice, *J Ethnopharmacol* **49**(1), 51-55 (1995)

Artemisia pallens Wall ex DC (Asteraceae) (Davana)

Artemisia pallens is used in Indian folk medicine for the treatment of diabetes mellitus. Oral administration of the methanol extract of aerial parts of the plant led to significant blood glucose lowering effect in glucose-fed hyperglycaemic and alloxan-induced diabetic rats. This effect of the extract was dose dependent and significant at 100 mg/kg level in glucose-fed rats. In fasted normal rats, the extract caused a moderate hypoglycaemic effect at a higher dose (1000 mg/kg). The aqueous extract was inactive.

Subramoniam A, P Pushpagandan, S Rajasekharan, DA Evans, PG Latha, R Valsaraj; Effects of *Artemisia pallens* Wall. on blood glucose levels in normal and alloxan-induced diabetic rats, *J Ethnopharmacol* **50**(1), 13-17 (1996).

Artemisia santonicum Linn. (Asteraceae)

Administration of an aqueous extract of *A. santonicum* (2 ml/kg; 0.42 g/kg) in normal and alloxan-induced diabetic rabbits significantly reduced blood glucose levels 6 h after administration. This activity was consistent and time-dependent.

Korkmaz H, A Gurdal; Effect of *Artemisia santonicum* L. on blood glucose in normal and alloxan-induced diabetic rabbits, *Phytother Res* **16**(7), 675-76 (2002)

Artemisia sphaerocephala Krasch (Asteraceae)

A new polysaccharide, composed of L-Ara, D-Xyl, D-Lyx, D-Man, D-Glc, D-Gal and isolated from the seeds of the plant, was administered orally for 4 weeks and the blood glucose changes were determined in fasted rats. The polysaccharide, at a dose of 200 mg/kg body weight, produced a significant decrease in blood glucose levels in diabetic rats. The effect on the plasma cholesterol was also significant in diabetic rats. A significant effect of the polysaccharide on plasma triglycerides in both normal and diabetic groups was also observed.

Zhang J, Y Huang, T Hou, Y Wang; Hypoglycaemic effect of *Artemisia sphaerocephala* Krasch seed polysaccharide in alloxan-induced diabetic rats, *Swiss Med Wkly* **136**(33-34), 529-32 (2006)

Artocarpus heterophyllus Lam (Moraceae)
(Jack fruit, H. Kathal)

Artocarpus heterophyllus is a species of tree of the mulberry family. The plant is native to India, Bangladesh, Philippines, Sri Lanka and Malay Peninsula. Jack fruits are edible.

The effect of hot-water extract of *A. heterophyllus* leaves on the glucose tolerance of normal human subjects and maturity-onset diabetic patients was evaluated. The extract significantly improved glucose tolerance in the normal subjects and the diabetic patients at an oral dose equivalent to 20 g/kg of the starting material.

Fernando MR, N Wickramasinghe, ML Thabrew, PL Ariyananda, FH Karunanayake; Effect of *Artocarpus heterophyllus* and *Asteracanthus longifolia* on glucose tolerance in normal human subjects and in maturity-onset diabetic patients, *J Ethnopharmacol* **31**(3), 277-82 (1991).

Asparagus adscendens Roxb. (Asparagaceae)
(S. Shweta musali, H. Safed Musli)

This is a thorny plant growing tall and erect. The rhizomes are 0.25-0.5 cm thick and white in colour. It is used as an aphrodisiac as well as to increase sperm count. Its use as a general tonic is also well known all over India. It is found in India, Afghanistan, and Iran. It grows abundantly in the forests of Uttar Pradesh, India.

An aqueous extract of *A. adscendens* induced a significant non-toxic increase in glucose-dependent insulinotropic actions in the clonal pancreatic *beta* cell line, BRIN-BD11. The extract also produced an increase in glucose uptake in 3T3-L1 adipocytes and a decrease in starch digestion *in vitro*. It was thus observed that the extract of

A. adscendens. stimulates insulin secretion, insulin action and inhibits starch digestion.

Mathews JN, PR Flatt, YH Abdel Wahab; *Asparagus adscendens* (Shweta musali) stimulates insulin secretion, insulin action and inhibits starch digestion, *Br J Nutr* **95**(3), 576-81 (2006)

Asparagus racemosus Willd.(Asparagaceae) (S & H. Shatavari)

It is a creeper that contains adventitious root system with numerous tuberous roots. These tuberous roots after proper processing and drying are used as medicine in Ayurveda, with the name of Shatavari. It is considered to be the main Ayurvedic rejuvenating female tonic for overall health and vitality.

Asparagus racemosus root is known to reduce blood glucose in rats and rabbits. In order to locate the active fraction, ethanol extract of the roots of the plant was sequentially partitioned with solvents of increasing polarity and each fraction was tested for its insulin-secretion property. The ethanol extract and each of the hexane, chloroform and ethyl acetate partition fractions stimulated insulin secretion in isolated perfused rat pancreas, isolated rat islet cells and clonal *beta*-cells concentration-dependently. The stimulatory effects of these fractions were potentiated by glucose, 3-isobutyl-1-methyl xanthine, tolbutamide and depolarizing concentration of KCl and inhibited by diazoxide and verapamil. The findings reveal that constituents of *A. racemosus* root extracts have wide-ranging stimulatory effects on physiological insulinotropic pathways.

Hannan JM, L Marenah, L Ali, B Rokeya, PR Flatt, YH Abdel-Wahab; Insulin secretory actions of extracts of *Asparagus racemosus* root in perfused pancreas, isolated islets and clonal pancreatic *beta*-cells, *J Endocrinol* **192**(1), 159-68 (2007)

Asteracanthus longifolia (S. Kokilaksha) Nees (Acanthaceae)

An investigation was made to verify the hypoglycaemic property, attributed to the plant by Ayurvedic physicians and traditional medical practitioners in Sri Lanka. The effects of an aqueous extract of the whole plant of *A. longifolia* on fasting blood glucose level and glucose tolerance were studied using Sprague-Dawley rats. The extract significantly lowered the fasting blood glucose level and markedly improved the glucose tolerance of the rats. The hypoglycaemic effect, produced by a therapeutic dose (equivalent to 5 g/kg of plant material), was comparable to that produced by a therapeutic dose of tolbutamide. The magnitude of the hypoglycaemic effect was, however, found to vary with the dosage administered and the storage time of the prepared extract. The effect of hot-water extract of the whole plant on the glucose tolerance of normal human subjects and maturity-onset diabetic patients was evaluated. The extract significantly improved glucose tolerance in the normal subjects and the diabetic patients at an oral dose equivalent to 20 g/kg of the starting material (1, 2).

1. Fernando MR, N Wickramasinghe, ML Thabrew, EH Karunanayaka; A preliminary investigation of the possible hypoglycaemic activity of *Asteracanthus longifolia*, *J Ethnopharmacol* **27**(1-2), 7-14 (1989).
2. Fernando MR, N Wickramasinghe, ML Thabrew, PL Ariyananda, EH Karunanayake; Effect of *Artocarpus heterophyllus* and *Asteracanthus longifolia* on glucose tolerance in normal human subjects and in maturity-onset diabetic patients, *J Ethnopharmacol* **31**(3), 277-82 (1991).

Astragalus membranaceus (Fisch.) (Fabaceae /Papilionaceae) (Milk-vetch, Huang-Qi)

Root extract of the plant has been reported to significantly lower the blood glucose level of streptozotocin-induced diabetic rats (1).

Compounds that target the peroxisome proliferator-activated receptors (PPAR *alpha* and PPAR *gamma*) are used to correct dyslipidaemia and restore glycaemic balance. As most of the diabetic patients suffer from atherogenic lipid abnormalities, in addition to insulin resistance, ligands are required that can activate both these receptors and the extract of *A. membranaceus* served this purpose satisfactorily. Bioassay-guided fractionation of the plant extract resulted in the isolation of the isoflavones, formononetin, and calycosin as the PPAR-activating compounds. The results suggest the potential value of these isoflavones as anti-diabetic agents with the ability to regulate lipid metabolism (2).

1. ParK JH, BK Kim, MK Park, SY Cho, JS Lee, HK Han, CS Jeong, KH Jung' Anti-diabetic activity of herbal drugs, *Korean J Pharmacogn* **28**(2), 72-74 (1997).
2. Shen P, MH Liu, TY Ng, YH Chan, EL Yong; Differential effects of isoflavones, from *Astragalus membranaceus* and *Pueraria thomsonii*, on the activation of PPAR *alpha*, PPAR *gamma*, and adipocyte differentiation *in vitro*, *J Nutr* **136**(4), 899-905 (2006).

Atractylodes japonica Koidz. ex Kitam. (Asteraceae/Compositae)

The rhizome of the plant is commonly used in Chinese and Korean herbal medicine. The glycans isolated from the rhizome exhibited hypoglycaemic activity. [See glycans in Addendum]

Konno C, Y Suzuki, K Oishi, E Munakata, H Hikino; Isolation and hypoglycaemic activity of atractans A, B and C, glycans of *Atractylodes japonica* rhizomes, *Planta Med* **No. 2**, 102-03 (1985).

Atractylodes macrocephala Koidz (Asteraceae)
(Baizhu in Chinese)

AMP-B, a complex polysaccharide isolated from the water extract of *A. macrocephala* roots, was found to be composed of 50.3% neutral polysaccharide, 40.4% uronic acid and 11.5% protein. The neutral polysaccharide is composed of glucose, galactose, mannose, arabinose and rhamnose in a molar ratio of 3.0:2.5:1.3:3.5:1.0. The polysaccharide was found to reduce blood glucose level in alloxan-induced diabetic rats markedly at doses of 50, 100 and 200 mg/kg, p.o, but no effect was observed in normal rats. AMP-B was found to recover pancreas damage of diabetic rats induced by alloxan.

Shan JJ, GY Tian; Studies on physico-chemical properties and hypoglycaemic activity of complex polysaccharide AMP-B from *Atractylodes macrocephala* Koidz,, *Yao Xue Xue Bao* **38**(6), 438-41 (2003) [Article in Chinese].

Atriplex halimus Linn. (Amaranthaceae)
(Mediterranean saltbush)

Atriplex halimus is a fodder shrub, native to Europe. Hypoglycaemic effect of salt bush and insulin-potentiating effect of its ash were studied (1-3).

1. Aharonson Z, J Shani, FG Sulman; Hypoglycaemic effect of the salt bush (*Atriplex halimus*)—a feeding source of the sand rat (*Psammomys Obesus*), *Diabetologia* **5**(6), 379-83 (1969)
2. Shani J, Z, Aharonson FG Sulman, W Mertz, G Frenkel, PF Kraicer; Insulin-potentiating effect of salt bush (*Atriplex halimus*) ashes, *Isr J Med Sci* **8**(6), 757-58 (1972)
3. Mertz W, EE Roginski, WA Gordon, WW Harrison, J Shani, FG Sulman; *In vitro* potentiation of insulin by ash from saltbush (*Atriplex halimus*), *Arch Int Pharmacodyn Ther* **206**(1), 121-28 (1973)

Avena sativa Linn. (Poaceae)
(Oats)

Avena sativa is a species of cereal grain. The seeds of this plant are used as food for people and as fodder for animals. Since oats are unsuitable for making bread on their own, they are often served as a porridge made from crushed or rolled oats or mixed with wheat flour to make breads and a variety of other baked goods,

Attempts were made to isolate hypoglycaemic compounds from oats (1). The influence of sterilization, drying and oat bran enrichment of pasta on glucose and insulin responses in healthy subjects and on the rate and extent of *in vitro* starch digestion were evaluated (2). Viscous polysaccharides are known to attenuate postprandial plasma glucose and insulin responses. The aqueous solution of the polysaccharide, present in oat gum, is highly viscous and, therefore, the dose-response to oat gum and the effect of viscosity on plasma glucose and insulin levels of healthy humans consuming 50 g glucose was studied. Increasing the dose of oat gum successively reduced the plasma glucose and insulin responses relative to a control without gum. It was further observed that reduction of viscosity of oat gum solution, by acid hydrolysis, reduced or eliminated the capacity to decrease postprandial glucose and insulin levels. The relationship shows that 79-96% of the changes in plasma glucose and insulin are attributable to viscosity, and that changes occur at relatively low doses and viscosities (3). The high amount of soluble *beta*-glucans in oats exerts beneficial effects on glucose tolerance and blood lipids. Diets containing oat extracts having soluble *beta*-glucans were found to improve glucose and insulin responses of moderately hypercholesterolemic men and women (4). The well-accepted oat bran concentrate bread products improved glycaemic, insulinemic, and lipidemic responses (5). The effects of different oat processing techniques were studied on the plasma glucose and insulin response in horses. The study indicated that the glucose and insulin responses are not clearly altered by the different types of oat processing. However, these responses tended to be lower in thermally treated oats when compared with untreated or finely ground oats (6). Yeast-leavened oat breads with high or low molecular weight *beta*-glucan do not differ in their effects on blood concentrations of lipids, insulin, or glucose in humans (7).

1. Limanski M, E Udolf; Attempted analysis of hypoglycaemic compounds obtained from oats, *Pol Tyg Lek* (Wars) **10**(30), 996-97 (1955) [Article in Polish]
2. Holm J, B Koellreutter, P Wursch; Influence of sterilization, drying and oat bran enrichment of pasta on glucose and insulin responses in healthy subjects and on the rate and extent of *in vitro* starch digestion, *Eur J Clin Nutr* **46**(9), 629-40 (1992)
3. Wood PJ, JT Braaten, FW Scott, KD Riedel, MS Wolynetz, MW Collins; Effect of dose and modification of viscous properties of oat gum on plasma glucose and insulin following an oral glucose load, *Br J Nutr* **72**(5), 731-43 (1994)
4. Hallfrisch J, DJ Scholfield, KM Behall; Diets containing soluble oat extracts improve glucose and insulin responses of moderately hypercholesterolemic men and women, *Am J Clin Nutr* **61**(2), 379-84 (1995)
5. Pick ME, ZJ Hawrysh, MI Gee, E Toth, ML Garg, RT Hardin; Oat bran concentrate bread products improve long-term control of diabetes: a pilot study, *J Am Diet Assoc* **96**(12), 1254-61 (1996)
6. Vervuert I, M Coenen, C Bothe; Effects of oat processing on the glycaemic and insulin responses in horses, *J Anim Physiol Anim Nutr* (Berl) **87**(3-4), 96-104 (2003)
7. Frank J, B Sundberg, A Kamal-Eldin, B Vessby, P Aman; Yeast-leavened oat breads with high or low molecular weight *beta*-glucan do not differ in their

effects on blood concentrations of lipids, insulin, or glucose in humans, *J Nutr* **134**(6), 1384-88 (2004)

Averrhoa bilimbi Linn. (Oxalidaceae) (Cucumber tree, Bilimbi)

Bilimbi is cultivated throughout Indonesia; in the Philippines; Sri Lanka and Myanmar. It is very common in Thailand, Malaya and Singapore; and found across the plains of India,

The effects of alcoholic extract of the leaves and stems of *A. bilimbi* and aqueous extract of its fruits were examined on the blood sugar and food intake of streptozotocin-induced diabetic rats. Intra-peritoneal injection of the alcoholic extract (0.3g/kg b.w.) over a 7 day period significantly reduced blood sugar level and food intake of streptozotocin-induced diabetic rats but aqueous extract of the fruits was only capable of reducing blood sugar level (1).

Pushparaj and his coworkers studied the hypoglycaemic and hypolipidaemic activities of an ethanol extract of *A. bilimbi* leaves as well as of its different solvent-soluble fractions in streptozotocin-induced diabetic rats (2, 3). The optimum hypoglycaemic dose of the ethanol extract was determined to be 125 mg/kg by oral glucose tolerance test in both normal and streptozotocin-induced diabetic rats. Repeated administration (twice a day) of this extract at this dose to diabetic rats for a period of 2 weeks significantly lowered blood glucose and blood triglycerides, when compared with the vehicle (distilled water)-treated group. The effect was comparable to metformin (500 mg/kg). *A. bilimbi* extract also significantly increased the HDL-cholesterol concentrations. Among the different solvent-soluble fractions, obtained by partitioning of the ethanol extract, only the water and butanol-soluble fractions produced significant blood glucose-lowering effect in the diabetic rats. On day 7 and day 14 in a two-week study, only these two fractions lowered the fasting blood glucose concentration significantly when compared with the vehicle (distilled water). While both these fractions significantly increased serum insulin level when compared to that in the vehicle-treated rats on day zero, it was only the water-soluble fraction that significantly lowered hepatic glucose-6-phosphatase activity. The work was extended to study the effects of different fractions in high fat diet fed-streptozotocin-induced diabetic rats and it was concluded that the water-soluble fraction is more potent than other solvent-soluble fractions in the amelioration of hyperglycaemia and hyperlipidaemia in high fat diet fed-streptozotocin-induced diabetic rats and that *A. bilimbi* is a potential source for the isolation of new orally active agent(s) for anti-diabetic therapy (4).

1. Tan BKH, P Fu, PW Chow, A Hsu; Effects of *Averrhoa bilimbi* on blood sugar and food intake in streptozotocin-induced diabetic rats, *Phytomedicine* **3**(Suppl.1), 271 (1996/97)

2. Pushparaj P, CH Tan, BK Tan; Effects of *Averrhoa bilimbi* leaf extract on blood glucose and lipids in streptozotocin-diabetic rats, *J Ethnopharmacol* **72**(1-2), 69-76(2000).

3. Pushparaj P, BK Tan, CH Tan; The mechanism of hypoglycaemic action of the semi-purified fractions of *Averrhoa bilimbi* in streptozotocin-diabetic rats, *Life Sci* **70**(5), 535-47 (2001).

4. Tan BK, CH Tan, Pushparaj PN; Anti-diabetic activity of the semi-purified fractions of *Averrhoa bilimbi* in high fat diet fed-streptozotocin-induced diabetic rats, *Life Sci* **76**(24), 2827-39 (2005).

Averrhoa carambola Linn. (Oxalidaceae)
(Star fruit, Coromandel gooseberry, H. Kamranga, Kamarakh)

It is a species of tree native to Indonesia, India and Sri Lanka and is popular throughout Southeast Asia. It is commercially grown in many countries including the United States (Florida and Hawaii). The pomace of *A. carambola* was found to possess a high level of insoluble fibre-rich fractions, mainly composed of pectic substances and hemicellulose. The water-holding capacities, swelling properties, and cation-exchange capacities of these fibre-rich fractions were significantly higher than those of cellulose. The apparent abilities of these fibre-rich fractions to adsorb glucose and reduce amylase activity implied that they might help control postprandial serum glucose. The consumption and application of the insoluble fibre-rich fractions of *A. carambola* as low-calorie bulk ingredients were recommended.

Chau CF, CH Chen, MH Lee; Characterization and physicochemical properties of some potential fibres derived from *Averrhoa carambola, Nahrung* **48**(1), 43-46 (2004).

Azadirachta indica A. Juss (Meliaceae) Syn. *Melia azadirachta* L.
(S. Nimba, H. Neem)

Azadirachta indica (Neem) is a tree in the mahogany family, Meliaceae and is native to Bangladesh, India, Myanmar, and Pakistan growing in tropical and semi-tropical regions. Because of various medicinal properties of *A. indica,* it is also widely cultivated and naturalized outside its native range.

Different parts of the plant (leaves, bark, root, seed etc.) were tested for their putative hypoglycaemic and anti-diabetic activities by different groups of workers. Researchers, using different experimental protocols and different experimental animals, were almost unanimous in confirming the anti-diabetic and hypoglycaemic activity of the extracts of different parts of the plant. The findings are summarised in the sequel.

Aqueous extract of *A. indica* leaves, prepared by boiling fresh tender leaves (100g) with distilled water (200 ml) for 2 h, showed hypoglycaemic and anti-hyperglycaemic effects. It significantly decreased the blood sugar levels and prevented adrenaline and glucose-induced hyperglycaemia (1). Oral administration of an aqueous extract of *A. indica* leaves produced hypoglycaemia in normal rats. A decrease in blood sugar level was also noticed in diabetic rats (6). Daily oral administration of neem leaf extract (100, 200 and 400 mg/kg b.w) for 28 days to alloxan (140mg/kg b.w., single dose)-induced diabetic rabbits significantly decreased their blood sugar levels (15, 16). Pretreatment with *A. indica* leaf extract two weeks before the administration of alloxan in rabbits only partially prevented the rise in blood glucose levels as compared to control diabetic animals. The effect, however, was more pronounced in diabetic animals in which the plant drug was administered for four weeks after induction of diabetes by alloxan. Similar effect was also observed with neem seed oil (14). Treatment of diabetic rats with an aqueous extract of fresh leaves of *A. indica* at a dose of 250 mg/kg body weight for 16 weeks resulted in gradual but significant fall in blood glucose level and improvement in serum total and LDL-cholesterol and triacylglycerol. The treatment also showed improvement in body weight and reversed retinopathy (17).

Chattopadhyay studied the possible mechanism of anti-hyperglycaemic effect of *Azadirachta indica* leaf extract. *A. indica* leaf extract, in itself, was found to have no action on peripheral utilization of glucose or on hepatic glycogen but the reduction in peripheral utilization of glucose and glycogenolytic effect due to epinephrine action was blocked by the leaf extract almost completely in diabetic rabbits and to a certain extent in normal ones. *A. indica* leaf extract was also found to block significantly the inhibitory effect of serotonin on insulin secretion mediated by glucose. The results have been discussed (8, 12). The author also made a comparison of blood sugar lowering activity of four important medicinal plants, *viz, Azadirachta indica, Gymnema sylvestre, Catharanthus roseus* and *Ocimum sanctum* and observed *A. indica* leaf extract to have the most potent blood sugar-lowering activity followed by *C. roseus, G. sylvestre* and *O. sanctum* (11).

Hypoglycaemic activity of different extracts of *Melia azadirachta* bark was tested in normal and alloxanised albino rats and only the aqueous extract of the bark showed significant hypoglycaemic activity (9).

Neem oil (2.5 ml) and nimbidin (200 mg/k b.w.), a bitter constituent of the plant, have been reported to exhibit significant hypoglycaemic activity in rabbits at the 6th hour after feeding (2). Hypoglycaemic activity of neem oil (*A. indica* seed oil) was studied in normal fasting rabbits as well as in glucose loaded and adrenaline-induced diabetic rabbits. Neem oil lowered blood sugar level of fasting normal rabbits. It also inhibited the rise of blood sugar in glucose-loaded animals and exerted an inhibitory effect in adrenaline-induced hyperglycaemic rabbits (3, 4). The effects of petroleum ether extracts of neem seed kernel and of seed husk on body and organ weight were studied in normal and diabetic rats. Oral administration of seed kernel extract (2 mg/kg b.w.) daily for 28 days significantly increased the body weight compared to the diabetic control. The treatment also reversed the observed decreases in the weight of spleen, heart, liver and testes, induced by streptozotocin-injection. A single dose of seed kernel extract (2.0 mg/kg b.w) administered after a glucose load (4ml/kg b.w. of 25% solution) was found to be effective in lowering the blood glucose level. Petroleum ether extract of seed husk was effective at a smaller dose (0.9 mg/kg b.w.). Treatment of insulin dependent diabetic rats (induced by sterptozotocin) with seed husk and seed kernel extracts at these dose levels for 28 days, significantly lowered their blood glucose levels, the effect was significant on 7th day for kernel extract, and on 14th day for husk extract (19). Both seed kernel and husk extracts prevented oxidative stress caused by streptozotocin in heart and erythrocytes. However, no such preventive effect was observed on renal and hepatic toxicity (20). Nimbela (a neem oil product) acted as a synergist with most of the oral anti-diabetics and helped to gradually reduce their intake (5). Medicinal uses of neem oil for the treatment of diabetes and atherosclerosis have also been reported (7).

Administration of neem kernel powder alone (500 mg/kg) and in combination with glibenclamide (0.25 mg/kg) to alloxan-induced diabetic rabbits for 30 days significantly decreased the concentration of serum lipids, blood glucose and activities of serum enzymes like alkaline phosphatase, acid phosphatase, lactate dehydrogenase, liver glucose 6-phosphatase and HMG CoA reductase. The changes observed were significantly greater when the treatment was given with neem kernel powder and glibenclamide than with neem kernel powder alone (10). Administration of an alcoholic extract of *A. indica* to alloxan-induced diabetic rabbits, once daily for four weeks, significantly improved their blood glucose and lipid profiles (13).

Clinical investigation with patients of type-2 diabetes mellitus indicated that *Azadirachta indica* has significant hypoglycaemic activity in high dose and can be successfully combined with oral hypoglycaemic agents in type-2 diabetic patients whose diabetes is not controlled by these agents (21).

The effects of administration of a combination water extracts (200 mg/kg b.w., once a day for 8 weeks) of *A. indica* leaves and *Abroma augusta* roots to alloxan-induced diabetic rats were studied. The treatment showed significant lowering of blood sugar level in fasted rats, resulted in a significant lowering of serum lipids and also decreased the formation of lipid peroxides and increased the activities of antioxidant enzymes (superoxide dismutase, catalase, glutathione peroxidase, and glutathione transferase) in erythrocytes. The treatment also prevented the decrease in body weight. The findings revealed that the combination of water extracts of the two drugs were more effective hypoglycaemic agent than when given alone (18).

1. Satyanarayana Murty K, D Narayana Rao, D Krishna Rao, LB Gopalakrishna Murty; A preliminary study on hypoglycaemic and anti-hyperglycaemic effects of *Azadirachta indica, Indian J Pharmacol* **10**(3), 247-50 (1978).

2. Pillai NR, G Santhakumari; Hypoglycaemic activity of *Melia azadirachta* Linn. (Neem), *Indian J Med Res* **74**(Dec), 931-33 (1981)
3. Sharma MK, AK Khare, H Feroz; Effect of neem oil on blood sugar levels of normal hyperglycaemic and diabetic animals,·*Nagarjun* **26**(10),247-50 (1983).
4. Sharma MK, AK Khare, H Feroz; Effect of neem oil on blood sugar levels in normal hyperglycaemic and diabetic animals, *Indian Med Gaz* **117**(11), 380-83 (1983)
5. Bhargava AK; Neem oil as a synergist to anti-diabetic drug for management of secondary hyperglycaemia, *Neem Newsletter* **4**(3), 31-32 (1987).
6. El-Hawary ZM, TS Kholief; Biochemical studies on some hypoglycaemic agents: (1) Effect of *Azadirachta indica* leaf extract, *Arch Pharmacol Res* **13**(1), 108-12 (1990).
7. Dixit VP, Prabha Jain, AK Purohit; Medicinal uses of Neem (*Azadirachta indica*) in fertility regulation, diabetes and atherosclerosis, *Recent Med Aromatic & Spice Crops, Today & Tomorrow,* New Delhi, India, **2**, 463-71 (1992).
8. Chattopadhyay RR, Possible mechanism of anti-hyperglycaemic effect of *Azadirachta indica* leaf extract, Part IV, *Gen Pharmacol* **27**(3), 431-34 (1996).
9. Bharti, RH Singh, JPN Chansouria; Hypoglycaemic activity of *Melia azadirachta* Linn. bark, *J Res Ayurveda Siddha* **17**(3-4), 162-68 (1996)
10. Bopanna KN, J Kannan, S Gadgil, R Balaraman, SP Rathod; Anti-diabetic and anti-hyperlipaemic effects of neem seed kernel powder on alloxan diabetic rabbits, *Indian J Pharmacol* **20**, 162-67 (1997).
11. Chattophadhyay RR, A comparative evaluation of some blood sugar lowering agents of plant origin, *J Ethnopharmacol* **67**(3), 367-72 (1999)
12. Chattophadhyay RR, Possible mechanism of anti- hyperglycaemic effect of *Azadirachta indica* leaf extract: part V, *J Ethnopharmacol* **67**(3), 373-76 (1999).
13. Kaushik A, KK Saxena, VK Srivastava, A Kumar, VS Singh; Effect of alcoholic extract of *Azadirachta indica* (neem) on blood glucose and lipid profile in experimentally induced diabetes mellitus, *Indian J Pharmacol* **31**(1), 56 (1999).
14. Khosla P, S Bhanwra, J Singh, S Seth, RK Srivastava; A study of hypoglycaemic effects of *Azadirachta indica* (Neem) in normal and alloxan diabetic rabbits, *Indian J Physiol Pharmacol* **44**(1), 69-74 (2000).
15. Gossain R, I Devi; Effect of *Azadirachta indica* on blood glucose and lipid profile in alloxan-induced diabetes in rabbits, *National Seminar on the Frontiers of Research & Development in Medicinal Plants*, CIMAP, Lucknow, **Abst. No. 241**, Sept.16-18, 2000
16. Gossain R, Indira Devi; Effect of *Azadirachta indica* on blood glucose and lipid profile in alloxan-induced diabetes in rabbits, *J Sci & Pharm* **3**(1), 16-20 (2002)
17. Ali Hussain HEM; Reversal of diabetic retinopathy in streptozotocin-induced

diabetic rats using traditional Indian anti-diabetic plant, *Azadirachta indica*, *Indian J Clin Biochem* **17**(2), 115-23(2002)

18. Eshrat Halim M; Lowering of blood sugar by water extract of *Azadirachta indica* and *Abroma augusta* in diabetic rats, *Indian J Exp Biol* **41**(6), 636-40 (2003)
19. Gupta S, PK Gupta, M Kataria; Hypoglycaemic effect of petroleum ether extract of neem (*Azadirachta indica*) seed husk and kernel in streptozotocin-induced diabetic rats, *Toxicol International* **10**(1), 41-46 (2003)
20. Gupta S, M Kataria, PK Gupta, S Murganandan, RC Yashroy; Protective role of extracts of neem seeds in diabetes caused by streptozotocin in rats, *J Ethnopharmacol* **90**(2-3), 185-89 (2004).
21. Waheed A, GA Miana, SI Ahmad; Clinical investigation of hypoglycaemic effect of seeds of *Azadirachta indica* in type-2 (NIDDM) diabetes mellitus, *Pak J Pharm Sci* **19**(4), 322-25 (2006)

Azorella compacta Phil. (Apiaceae/Umbelliferae) (Yareta, llareta)

Azorella compacta is a tiny flowering plant in the family Apiaceae, native to South America, in Peru, Bolivia, Chile and Argentina. *A. compacta* is a slow-growing dwarf mat-forming plants growing in high altitude.

Aqueous or ethanol infusions of *A. compacta* are used as anti-diabetic in some regions of Chile. The diterpenic compounds, mulinolic acid, azorellanol, and mulin-11,13-dien-20-oic acid, isolated from the plant were tested for their possible anti-diabetic activity. Two injections of the first two compounds to streptozotocin-induced diabetic rats significantly decreased the glycaemic levels of the diabetic animals very close to those reached by chlorpropamide injection, but no effect was detected in animals treated with mulin-11,13-dien-20-oic acid. Again, while injection of azorellanol elevated blood serum insulin level of diabetic rats, no change in serum insulin level was effected by mulinolic acid. The results justify the use of this plant in Chile as an anti-hyperglycaemic drug. Azorellanol was considered to act on the *beta* cells of pancreatic islets while mulinolic acid might act upon glucose utilization in the liver.

Fuentes NL, H Sagua, G Morales, J Borquez, AS Martin, J Soto, LA Loyola; Experimental anti-hyperglycaemic effect of diterpenoids of llareta *Azorella compacta* (Umbelliferae) Phil in rats, *Phytother Res* **19**(8), 713-16 (2005).

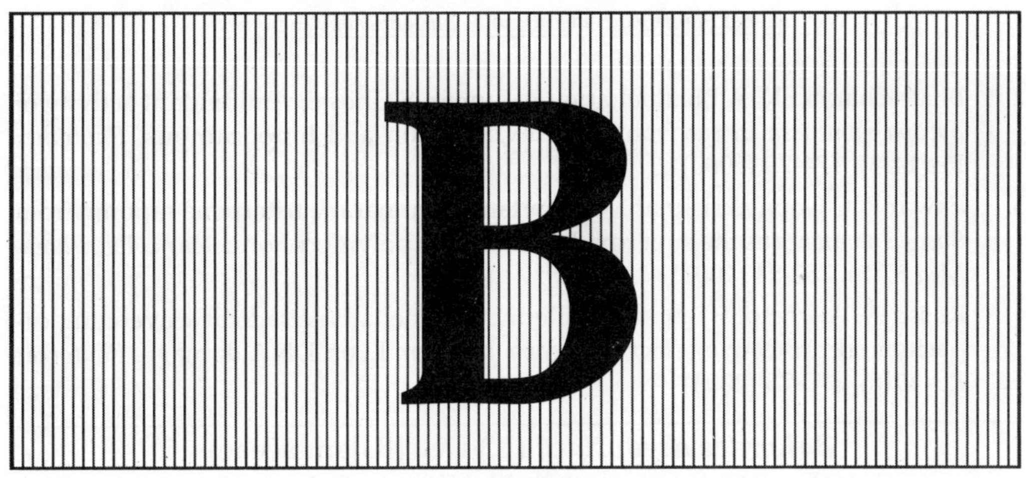

Baccharis genistelloides (Lam.) Pers. (Asteraceae) (Carqueja)

Baccharis genistelloides is a perennial green herb that grows nearly vertical and produces yellowish-white flowers at the top of the plant. It is found throughout the Amazon rainforest in Peru, Brazil, and Colombia, as well as in tropical parts of Argentina, Paraguay, and Uruguay. Indigenous peoples of the rainforest have utilized this herb for centuries to cure common ailments like diabetes, stomach ulcers, angina, poor blood circulation etc.

The treatment of healthy animals with the aqueous extract of *B. genistelloides* (4.2 mg/kg) reduced the body weight, serum glucose and triglyceride levels.

Coelho MG, PA Reis, VB Gava, PR Marques, CR Gayer, GA Laranja, I Felzenswalb, KC Sabino; Anti-arthritic effect and subacute toxicological evaluation of *Baccharis genistelloides* aqueous extract, *Toxicol Lett* **154**(1-2), 69-80 (2004)

Bacopa monnieri Linn. (Scrophulariacea) (Water hyssop, H. Brahmi)

Bacopa monnieri is a perennial, creeping herb, found in wetlands and muddy shores. It commonly grows in marshy areas throughout India, Nepal and Sri Lanka. It is also found in China and Vietnam.

It is well known that oxidative stress is involved in the pathogenesis of diabetes and its complications. The therapeutic potential of antioxidants for the treatment of diabetes is also well documented. *B. monnieri* is one such plant, the antioxidant and free radical scavenging property of which has been reported in a number of publications (1-4).

1. Tripathi YB, S Chaurasia, E Tripathi, A Upadhyay, GP Dubey; *Bacopa monniera* Linn. as an antioxidant: mechanism of action, *Indian J Exp Biol* **34**(6), 523-26 (1996)

2. Bhattacharya SK, A Bhattacharya, A Kumar, S Ghosal; Antioxidant activity of *Bacopa monniera* in rat frontal cortex, striatum and hippocampus, *Phytother Res* **14**(3), 174-79 (2000)

3. Pawar R, C Gopalakrishnan, KK Bhutani; Dammarane triterpene saponin from *Bacopa monniera* as the superoxide inhibitor in polymorphonuclear cells., *Planta Med* **67**(8), 752-54 (2001)

4. Russo A, AA Izzo, F Borrelli, M Renis, A Vanella Free radical scavenging capacity and protective effect of *Bacopa monniera* L. on DNA damage, *Phytother Res* **17**(8), 870-75 (2003)

Balanites aegyptiaca (L.) Del. (Balanitaceae) (Egyptian myrobalan, H. Hingan, S. Ingudi)

Balanites aegyptiaca is a multi-branched, spiny shrub with dark green leaves. Its flower buds are ovoid and fruits are ellipsoid with hard stone seeds. The seeds are used for rosary beads and necklaces.

Oral administration of an aqueous extract of mesocarps of the fruits of *B. aegyptiaca* exhibited a prominent anti-diabetic activity in streptozotocin-induced diabetic mice. Four steroidal saponins, built on furost-5-ene-3β,22, 26-triol system and isolated from the active fraction of the extract, were fully identified. While individual saponins failed to show any anti-diabetic activity, a recombination of these saponins resulted in a significant activity.

Kamel MS, K Ohtani, T Kurokawa, MH Assaf, MA el-Shanawany, AA Ali, R Kasai, S Ishibashi, O Tanaka; Studies on *Balanites aegyptiaca* fruits, an anti-diabetic Egyptian folk medicine, *Chem Pharm Bull* (Tokyo) **39**(5), 1229-33 (1991).

Barleria lupulina Lindl. (Acanthaceae) (Hophead Philippine violet)

Barleria lupulina is an erect shrub, possibly native to Mauritius, but naturalized in other tropical areas. Based on folkloric reports of its use for the treatment of diabetes, methanol extract of aerial parts of the plant was tested for its putative anti-diabetic activity. Oral administration of the extract at doses of 100, 200 and 300 mg/kg exerted significant anti-hyperglycaemic effect in streptozotocin-induced hyperglycaemia in rats (1). The anti-hyperglycaemic efficacy was observed from 4 h after its administration up to 12 h.; a maximum activity at 12 h after administration was observed with a dose of 200 mg/kg b.w. The reduction of blood glucose level was comparable to the standard drug glibenclamide (10 mg/kg b.w.) when the extract was administered to streptozotocin-induced diabetic rats at a dose of 300 mg/kg b.w. The methanol extract of the aerial parts of the plant was thus found to exhibit a pronounced blood glucose-lowering potential in streptozotocin-induced hyperglycaemic rats and provided a pharmacological support to the traditional claims of its anti-diabetic activity. (2).

1. Suba V, T Murugesan, RB Rao, L Ghosh, M Pal, SC Mandal, BP Saha; Anti-diabetic potential of *Barleria lupulina* extract in rats, *Fitoterapia* **75**(1) (2004) 1-4, **75**(3-4), 4-6 (2004)
2. Suba V, T Murugesan, G Arunachalam, SC Mandal, BP Saha; Anti-diabetic potential of *Barleria lupulina* extract in rats, *Phytomedicine* **11**(2-3), 202-05 (2004).

Barleria prionitis Linn. (Acanthaceae) (Porcupine flower)

Barleria is a hardy, prickly shrub, which is well adapted to the tropic of northern Australia. It is regarded as a weed that threatens biodiversity and causes other environmental damage.

Aqueous and alcoholic extracts of leaf and root of the plant (200 mg/kg) caused a significant fall in blood glucose level in alloxan-induced diabetic rats. The extract was almost equipotent to chlorpropamide in its ability to reduce blood sugar levels.

Geetham M, AK Wahi; Anti-diabetic activity of *Barleria prionitis* Linn., *J Nat Remedies* **1**(1), 64-66 (2001)

Bauhinia candicans Benth (Fabaceae Caesalpiniaceae)

The plant is native to Argentina, Bolivia, Brazil, Paraguay and Uruguay and has been introduced in South Africa. In spring season, the plant produces beautiful white fragrant flowers, which cover the entire plant at least for 3 weeks. *Bauhinia candicans* is a Chilean popular medicine for the treatment of diabetes (1).

The methanol extract of the leaves of *B. candicans* was fractionated by partitioning with different solvents and the effect of each fraction was studied in experimentally-induced diabetic rabbits. The crude extract (8 mg/kg) showed hypoglycaemic activity and reduced urinary glucose excretion. Among the fractions, the highest activity was exhibited by the butanol-soluble fraction, which reduced plasma glucose level in normal, as well as, in glucose loaded rabbits. The increase in peripheral metabolism of glucose by *B. candicans* leaf extract was suggested (2). A butanol extract of dried leaves of the plant showed, *in vitro*, a stimulatory effect of glucose uptake in isolated gastric glands of normal and alloxan-induced diabetic rabbits. The extract produced a dose-dependent effect and was similar to the effect of insulin. It was suggested that the compounds present in the extract efficiently increase glucose transport at the basolateral side of isolated gastric glands (3).

1. Lemus I, R Garcia, E Delvillar, G Knop; Hypoglycaemic activity of four plants used in Chilean popular medicine, *Phytother Res* **13**(2), 91-94 (1999)
2. Fuentes O, P Arancibia-Avila, J Alarcon; Hypoglycaemic activity of *Bauhinia candicans* in diabetic induced rabbits, *Fitoterapia* **75**(6), 527-32 (2004).

3. Fuentes O, J Alarcon; *Bauhinia candicans* stimulation of glucose uptake in isolated gastric glands of normal and diabetic rabbits, *Fitoterapia* 77(4), 271-75 (2006)

Bauhinia cheilandra (Bowgarb Steudel. (Caesalpiniaceae / Fabaceae

In glucose loaded and alloxan-induced diabetic rats, methanol extract of the leaves of *B. cheilandra*, at doses of 300, 600, and 900 mg/kg, showed statistically significant hypoglycaemic activity.

Almeida ER, MC Guedes, JF Albuquerque, H Xavier; Hypoglycaemic effect of *Bauhinia cheilandra* in rats, *Fitoterapia* 77(4), 276-78 (2006)

Bauhinia forficata Link (Fabaceae Leguminosae) (Brazilian Orchid-Tree, "paw-of-cow")

Bauhinia forficata is widely used in Brazilian folk medicine for the treatment of diabetes mellitus. The effects of using *B. forficata* leaf decoction (150 g leaf/l water; 35.2±7.8 ml/100 g body weight mean daily dose) as a drinking-water substitute for about 1 month on streptozotocin-induced diabetic male Wistar rats were investigated. The streptozotocin-induced diabetic rats, treated with the decoction, showed a significant reduction in serum and urinary glucose and urinary urea levels as compared to the diabetic control but no difference was observed between decoction-treated and untreated non-diabetic rats. The improvement in carbohydrate metabolism seen in the rats treated with *B. forficata* decoction does not appear to be linked to the inhibition of glycogenolysis or the stimulation of glycogenesis nor does it appear to act in a way similar to insulin or the sulfonylureas, although it may act by the inhibition of neoglycogenesis in a manner similar to that of the biguanides (1).

The effect of n-butanol-soluble fraction of *B. forficata* leaves on the serum glucose levels of experimentally induced diabetic rats was studied. Oral administration of n-butanol fraction led to a significant blood glucose-lowering effect in normal and diabetic rats. However, in glucose-fed hyperglycaemic normal rats, the maximum dose of this fraction failed to decrease blood glucose levels. The maximum effect of n-butanol fraction was detected at 1 h with a dose of 800 mg/kg in diabetic animals and this profile was maintained for the next 3 h. (2).

The anti-diabetic activity of aqueous, ethanol and hexane extracts of *B. forficata* was investigated in a model of alloxan-induced diabetic rats. Oral administration of the extracts daily for 7 days at doses of 200 and 400 mg/kg, 48 h after alloxan injection (60 mg/kg, i.v.) showed significant reductions in plasma glucose, triglycerides, total cholesterol and HDL-cholesterol as compared to the diabetic controls. The activity was comparable to that of glibenclamide. The results suggest the validity of the clinical use of *B. forficata* in the treatment of diabetes mellitus type-2 (3).

The repercussions of diabetes on the defence system against oxidative stress in pregnant female rats and the influence of the treatment with *B. forficata* extract on the antioxidant system, glycaemic control, hepatic glycogen, etc. was studied. Virgin female Wistar rats were injected with 40 mg/kg streptozotocin before mating. An aqueous extract of *B. forficata* leaves was administered to non-diabetic and diabetic pregnant rats in 3 doses; 500 mg/kg from 0 to 4th day of pregnancy, 600 mg/kg from 5th to 14th day and 1000 mg/kg from 15th to 20th day. Biochemical measurement of maternal blood sample and liver indicated that the diabetic pregnant rats were hyperglycaemic, hyperlipaemic, hypertriglyceridaemic, hypercholesterolaemic and hyperuricaemic with a low level of reduced glutathione and superoxide dismutase. Treatment with *B. forficata* extract increased hepatic glycogen, decreased uric acid concentration and increased GSH activity. It was from this last observation that the authors suggested that the plant might have some action on antioxidant defence system (4).

Kaempferitrin (kaempferol-3,7-O-α-dirhamnoside), the major flavonol constituent of n-butanol-soluble fraction of *B. forficata,* showed positive blood glucose-lowering effect in normal and alloxan-induced diabetic rats. While in normal rats, blood glucose lowering was observed only with the higher dose of kaempferitrin (200 mg/kg) at 1 h after treatment, in diabetic rats the hypoglycaemic effect was evident at all doses tested (50, 100, and 200 mg/kg), and this profile was maintained throughout the period studied. Kaempferitrin, however, failed to decrease blood glucose levels in glucose-fed hyperglycaemic normal rats. The antioxidant properties of kaempferitrin and its action against reactive oxygen species were evaluated *in vitro.* The compound showed high reactivity with 1,1-diphenyl-2-picryl hydrazyl, inhibited myeloperoxidase activity and decreased lipid per-oxidation. The long-term effect of kaempferitrin on glycaemia in diabetic rats as well as the *in vitro* effect of this compound on ^{14}C-D-glucose uptake and ^{14}C-leucine incorporation into protein in normal rat soleus muscle was studied. Kaempferitrin was found to stimulate the glucose uptake percentile, as efficiently as insulin in muscle from normal rats. It did not have any effect on protein synthesis in muscle from normal and diabetic animals. However, the protein synthesis in the kaempferitrin-treated groups was maintained at the same level as the respective controls. Thus, the hypoglycaemic effect and the prompt efficiency of the kaempferitrin in stimulating [U-^{14}C]-2-deoxy-D-glucose uptake in muscle, constitute the first evidence to indicate that the acute effect of this compound on blood glucose lowering may occur as a consequence of the altered intrinsic activity of the glucose transporter not involving directly the synthesis of new carriers (5, 6).

The effects of a *Bauhinia forficata* aqueous extract upon hyperglycaemia, glycogenolysis, increase of plasma catecholamines, lethality and changes in serum insulin and plasma electrolytes, induced by *Tityus serrulatus* scorpion venom, were studied and compared with the effects of the regular insulin therapy. The extract failed to reduce intense glycogenolysis and the release of catecholamines and did not stimulate the release of endogenous insulin, although caused changes in the electrolyte plasma levels similar to insulin. The extract and insulin were found to antagonize some effects of the scorpion venom but their use should be avoided in the treatment of *Tityus serrulatus* envenoming, since they enhance the lethality of the venom (7).

1. Pepato MT, EH Keller, AM Baviera, IC Kettelhut, RC Vendramini, IL Brunetti; Anti-diabetic activity of *Bauhinia forficata* decoction in streptozotocin-diabetic rats, *J Ethnopharmacol* **81**(2), 191-97 (2002)
2. Silva FR, B Szpoganicz, MG Pizzolatti, MA Willrich, E de-Sousa; Acute effect of *Bauhinia forficata* on serum glucose levels in normal and alloxan- induced diabetic rats, *J Ethnopharmacol* **83**(1-2), 33-37 (2002)
3. Lino Cde S, JP Diogenes, BA Pereira, RA Faria, M Andrade Neto, RS Alves, MG de-Queiroz, FC de-Sousa, GS Viana; Anti-diabetic activity of *Bauhinia forficata* extracts in alloxan-diabetic rats, *Biol Pharm Bull* **27**(1), 125-27 (2004).
4. Damasceno DC, GT Volpato, M Calderon Ide, R Aguilar, MV Rudge; Effect of *Bauhinia forficata* extract in diabetic pregnant rats: maternal repercussions, *Phytomedicine* **11**(2-3), 196-201 (2004).
5. de-Sousa E, L Zanatta, I Seifriz, TB Creczynski-Pasa, MG Pizzolatti, B Szpoganicz, FR Silva; Hypoglycaemic effect and antioxidant potential of kaempferol-3,7-O-(*alpha*)-dirhamnoside from *Bauhinia forficata* leaves, *J Nat Prod* **67**(5), 829-32 (2004).
6. Jorge AP, H Horst, E de-Sousa, MG Pizzolatti, FR Silva; Insulinomimetic effects of kaempferitrin on glycaemia and on ^{14}C-glucose uptake in rat soleus muscle, *Chem Biol Interact* **149**(2-3), 89-96 (2004).
7. Vasconcelos F, SV Sampaio, MA Garofalo, LF Guimaraes, JR Giglio, EC Arantes; Insulin-like effects of *Bauhinia forficata* aqueous extract upon *Tityus serrulatus* scorpion envenoming, *J Ethnopharmacol* **95**(2-3), 385-92 (2004).

Bauhinia megalandra Griseb. (Fabaceae / Leguminosae)

In vitro testing with rat liver slices showed that an aqueous extract of *B. megalandra* leaves caused a decrease (nearly 50%) in glucose production from lactate or fructose. The result suggests that the main effect of the extract is the inhibition of glucose-6-phosphate transporter (T_1) of the microsomal glucose-6-phosphatase system, however, an inhibition of T_3 was not ruled out. The inhibition of glucose-6-phosphotase might explain the decrease in neoglucogenic capacity of the liver slices, which, in turn, explains the reduction of glucose levels in diabetic patients (1).

Aqueous extract of *B. megalandra* leaves was able to inhibit the intestinal glucose absorption in a concentration-dependent way. The extract drastically reduced the ^{14}C-glucose uptake by enterocyte brush border membrane vesicles. Oral administration of the extract simultaneously with glucose improved the glucose tolerance with a significant reduction of the 30-min peak but the extract failed to show any effect on the glucose tolerance when glucose was administrated subcutaneously (2).

The anti-hyperglycaemic activity of eight flavonoids, isolated from the methanol extract of *B. megalandra* fresh leaves, was evaluated by rat liver microsomal glucose-6-phosphatase bioassay. All the flavonoids assayed showed an inhibitory effect on the intact microsomal glucose-6-phosphatase: The highest inhibitory activity was shown by quercetin 3-O- α-(2″galloyl) rhamnoside and kaempferol 3-O-α-(2″galloyl) rhamnoside (3).

1. Gonzalez-Mujica F, N Motta, A Becerra; Inhibition of hepatic neoglucogenesis and glucose-6-phosphatase by aqueous extract of *Bauhinia megalandra* leaves, *Phytother Res* **12**(4), 291-93 (1998)
2. Gonzalez-Mujica F, N Motta, AH Marquez, J Capote-Zulueta; Effects of *Bauhinia megalandra* aqueous leaf extract on intestinal glucose absorption and uptake by enterocyte brush border membrane vesicles, *Fitoterapia* **74**(1-2), 84-90 (2003).
3. Estrada O, M Hasegawa, F Gonzalez-Mujica, N Motta, E Perdomo, A Solorzano, J Mendez, B Mendez, EG Zea; Evaluation of flavonoids from *Bauhinia megalandra* leaves as inhibitors of glucose-6-phosphatase system, *Phytother Res* **19**(10), 859-63 (2005).

Bauhinia variegata Linn. (Fabaceae) (Orchid tree, "Mororo")

Bauhinia variegata is a very popular ornamental tree in subtropical and tropical climates, grown for its scented flowers. It is widely utilized in popular medicine as an anti-diabetic agent in Brazil and has been shown to have an insulin-like protein in its leaves. A chloroplast protein with a molecular mass similar to that of bovine insulin was extracted from the leaves of the plant. The activity of this insulin-like protein (0.48 mg/ml) on serum glucose levels of four-week-old Swiss albino (CF1) diabetic mice was similar to that of commercial swine insulin used as control. Its activity on alloxan-induced mice also showed that it has insulin-like properties. The presence of an insulin-like protein in chloroplasts indicates its involvement in carbohydrate metabolism and suggests that insulin-signaling pathways have been conserved through evolution.

Azevedo CR, FM Maciel, LB Silva, AT Ferreira, M da Cunha, OL Machado, KV Fernandes, AE Oliveira, J Xavier-Filho; Isolation and intracellular localization of insulin-like proteins from leaves of *Bauhinia variegata*, *Braz J Med Biol Res* **39**(11), 1435-44 (2006)

Belamcanda chinensis (L) DC. (Indaceae) (Leopard lily)

Aldose reductase is known to play a key role in diabetic complications. Twelve phenolic compounds including some isoflavonoids were isolated from the rhizomes of the plant and these were tested for their effects on rat lens aldose reductase. Of the isoflavonoids, tectoridin and tectorigenin exhibited the highest aldose reductase inhibitory potency for dl-glyceraldehyde as a substrate. Oral administration of these compounds (100 mg/kg for 10 consecutive days) to strptozotocin-induced diabetic rats caused a significant inhibition of sorbitol accumulation in the tissues such as lens, sciatic nerves, and red blood cells. Tectorigenin was found to be more potent than tectoridin.

Jung SH, YS Lee, S Lee, SS Lim, YS Kim, KH Shin; Isoflavonoids from the rhizomes of *Belamcanda chinensis* and their effects on aldose reductase and sorbitol accumulation in streptozotocin-induced diabetic rat tissues, *Arch Pharmacal Res* **25**(3), 306-12 (2002)

Berberis vulgaris Linn. (Berberidaceae) (European barberry)

It is a shrub, native to central and southern Europe, northwest Africa and western Asia. The plant, other than its fruits and seeds, is mildly poisonous. Its most important constituent, berberine, is known to have a number of therapeutical effects including anti-hyperglycaemic effects. Cannabisin G and (±)-lyoniresinol, isolated from the root bark of the plant, exhibited a hydroxyl radical-scavenging activity. Treatment of rat model of T2DM with berberine for 4 weeks displayed significant hypolipidemic, hypoglycaemic, and insulin sensitizing functions. It showed an exciting anti-diabetic efficacy in this study and it is considered to be of great value for the treatment of type-2 diabetes.

Zhang W, YC Xu, FJ Guo, Y Meng, ML Li; Anti-diabetic effects of cinnamaldehyde and berberine and their impacts on retinol-binding protein 4 expression in rats with type-2 diabetes mellitus, *Chin Med J* (Engl) **121**(21), 2124-28 (2008)

Bergenia ciliata Moench (Saxifragaceae)

Bergenia is a genus of flowering plants, native to central Asia, from Afganistan to China. *B. ciliata* has been employed in folklore medicine to treat symptoms of diabetes mellitus. All the extracts except chloroform extract of root and leaves of *B. ciliata* were found to possess hypoglycaemic activity in streptozotocin-induced diabetic rats. The plant was, however, found to elicit severe toxicity in experimental animals. The symptoms of toxicity in intracutaneous test were erythema and oedema, whereas acute systemic toxicity that was frequently observed were breathing problem and initiations of diarrhoea with blood in stool of experimental model.

Islam M, I Azhar, K Usmanghani, MA Gill, A Ahmad, Shahabuddin; Evaluation of *Bergenia ciliata, Pak J Pharm Sci* **15**(1), 15-33 (2002).

Beta vulgaris Linn. (Chenopodiaceae) (Sugar beet, H. Chukandar)

Beta vulgaris is a native of South Europe, where it is extensively cultivated as an article of food and especially for the production of sugar. Beet is now cultivated in different parts of the world. Betavulgarosides II, III, and IV (oleanolic acid oligoglycosides), isolated from sugar beet, were found to exhibit hypoglycaemic activity in an oral glucose tolerance test in rats.

Yoshikawa M, T Murakami, M Kadoya, H Matsuda, O Muraoka, J Yamahara, N Murakami; Medicinal foodstuff. III. Sugar beet. (1): Hypoglycaemic oleanolic acid oligoglycosides, betavulgarosides I, II, III, and IV from the root of *Beta vulgaris* L (Chenopodiaceae), *Chem Pharm Bull* (Tokyo) **44**(6), 1212-17 (1996).

Beta vulgaris L. var. ***cicla*** (L.) Koch (Chenopodiaceae) (Chard)

Chard is one of the plants that are used as hypoglycaemic agents by diabetic patients in Turkey. The effect of feeding chard on diabetes-induced impairments in rat skins was investigated. Uncontrolled induced diabetes caused significant increases in non-enzymatic glycosylation of skin proteins, lipid peroxidation and blood glucose. Administration of chard extract inhibited these effects except the increase in lipid peroxidation. The results of the investigation indicated that the use of chard might be effective in preventing or at least retarding the development of some diabetic complications (1).

An investigation was taken up to study whether chard, used in folk remedies for decreasing blood glucose levels, affects pancreatic *beta* cells and blood glucose. While in the diabetic group, a decrease in the number of *beta* cells of Langerhans islets and in the secretory materials was observed, in the diabetic group receiving chard extract, an increase in the number of *beta* cells of Langerhans islets and in the secretory granules was noted. The extract, while having no effect on blood glucose and body weight in the normal animals, reduced the blood glucose value in streptozotocin-induced hyperglycaemic animals. But, in a diabetic group given chard, the body weight significantly increased in comparison to the diabetic group. Maximum reduction in blood glucose levels was observed on the 42nd day. From the morphological and biochemical results obtained, it was concluded that the extract of this plant, when administered by gavage, might reduce blood glucose levels by regeneration of the *beta* cells (2).

In diabetes mellitus, increased free radical formation raises the incidence of atherosclerosis and cardiovascular diseases. The effect of feeding chard on diabetes-induced free radical-mediated injury in rat aorta and heart tissues was studied. The results of the present study indicated that the increase of lipid peroxidation and decrease of glutathione levels in both aorta and heart tissues of the streptozotocin-induced diabetic rats were reversed by treatment with chard extract (2 g/kg) for28 days (3).

The effects of chard extract on serum urea and creatinine concentrations and on kidney tissue in normal and streptozotocin-induced diabetic rats were studied. Significant degenerative changes in kidney tissue of diabetic rats were observed, but in the group given chard extract (2 g/kg, 28 days) the morphology of kidney tissue was found to be nearly the same as the controls. The increase in serum urea and creatinine levels in the diabetic groups was significantly reduced by treatment with chard extract, which is thus able to confer a protective effect on the kidney of diabetic rats (4).

1. Tunali T, A Yarat, R Yanardag, F Ozcelik, O Ozsoy, G Ergenekon, N Emekli; The effect of chard (*Beta vulgaris* L. var. *cicla*) on the skin of streptozotocin induced diabetic rats, *Pharmazie* **53**(9), 638-40 (1998)
2. Bolkent S, R Yanardag, A Tabakoglu-Oguz, O Ozsoy-Sacan; Effects of chard (*Beta vulgaris* L. var. *cicla*) extract on pancreatic β cells in streptozotocin-diabetic rats: a morphological and biochemical study, *J Ethnopharmacol* **73**(1-2), 251-59 (2000).
3. Sener G, O Sacan, R Yanardag, G Ayanoglu-Dulger; Effects of chard (*Beta vulgaris* L. var. *cicla*) extract on oxidative injury in the aorta and heart of streptozotocin-diabetic rats, *J Med Food* **5**(1), 37-42 (2002).
4. Yanardag R, S Bolkent, O Ozsoy-Sacan, O Karabulut-Bulan; The effects of chard (*Beta vulgaris* L. var. *cicla*) extract on the kidney tissue, serum urea and creatinine levels of diabetic rats, *Phytother Res* **16**(8), 758-61 (2002).

Bidens pilosa Linn. (Asteraceae)
(Broom stick)

Bidens pilosa is a plant of the Asteraceae family. It is considered a weed in some tropical habitats. However, in some parts of the world it is also used as a source of food.

A number of phytochemicals (aliphatic compounds, fatty acids, steroids, triterpenoids and their glycosides) were isolated from different solvent extracts of the plant material. The plant extract showed non-significant decrease in blood glucose level (1).

The hypoglycaemic activity of an aqueous ethanol extract, prepared from *Bidens pilosa,* was studied in healthy and alloxan-diabetic mice. The extract significantly diminished glycaemia (13.8%) in healthy mice at 4h and significantly decreased the blood sugar levels in mildly diabetic mice at 4h after intra-peritoneal administration (2).

A butanol-soluble fraction of *B. pilosa* suppressed the development of diabetes, helped maintain levels of blood sugar and insulin in non-obese diabetic mice in a dose-dependent manner. The extract also elevated the serum imunoglobulin IgE levels regulated by Th2 cytokines in non-obese diabetic mice. Using an *in vitro* T cell differentiation assay, it was observed that the butanol fraction inhibited the differentiation of naive helper T (Th0) cells into Th1 cells but enhanced their transition into type II helper T (Th2) cells. The polyacetylenic compounds [2-β-D-glucopyranosyloxy-1-hydroxy-5(*E*)-tridecene-7,9,11-triyne and 3-β-D-glucopyranosyloxy-1-hydroxy-6(*E*)-tetradecene-8,10,12-triyne], present in butanol-soluble fraction of *B. pilosa*, are capable of modulating the differentiation of helper T cells and prevent autoimmune diabetes in non-obese diabetic mice (3),

1. Sarg TM, AM Ateya, NM Farrag, FA Abbas; Constituents and biological activity of *Bidens pilosa* L. grown in Egypt, *Acta Pharm Hung* **61**(6), 317-23 (1991)
2. Alarcon-Aguilar FJ, R Roman-Ramos, JL Flores-Saenz, F Aguirre-Garcia; Investigation on the hypoglycaemic effects of extracts of four Mexican medicinal plants in normal and alloxan-diabetic mice, *Phytother Res* **16**(4), 383-86 (2002).
3. Chang SL, CL Chang, YM Chiang, RH Hsieh, CR Tzeng, TK Wu, HK Sytwu, LF Shyur, WC Yang; Polyacetylenic compounds and butanol fraction from *Bidens pilosa* can modulate the differentiation of helper T cells and prevent autoimmune diabetes in non-obese diabetic mice, *Planta Med* **70**(11), 1045-51 (2004).

Bidens pilosa L. var. ***radiata*** Sch. Bip. (Asteraceae)

Two known polyacetylenic glucosides (2-β-D-glucopyranosyloxy-1-hydroxy-5(*E*)-tridecene-7,9,11-triyne and 3-β-D-glucopyranosyloxy-1-hydroxy-6(*E*)-tetradecene-8,10,12-triyne) were isolated from the aqueous alcohol extract of the aerial parts of *B. pilosa* var. *radiata*. Administration of a (3:2) mixture of these two polyacetylenic glucosides resulted in a significant drop in blood glucose level in C57 BL/Ks-db/db mice.

Ubillas RP, CD Mendez, SD Jolad, J Luo, SR King, TJ Carlson, DM Fort; Antihyperglycaemic acetylenic glucosides from *Bidens pilosa, Planta Med* **66**(1), 82-83 (2000)

Biophytum sensitivum (L.) DC.(Oxalidaceae)

Biophytum sensitivum is a plant, native to China, Indian subcontinent, Thiland and Malaysia and is used as a Nepalese folk medicine for the treatment of hyperglycaemic patients. Its hypoglycaemic effect was studied in alloxan-induced diabetic male rabbits of different severities; sub-diabetic (alloxan recovered), mild diabetic and severely diabetic. Following administration of a single dose of the leaf extract of the plant, a fall in glucose values by 25.9% and 27.4%, respectively after 1 hour and 2.5 hour, was observed in the sub-diabetic rabbits. The corresponding fall in glucose values were 36.9% and 37.7% in the mild diabetic rabbits. Improved response of oral glucose tolerance test was also observed in sub-diabetic and mild diabetic animals. More significant improvements occurred following one week of the above treatment. The significant hypoglycaemic effect of the plant material is possibly due to pancreatic *beta*-cell stimulating action (1).

An acute effect of the leaf extract of the plant on fasting plasma glucose levels and serum insulin response was examined in non-diabetic and alloxan-induced diabetic rabbits. A single administration of the leaf extract (200 mg/kg b.w.) to 16h fasted non-diabetic rabbits brought about a 16.1% fall in fasting plasma glucose level at the end of 1 and 2 h, and this hypoglycaemic effect lasted for 6h. Serum insulin levels also showed a significant rise in the treated animals, which suggested a pancreatic mode of action of *B. sensitivum*. The plant extract, however, failed to produce such hypoglycaemic or serum insulin response in alloxan-induced diabetic rabbits. However, the administration of the above dose of the leaf extract attenuated the plasma glucose response to oral administration of glucose (3 g/kg b.w.) load. The serum insulin levels in the treated animals showed a rise at the end of 2 and 6 h. From the observations, it was surmised that the hypoglycaemic response of *B. sensitivum* might be mediated through stimulating the synthesis/release of insulin from the *beta* cells of Langerhans (2).

1. Puri D, N Baral; Hypoglycaemic effect of *Biophytum sensitivum* in the alloxan diabetic rabbits, *Indian J Physiol Pharmacol* **42**(3), 401-06 (1998).
2. Puri D; The insulinotropic activity of a Nepalese medicinal plant *Biophytum sensitivum*: preliminary experimental study, *J Ethnopharmacol* **78**(1), 89-93 (2001).

Bixa orellana Linn. (Bixaceae)
(Annatto)

Annatto (*Bixa orellana*) is native to tropical America and West Indies but is widely cultivated in Asia and Africa. It is a Caribbean folklore plant for the treatment of diabetes mellitus. Morrison and West studied the effect of the plant extract on blood sugar levels in anaesthetized dogs (1). The toxicity of the hyperglycaemia-inducing extract of *B. orellana* was also evaluated (2).

The red powdery extract from the seeds of *B. orellana*, which is generally used for colouring food items, is a folk remedy for the treatment of diabetes mellitus in the West Indies. Purification of the extract yielded *trans*-bixin [(2*E*, 4*E*, 6*E*, 8*E*, 10*E*, 12*E*,14*E*, 16*E*, 18*E*)-4,8,13,17-Tetramethyl-2,4,6,8,10,12,14,16,18-eicosano nonaene dioic acid monomethyl ester], a red-brown carotenoid acid ester, which caused hyperglycaemia in anaesthetised mongrel dogs. Electron microscopic examination revealed damage to mitochondria and endoplasmic reticulum mainly in liver and pancreas. When dogs were fed on a diet fortified with riboflavin, there was neither demonstrable tissue damage nor associated hyperglycaemia. The findings point to the possible role of plant extracts/food additives in the development of diabetes mellitus especially in the undernourished state (3).

Based on preliminary investigations, the plant extract was found to exhibit hypoglycaemic properties. With an objective of isolating the hypoglycaemic principle(s) from the crude extract, it was subjected to chromatographic fractionations, which resulted in the isolation of an oil-soluble, partially purified "annatto" extract. This semi-purified fraction caused a decrease in blood glucose level of test animals 1 h after administration. This hypoglycaemia persisted for an additional hour when the oral glucose tolerance test was performed on dogs treated with annatto and compared with the control. There was an increase in plasma insulin level in comparison to the control. Insulin receptor studies, done on mononuclear leucocytes and erythrocytes, obtained from blood taken 1 h after administration of the drug, showed that there was an increase in the percentage of receptor binding when compared with the control. Insulin affinity results showed that there was an increase in mononuclear leucocytes for the annatto treated dogs compared to the control. From the results of detailed investigation, it was inferred that annatto was responsible for the hypoglycaemic activity seen in the dogs and that it was mediated by an increase in plasma insulin concentration as well as by an increase in insulin binding on the insulin receptor due to elevated affinity of the ligand for the receptor (4).

1. Morrison EY, ME West; The effect of *Bixa orellana* (annatto) on blood sugar levels in the anaesthetized dog, *West Indian Med J* **34**(1), 38-42 (1985).
2. Morrison EY, S Smith-Richardson, M West, SE Brooks, K Pascoe, C Fletcher; Toxicity of the hyperglycaemic-inducing extract of the annatto (*Bixa orellana*) in the dog, *West Indian Med J* **36**(2), 99-103 (1987).
3. Morrison EY, H Thompson, K Pascoe, M West, C Fletcher; Extraction of an hyperglycaemic principle from the annatto (*Bixa orellana*), a medicinal plant in the West Indies, *Trop Geogr Med* **43**(1-2), 184-88 (1991).
4. Russell KR, EY Morrison, D Ragoobirsingh, The effect of annatto on insulin binding properties in the dog, *Phytother Res* **19**(5), 433-36 (2005).

Blighia sapida KD Koenig (Sapindaceae) (Ackee)

The plant is native to tropical West Africa but cultivated sporadically throughout the tropics, particularly in Jamaica. It yields fruits as red, yellow or orange capsules, 2-4 inches long, opening at maturity, with 3 cream coloured arils, each tipped with a black seed. Unripe fruits of Jamaican ackee tree are reported to contain hypoglycin. The hypoglycaemic and toxic effects of this compound have been reviewed (1). The death of forty children after consumption of unripe arils of *B. sapida* in May-June, 1984, prompted an experimental study of the toxicity of hypoglycin A, present in the arils. The study with rats showed that the toxicity of hypoglycin A is raised by starvation. It was further observed that daily ingestion of infra-toxic doses produce a cumulative and delayed hypoglycaemic effect that can be lethal. The ripe arils that contain less hypoglycin A could produce this cumulative and delayed effect on starving children (2). The ripe ackee fruit is used traditionally in Jamaican cooking. However, unripe fruits are toxic and cause severe hypoglycaemia leading to severe convulsions and even death (3).

1. Sherratt HSA; Hypoglycin, the famous toxin of the unripe Jamaican ackee fruit, *Trends Pharmacol Sci* **7**(5), 186-91 (1986)
2. Foungbe S, Y Naho, C Declume; Experimental study of the toxicity of arillus from *Blighia sapida* (Sapindaceae) in relation with intoxication of children in Katiola (Cote-dinvoire), *Ann Pharm Fr* **44**(6), 509-15 (1986)
3. Olin BR; Ackee: a monograph, *Lawrence Reviews of Natural Products*, May, pp 1-2 (1992).

Boerhaavia diffusa Linn. (Nyctaginaceae) (Hog weed, S. Punarnava, H. Snathikari)

An aqueous extract of *B. diffusa* leaves showed a non-dose dependent hypoglycaemic activity. The hypoglycaemic activity at a dose of 200 mg/kg was more than that observed at a dose of 400 mg/kg (1). Administration of *B, diffusa* root extract (150 mg/kg, daily for 15 days) to male and female mice decreased the concentrations of one or both the thyroid hormones (triiodothyronine and thyroxine). The extract also lowered serum glucose concentration indicating that the hypoglycaemic activity of the plant extract might have been mediated through the inhibition of thyroid functions (2).

A significant decrease in blood glucose and significant increase in plasma insulin levels were observed in normal and alloxan induced diabetic rats, treated with daily oral administration of *B. diffusa* leaf extract (200 mg/kg) for 4 weeks. It also resulted in a significant reduction of glycosylated haemoglobin and an increase in total haemoglobin level. Administration of *B. diffusa* leaf extract in normal and diabetic rats significantly increased the activities of the hepatic enzymes such as hexokinase and significantly decreased those of glucose-6-phosphatase, fructose-1,6-bisphosphatase. Rats treated with *B. diffusa* leaf extract showed significant improvement in glucose tolerance. The effect of the plant extract was more pronounced than that of glibenclamide (3), Hyperlipidaemia is an associated complication of diabetes mellitus. Oral administration of *B. diffusa* leaf extract at 200 mg/kg of body weight for 4 weeks resulted in a significant reduction in serum and tissue cholesterol, free fatty acids, phospholipids, and triglycerides. In fact, *B. diffusa* leaf extract supplementation was found to be more effective than glibenclamide in the treatment of diabetic rats (4). The treatment also resulted in a significant reduction in thiobarbituric acid reactive substances and hydroperoxides, with a significant increase in reduced glutathione, superoxide dismutase, catalase, glutathione peroxidase and glutathione-S-transferase in liver and kidney of alloxan induced diabetic rats (5).

1. Chude MA, OE Orisakwe, OJ Aponue, KS Gamaniel, OH Vongtau, E Oki; Hypoglycaemic effect of the aqueous extract of *Boerhaavia diffusa* leaves, *Indian J Pharmacol* **33**(3), 215-16 (2001)
2. Gholap S, A Kar; Relative efficacy of three Indian medicinal plants in the regulation of serum thyroid hormones and glucose concentration in male and female nice, *J Med Arom Plant Sci* **24**(4), 1002-05 (2002)
3. Pari L, M Amarnath Satheesh; Anti-diabetic activity of *Boerhaavia diffusa* L.: effect on hepatic key enzymes in experimental diabetes, *J Ethnopharmacol* **91**(1), 109-13 (2004).
4. Pari L, M Amarnath Satheesh; Anti-diabetic effect of *Boerhavia diffusa*: effect on serum and tissue lipids in experimental diabetes, *J Med Food* **7**(4), 472-76 (2004).
5. Satheesh MA, L Pari; Antioxidant effect of *Boerhavia diffusa* L. in tissues of alloxan induced diabetic rats, *Indian J Exp Biol* **42**(10), 989-92 (2004).

Bombax ceiba Linn. (Malvaceae)
(Cotton tree, S. Salmali, H. Shimul)

Bombax ceiba is a tropical tree with straight tall trunk with spikes. The leaves fall in the winter and the tree is covered with red flowers with 5 petals in the spring before green leaves reappear. Its fruits burst and produce fibres like cotton. These fibres are used for making pillows. The tree might be from India but widely planted in Malaysia, Indonesia, South China, and Taiwan.

Shamimin, a flavonol C-glucoside from *B. ceiba* leaves, showed significant hypoglycaemic activity at 500 mg/kg in Sprague-Dawley rats. Further studies revealed that shamimin did not cause any mortality in mice at the dose of 1 g/kg but in rats 500 mg/kg was a lethal dose.

Saleem R, M Ahmad, SA Hussain, AM Qazi, SI Ahmad, MH Qazi, M Ali, S Faizi, S Akhtar, SN Husnain; Hypotensive, hypoglycaemic and toxicological studies on the flavonol C-glycoside shamimin from *Bombax ceiba, Planta Med* **65**(4), 331-34 (1999).

Borassus flabellifer **Linn. (Arecaceae)**
(Palmyra palm, Toddy Palm, S. Tala, H. Tar)

Borassus flabellifer, the Asian palmyra palm or Toddy palm is robust and tall. Its large trunk resembles that of the cocoanut tree and is ringed with leaf scars. It grows wild from the Persian Gulf to the Cambodian-Vietnamese border and is commonly cultivated in India, Southeast Asia, Malaysia and occasionally in other warm regions including Hawaii and southern Florida. The coconut-like fruits are three-sided when young, becoming rounded when mature. The outer covering of ripe fruit is smooth, thin, leathery, and brown, turning nearly black after harvest. The chief product of Toddy Palm is the sweet sap (toddy) obtained by tapping the tip of the inflorescence, The concentrate of the sap yields jaggery, which is much more nutritious than crude cane sugar,

Ethanol extract of the roots of female palm (*B. flabellifer*) produced hypoglycaemic and hypocholesterolemic effects but the effects were not dose dependent (1).

Oral administration of methanol extract of the male flowers of *B. flabellifer* was found to inhibit the increase of serum glucose levels in sucrose-loaded rats at a dose of 250 mg/kg. Six new spirostane-type steroid saponins, borassosides A-F, were isolated from this extract and their structures were determined. Dioscin, the principal steroid saponin, of the extract, was found to inhibit the increase of serum glucose levels in sucrose-loaded rats at a dose of 50 mg/kg, p.o. (2).

1. Ravishankar B, HG Makwana, RB Nair, NP Vijayan, CK Sasikala, VN Saraswathy, S Sulochana; Some pharmacological studies on female palm of *Borassus flabellifer* Linn. (Palmyra palm), *J Res Ayur Siddha* **10**(1-2), 75-86 (1989)
2. Yoshikawa M, F Xu, T Morikawa, Y Pongpiriyadacha, S Nakamura, Y Asao, A Kumahara, H Matsuda; Medicinal flowers. XII.(1)) New spirostane-type steroid saponins with antidiabetogenic activity from *Borassus flabellifer*, *Chem Pharm Bull* (Tokyo) **55**(2), 308-16 (2007)

Bougainvillea spectabilis **Willd (Nyctaginaceae)**
(Bougainvillea)

Bougainvillea is a genus of flowering plant, named after Louis Antoine de Bougainville, an admiral in the French Navy who discovered the plant in Brazil in 1768. This ornamental vine is native to Brazil but it has been naturalised in most countries with warm climates.

Bougainvillea spectabilis is a traditional anti-diabetic plant and the water-soluble fractions from different solvent extracts of the plant exhibited blood sugar lowering effect in diabetic rats (1).

Administration of pinitol, isolated from the alcoholic extract of the plant, at a dose level of 0.01g/kg effected a significant fall in blood sugar in normal, fasted and alloxan-induced diabetic albino mice. Glucose tolerance test also indicated its hypoglycaemic effect (2).

Oral administration of the leaf juice (1g leaf = 1 ml juice) at the dose of 1 ml/kg b.w./d for 14 consecutive days significantly lowered the hyperglycaemic response with 45 percent reduction of blood sugar levels in alloxan-induced diabetic rabbits. Increase in liver and muscle glycogen with repeated administration of leaf juice in alloxan-induced diabetic rats indicated its profound hypoglycaemic activity (3,4). Oral administration of alcoholic extract of *B. spectabilis* leaves to streptozotocin-induced diabetic rats caused significant reduction of blood sugar level, elevation of liver glycogen and significant increase of insulin level of treated animals (5).

D-pinitol, the active principle of the plant, is claimed to exert insulin-like effects. In order to verify this claim, the effects of D-pinitol on glucose homeostasis in animal models of diabetes, and on glucose transport by cultured muscle cells were studied. In streptozotocin-induced diabetic mice, D-pinitol (100 mg/kg p.o.) acutely decreased hyperglycaemia at 6 h. A similar decrease in plasma glucose level was observed after intra-peritoneal administration of D-pinitol (100 mg/kg). Insulin concentrations and the rate of insulin-induced disappearance of glucose were not altered by D-pinitol (100 mg/kg p.o.) Chronic administration of D-pinitol (100 mg/kg i.p. twice daily for 11 days) to streptozotocin-induced diabetic mice maintained a reduction in plasma glucose concentrations. In normal non-diabetic and severely insulin resistant ob/ob mice, D-pinitol (100 mg/kg p.o) did not significantly affect plasma glucose or insulin during acute studies. Incubation of L6 muscle cells with D-pinitol (10^{-3} M) increased basal 2-deoxyglucose uptake by 41% after 10 min and by 34% after 4 h. The effect of D-pinitol was inhibited by phosphatidylinositol 3-kinase inhibitor LY294002. D-pinitol did not increase insulin-stimulated 2-deoxyglucose uptake by L6 cells. The results of the study support the view that D-pinitol can exert an insulin-like effect to improve glycaemic control in hypoinsulinaemic streptozotocin-induced diabetic mice (6).

The administration of 50% ethanol extract of *B. spectabilis* bark to streptozotocin-induced diabetic rats for 30 days reversed the effects of sterptozotocin and caused significant decrease in blood glucose and lipid levels. A decrease in blood glucose level with concomitant increase in liver glycogen level in diabetic animals, treated with the extract, suggests that the anti-hyperglycaemic activity of the extract is due to increased uptake of glucose for the formation of glycogen by enhanced glycogenesis (7).

1. Sarker S, PC Das, G Podder; Hypoglycaemic activity of *Bougainvillea spectabilis* in streptozozotocin (STZ)-induced diabetic rats, *J Inst Chem.,* Calcutta **58**(Pt. 1), 31-32 (1986)

2. Narayanan CR, DD Joshi, AM Majumdar, VV Dhekne; Pinitol - a new anti-diabetic compound from the leaves of *Bougainvillea spectabilis, Curr Sci* **56**(3), 139-41 (1987).

3. Deshmukh AA, VP Vadlamudi, KR Wagh; Hypoglycaemic activity of *Bougainvillea spectabilis, Probe* **31**(3), 254-56 (1992).

4. Deshmukh AA, VP Vadlamudi, KR Wagh, MJ Qureshi; Nature of hypoglycaemic action of leaf juice of *Bougainvillea spectabilis, Indian J Indigenous Med* **8**(2), 65-66 (1992).

5. Banerjee R, BB Patra, J Das, PC Das, S Mondal, A Chatterjee; Evaluation of hypoglycaemic properties of alcoholic extract of *Bougainvillea spectabilis* on experimental animal model, *Int Seminar Trad Med,* Calcutta, November 7-9, p. 137 (1992).

6. Bates SH, RB Jones, CJ Bailey; Insulin-like effect of pinitol, *Br J Pharmacol* **130**(8), 1944-48 (2000)

7. Purohit A, A Sharma; Anti-diabetic efficacy of *Bougainvillea spectabilis* bark extract in streptozotocin-induced diabetic rats, *J Cell Tissue Res* **6**(1), 537-540 (2006)

Boussingaultia baselloides Kunth (Basellaceae) (H. Nar Sundar).

Boussingaultia baselloides is a South American species of ornamental succulent vine, commonly known as the madeira-vine. Boussingoside A1, a triterpene glycoside, isolated from the methanol extract of the leaves of the plant, exhibited very strong hypoglycaemic activity in rats.

Espada A, J Rodriguez, CM Villaverde, R Riguera; Hypoglycaemic triterpenoid saponins from *Boussingaultia baselloides, Canad J Chem* **68**(11), 2039-44 (1990)

Bouvardia terniflora Salisb. (Rubiaceae)

The administration of chloroform extract of *B. terniflora* (300 mg/kg) to diabetic mice decreased the blood glucose level by 58.56%. The extract, administered to normal mice, reduced blood glucose levels by 33.42 %. The hypoglycaemic effect of the plant extract, used in traditional medicine for treatment of diabetes was confirmed.

Perez-Gutierrez RM, C Perez-Gonzalez, MA Zavala-Sanchez, S Perez- Gutierrez; Hypoglycaemic activity of *Bouvardia terniflora, Brickellia veronicaefolia,* and *Parmentiera edulis, Salud Publica Mex* **40**(4), 354-58 (1998) [Article in Spanish].

Brassica juncea (L.) Czern (Brassicaceae) (Indian mustard, H. Sarso, Rai)

Cultivars of *Brassica juncea* are grown as green vegetables and the production of oilseed. The seeds are also consumed in India as a spice in various food items and also used by diabetics in India,

Effect of *Brassica juncea* on carbohydrate metabolism was studied using rats as experimental animals and it was found to exhibit significant hypoglycaemic action. Administration of the plant drug caused an increase in the concentration of hepatic glycogen, obviously due to glycogenesis. The increased activity of glycogen synthetase, and the decreased activity of glycogen phosphorylase and gluconeogenic enzymes are considered to be mechanisms for its hypoglycaemic effect (1).

The hypoglycaemic and anti-hyperglycaemic activity of various strengths (5, 10 and 15%) of *B. juncea* seed diet was studied in alloxan and streptozotocin-induced diabetes in albino rats. In addition, key enzymes of carbohydrate metabolism and hepatic glycogen content were also assessed to understand the mechanism of action. *B. juncea* seed diet (10 and 15%) showed significant anti-hyperglycaemic effect in alloxan but not in streptozotocin-induced diabetic rats. It also failed to modulate the hepatic glycogen content and enzyme activities (2).

Antioxidant effects of isorhamnetin 3,7-di-O-β-D-glucopyranoside, isolated from mustard leaf, were studied in streptozotocin-induced diabetic rats. Oral administration of this flavone glycoside (10 or 20 mg/kg b.w. for 10 days) to diabetic rats significantly reduced serum levels of glucose and 5-hydroxymethyl furfural (5-HMF), which is an indicator of oxidative stress. The levels of thiobarbituric acid reactive substances (TBARS) in serum, liver and kidney mitochondria also declined significantly in a dose-dependent manner. Intra-peritoneal administration of isorhamnetin diglucoside reduced these levels only slightly. Isorhamnetin showed potent antioxidant activity *in vitro*. In addition, intra-peritoneal administration of isorhamnetin reduced serum glucose, 5-HMF, and TBARS suggesting that the diglucoside is first metabolised *in vivo* to isorhamnetin, which plays an important role as an antioxidant (3).

Brassica juncea seeds, was assessed in a fructose-mediated non-genetic model of insulin resistance. Feeding of fructose rich diet for 30 days resulted in a rise of blood glucose by 29.4%, insulin by 101.2% and cholesterol by 26.7% indicating development of insulin resistance. However, feeding of a fructose diet containing 10% *Brassica juncea* seed powder for 30 days significantly decreased fasting serum glucose, insulin and cholesterol levels but did not normalize them. From the results of the present study it was inferred that *Brassica juncea* seeds might play a role in the management of pre-diabetic state of insulin resistance and should be promoted for use in patients prone to diabetes (4).

1. Khan BA, A Abraham. S Leelamma; Hypoglycaemic action of *Murraya koenigii* (curry leaf) and *Brassica juncea* (mustard): mechanism of action, *Indian J Biochem Biophys* **32**(2), 106-08 (1995).
2. Grover JK, S Yadav, V Vats; Hypoglycaemic and anti-hyperglycaemic effect of *Brassica juncea* diet and their effect on hepatic glycogen content and the key enzymes of carbohydrate metabolism, *Mol Cell Biochem* **241**(1-2), 95-101 (2002).

3. Yokozawa T, HY Kim, EJ Cho, JS Choi, HY Chung; Antioxidant effects of isorhamnetin 3,7-di-O-b-D-glucopyranoside isolated from mustard leaf (*Brassica juncea*) in rats with streptozotocin-induced diabetes, *J Agric Food Chem* **50**(19), 5490-95 (2002)

4. Yadav SP, V Vats, AC Ammini, JK Grover; *Brassica juncea* (Rai) significantly prevented the development of insulin resistance in rats fed fructose-enriched diet, *J Ethnopharmacol* **93**(1), 113-16 (2004).

Brassica napus **Linn. (Brassicaceae)** (Rape seed)

Rapeseed is grown for the production of animal feed, vegetable oil for human consumption, and also for production of biodiesel. Leading producers of rapeseed include the Europian Union, Canada, the United States, Australia, China and India.

Rapeseed pollens have been reported to reduce blood glucose levels in rats, fed on a high lipid diet.

Samochowiec L, J Wojcieki; Effect of pollen on serum and liver lipids in rats fed on a high lipid diet, *Herba Pol* **27**(4), 333-39 (1981).

Brassica oleracea* var. *capitata Linn.(Brassicaceae/Cruciferae) (Cabbage, H. Pattagobi)

The hypoglycaemic activity of cabbage oil, obtained by cold extraction of dried and sliced leaves with diethyl ether, was studied in streptozotocin-induced diabetic rats with blood sugar above 160 mg/100 ml. The oil significantly reduced blood sugar, serum and liver cholesterol, serum, liver and kidney glycerides and total liver lipids of rats. The hypoglycaemic activity of cabbage oil was compared with insulin and the activity was considered to be due to the presence of sulphur-containing compounds in the oil.

Tarfa SP, PK Josephm KT Augusti, Preliminary studies on the anti-diabetic effects of cabbage (*Brassica oleracea* var. *capitata* L.) on streptozotocin diabetic rats, *Curr Sci* **57**(1), 32-33 (1988).

Brassica oleracea* L. var. *caulorapa **DC.** Syn. *B. oleracea* var *gongylodes* L (Knaol khol H. Ganth gobi)

Oral administration of the aqueous extract of *B. oleracea* var. *gongylodes* stem to normal and alloxan-induced diabetic rats significantly lowered their blood glucose levels (1). The anti-diabetic and antioxidant effect of *B. oleracea* var. *caulorapa*, which is used as a vegetable, was studied in NIDDM subjects. Twenty patients were divided into two groups, control and experimental. The diets of experimental patients were supplemented with knol khol (50g/day) for a period of 8 weeks.

Knol khol therapy significantly improved the glycaemic control, brought down lipid peroxidation in erythrocytes, plasma and urine, and significantly elevated the activity of glutathione reductase and glutathione-S-transferase. The treatment also brought down the activity of catalase in erythrocytes. The findings confirmed the anti-diabetic and antioxidant activity of knol khol (2).

1. Srinivas P, PA Paul; Hypoglycaemic activity of *Brassica oleracea* var *gongylodes* in normal and diabetic rats, *Fitoterapia* **64**(4), 301-03 (1993)

2. Andallu B, A Haripriya, R Vijayadurga; Anti-diabetic and antioxidant role of knoll khol (*Brassica oleracea* var. *caulorapa*) in NIDDM subjects, *Nutr Soc, India,* 35th Annual Meeting NIN, Hyderabad, p. 41 December 12-13, 2003

Brickellia veronicaefolia Ell. (Asteraceae)

Brickellia is a genus of plants in the sunflower family and is native to the American southwest, especially Texas. The plant contains high amounts of essential oil, and germacrene D, a natural insecticide.

Intra-peritoneal administration of hexane extract of *B. veronicaefolia* (300 mg/kg) to alloxan-induced diabetic mice decreased the blood glucose level by 72.13%. In normal mice, the reduction of blood glucose level was 39.84%. The hypoglycaemic effect of the plant extract, used in traditional medicine for diabetes treatment, is confirmed (1).

Hypoglycaemic activity-guided fractionation of the chloroform extract of the leaves of the plant led to the isolation of 5, 7,3'-trihydroxy-3,6,4'-trimethoxyflavone. The isolated flavone was tested for hypoglycaemic activity in normal and alloxan-induced diabetic CD1 mice. The flavone produced a significant hypoglycaemic effect in normal as well as in diabetic mice. It was found to be slow and less effective than tolbutamide (2). The antioxidant and free radical scavenging activities of this flavone were also studied (3).

1. Perez-Gutierrez RM, C Perez-Gonzalez, MA Zavala-Sanchez, S Perez-Gutierrez; Hypoglycaemic activity of *Bouvardia terniflora, Brickellia veronicaefolia,* and *Parmentiera edulis, Salud Publica Mex* **40**(4), 354-58 (1998) [Article in Spanish].

2. Perez RM, H Cervantes, MA Zavala, J Sanchez, S Perez, C Perez; Isolation and hypoglycaemic activity of 5,7,3'-trihydroxy-3,6,4'-trimethoxyflavone from *Brickellia veronicaefolia, Phytomedicine* 7(1), 25-29 (2000)

3. Perez G RM, SR Vargas, MFJ Martinez, RI Cordova, Antioxidant and free radical scavenging activities of 5,7,3'-trihydroxy-3,6,4'-trimethoxyflavone from *Brickellia veronicaefolia. Phytother Res* **18**(5), 428-30 (2004)

Bridelia ferruginea Benth (Phyllanthaceae / Euphorbiaceae)

B. ferruginea is used in African traditional medicine to cure a variety of ailments including diabetes. Infusion of *B. ferruginea* leaves lowered the blood sugar level of 8 diabetic patients from average 250 mg% to 120 mg% in 2 weeks. However, hyperglycaemia reappeared after the drug was withdrawn. Alcoholic and aqueous extracts of the plant significantly lowered the fasting blood sugar of normal rats but failed to adequately protect the animals against alloxan-induced diabetes. Flavonoids and biflavonoids based on apigenin and kaempferol moieties together with their O- and C-glycosides were isolated from the methanol extract of the leaves of the plant (1). Quercetin-3-neohesperidoside, isolated from the leaves of the plant, was found to reduce the blood sugar levels of fasting New Zealand white rabbits. The effect of this flavone glycoside was compared with those of glibenclamide, insulin and chlorpropamide. The onset and duration of action of this drug was comparable to that of glibenclamide but differed from the others (2). The flavonoid content of leaf extract of the plant was 0.015% based on rutin. The tablets of leaf extract showed a very long shelf life of 96 years. Tablets of *B. ferruginea* (25 mg/kg) lowered the blood glucose level of normal healthy rabbits by about 40 percent (3).

1. Iwu MM; The hypoglycaemic properties of *Bridelia ferruginea, Fitoterapia* **54**(6), 243-48 (1983).
2. Addae-Mensah I, RW Munenge; Quercetin-3-neohesperidoside (rutin) and other flavonoids as the active hypoglycaemic agents of *Bridelia ferruginea, Fitoterapia* **60**(4), 359-62 (1989).
3. Onunkwo GC, PA Akah, OK Udeala; Studies on ferruginea leaves (1) Stability and hypoglycaemic actions of the leaf extract tablets, *Phytother Res* **10**(5), 418-20 (1996)

Bryonia alba Linn. (Cucurbitaceae)
(Black-berried white bryony)

The action of *B. alba* root extract on lipid peroxidation in microsomes and on fatty acid composition of individual lipid fractions in the liver of alloxan-induced diabetic rats was examined. Administration of *B. alba* extract was found to produce an appreciably normalizing effect on the biochemical indices of liver function (1).

Hypoglycaemic action of trihydroxy-unsaturated fatty acids, present in *B. alba,* was studied in alloxan-induced diabetes by Russian workers (2). These workers showed, in a later publication (3), how lipid metabolism, which is severely disordered in alloxan-induced diabetic rats, is restored by administration of trihydroxyoctadecadienoic acids (0.05 mg/kg/day for 15 days. i.m.), obtained from the roots of *B. alba.* The C_{18}- fatty acids, isolated from the plant, were a mixture of 12,13,16-trihydroxy-9*Z*,14*E*-octadecadienoic acid, 12,15,16-trihydroxy-9*Z*,13*E*-octadecadienoic acid, 9,10, 13-trihydroxy-11*E*,15*Z*-octadecadienoic acid and 9,12,13-

trihydroxy-10*E*,14Z-octadecadienoic acid. From the results of detailed investigation, it was concluded that C_{18}- acids from *B. alba* were capable of correcting major metabolic abnormalities typical of severe diabetes mellitus.

1. Karagezian KG, GS Vartanian, AG Panosiàn; Effect of an extract from the roots of bryony (*Bryonia alba*) on lipid peroxidation in the liver of rats with alloxan diabetes, *Biull Eksp Biol Med* **92**(8), 35-37 (1981) [Article in Russian].
2. Panosian AG, GM Avetisian, KG Karagezian, GS Vartanian, GKh Buniatian; Hypoglycaemic action of *Bryonia alba* L. unsaturated fatty trihydroxy acids in alloxan diabetes, *Dokl Akad Nauk* **256**(5), 1267-69 (1981) [Article in Russian].
3. Karagezian KG, GS Vartanian, MI Agadjanov, AG Panosian; JR Hoult; Restoration of the disordered glucose-fatty acid cycle in alloxan-diabetic rats by trihydroxyoctadecadienoic acids from *Bryonia alba*, a native Armenian medicinal plant, *Planta Med* **64**(5),417-22 (1998).

Bryophyllum pinnatum (Lam.) Oken, (Crassulaceae) (Air plant. Canterbury bells)

There are about 20 to 30 *Bryophyllum* species, native originally of South Africa, Madagascar, Australia and Asia. This group of plants is notable for growing small plantlets on the fringes of the leaves. These plantlets eventually drop off and develop roots. Nowadays, *Bryophyllum* species are deliberately cultivated in many parts of the tropics for their attractiveness and interesting reproduction.

Investigation was made to scientifically verify the validity of the ethnomedical uses of *B. pinnatum* leaves for its anti-nociceptive, anti-inflammatory and anti-diabetic properties. Aqueous extract of *B. pinnatum* leaves (25-800 mg/kg p.o. or ip) caused significant hypoglycaemia in rats. The different flavonoids, polyphenols, triterpenoids and other chemical constituents of the herb are speculated to account for the observed anti-diabetic properties of the plant.

Ojewole JA; Anti-nociceptive, anti-inflammatory and anti-diabetic effects of *Bryophyllum pinnatum* (Crassulaceae) leaf aqueous extract, *J Ethnopharmacol* **99**(1), 13-19 (2005)

Buddleja officinalis Maxim. (Scrophulariaceae / Buddleiaceae)

The inhibitory effect of a 70% methanolic extract of the flowers of *B. officinalis* was tested on unpurified rat lens aldose reductase, an enzyme involved in the complications of diabetes. The extract showed significant inhibition. It is suggested that the inhibitory effect of *B. officinalis* flowers on aldose reductase is partially attributable to the flavonols or their glycosides, present in the flowers.

Matsuda H, H Cai, M Kubo, H Tosa, M Iinuma; Study on anti-cataract drugs from natural sources. II. Effects of *Buddlejae flos* on *in vitro* aldose reductase activity, *Biol Pharm Bull* **18**(3), 463-66 (1995)

Bumelia sartorum Mart (Sapotaceae) (Obtuse leaf jungleplum)

Bumelia sartorum is distributed throughout the tropics of South America and also found in Mexico. The plant has been mentioned in Brazilian folklore for its use in the treatment of diabetes mellitus.

An ethanol extract of root bark of *B. sartorum* elicited hypoglycaemic effect in normal and alloxan-induced diabetic rats. The extract was also found to alter glucose tolerance in diabetic rats, enhance glucose uptake in skeletal muscle and inhibit glycogenolysis in the liver. Based on these observations, it was inferred that the hypoglycaemic effect of the extract was possibly due to an enhanced secretion of insulin from the islets of Langerhans or an increased utilization of glucose by peripheral tissues. Bassic acid, a constituent of the extract, was proved to be responsible for the hypoglycaemic activity. This triterpene acid elicited significant hypoglycaemic activity in alloxan-induced diabetic rats. It also altered the pattern of glucose tolerance in these animals and increased plasma insulin levels. Further, treatment with this acid increased significantly the glucose uptake process and glycogen synthesis in isolated rat diaphragm. The hypoglycaemic activity of bassic acid may be mediated through enhanced secretion of insulin from the pancreatic β-cells (1, 2)

1. Almeida RN, JM Filho, SR Naik; Chemistry and pharmacology of an ethanol extract of *Bumelia sartorum, J Ethnopharmacol* **14**(2-3), 173-85 (1985).
2. Naik SR, JM Barbosa Filho, JN Dhuley, V Deshmukh; Probable mechanism of hypoglycaemic activity of bassic acid, a natural product isolated from *Bumelia sartorum, J Ethnopharmacol* **33**(1-2), 37-44 (1991)

Butea monosperma (Lam) Taub (Fabaceae) (Syn. *Butea frondosa*) (Flame of the Forest, H. Palash)

Butea monosperma is native to tropical southern Asia, from Pakistan, India, Nepal, Sri Lanka, Myanmar, Thailand, Laos, Cambodia, Vietnam, Malaysia and western Indonesia. It is a medium sized tree that yields 2.5 cm long, bright orange-red flowers.

The anti-hyperglycaemic activity of an ethanol extract of *Butea monosperma* was studied in glucose-loaded and alloxan-induced diabetic rats. Oral administration of a single dose of the extract (200 mg/kg) significantly improved glucose tolerance and caused reduction in blood glucose level in alloxan-induced diabetic rats. Oral administration of the extract at the same dose once daily for two weeks significantly reduced blood glucose, serum cholesterol and improved HDL-cholesterol and albumin as compared to diabetic control group.

Somani R, S Kasture, AK Singhai; Anti-diabetic potential of *Butea monosperma* in rats, *Fitoterapia* **77**(2), 86-90 (2006)

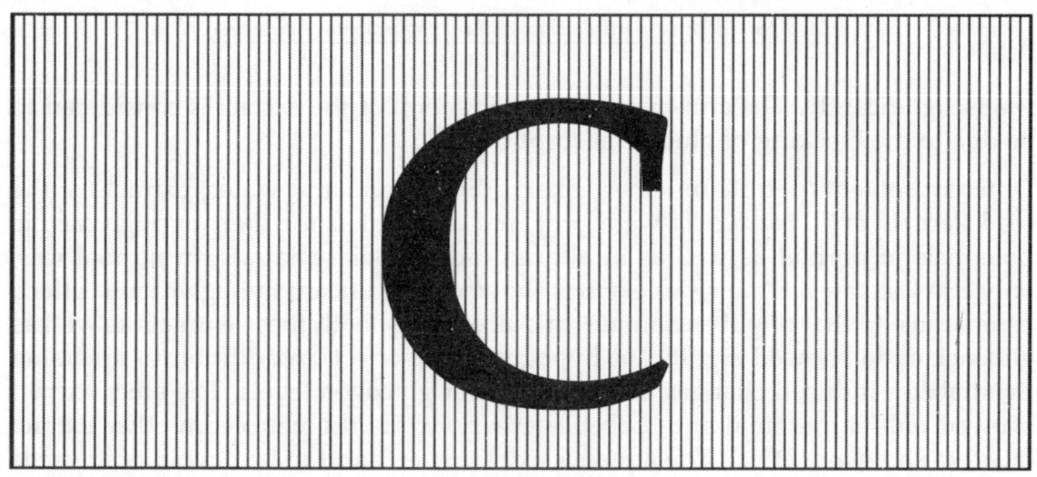

Caesalpinia bonducella Fleming (Fabaceae/Leguminosae)

Caesalpinia bonducella is widely distributed throughout the coastal region of India and the tribal people of Andaman and Nicober Island use this plant for controlling blood sugar. It is also used as a folklore medicine in the Caribbean Islands for the management of diabetes.

Administration of *C. bonducella* seed powder (1.5g/kg, only once per os), significantly decreased the blood glucose level of rabbits after 12 h of administration. In diabetic rabbits, the drug produced anti-hyperglycaemic effect within 3 days when given at the same dose for 10 days (1). Hypoglycaemic, anti-hyperglycaemic and hypolipidemic activities of the aqueous and 50% ethanol extracts of *C. bonducella* seeds were studied in normal and streptozotocin-induced diabetic rats. In normal rats, both the extracts exhibited hypoglycaemic activity as early as 4 h after administration at a dose of 100 mg/kg; the effect produced by the aqueous extract was, however, of prolonged duration as compared to ethanol extract. In diabetic rats, both the extracts produced significant anti-hyperglycaemic effect from day 5 onwards. *C. bonducella* seeds were thus found to possess an anti-diabetic principle, which can be useful for the treatment of diabetes (2). Chakrabarti and co-workers studied the effects of aqueous and ethanol extracts of the seeds of this plant in both type-1 and type-2 diabetes mellitus using Long Evans rats and observed significant blood sugar lowering effect in type-2 diabetic model. The mechanism of action was also studied (5). The hypoglycaemic activity of different extracts from *C. bonducella* in chronic type-2 diabetic model was evaluated along with insulin secretagogue activity of five fractions isolated from the *C. bonducella* seed kernel. Both the aqueous and ethanol extracts showed potent hypoglycaemic activity in chronic type-2 diabetic model. Two fractions BM 169 and BM 170 B could increase secretion of insulin from isolated islets (6). Oral administration of the seed extract of *Caesalpinia bonducella* (300 mg/kg) produced significant anti-hyperglycaemic action in alloxan induced hyperglycaemic rats. It also lowered blood urea nitrogen levels significantly. The anti-hyperglycaemic action of the extract is considered to be due to the blocking of glucose absorption (7).

Different solvent (petroleum ether, ether, ethyl acetate and water) extracts of the seed kernels of *C. bonducella* were prepared and tested for their hypoglycaemic potentials in normal as well as in alloxan induced diabetic rats. In normal rats, only ethyl acetate and aqueous extracts showed a significant hypoglycaemic effect, comparable to that of glibenclamide. In diabetic rats, both these extracts as well as glibenclamide showed significant hypoglycaemic effect, in addition to reversing the diabetes-induced changes in lipid and liver glycogen levels. The ether extract showed only a marginal anti-diabetic activity, while the petroleum ether extract failed to show any effect. The aqueous extract was found to be devoid of any free radical scavenging activity, but the ethyl acetate extract showed a maximum of 49% activity at the end of 1 hour (4). However, a suspension of powdered seed kernel of *C. bonducella*, growing in Dar es Salaam, Tanzania, failed to show any hypoglycaemic activity (3).

1. Rao VV, SK Dwivedi, D Swarup; Hypoglycaemic effect of *Caesalpinia bonducella* in rabbits, *Fitoterapia* **65**(3), 245-47 (1994)
2. Sharma SR, SK Dwivedi, D Swarup; Hypoglycaemic, anti-hyperglycaemic and hypolipidaemic activities of *Caesalpinia bonducella* seeds in rats, *J Ethnopharmacol* **58**(1), 39-44 (1997).
3. Moshi MJ, V Nagpa; Effect of *Caesalpinia bonducella* seeds on blood glucose in rabbits, *Pharmaceut Biol* **38**(2), 81-86 (2000)
4. Sudeep Parameshwar, KK. Srinivasan, C Mallikarjuna Rao; Oral anti-diabetic activities of different extracts of *Caesalpinia bonducella* seed kernels, *Pharmaceut Biol* **40**(8), 590-95 (2002)
5. Chakrabarti S, TK Biswas, B Rokeya, L Ali, M Mosihuzzaman, N Nahar, AK Khan, B Mukherjee; Advanced studies on the hypoglycaemic effect of *Caesalpinia bonducella* F. in type 1 and 2 diabetes in Long Evans rats, *J Ethnopharmacol* **84**(1), 41-46 (2003).
6. Chakrabarti S, TK Biswas, T Seal, B Rokeya, L Ali, AK Azad Khan, N Nahar, M Mosihuzzaman, B Mukherjee; Anti-diabetic activity of *Caesalpinia bonducella* F. in chronic type-2 diabetic model in Long-Evans rats and evaluation of insulin secretagogue property of its fractions on isolated islets, *J Ethnopharmacol* **97**(1), 117-22 (2005)
7. Kannur DM, VI Hukkeri, KS Akki; Anti-diabetic activity of *Caesalpinia bonducella* seed extracts in rats, *Fitoterapia* **77**(7-8), 546-49 (2006).

Caesalpinia ferrea Mart ex Tul. (Caesalpinaceae/ Fabaceae/ Leguminosae) (Brazillian Ironwood, 'Juca')

Caesalpinia ferrea, called 'Juca', is one of the medicinal plants in Brazil used for the treatment of diabetes. Ellagic acid and 2-(2,3,6-trihydroxy-4-carboxyphenyl) ellagic acid, isolated from the fruits of this plant, have been recognized as aldose reductase inhibitors, which are known to prevent eye and nerve damage in diabetes. While inhibitory activity of both the acids against aldose reductase was tested *in vitro,* only ellagic acid was tested *in vivo.* An aldose reductase catalyzes the reduction of glucose to sorbitol and a measurement of the accumulation of sorbitol may be suitably utilized to know the inhibitory activity of a compound. Both the acids significantly and dose-dependently inhibited sorbitol accumulation in erythrocytes, eye lens and sciatic nerve under incubating with glucose *in vitro.* Ellagic acid at a dose of 75 mg/kg/d showed the most potent inhibition of sorbitol accumulation in erythrocytes, lens and sciatic nerve *in vivo.* An aldose reductase inhibitor is generally used to prevent eye and nerve damage in diabetes. The fruit of *Caesalpinia ferrea* might, therefore, be able to relieve diabetic complications.

Ueda H, K Kawanishi, M Moriyasu; Effects of ellagic acid and 2-(2,3,6-trihydroxy-4-carboxyphenyl) ellagic acid on sorbitol accumulation *in vitro* and *in vivo, Biol Pharm Bull* **27**(10), 1584-87 (2004).

Caesalpinia species

Brazilin is a red pigment obtained from the wood of several South American species of *Caesalpinia* and it is a close relative of the blue-black dye haematoxylin. Of the different *Caesalpinia* species that are known to yield brazilin, brazilwood (*C. echinata*) and sappanwood (*C. sappan*) are important. The sappanwood is found in India, Malaysia, and Sri Lanka.

Brazilin was found to have hypoglycaemic action and increased glucose metabolism in experimental animals. Brazilin also increased basal glucose transport in 3T3-L1 fibroblasts and adipocytes. However, insulin-stimulated glucose transport was not affected by brazilin. Auto-phosphorylation of insulin receptor was not affected by brazilin treatment in 3T3-L1 fibroblasts. Brazilin decreased the protein kinase C activity in 3T3-L1 fibroblasts and adipocytes (1). The action of brazilin on gluconeogenesis and ketogenesis in isolated rat hepatocytes was studied in order to elucidate the mechanism of hypoglycaemic action of brazilin. Brazilin decreased gluconeogenesis at 100 μM in hepatocytes isolated from diabetic rats and also decreased basal and glucagon-induced gluconeogenesis in hepatocytes from normal rats. Fatty acids-induced gluconeogenesis was significantly reduced by brazilin. The results of detailed investigation suggest that a decreased gluconeogenic flux in hepatocytes might at least partly contribute to the hypoglycaemic effects of brazilin (2).

1. Kim YM, SG Kim, LY Khil, CK Moon; Brazilin stimulates the glucose transport in 3T3 L1 cells, *Planta Med* **61**(4), 297-301 (1995)

2. Won HS, J Lee, LY Khil, SH Chae, MY Ahn, RH Lee, JH Chang, YC Kim, CK Moon; Mechanism of action of Brazilin on gluconeogenesis in isolated rat hepatocytes, *Planta Med.* **70**(8), 740-44 (2004).

Cajanus cajan (L.) Millsp. (Fabaceae)
(Pigeon pea, Red gram, H. Arhar, Toor, S. Adhaki)

Red gram is an important legume crop and the Indian subcontinent, Eastern Africa and Central America are the world's three main red gram producing regions. Red gram juice (2 ml filtered juice from fresh raw seeds) was found to be hypoglyaemic and hypocholesterolaemic when tested in 40 alloxan-induced diabetic male albino rats. The juice also reduced blood urea level (1). The effects of roasted and un-roasted seeds of *C. cajan* on serum glucose levels of normal and alloxan-induced diabetic mice were studied. Single doses of un-roasted seeds, on administration to normal as well as alloxanized mice, showed significant reduction in the serum glucose levels after 1-2h and a significant rise at 3h. In case of roasted seeds, on other hand, there was a significant increase in serum glucose levels during 3 h experimental period. It was, therefore, concluded that roasting of seeds at high temperature for half an hour resulted in the total loss of hypoglycaemic principle but not the hyperglycaemic principle present in the seeds (2).

1. Giri J, B Suganthi, S Kowsalya; Effect of red gram (*Cajanus cajan*) on blood glucose level in diabetic rats, *Indian J Nutr Diet* **23**(4), 82-87 (1986)

2. Amalraj T, S Ignacimuthu; Hypoglycaemic activity of *Cajanus cajan* (seeds) in mice, *Indian J Exp Biol* **36**(10), 1032-33 (1998).

Calamintha officinalis Moench (Lamiaceae Labiatae)
(Basil Thyme)

Calamint belongs to a genus closely related to both the Thymes and to Catnep and Ground Ivy. It contains a camphoraceous, volatile, stimulating oil in common with the other mints.

The effects of an aqueous extract of the aerial parts of *C. officinalis,* (after a single dose or daily oral administration for 15 days,) on plasma blood glucose concentrations and on basal insulin levels in normal and streptozotocin-induced diabetic rats were studied. The plant extract showed hypoglycaemic effect with no change in basal plasma insulin concentrations in both normal and streptozotocin-induced diabetic rats. The underlying mechanism, therefore, appears to be independent of insulin secretion.

Lemhadri A, NA Zeggwagh, M Maghrani, H Jouad, JB Michel, M Eddouks; Hypoglycaemic effect of *Calamintha officinalis* Moench. in normal and streptozotocin-induced diabetic rats, *J Pharm Pharmacol* **56**(6), 795-99 (2004)

Calendula officinalis Linn (Asteraceae) (English Marigold, Pot Marigold)

The leaves and petals of Pot Marigold are edible. The petals are often used as a substitute for saffron and to garnish dishes. The methanol extract of the flowers of *C. officinalis* and its n-butanol-soluble fraction showed hypoglycaemic effect, inhibitory activity on gastric emptying, and gastroprotective effect. The principal saponin constituents, glycosides A, B, C, D, and F, isolated from the butanol-soluble fraction, exhibited potent inhibitory effects on an increase in serum glucose levels in glucose-loaded rats. Some structure-activity relationships have also been discussed.

Yoshikawa M, T Murakami, A Kishi, T Kageura, H Matsuda; Medicinal flowers. III. Marigold. (1): hypoglycaemic, gastric emptying inhibitory, and gastroprotective principles and new oleanane-type triterpene oligoglycosides, calendasaponins A, B, C, and D, from Egyptian *Calendula officinalis*, *Chem Pharm Bull* (Tokyo) **49**(7), 863-70 (2001)

Calligonum comosum L'Herit (Polygonaceae) (West African: Mauritania)

This plant is found in sandy areas of the North African desert. It is also found on the desert sands of the Middle East and also on the Rajputana desert of western India. Oral administration of an aqueous extract of the plant to albino rats produced a hypoglycaemic effect, indicated by a decrease in blood sugar level. Diabetic state of rats was alleviated by treatment with the extract (300 mg/kg b.w.).

El-Hawary ZM, TS Kholief; Biochemical studies on some hypoglycaemic agents: (2) Effect of *Calligonum comosum* extract, *Arch Pharmacal Res* **13**(1), 113-16 (1990).

Camellia sinensis (L) Kuntze (Theaceae) (Tea plant, H. Cha)

Camellia sinensis is the tea plant, the leaves and leaf buds of which are used to produce tea. Different varieties of tea (white tea, green tea, oolong tea and black tea) are all harvested from this species, but are processed differently to attain different levels of oxidation.

Shimizu and co-workers studied the hypoglycaemic constituents of Japanese tea (1) while Gomes and co-workers evaluated the effect of the hot water extract of black tea on streptozotocin-induced diabetes in rats and found it to possess both preventive and curative effects on experimentally produced diabetes in rats, like green tea (2).

An aqueous solution of polyphenols of green tea was found to inhibit lipid peroxidation and scavenge hydroxyl and superoxide radicals *in vitro*. Green tea polyphenols were found to reduce serum glucose level in alloxan-induced diabetic rats significantly at a dose level of 100 mg/kg b.w. Continued daily administration of the polyphenols (50 and 100 mg/kg b.w.) for 15 days reduced the elevated serum glucose level, produced by alloxan administration. Elevated levels of hepatic and renal enzymes, produced by alloxan, were also reduced by green tea polyphenols. The increased serum lipid peroxidation and decreased liver glycogen levels, observed after alloxan administration, were reversed by treatment with green tea polyphenols. Tea polyphenol treated group also showed increased antioxidant potential as seen from improvements in superoxide dismutase and glutathione levels (5). It has been suggested that green tea consumption prevents type-2 diabetes. Green tea was found to promote glucose metabolism in healthy human volunteers in oral glucose tolerance tests. It lowered blood glucose levels in diabetic db+/db+ mice and streptozotocin-induced diabetic mice 2-6 h after administration at 300 mg/kg without affecting serum insulin level. It was also demonstrated for the first time that a certain serum protein might be involved in the anti-hyperglycaemic effect of green tea (7). The effect of green tea on glucose tolerance and insulin sensitivity was tested in Sprague-Dawley rats. Substitution of drinking water (deionised distilled water) of control rats by green tea (solution of 0.5 mg lyophilised green tea in deionised distilled water) in experimental animals for a period of 12 weeks lowered their fasting plasma glucose levels, insulin, triglyceride and free fatty acids. Insulin-stimulated glucose uptake of, and insulin binding to adipocytes were significantly increased in the green tea group. Results demonstrated that green tea enhances insulin sensitivity and that polyphenols are the active components (8).

Epigallocatechin 3-gallate, the major green tea polyphenolic constituent has been reported to mimic the cellular effects of insulin including the reductive effect on the gene expression of rate-limiting gluconeogenic enzymes in a cell culture system. Administration of green tea, that contains this polyphenolic constituent, caused a reduction in the level of mRNAs for gluconeogenic enzymes, phosphoenolpyruvate carboxykinase and glucose-6-phosphatase in the mouse liver. Epigallocatechin 3-gallate alone was also found to down-regulate the gene expression of these enzymes. The observations support the idea that green tea intake may be beneficial in the prevention of diabetes mellitus (10). Effect of long-term oral administration of green tea extract on weight gain and glucose tolerance in Zucker diabetic rats was studied but no significant difference was observed (11).

Tea polyphenols, in addition to their protective effect against oxidative damage, have been shown to increase insulin activity. In an epididymal fat cell assay, tea, as it is normally consumed, was shown to increase insulin activity more than 15-fold *in vitro*. Black, green, and oolong teas, that contain leaves of *C. sinensis*, were all shown to increase insulin activity. High-performance liquid chromatographic fractionation of tea extracts showed that the majority of the insulin-potentiating activity for green and oolong teas was due to epigallocatechin gallate. In addition to epigallocatechin gallate, tannins, theaflavins, and other undefined compounds were responsible for insulin-potentiating activity of black tea. However, of all these compounds, the greatest activity was due to epigallocatechin gallate followed by epicatechin gallate, tannins, and theaflavins. It was further shown that while addition of lemon to the tea did not affect the insulin-potentiating activity, addition of milk significantly decreased the insulin-potentiating activity (6). African black tea extract significantly showed suppressive effect of the elevation of blood glucose on oral glucose tolerance test of 8 week-old KK-A(y)/TaJcl mice. Long-term treatment with black tea extract showed significant suppression of post-prandial blood glucose and obesity (12).

Bio-tea was prepared by fermenting black tea decoction with a culture containing *Saccharomyces ludwigii* and *Acetobacter xylinum*. Administration of bio-tea (1.71 ml/kg) to normal albino mice caused hypoglycaemia after 30 min with maximum effect after 2 hour and became normal beyond 8 hr. In alloxan-induced diabetic albino mice, repeated treatment with bio-tea for three days brought about a significant fall in mean blood sugar level. Hypoglycaemic effect was persistent in alloxan-induced diabetic mice. Effect on glucose tolerance test showed a significant fall of blood sugar level of bio-tea treated animals after 1 h of glucose treatment (3).

Coarse tea contained a significant amount of polysaccharide complex. When 7 weeks old C57BL/8 mice were injected with this polysaccharide complex, the levels of blood glucose in normal and hyperglycaemic model mice decreased significantly (4).

Oral administration of vanadate exhibits a strong hypoglycaemic effect but it suffers from toxic side effects like life-threatening diarrhoea. In view of potent anti-diarrhoeal effects of tea, the potential of suspending vanadate in a tea decoction was studied to reduce the diarrhoeal action of vanadate. Streptozotocin-induced diabetic rats were orally gavaged with vanadate suspended in water or in the tea decoction, or with the tea extract alone and their blood glucose levels were assessed daily over 11 weeks. Both the vanadate/water and vanadate/tea solutions acutely reduced blood glucose but the majority of vanadate/water-treated rats developed diarrhoea and mortality rates approached 40%. Vanadate/tea-treated diabetic rats experienced no diarrhoea or mortality and liver and kidney analyses were normal. Animals, treated with vanadate/tea, retained blood glucose levels below 10 mmol/L for about 24 consecutive days without subsequent treatments. Cataract formation was completely prevented. Because of its long-lasting effects, and lack of side effects, vanadate/tea represents a potentially important alternative therapy for an insulin-deficient diabetic state (9).

1. Shimizu M, S Wada, T Hayashi, M Arisawa, K Ikegaya, S Ogaku, S Yano, N Morita; Studies on hypoglycaemic constituents of Japanese tea, *Yakugaku Zasshi* **108**(10), 964-70 (1988) [Article in Japanese]

2. Gomes A, JR Vedasiromoni, M Das, RM Sharma, DK Ganguly; Anti-hyperglycaemic effect of black tea (*Camellia sinensis*) in rat, *J Ethnopharmacol* **45**(3), 223-26 (1995)

3. Shenoy KC; Hypoglycaemic activity of bio-tea in mice, *Indian J Exp Biol* **38**(3), 278-79 (2000)

4. Dongfeng W, W Chenghong, L Jun, Z Guiwen; Components and activity of polysaccharides from coarse tea, *J Agric Food Chem* **49**(1), 507-10 (2001)

5. Sabu MC, K Smitha, R Kuttan; Anti-diabetic activity of green tea polyphenols and their role in reducing oxidative stress in experimental diabetes, *J Ethnopharmacol* **83**(1-2), 109-16 (2002).

6. Anderson RA, MM Polansky; Tea enhances insulin activity, *J Agric Food Chem* **50**(24), 7182-86 (2002).

7. Tsuneki H, M Ishizuka, M Terasawa, JB Wu, T Sasaoka, I Kimura; Effect of green tea on blood glucose levels and serum proteomic patterns in diabetic (db/db) mice and on glucose metabolism in healthy humans, *BMC Pharmacol* **4**, 18 (2004).

8. Wu LY, CC Juan, LT Ho, YP Hsu, LS Hwang; Effect of green tea supplementation on insulin sensitivity in Sprague-dawley rats, *J Agric Food Chem* **52**(3), 643-48 (2004)

9. Clark TA, CE Heyliger, AL Edel, DP Goel, GN Pierce; Co-delivery of a tea extract prevents morbidity and mortality associated with oral vanadate therapy in streptozotocin-induced diabetic rats, *Metabolism* **53**(9), 1145-51 (2004).

10. Koyama Y, K Abe, Y Sano, M Njelekela, Y Shop, Y Hara, M Isemura; Effects of green tea on gene expression of hepatic gluconeogenic enzymes *in vivo*, *Planta Med* 70(11), 1100-02 (2004)

11. Janle EM, C Portocarrero, Y Zhu, Q Zhou; Effect of long-term oral administration of green tea extract on weight gain and glucose tolerance in Zucker diabetic (ZDF) rats, *J Herb Pharmacother* **5**(3), 55-65 (2005)

12. Shoji Y, H Nakashima; Glucose-lowering effect of powder formulation of African black tea extract in KK-A(y)/TaJcl diabetic mouse, *Arch Pharm Res* **29**(9), 786-94 (2006)

Canavalia ensiformis (L.) D.C (Fabaceae)
(Jack-bean)

Jack-bean is a legume which is used for animal fodder and human nutrition, especially in Brazil. Canatoxin, the toxic protein purified from *C. ensiformis* seeds, has been shown to release insulin from isolated rat pancreatic islets. This effect is time and dose dependent and occurs in the absence as well in the presence of glucose, but is markedly reduced at lower temperatures. At 1-2 μM, the insulinotropic effect of canatoxin is equivalent to that of 20 mM glucose. That the stimulatory effect of canatoxin is not caused by a toxic or lytic effect of the toxin on the islets is evident from the observation that the islets once exposed to this toxin are able to respond to a new insulinotropic stimulus. From the results of the detailed investigation, it was inferred that canatoxin might act on islets through the same pathway as that used by glucose. Canatoxin was shown to induce serotonin release from rabbit platelets and insulin release from isolated pancreatic islets, both of which were inhibited by lipoxygenase inhibitors (1, 2).

The hyperinsulinemia produced by canatoxin was both time and dose dependent and lasted only about 30 min, while the fall in blood glucose levels was long lasting. The hyperinsulinemic response to canatoxin was greater in females than in males but no difference was noted in the hypoglycaemia. Pretreatment of rats with naloxone, naltrexone, atropine or hexamethonium abolished both the hyperinsulinemia and the hypoglycaemia. These data suggest that these phenomena are influenced by opioids and depend on parasympathetic stimulation (3).

1. Barja-Fidalgo C, JA Guimaraes, CR Carlini; Canatoxin, a plant protein, induces insulin release from isolated pancreatic islets, *Endocrinology* **128**(2), 675-79 (1991)
2. Barja-Fidalgo C, JA Guimaraes, CR Carlini; Lipoxygenase-mediated secretory effect of canatoxin the toxic protein from *Canavalia ensiformis* seeds, *Toxicon* **29**(4-5), 453-59 (1991).
3. Ribeiro-DaSilva G, JF Prado; Increased insulin circulating levels induced by canatoxin in rats, *Toxicon* **31**(9), 1131-36 (1993).

Cannabis sativa Linn. (Cannabaceae)
(Mrijuana, S. Ganjika, H. Ganja)

Cannabis, also known as marijuana, is a psychoactive product of the plant, *Cannabis sativa*. Δ^9- Tetrahydrocannabinol is one of the psychoactive molecules that produce the "high" associated with marijuana.

A study, conducted by Singh and co-workers, indicates that chronic use of cannabis does not produce serious harmful effects in human subjects. Moreover, the hypotensive and hypoglycaemic properties of cannabis make it useful in cases of diabetic hypertension.

Singh N, S Vrat, B Ali, KP Bhargava; Assessment of biological effects of chronic use of Cannabis (Marihuana) in human subjects, *Q J Crude Drug Res* **19**(2-3), 81-91 (1981)

Capparis decidua (Forssk.) Edgew. (Capparaceae)
(H. Karir)

Capparis decidua is a small much-branched tree of the Thar desert and other arid regions in southern Asia. Its pink fleshy berries are readily eaten by birds. The spicy fruits are also used for preparing vegetables, curry and fine pickles. *Capparis decidua* powder is known as a hypoglycaemic agent and its effect on lipid peroxidation (LPO) and the antioxidant defense system was assessed in rat tissues. The increased levels of blood glucose in diabetes produce superoxide anions and hydroxyl radicals in the presence of transition metal ions which cause oxidative damage to cell membranes. The heart tissue showed an increased lipid peroxidation in diabetic rats while no significant change was observed in the liver and kidney. A lowering of lipid peroxidation was observed by treatment with *C. deciduas* powder and this effect was better than insulin-treated rats. The superoxide dismutase activity increased in the heart and kidneys in the diabetic group of rats but treatment with *C. decidua* decreased this activity in the liver and kidney. Total and Se-dependent glutathione peroxidase in the heart was markedly lowered in diabetic rats, which recovered with insulin as well as with *C. decidua* treatment. The increase in glutathione peroxidase and catalase activity with *C. decidua* treatment may lower H_2O_2 toxicity and reduce oxidative stress in diabetes. Like insulin, *C. decidua* also decreased glutathione reductase activity in the kidney and heart, which resulted in the decrease in glutathione content in these tissues. The increase in glucose-6-phosphate dehydrogenase in the kidney and heart of diabetic rats decreased with *C. decidua* treatment. The results of the investigation suggested that *C. deciduas* possessed both anti-diabetic and anti-oxidative activity.

Yadav P, S Sarkar, D Bhatnagar; Action of *Capparis decidua* against alloxan-induced oxidative stress and diabetes in rat tissues, *Pharmacol Res* **36**(3), 221-28 (1997)

Capparis spinosa Linn. (Capparaceae)
(Caper berry)

The caper is a perennial spiny shrub, native to the Mediterranean region. It grows wild on walls or in rocky coastal areas. The plant is best known for its edible bud and fruit (caper berry), which are usually consumed as pickles. The hypoglycaemic effect of an aqueous extract of *C. spinosa* fruit was studied in normal and streptozotocin-induced diabetic rats. Oral administration of a single dose of the aqueous extract of *C. spinosa* (20 mg/kg) produced a significant decrease in blood glucose level in streptozotocin-induced diabetic rats and the blood glucose level was nearly normalised 2 weeks after daily repeated oral administration of the extract. No highly significant change in blood glucose level was noticed in normal rats after both acute and chronic treatments with the extract. No change was also observed in basal plasma insulin concentration after treatment with *C. spinosa* fruit extract in either normal or streptozotocin-induced diabetic rats indicating the observed hypoglycaemic activity to be independent of insulin secretion. Aqueous extract of *C. spinosa* was thus found to exhibit a potent anti-hyperglycaemic activity in streptozotocin-induced diabetic rats without affecting basal plasma insulin concentrations.

Eddouks M, A Lemhadri, JB Michel; Caraway and caper: potential anti-hyperglycaemic plants in diabetic rats, *J Ethnopharmacol* **94**(1), 143-48 (2004).

Capsicum annuum Linn. (Solanaceae) (Chili pepper, Cayenne pepper)

Capsicum annuum is a domesticated species of the plant genus *Capsicum*, native to Mexico. Of the different *Capsicum* species, *C. annuum* and *C. frutescens* are generally recognized as safe for human consumption as spices. *Capsicum annuum* is used in sweet bell peppers, paprika, pimento, and other red pepper products.

C. annuum extract, prepared by suspending a powder of dried whole fruits in normal saline, caused a dose dependent decrease in fasting blood glucose level of rats. Pre-treatment with the capsicum (500 mg/kg) either orally or intraperitoneally, significantly altered the shape of oral glucose curves. The peak glucose level after the oral glucose load was significantly decreased. The lowering of blood glucose concentrations, produced by *C. annuum*, may involve inhibition of intestinal glucose transport and its action upon the systemic glucose metabolism in the liver.

Monsereenusorn Y; Effect of *Capsicum annuum* on blood glucose level, *Q J Crude Drug Res* **18**(1), 1-7 (1980)

Capsicum frutescens Linn. (Solanaceae) (Capsicum, H. Lal Mirch)

Unlike *C. annuum*, *Capsicum frutescens* is a short-lived perennial with woody stems. It is used in tabasco, tabasco sauce, and other red chili pepper.

Capsicum frutescens is used for the treatment of diabetes by traditional healers in Jamaica. Capsaicin, its active principle, was isolated and tested for its putative anti-diabetic activity. While in an earlier publication, Babu and Srinivasan (1) observed that feeding 15 mg% capsaicin diet to streptozotocin-induced diabetic albino rats did not significantly improve the metabolic status in diabetic condition, Tolan and co-workers (2, 3) observed that capsaicin caused a decrease in blood glucose level, an increase in plasma insulin level and a decrease in the percentage receptor binding for the capsaicin-treated dogs when compared with the control, 2.5 h after the administration of the drug. From the results of the investigation, it was inferred that capsaicin is responsible for the hypoglycaemic episodes seen in the dogs and that it also causes an increase in insulin secretion which leads to a reduction of insulin binding on the insulin receptors.

Animal and some human studies have indicated that the consumption of chili-containing meals attenuate postprandial hyperinsulinemia (4).

1. Babu PS, K Srinivasan; Influence of dietary capsaicin and onion on the metabolic abnormalities associated with streptozotocin induced diabetes mellitus, *Mol Cell Biochem* **175**(1-2), 49-57 (1997).

2. Tolan I, D Ragoobirsingh, EY Morrison; The effect of capsaicin on blood glucose, plasma insulin levels and insulin binding in dog models, *Phytother Res* **15**(5), 391-94 (2001).
3. Tolan I, D Ragoobirsingh, EY Morrison; Isolation and purification of the hypoglycaemic principle present in *Capsicum frutescens, Phytother Res* **18**(1), 95-96 (2004)
4. Ahuja KD, IK Robertson, DP Geraghty, MJ Ball; Effects of chili consumption on postprandial glucose, insulin, and energy metabolism, *Am J Clin Nutr* **84**(1), 63-69 (2006)

Caralluma attenuata Wight (Apocynaceae)

Butanol extract of *Caralluma attenuata,* at the oral dose of 250 mg/kg, showed statistically significant and considerable anti-hyperglycaemic activity in glucose loaded and alloxan-induced diabetic rats (1). Phytochemical and anti-diabetic studies on this plant were also conducted (3).

Jayakar and co-workers (2) observed that both aqueous and alcoholic extracts of *C. attenuata* (100 mg/kg) reduced the blood glucose level of both normal and alloxan-induced diabetic rats 3 h after oral administration.

1. Venkatesh S, GD Reddy, RM Reddy, M Ramesh, AV Rao; Anti-hyperglycaemic activity of *Caralluma attenuata, Fitoterapia* **74**(3), 274-79 (2003).
2. Jayakar B, B Rajkapoor, B Suresh; Effect of *Caralluma attenuata* in normal and alloxan induced diabetic rats, *J Herb Pharmacother* 4(1), 35-40 (2004).
3. Venkatesh, S; Phytochemical and anti-diabetic studies on *Helicteres isora* Linn. and *Caralluma attenuata* Wight, *Indian J Pharmaceut Edu* **39**(4), 221-22 (2005)

Caralluma edulis (Edgew) Benth. (Apocynaceae)

Caralluma edulis is a succulent species in the plant family Apocynaceae. Its leaves and stems are eaten in North Africa.

The powdered roots of *Caralluma edulis,* administered in doses of 2, 3 and 4 g/kg body-weight, to normal and alloxan-diabetic rabbits did not show any significant hypoglycaemic effect.

Wadood A, N Wadood, SA Shah; Effects of *Acacia arabica* and *Caralluma edulis* on blood glucose levels of normal and alloxan diabetic rabbits, *J Pak Med Assoc* **39**(8), 208-12 (1989)

Caralluma tuberculata N.E. Brown (Apocynaceae) (Pamanghi)

Hypoglycaemic activity of the fresh juice of *Caralluma tuberculata* was studied in normoglycaemic, hyperglycaemic and alloxan-induced diabetic rats. Fresh juice of the plant (2ml/200g b.w.) significantly reduced the blood glucose concentration in animals, previously loaded with glucose (2g/kg). A significant reduction of blood glucose level was also observed in alloxan-induced diabetic rats.

Ahmad MM, M Moin-ud-din Shaikh; Improvement in glucose tolerance by *Caralluma tuberculata, Acacia nilotica, Papavar somniferum, Pakistan J Zoology* **21**(4), 325-32 (1989)

Carissa edulis (Forssk.) Vahl (Apocynaceae)
(Natal plum, S. Mutsamviringa)

Carissa edulis is widespread in tropical Africa, Asia from Yemen to India and Thailand and the Indian Ocean islands. Treatment of streptozotocin-induced diabetic rats with ethanol extract of *C. edulis* leaves significantly reduced the blood glucose level during the first three hours of treatment. In normal rats, the treatment produced insignificant changes in blood glucose levels compared to glibenclamide.

El-Fiky FK, MA Abou Karam, EA Afify; Effect of *Luffa aegyptiaca* (seeds) and *Carissa edulis* (leaves) extracts on blood glucose level of normal and streptozotocin diabetic rats, *J Ethnopharmacol* **50**(1), 43-47 (1996)

Carum carvi Linn. (Apiaceae)
(Caraway)

Carum carvi is a Eurasian plant with small white flowers yielding aromatic caraway seed. The hypoglycaemic effect of an aqueous extract of *C. carvi* was studied in normal and streptozotocin-induced diabetic rats. Oral administration of a single dose or 14 daily doses of the aqueous extract of *C. carvi* (20 mg/kg) produced a significant decrease in blood glucose level in streptozotocin-induced diabetic rats. The blood glucose levels were nearly normalised 2 weeks after daily repeated oral administration of the extract. No significant change in blood glucose level was noticed in normal rats after both acute and chronic treatments with the extract. No change was also observed in basal plasma insulin concentration after treatment with *C. carvi* extract in either normal or streptozotocin-induced diabetic rats indicating that the observed hypoglycaemic activity is independent of insulin secretion. Aqueous extract of *C. carvi* was thus found to exhibit a potent anti-hyperglycaemic activity in streptozotocin-induced diabetic rats without affecting basal plasma insulin concentrations.

Eddouks M, A Lemhadri, JB Michel; Caraway and caper: potential anti-hyperglycaemic plants in diabetic rats, *J Ethnopharmacol* **94**(1), 143-48 (2004).

Casearia esculenta Roxb. (Samydaceae / Flacourtiaceae) (H. Saptarangi, S. Saptacakrah)

Casearia esculenta is an indigenous anti-diabetic drug, which is popularly used in rural South India. The roots are especially claimed to be efficacious in milder chronic diabetic cases. It is also used in some commercial Ayurvedic formulations.

Gupta and co-workers (1) studied the anti-diabetic effect of the plant. Prakasam and co-workers studied the various aspects of the anti-diabetic efficacy of the root extract of the plant (2-7). Administration of an aqueous extract of *C. esculenta* root (300 mg/kg b.w.) for 45 days resulted in a significant reduction in blood glucose and in a decrease of the activities of glucose-6-phosphatase and fructose-1,6-biphosphatase and an increase in the activity of liver hexokinase. The study confirmed the potent anti-hyperglycaemic activity of root extract of *C. esculenta* but showed it to be weaker than that of glibenclamide (2). In a short duration study on albino rats, an aqueous extract of *C. esculenta* was found to lower blood glucose in basal conditions and after a glucose load in normal rats. Maximum reduction in blood glucose was observed between 2-3 h at a dose level of 200 and 300 mg/kg body weight. Oral administration of the extract significantly reduced the blood sugar in streptozotocin-induced diabetic rats for 15 days. The extract was also found to reduce the increased plasma thiobarbituric acid reactive substances, hydroperoxides, ceruloplasmin and elevate the levels of reduced glutathione, vitamin C and vitamin E. The extract of *C. esculenta* was thus found to ameliorate biochemical changes induced by streptozotocin in diabetic rats (3, 4). The effect of *C. esculenta* root extract on oxidative stress-related parameters in streptozotocin-induced diabetic rats was also studied. Treatment of these rats with *C. esculenta* root extract (45 days) not only significantly decreased thiobarbituric acid reactive substances but remarkably improved tissue antioxidants status such as glutathione, ascorbic acid and *alpha*-tocopherol in liver and kidney. Further, the decreased activities of enzymatic antioxidants such as superoxide dismutase and catalase in diabetic rats returned to normal levels following treatment with *C. esculenta* root extract over a period of 45-days (6). The root extract of the plant also showed hypolipidaemic activity and administration of the extract of *C. esculenta* (300 mg/kg b.w.) for 45 days resulted in significant reduction in serum and tissue cholesterol, phospholipids, free fatty acids and triglycerides in streptozotocin-induced diabetic rats (5). The influence of the root extract of the plant on glycoprotein components in streptozotocin-induced diabetic rats was also studied. The massive elevation of glycoprotein components such as hexose, hexosamine, sialic acid and fucose in plasma and tissues of diabetic control and experimental animals caused by streptozotocin (50 mg/kg body weight) injection were reverted back to the normal values upon oral administration of *C. esculenta* root extract (200 and 300 mg/kg b.w.) for 45 days (7).

1. Gupta SS, SC Verma, VP Garg, P Khandelwal; Studies on the anti-diabetic

effects of *Casearia esculenta, Indian J Med Res* **55**(7), 754-63 (1967)

2. Prakasam A, S Sethupathy, KV Pugalendi; Antihyperglycaemic effect of *Casearia esculenta* root extracts in streptozotocin-induced diabetic rats, *Pharmazie* **57**(11), 758-60 (2002).
3. Prakasam A, S Sethupathy, KV Pugalendi; Effect of *Casearia esculenta* root extract on blood glucose and plasma antioxidant status in streptozotocin diabetic rats, *Polish J Pharmacol* **55**(1), 43-49 (2003)
4. Prakasam A, S Sethupathy, KV Pugalendi; Glycaemic control by *Casearia esculenta*—a short duration study in albino rats, *Pharmazie* **58**(1), 49-52 (2003)
5. Prakasam A, S Sethupathy, KV Pugalendi; Hypolipidaemic effect of *Casearia esculenta* root extracts in streptozotocin-induced diabetic rats, *Pharmazie* **58**(11), 828-32 (2003)
6. Prakasam A, S Sethupathy, KV Pugalendi; Anti-peroxidative and antioxidant effects of *Casearia esculenta* root extract in streptozotocin-induced diabetic rats, *Yale J Biol Med* **78**(1), 15-23 (2005)
7. Prakasam A, S Sethupathy, KV Pugalendi; Influence of *Casearia esculenta* root extract on glycoprotein components in streptozotocin diabetic rats, *Pharmazie* **60**(3), 229-32 (2005)

Cassia alata Linn. (Fabaceae)
(Candle Bush, Candlestick Plant)

It is a striking spring and summer bloomer with golden blooms that last for several weeks. It is native to Mexico but can be found in diverse habitats.

The oral effectiveness of *C. alata* leaf extract on streptozotocin-induced hyperglycaemic rats was studied and the results were compared with that of glibenclamide. The extract showed no effect on glucose levels in normoglycaemic animals but it reduced the blood sugar value in streptozotocin-induced hyperglycaemic animals (1).

The ethyl acetate extract of the leaves of *C. alata* showed hypoglycaemic activity at a dosage of 5 mg/20 g, mice.

1. Palanichamy S, S Nagarajan, M Devasagayam; Effect of *Cassia alata* leaf extract on hyperglycaemic rats, *J Ethnopharmacol* **22**(1), 81-90 (1988).
2. Villasenor IM, AP Canlas, MP Pascua, MN Sabando, LA Soliven; Bioactivity studies on *Cassia alata* Linn. leaf extracts, *Phytother Res* **16**(Suppl.1), S93-96 (2002).

Cassia auriculata Linn. (Fabaceae) (Avaram Senna, Avaram)

It is a legume tree that occurs in the dry regions of India and Sri Lanka. It is common along the sea coast and the dry zone in Sri Lanka.

An aqueous extract of *C. auriculata* leaves was found to lower the serum glucose level in normal rats; the maximum reduction at a dose of 200 mg/kg body weight at 4th hour was observed to be 31%. In alloxan-induced diabetic rats, chronic administration of the extract significantly reduced the serum glucose level from the third day till the end of the experiment. The extract was also found to inhibit the body weight reduction, induced by alloxan administration. Glucose uptake and glycogen deposition studies suggested that *C. auriculata* leaf extract has no direct insulin like effect, which can enhance the peripheral utilization of glucose (2).

C. auriculata flower extract, at doses of 0.15, 0.30 and 0.45 g/kg body weight for 30 days, suppressed the elevated levels of blood glucose and lipids in diabetic rats. It also significantly decreased blood glucose, glycosylated haemoglobin and gluconeogenic enzymes and increased plasma insulin, haemoglobin and hexokinase activity. The anti-hyperglycaemic effect of the aqueous extract of *C. auriculata* flowers suggests that enhanced gluconeogenesis during diabetes is shifted towards normal and that the extract enhances the utilization of glucose through increased glycolysis. The effect of *C. auriculata* flower extract was found to be more prominent than that of glibenclamide. The findings of the investigation indicated anti-hyperlipidaemic and anti-diabetic activity of the *Cassia auriculata* flowers (1, 3, 4).

Significant increase in the activities of superoxide dismutase, catalase, glutathione peroxidase, glutathione-S-transferase and reduced glutathione were observed in the brain of streptozotocin-induced diabetic rats on treatment with *C. auriculata* flower extract and glibenclamide. Both the treated groups showed significant decrease in thiobarbituric acid reactive substances and hydroperoxide formation in the brain, suggesting its role in protection against lipid peroxidation-induced membrane damage. The findings suggested possible anti-peroxidative role of *C. auriculata* flower extract (5).

Methanol extract of dried flowers of *Cassia auriculata* (Ranawara) was found to have a very strong *alpha*-glucosidase inhibitory activity *in vitro*, preferably on maltase and inhibited the maltase activity competitively. As a result, a single oral administration of methanol extract of *C. auriculata* flowers in Sprague-Dawley rats caused a significant and potent lowering of blood glycaemic response toward maltose ingestion at 30 min after a dosing of 5 mg/kg. The anti-hyperglycaemic effect of the extract was as potent as that of therapeutic drug, acarbose (6).

The effects of ethanol and aqueous extracts of *C. auriculata* whole plant on blood glucose, triglyceride, HDL-cholesterol and total cholesterol were studied in streptozotocin-induced neonatal diabetic rat models. Administration of an ethanol extract at a dose of 400 mg/kg and aqueous extract at doses of 250 and 500 mg/kg body weight for 28 days led to suppression of elevated glucose, cholesterol and triglyceride levels (7). A significant level of reduction in serum glucose, triglycerides and cholesterol and an increase in plasma insulin level were observed in alloxan-induced diabetic male Wister rats, treated with *C. auriculata* leaf and flower extracts (250 mg/kg b.w.). The authors suggested the use of these extracts in the management of diabetes and coronary heart disease (8).

1. Pari L, M Latha; Effect of *Cassia auriculata* flowers on blood sugar levels, serum and tissue lipids in streptozotocin diabetic rats, *Singapore Med J* **43**(12), 617-21 (2002).
2. Sabu MC, T Subburaju; Effect of *Cassia auriculata* Linn. on serum glucose level, glucose utilization by isolated rat hemidiaphragm, *J Ethnopharmacol* **80**(2-3), 203-06 (2002)
3. Pari L, M Latha; Anti-diabetic activity of *Cassia auriculata* flowers: Effect on lipid peroxidation in streptozotocin diabetic rats, *Pharmaceut Biol* **40**(7), 512-17 (2002)
4. Latha M, L Pari; Anti-hyperglycaemic effect of *Cassia auriculata* in experimental diabetes and its effects on key metabolic enzymes involved in carbohydrate metabolism, *Clin Exp Pharmacol Physiol* **30**(1-2), 38-43 (2003).
5. Latha M, L Pari; Preventive effects of *Cassia auriculata* L. flowers on brain lipid peroxidation in rats treated with streptozotocin, *Mol Cell Biochem* **243**(1-2), 23-28 (2003).
6. Abesundara KJ, T Matsui, K Matsumoto; *alpha*-Glucosidase inhibitory activity of some Sri Lanka plant extracts, one of which, *Cassia auriculata*, exerts a strong anti-hyperglycaemic effect in rats comparable to the therapeutic drug acarbose, *J Agric Food Chem* **52**(9), 2541-45 (2004).
7. Juvekar AR, GV Halade; Hypoglycaemic activity of *Cassia auriculata* in neonatal streptozotocin-induced non insulin dependent diabetes mellitus in rats, *J Nat Remedies* **6**(1), 14-18 (2006)
8. Uma Devi P, S Selvi, S Suja, K Selvam, P Chinnaswamy; Anti-diabetic and hypolipidaemic effect of *Cassia auriculata* in alloxan-induced diabetic rats, *Int J Pharmacol* **2**(6), 601-07 (2006)

Cassia fistula Linn. (Fabaceae)
(Golden shower tree, H. Amaltas)

The Golden Shower Tree is a flowering plant, native to southern Asia and widely found in Pakistan, India and Sri Lanka. Fistula flowers are golden yellow hanging in groups almost 12 inches in length. This Cassia is a summer bloomer starting as early as April. Widely grown as an ornamental plant, it is also an important herb used in many medicinal preparations.

The alcohol (95%) extract of the roots of *C. fistula* was shown to lower the blood sugar level up to 50 percent after 2 h when tested on fasted albino rats. The extract furnished 7-methylphyscion, betulinic acid and b-sitosterol (1).

Along with the other activities such as anti-tumour, antioxidant, hypoglycaemic, hepatoprotective, antibacterial, hypocholesterolaemic, and anti-diabetic activity, the healing potential of *C. fistula* provides a scientific rationale for the traditional use of this plant in the management of infected dermal wound (2).

1. Vaishnava MM, AK Tripathi, KR Gupta; Constituents of *Cassia fistula* roots, *Fitoterapia* **64**(1), 95 (1993).
2. Senthil Kumar M, R Sripriya, H Vijaya Raghavan, PK Sehgal; Wound healing potential of *Cassia fistula* on infected albino rat model, *J Surg Res* **131**(2), 283-89 (2006)

Cassia kleinii Wight & Arn (Fabaceae / Leguminosae)

Alcoholic extract of *Cassia kleinii* leaves exhibited concentration dependent anti-hyperglycaemic activity in glucose loaded rats. While the extract failed to show hypoglycaemic effect in fasted normal rats, it showed remarkable efficacy in alloxan-induced diabetic rats at a dose of 200 mg/kg.

Babu V, T Gangadevi, A Subramoniam; Anti-hyperglycaemic activity of *Cassia kleinii* leaf extract in glucose fed normal rats and alloxan-induced diabetic rats, *Indian J Pharmacol* **34**(6), 409-15 (2002)

Cassia tora Linn. (Fabaceae/Caesalpinaceae) (H. Chakvad, S. Chakramarda)

Naphthopyrone glucosides, cassiaside, rubrofusarin-6-O-β-D-gentiobioside and toralactone-9-O- β -D-gentiobioside, isolated from the seeds of *Cassia tora,* were found to inhibit formation of advanced glycation end products (1).

The inhibitory activity of *C. tora* anthraquinones, against advanced glycation end products (AGEs) formation and rat lens aldose reductase (RLAR) was evaluated by *in vitro* bioassays. Among the compounds, emodin and obtusifolin exhibited significant inhibitory activity on AGEs formation, while aurantio-obtusin, chryso-obtusin-2-O-β-D-glucoside and emodin showed a significant inhibitory activity on RLAR (2).

1. Lee GY, DS Jang, YM Lee, JM Kim, JS Kim; Naphthopyrone glucosides from the seeds of *Cassia tora* with inhibitory activity on advanced glycation end products (AGEs) formation, *Arch Farm Res* **29**(7), 587-90 (2006)
2. Jang DS, GY Lee, YS Kim, YM Lee, CS Kim, JL Yoo, JS Kim; Anthraquinones

from the seeds of *Cassia tora* with inhibitory activity on protein glycation and aldose reductase, *Biol Pharm Bull* **30**(11), 2207-10 (2007)

Castanospermum australe A.Cunn & C.Fraser ex Hook.(Fabaceae) (Australian chestnut)

Castanospermine, a substance derived from the Australian chestnut, was tested against a variety of commercially available glycosidases and found to be a potent inhibitor of almond emulsin *beta*-glucosidase. Fifty-percent inhibition of *beta*-glucosidase required about 10 μg/ml of castanospermine. Castanospermine also inhibited the lysosomal *alpha*-glucosidase, and this inhibition required comparable levels of alkaloid to that required for inhibition of *beta*-glucocerebrosidase (1). Daily injections of castanospermine, at levels of 0.5 mg/g of body weight, or higher, for 3 days decreased hepatic *alpha*-glucosidase to 40% of control values. In liver, both the neutral and the acidic *alpha*-glucosidase activities were inhibited, but the former was more susceptible. A marked decrease in the amount of glycogen in the cytoplasm was observed in animals receiving castanospermine at 1.0 mg or higher per g of body weight for 3 days (2).

1. Saul R, JP Chambers, RJ Molyneux, AD Elbein; Castanospermine, a tetrahydroxylated alkaloid that inhibits beta-glucosidase and beta-glucocerebrosidase, *Arch Biochem Biophys* **221**(2), 593-97 (1983)
2. Saul R, JJ Ghidoni, RJ Molyneux, AD Elbein; Castanospermine inhibits *alpha*-glucosidase activities and alters glycogen distribution in animals, *Proc Nat Acad Sci*, USA, **82**(1), 93-97 (1985)

Catha edulis (Vahl.) Endl (Celastraceae) (Bushman's tea, Khat)

Catha edulis is a flowering plant, native to tropical East Africa and the Arabian Peninsula. It is a sacred plant of the ancient Egyptians. World Health Organisation classified 'Khat' as a drug of abuse that can produce mild to moderate psychological dependence.

The effect of regular khat chewing on serum glucose and C-peptide levels was investigated both in healthy individuals and type-2 diabetic patients. The levels of glucose and C-peptide were insignificantly different between khat chewers and non-kat chewers in case of healthy individuals. In diabetic group, khat chewers showed a non-significant increase of glucose levels at 0, 1 and 2 h of khat chewing. However, the non-significant increase in serum glucose level at 1 h of khat chewing corresponded with a significant increase of serum C-peptide levels.

Saif-Ali R, A Al-Qirbi, A Al-Geiri, M Al-Habori; Effect of *Catha edulis* on plasma glucose and C-peptide in both type-2 diabetics and non-diabetics, *J Ethnopharmacol* **86**(1), 45-49 (2003)

Catharanthus roseus (L) G Don (Apocynaceae) (Madagascar periwinkle, H. Sadabahar)

Catharanthus roseus is native and endemic to Madagascar and has several synonyms (*Vinca rosea, Ammocallis rosea* and *Lochnera rosea*). In the wild, it is an endangered plant but it is widely cultivated and is naturalised in subtropical and tropical areas of the world. It is an evergreen subshrub and its flowers are white to dark pink in colour with a darker red centre. The plant is rich in alkaloids some of which are reported to be used by the pharmaceutical industry for the treatment of childhood leukemia, Hodgkin's disease, testicular cancer and cancerous tumors.

Dichloromethane:methanol (1:1) extract of leaves and twigs of *C. roseus,* exhibited hypoglycaemic activity in streptozotocin-induced diabetic rat model. Oral administration of the extract at a dose of 500 mg/kg for 7 and 15 days showed 48.6 and 57.6% hypoglycaemic activity, respectively. Prior treatment at the same dose for 30 days provided complete protection against streptozotocin challenge. The decreases of enzymic activities of glycogen synthase, glucose 6-phosphate-dehydrogenase, succinate dehydrogenase and malate dehydrogenase in liver of diabetic animals were almost normalized after treatment with the extract at a dose 500 mg/kg p.o. for 7 days. Increased levels of 2-thiobarbituric acid reactive substances, indicative of oxidative stress in diabetic rats, were also normalized by treatment with the extract (1).

The hypoglycaemic activity of the leaf juice of *C. roseus* was evaluated in normal and alloxan-induced diabetic rabbits. The leaf juice of *C. roseus* produced a dose-dependent reduction in blood glucose of both normal and diabetic rabbits (2, 3). The effect was found to be comparable to that of glibenclamide. The mode of action of the active compound(s) of *C. roseus was* possibly mediated through enhanced secretion of insulin from the *beta* cells of Langerhans or through extra-pancreatic mechanism (3).

Suspension cultures of *C. roseus* were established from three different cell lines (CWS, CWS-A, CWS-G) The cell extracts of CWS and CWS-A respectively, caused 71% and 86% decrease in blood sugar levels of diabetic rats. CWS-G, however, failed to show any anti-diabetic activity (1).

1. Benjamin BD, SM Kelkar, MS Pote, GS Kaklij, AT Sipahimalani, MR Heble; *Catharanthus roseus* cell culture: Growth, alkaloid synthesis and anti-diabetic activity, *Phytother Res* **8**(3), 185-86 (1994)
2. Singh SN, P Vats, S Suri, R Shyam, MM Kumria, S Ranganathan, K Sridharan; Effect of an anti-diabetic extract of *Catharanthus roseus* on enzymic activities in streptozotocin induced diabetic rats, *J Ethnopharmacol* **76**(3), 269-77 (2001).
3. Nammi S, MK Boini, SD Lodagala, RB Behara; The juice of fresh leaves of *Catharanthus roseus* Linn. reduces blood glucose in normal and alloxan diabetic rabbits, *BMC Compliment Altern Med* **3**, 4 (2003).

4. Satyanarayana S, GS Sarma, A Ramesh, K Sushruta, N Srinivas; Evaluation of herbal preparations for hypoglycaemic activity in normal and diabetic rabbits, *Pharmaceut Biol* **41**(6), 466-72 (2003)

Cecropia obtusifolia Loefl. (Urticaceae / Cecropiaceae) (Trumpet tree)

Cecropia is a genus of trees in the nettle family, Urticaceae. *Cecropia obtusifolia* is found in Columbia, Costa Rica, Mexico, and Panama. Oral administration of a single dose (90 and 150 mg/kg) of water extract of *C. obtusifolia* leaves lowered the plasma glucose levels in diabetic rats 3 h after administration. Similar effect was also observed with butanol extract at doses of 9 and 15 mg/kg and with glibenclamide, used as a reference drug, at a dose of 3 mg/kg. Chlorogenic acid (3-caffeoylquinic acid) and the flavone, isoorientin were the main constituents of the extracts (1). A single oral administration of methanol extract (1 g/kg) of the plant also showed a significant decrease in plasma glucose levels 2 and 4 h after the drug administration. This effect was correlated with the chlorogenic acid content of the plant extract (2).

1. Andrade-Cetto A, H Wiedenfeld; Hypoglycaemic effect of *Cecropia obtusifolia* on streptozotocin diabetic rats, *J Ethnopharmacol* **78**(2-3), 145-49 (2001)

2. Nicasio P, L Aguilar-Santamaria, E Aranda, S Ortiz, M Gonzalez; Hypoglycaemic effect and chlorogenic acid content in two *Cecropia* species, *Phytother Res* **19**(8), 661-64 (2005)

Cecropia peltata Linn. (Urticaceae / Cecropiaceae)) (Yagrumo Hembra)

Cecropia peltata is a native of West Indies. The stems of the tree are hollow and often inhabited by biting ants. Like *Cecropia obtusifolia, C. peltata* also showed significant hypoglycaemic effect and, in fact, it was superior to *C. obtusifolia*. The hypoglycaemic effect produced by different doses of *C. peltata* showed a linear relationship with chlorogenic acid content.

Nicasio P, L Aguilar-Santamaria, E Aranda, S Ortiz, M Gonzalez; Hypoglycaemic effect and chlorogenic acid content in two *Cecropia* species, *Phytother Res* **19**(8), 661-64 (2005)

Cedronella canariensis (L.) Willd. ex Webb & Bethel. (Lamiaceae) (Balm of Gilead)

It is a perennial herbaceous plant native to N. Africa and Canary Islands. The leaves consisting of 3 leaflets are rather uncharacteristic to the family, Lamiaceae. Chloroform extract of the aerial parts of the plant showed a significant hypoglycaemic and diuretic effect.

Lopez-Garcia RE, Martin Herrera, V Darias, RM Rabanal; ,Study of the hypoglycaemic, diuretic and cardiovascular activity of *Cedronella canariensis* var. *canariensis* (L) W.& B, *Phytother Res* **10**(6), 541-43 (1996)

Ceiba pentandra L. Gaertn (Malvaceae / Bombacaceae) (Kapok, Silk cotton tree)

Ceiba pentandra is a majestic tropical tree with giant umbrella-shaped crown. They are among the tallest trees in the tropical forest reaching as high as 60 m in rainforests of the Amazon. *C, pentandra* is native to Mexico, South America and also to tropical West Africa.

C, pentandra is claimed to be anti-diabetic by traditional medical practitioners of Nigeria. To verify the validity of this claim, aqueous extract of *C. pentandra* bark was administered *ad libitum* in drinking water to the experimentally diabetic rats for 28 days. Administration of the bark extract caused a statistically significant reduction in plasma glucose level in streptozotocin-induced diabetic rats. The extract appeared to be non-toxic from biochemical studies.

Ladeji O, I Omekarah, M Solomon; Hypoglycaemic properties of aqueous bark extract of *Ceiba pentandra* in streptozotocin-induced diabetic rats, *J Ethnopharmacol* **84**(2-3), 139-42 (2003).

Celosia argentea Linn. (Amaranthaceae) (Plumed cockscomb, Woolflowers, H. Safed Murga)

Celosia argentea, commonly known as plumed cockscomb, is a plant of tropical origin, and is known for very bright colours of its flowers. Seeds of *C. argentea* are used in Indian folk medicine for the treatment of diabetes mellitus. Alcoholic extract of *C. argentea* seeds was found to reduce the increase of blood glucose in alloxan-induced diabetic rats. Chronic administration of the extract for two weeks significantly reduced the blood glucose in alloxan-induced diabetic rats. The extract also prevented a decrease in body weight in alloxan-induced diabetic rats.

Ventrichelvan T, M Jegadeesan, BA Devi; Anti-diabetic activity of alcoholic extract of *Celosia argentea* Linn. seeds in rats, *Biol Pharm Bull* **25**(4), 526-28 (2002).

Centaurea aspera Linn. (Asteraceae / Compositae) (Star thistle)

It is a thistle-like flowering plant, common in some European countries.

Two aqueous extracts of *C. aspera* flowers, prepared under different conditions, were tested for hypoglycaemic activity in normal and alloxan-induced diabetic rats. Oral and chronic administration of both extracts were found to exert a significant hypoglycaemic effect in diabetic rats, but only the extract, obtained by exhaustive extraction with hot water, displayed an acute hypoglycaemic activity in normal animals. The hypoglycaemic activity of flower extracts was compared against glibenclamide as a standard.

Masso JL, T Adzet; Hypoglycaemic activity of *centaurea aspera* L, *Rev Esp Fisiol* **32**(4), 313-16 (1976) [Article in Spanish]

Centaurea corcubionensis Lainz (Asteraceae)

The hypoglycaemic activity of *Centaurea corcubionensis* was studied in normoglycaemic and hyperglycaemic rats. Infusions of leaves and flowers of the plant (5g/kg) significantly lowered blood glucose levels and increased circulating insulin levels. It also induced heavy release of insulin from islets of Langerhans, isolated from rat pancreas. Infusions induced a significant fall in glycaemia levels in rats with glucose-induced hyperglycaemia, but had no effect on alloxan-diabetic animals.

Chucla MT, M Lamela, A Gato, I Cadavid; *Centaurea corcubionensis*: a study of its hypoglycaemic activity in rats, *Planta Med* **54**(2), 107-09 (1988)

Centaurea phyllocephala Boiss (Asteraceae)

The use of this plant as an anti-diabetic agent in folklore medicine could not be justified. Investigations on various extracts of *C. phyllocephala* revealed that basal plasma glucose concentration and plasma glucose response to glucose load were either elevated or unchanged by the i.v. administration of these extracts in anaesthetized rats or by ip or oral administration of the extracts in conscious rats.

Twaij HA, A Kery, NK Al-Khazraji; Some pharmacological, toxicological and phytochemical investigations on *Centaurea phyllocephala*, *J Ethnopharmacol* **9**(2-3), 299-314 (1983)

Centaurea species

The hypoglycaemic action of the *Centaurea* species was studied and its active peptides were fractionated.

Viguera JM, A Casabuena; The hypoglycaemic action of the *Centaurea* species, IV: Fractionation of active peptides with ammonium sulphate, *Farmacognosia* **25**(3), 89-102 (1965) [Article in Spanish]

Cephalandra indica Naud (Cucurbitaceae) (Ivy gourd, S. Bhimba, H. Kunduru)

Cephalandra indica (Syn. *Coccinia indica*) is a climbing shrub, flowering throughout the year and common in hedges. Ripe fruits are edible; raw or green fruits are used in curries. It has been listed as an effective plant drug for the treatment of diabetes mellitus (1). It showed glycaemic control in NIDDM patients, who did not respond to diet therapy alone. Results of investigation with NIDDM patients of both sexes and of different age groups revealed that *C. indica* possesses moderate blood sugar lowering effect, which increases with the increase in duration of treatment (2).

See *Coccinia indica* for further reports.

1. Kapoor RK; Diabetes mellitus, *Indian J Homoeopath* **19**(3), 114-20 (1984)
2. Banerjee A, P Ray, A Roy, R Ray; Clinical evaluation of *Cephalandra indica* (Telakucha) in diabetes mellitus, *Int Conf Curr Prog Med Aromatic Pl Res*, Calcutta, India p. 135, Dec 30, 1994-Jan 1, 1995.

Cichorium intybus Linn. (Asteraceae)
(Common chicory)

Common chicory (*Cichorium intybus*) is a perennial herb with blue or lavender flowers. Native to Europe, it was naturalised in North America where it has become common roadside plant. The baked and ground roots of the plant are used as a coffee substitute and additive. Its use as a coffee additive is still very popular in India.

The anti-diabetic activity of the methanol extract of the roots of the plant was examined in streptozotocin-induced diabetic rats and it showed a significant reduction of blood glucose levels.

Ki CG, DS Yim, SY Lee; Biological activities of the root of *Cichorium intybus*, *Nat Prod Sci* 5(4), 155-58 (1999)

Chamaemelum nobile (L.) All. (Asteraceae / Compositae)
(Roman Chamomile)

Chamaemeloside, a 3-hydroxy-3-methylglutaric acid-containing flavonoid glucoside, was isolated from the plant. Chamaemeloside showed hypoglycaemic activity *in vivo* and the activity was comparable to that of free 3-hydroxy-3-methylglutaric acid. An improved isolation scheme for obtaining chamaemeloside from *C. nobile* was presented (1).

Oral administration of a single dose of *C. nobile* aqueous extract (20mg/kg b.w.) reduced blood glucose levels 6h after administration in normal and streptozotocin-induced diabetic rats. Similar reduction in blood glucose level was observed after 15 days of treatment. Basal plasma insulin concentrations were found to remain unchanged after treatment in both normal and streptozotocin-induced diabetic rats. *C. nobile* was thus shown to exhibit a significant hypoglycaemic effect in normal and streptozotocin-induced diabetic rats without affecting basal plasma insulin concentrations (2).

1. Konig GM, AD Wright, WJ Keller, RL Judd, S Bates, C Day; Hypoglycaemic

activity of an HMG-containing flavonoid glucoside, chamaemeloside, from *Chamaemelum nobile, Planta Med* **64**(7), 612-14 (1998)

2. Eddouks M, A Lemhadri, NA Zeggwagh, JB Michel; Potent hypoglycaemic activity of the aqueous extract of *Chamaemelum nobile* in normal and streptozotocin-induced diabetic rats, *Diabetes Res Clin Pract* 67(3), 189-95 (2005)

Chlorophytum borivilianum Santapau & Fernandes (Agavaceae / Liliaceae) (H. Safed Musli)

Chlorophytum borivilianum is eaten as a leaf vegetable in some parts of India, and its roots are used medicinally as a sex tonic under the name safed moosli. It is a very popular herb in traditional Indian medicine and is a member of a group of herbs used as 'Rasayan' or adaptogen.

A fructo-oligosaccharide, isolated from *C. borivilianum* and fully characterised by chemical and spectral analysis, showed significant anti-diabetic activity along with moderate antioxidant activity in streptozotocin-induced diabetic animals. The plant extract also showed similar activity.

Narasimhan S, R Govindarajan, V Madhavan, M Thakur, VK Dixit, S Mehrotra, KP Madhusudanan; Action of (2α1) fructo-oligopolysaccharide fraction of *Chlorophytum borivilianum* against streptozotocin-induced oxidative stress, *Planta Med* **72**(15),1421-24 (2006)

Cicer arietinum L. (Fabaceae) (Chickpea, H. Chana, S. Chanaka)

Compared with a wheat-based meal, a single chickpea-based meal led to a lesser response in plasma glucose and insulin concentrations, but this was not translated into long-term improvement in insulin sensitivity, at least in healthy subjects (1). Insulin and satiety responses of chickpea flour bread were compared with those of extruded chickpea flour bread. Both breads demonstrated acceptable palatability but while chickpea flour bread demonstrated some hypoglycaemic effect compared to white bread, neither chickpea flour bread nor extruded chickpea flour bread demonstrated effects on satiety or food intake. The hyperinsulinaemic effect of chickpea flour bread observed in this study requires further investigation (2).

1. Nestel P, M Cehun, A Chronopoulos; Effects of long-term consumption and single meals of chickpeas on plasma glucose, insulin, and triacylglycerol concentrations, *Am J Clin Nutr* **79**(3), 390-95 (2004)

2. Johnson SK, SJ Thomas, RS Hall; Palatability and glucose, insulin and satiety responses of chickpea flour and extruded chickpea flour bread eaten as part of a breakfast, *Eur J Clin Nutr* **59**(2), 169-76 (2005)

Cimicifuga dahurica Maxim. (Ranunculaceae) (Sheng-ma)

The plant is native to Siberia, Mongolia, China and Japan. The leaves of this species have unusual heart-shaped bases. The plant is used for the treatment of dental woes, herpes sores and headache. Isoferulic acid, isolated from the rhizome of *C. dahurica*, was shown to exhibit anti-hyperglycaemic activity *in vivo*. An anti-hyperglycaemic action of isoferulic acid in spontaneously diabetic rats, similar to type-1 diabetes, was presented.

Liu IM, TC Chi, FL Hsu, CF Chen, JT Cheng; Isoferulic acid as active principle from the rhizoma of *Cimicifuga dahurica* to lower plasma glucose in diabetic rats, *Planta Med* **65**(8), 712-14 (1999).

Cinnamomum cassia Blume (Lauraceae) (Cassia, Chinese cinnamon)

It is an evergreen tree native to China and Vietnam. Like its close relative, *Cinnamomum zeylanicum*, also known as "true cinnamon", it is used primarily for its aromatic bark, which is used as a spice,

The effects on blood glucose and plasma insulin levels in rats under the influence of *Cinnamomum cassia* bark or extract were studied. The *C. cassia* extract was slightly more efficacious than the equivalent amount of *C. cassia* bark. A decrease in blood glucose levels was observed in a glucose tolerance test, but it was not obvious in rats that were not challenged by a glucose load. It elevated plasma insulin levels and the effect was direct since a stimulatory *in vitro* effect of insulin release from INS-1 cells (an insulin secreting cell line) was observed (1).

The effects of cinnamon supplementation on insulin sensitivity, glucose tolerance and blood lipid profile were studied in postmenopausal patients with type-2 diabetes. From the results of the investigation, it was inferred that cinnamon supplementation (1.5 g/d) does not improve whole-body insulin sensitivity or oral glucose tolerance and does not modulate blood lipid profile in postmenopausal patients with type-2 diabetes (2). The anti-diabetic effect of *C. cassia* extract was studied in a type-2 diabetic animal model (C57BIKsj db/db). Administration of cinnamon extract for 6 weeks decreased the blood glucose concentration in a dose-dependent manner. It significantly increased serum insulin and HDL-cholesterol levels and decreased the concentration of triglycerides, total cholesterol and intestinal *alpha*-glycosidase activity (3).

Investigation was made to clarify the mechanism of the anti-diabetic activities of the bark extract of *C. cassia*. Treatment of mice with streptozotocin resulted in hyperglycaemia and hypoinsulinaemia but these diabetogenic effects of streptozotocin were completely prevented when mice were pre-treated with *C cassia* bark extract. The inhibitory effect of the extract on streptozotocin-induced hyperglycaemia was mediated through the suppression of induced nitric oxide synthase (iNOS) expression, which in turn appeared to involve the inhibition of NF-*kappa* B activation (4).

1. Verspohl EJ, K Bauer, E Neddermann; Anti-diabetic effect of *Cinnamomum cassia* and *Cinnamomum zeylanicum in vivo* and *in vitro*, *Phytother Res* **19**(3), 203-06 (2005)
2. Vanschoonbeek K, BJ Thomassen, JM Senden, WK Wodzig, LJ van-Loon; Cinnamon supplementation does not improve glycaemic control in postmenopausal type-2 diabetes patients, *J Nutr* **136**(4), 977-80 (2006)
3. Kim SH, SH Hyun, SYChoung; Anti-diabetic effect of cinnamon extract on blood glucose in db/db mice, *J Ethnopharmacol* **104**(1-2), 119-23 (2006)
4. Kwon KB, EK Kim, ES Jeong, YH Lee, YR Lee, JW Park, DG Ryu, BH Park; Cortex cinnamomi extract prevents streptozotocin- and cytokine-induced *beta*-cell damage by inhibiting NF-*kappa* B, *World J Gastroenterol* **12**(27), 4331-37 (2006)

Cinnamomum tamala (Buch-Ham) Nees &Eberm (Lauraceae) (H. Tejpat)

Cinnamomum tamala is a moderate sized evergreen tree, which is the source of tejpat leaves. It is distributed in tropical and sub-tropical Himalayas, Khasi and Jaintia hills and also in Bangladesh. The leaves of the plant were found to exhibit hypoglycaemic activity in non-insulin dependent diabetic patients (1). Oral administration of an ethanol (50%) extract of *C. tamala* leaves significantly lowered the plasma glucose levels in normoglycaemic and streptozotocin-induced hyperglycaemic rats. The extract also showed anti-hypercholesterolaemic and anti-hypertriglyceridaemic activity in streptozotocin-induced diabetic rats (2).

1. Chandola HM, SN Tripathi, KN Upupa; Hypoglycaemic response of *C. tamala* in patients of maturity onset (insulin independent) diabetes, *J Res Ayur Siddha* **1**(2), 275-290 (1980)
2. Sharma SR, SK Dwivedi, D Swarup; Hypoglycaemic and hypolipidaemic effects of *Cinnamomum tamala* Nees leaves, *Indian J Exp Biol* **34**(4), 372-74 (1996)

Cinnamomum zeylanicum Breyne (Lauraceae) (True cinnamon, Ceylon Cinnamon, H. Dalchini)

Cinnamon (*C. zeylanicum*) is an ancient spice and it has a more delicate aroma than the Chinese variety (*C. aromaticum* or *C. cassia*). The major constituents of the essential oil of cinnamon bark are cinnamaldehyde and and eugenol.

Cinnamon extract has been shown to potentiate the action of insulin in isolated adipocytes. Using isolated rat epididymal adipocytes, the effect of cinnamon extract on the influence of bovine serum albumin on insulin activity was studied. Albumin at 0.01-0.1% decreased the insulin stimulatory effects of cinnamon. It was, therefore, suggested that the effects of albumin be assessed when evaluating the insulin-enhancing effects of other substances using isolated adipocytes (1).

The possible effects of cinnamon extract on insulin function were tested in the insulin-dependent utilization of glucose using a rat epididymal adipocyte assay and cinnamon was proved to be the most bioactive product of the 49 herbs and spices used. The glucose oxidation enhancing bioactivity of cinnamon was, however, lost by treatment with poly(vinylpyrrolidone), indicating the phenolic nature of the active phytochemicals (2).

Water extract of *C. zeylanicum* bark significantly reduced blood glucose value at 1h during glucose tolerance test. When diabetic animals with fasting blood glucose were treated with cinnamon extract (200 mg/kg, b.w.) once daily for 2 weeks, the fasting blood glucose level came down (7).

A hydroxychalcone polymer, derived from cinnamon, was found to function like insulin in 3T3-LI adipocytes. Treatment with the chalcone polymer stimulated glucose uptake and glycogen synthesis to a level similar to insulin. Like insulin, it also activated glycogen synthase and inhibited glycogen synthase kinase-3-*beta* activities. Analysis of the insulin receptor demonstrated that the receptor was phosphorylated upon exposure to this chalcone polymer of cinnamon, which, in turn, supported that the insulin cascade was triggered by the chalcone polymer. The responses observed using the dual treatment of chalcone polymer and insulin indicated synergism between the two compounds. The chalcone polymer of cinnamon was thus proved to mimic the effects of insulin and it may be useful in the treatment of insulin resistance (3). Water-soluble polyphenol polymers from cinnamon that increase insulin-dependent *in vitro* glucose metabolism and display antioxidant activity were isolated and characterized by NMR and mass spectral analysis. The polymers were composed of monomeric units with a molecular mass of 288. Two trimers with a molecular mass of 864 and a tetramer with a mass of 1152 were isolated. These polyphenolic polymers (doubly linked procyanidin oligomers of the catechins and/or epicatechins), present in cinnamon, were found to function as antioxidants, potentiate insulin action, and were beneficial in the control of glucose intolerance and diabetes (5). The effects of three concentrations (0.2, 0.3, and 0.4 mg/ml) of a cinnamon extract on glucose uptake and adiponectin secretion in 3T3-L1 adipocytes were examined in the presence and absence of 0.5 nM and 50 nM insulin. The study indicates that although 0.2 mg/ml cinnamon extract has insulin-mimetic action in 3T3-adipocytes in terms of glucose uptake, secretion of the anti-diabetic hormone adiponectin is adversely affected (9).

Like *Cinnamomum cassia,* C. *zeylanicum* also decreased the blood glucose levels observed in a glucose tolerance test but the former was more potent than the latter (8).

Cinnamon was shown to potentiate the insulin effect through upregulation of the glucose uptake in cultured adipocytes. Cinnamon extract was found to improve insulin action *via* increasing glucose uptake *in vivo,* at least in part through enhancing the insulin-signaling pathway in skeletal muscle (4). It was further shown that cinnamon extract prevents the insulin resistance induced by a high-fructose diet, at least in part, by enhancing insulin signaling and possibly *via* the NO pathway in skeletal muscle (6). A study was designed to investigate whether cinnamon bark extract mitigates the adverse effects of fructose loading on glucose metabolism and lipid profile in rats. The findings of the study indicate the improvement of glucose metabolism *in vivo* by cinnamon bark extract in fructose-fed rats. The extract also prevented the hyperlipidaemia observed in fructose-fed rats and improved glucose tolerance (10).

1. Berrio LF, MM Polansky, RA Anderson; Insulin activity: stimulatory effects of cinnamon and brewer's yeast as influenced by albumin, *Horm Res* **37**(6), 225-29 (1992)

2. Broadhurst CL, MM Polansky, RA Anderson; Insulin-like biological activity of culinary and medicinal plant aqueous extracts *in vitro, J Agric Food Chem* **48**(3), 849-52 (2000)

3. Jarvill-Taylor KJ, RA Anderson, DJ Graves; A hydroxychalcone derived from cinnamon functions as a mimetic for insulin in 3T3-L1 adipocytes, *J Am Coll Nutr* **20**(4), 327-36 (2001)

4. Qin B, M Nagasaki, M Ren, G Bajotto, Y Oshida Y Sato; Cinnamon extract (traditional herb) potentiates *in vivo* insulin-regulated glucose utilization *via* enhancing insulin signaling in rats, *Diabetes Res Clin Pract* 62(3), 139-48 (2003).

5. Anderson RA, CL Broadhurst, MM Polansky, WF Schmidt, A Khan, VP Flanagan, NW Schoene, DJ Graves; Isolation and characterization of polyphenol type-A polymers from cinnamon with insulin-like biological activity, *J Agric Food Chem* **52**(1), 65-70 (2004)

6. Qin B, M Nagasaki, M Ren, G Bajotto, Y Oshida Y Sato; Cinnamon extract prevents the insulin resistance induced by a high-fructose diet, *Horm Metab Res* 36(2), 119-25 (2004).

7. Prachi A, KY Murali, PS Murthy, V Tandon, Ramesh Chandra; Preliminary studies on the anti-diabetic effect of *Cinnamomum zeylanicum, Chemistry Biology Interface: Synergistic New Frontiers,* p. 25-27, Nov. 21-26, 2004, New Delhi, India

8. Verspohl EJ, K Bauer, E Neddermann; Anti-diabetic effect of *Cinnamomum cassia* and *Cinnamomum zeylanicum in vivo* and *in vitro, Phytother Res* **19**(3), 203-06 (2005).

9. Roffey B, A Atwal, S Kubow; Cinnamon water extracts increase glucose uptake but inhibit adiponectin secretion in 3T3-L1 adipose cells, *Mol Nutr Food Res* **50**(8), 739-45 (2006)

10. Kannappan S, T Jayaraman, P Rajasekar, MK Ravichandran, CV Anuradha; Cinnamon bark extract improves glucose metabolism and lipid profile in the fructose-fed rat, *Singapore Med J* **47**(10), 858-63 (2006)

Cirsium pascuarense (H. B. K.) Spreng (Asteraceae)

Intra-peritonial administration of the hexane extract of *C. pascuarense* (100, 150 and 200 mg/kg) produced a significant hypoglycaemic effect in normal as well as in diabetic mice. The extract also altered glucose tolerance in alloxan-induced diabetic rats. Chloroform and methanol extracts of the plant did not produce any significant change in blood glucose levels.

Perez-Gutierrez RM, E Ramirez, R Vargas; Effect of *Cirsium pascuarense* on blood glucose levels of normoglycaemic and alloxan-diabetic mice, *Phytother Res* **15**(6), 552-54 (2001).

Cissus sicyoides Linn. (Vitaceae)
(Princess vine)

Cissus sicyoides is an exotic vine, native to tropical Mexico, Central America, and the Caribbean islands. It is a medicinal plant of Brazil and is used for the treatment of several diseases, particularly diabetes. In order to verify the anti-diabetic effects of the plant, its leaf decoctions were administered over extended periods to normal and streptozotocin-induced diabetic rats and the physiological and metabolic parameters that are altered in diabetic animals were studied with a parallel treatment with insulin. The treatment with the decoction significantly reduced the intake of both food and fluid and the volume of urine excreted, as well as the levels of blood glucose, urinary glucose and urinary urea, in comparison with controls. The fact that normal animals treated with *C. sicyoides* exhibited no changes in any of the measured parameters suggests that its mode of action in diabetic animals does not resemble those of sulphonylurea or insulin. It may, however, act in a way similar to biguanide, *via* inhibition of gluconeogenesis (1).

In another experiment, it was shown that the daily treatment of diabetic rats with aqueous extract prepared from fresh leaves of *C. sicyoides* for 7 days (100 and 200 mg/kg, p.o.) significantly decreased blood glucose levels as compared to the same groups before the plant drug treatment. While no changes were seen in total cholesterol levels, a significant decrease was observed in plasma triglyceride levels, in the alloxan-induced diabetic rats after the plant drug treatment with both doses, as compared to the same groups before treatment. Significant decreases in blood glucose (25%) and triglyceride (48%) levels were also observed in the alloxan-induced diabetic rats after 4 days treatment with the plant drug (200 mg/kg, p.o.). The results point out the potential benefit of the plant extract and justify its use in the treatment of type-2 diabetes mellitus (2).

1. Pepato MT, AM Baviera, P Perez Mda, C Kettelhut Ido, IL Brunetti; *Cissus sicyoides* (princess vine) in the long-term treatment of streptozotocin-diabetic rats, *Biotechnol Appl Biochem* **37**(Pt 1), 15-20 (2003).

2. Viana GS, AC Medeiros, AM Lacerda, LK Leal, TG Vale, FJ Matos; Hypoglycaemic and anti-lipemic effects of the aqueous extract from *Cissus sicyoides*, *BMC Pharmacol* **4**, 9 (2004)

Citrullus colocynthis (L) Schrad. (Cucurbitaceae) (Colocynth, Bitter apple)

The colocynth is a viny plant, native to the Mediterranean basin and Asia, especially Turkey. Its fruit, which is lemon-sized, yellowish, spongy, and extremely bitter, is a powerful hepatic stimulant and cathartic. It is used as a strong laxative. Its seed, which is edible but similarly bitter, and rich in fat and protein, is eaten whole or used as an oilseed.

Infusions of *C. colocynthis* fruits are traditionally used as anti-diabetic medication in Mediterranean countries. In order to verify the putative anti-diabetic activity of this plant drug, different extracts of *C. colocynthis* seed as well β-pyrazol-1-ylalanine, the major free amino acid present in the seeds, were tested *in vitro* in the isolated rat pancreas and isolated rat islets in the presence of 8.3 mM glucose. All tested extracts, when perfused for 20 min at 0.1 mg/ml, immediately and significantly stimulated insulin secretion but this effect was transient. In addition, the purified extract induced a clear dose-dependent increase in insulin release from isolated islets. Moreover, a significant and persistent increase in pancreatic flow rate appeared during perfusions of all the fractions. An insulinotropic effect of the plant drug partially account for the anti-diabetic activities of these fruits (1)

In normal rabbits, oral administration of an aqueous extract of the rind of *C. colocynthis* (300 mg/kg) produced a significant reduction in plasma glucose after 1 h and highly significant reduction after 2, 3 and 6 h. Phytochemical screening revealed that the rind of *C. colocynthis* and its aqueous extract contains tertiary and quaternary alkaloids, glycoside and saponin components. The hypoglycaemic effects of these components, given orally at a dose of 50 mg/kg, were studied in normoglycaemic rabbits. The alkaloid fraction did not significantly lower the blood glucose levels while the glycoside fraction significantly lowered the fasting glucose levels after 2 and 3 h and highly significantly after 6 h. The effect was more pronounced with saponin fraction. Graded doses (10, 15 and 20 mg/kg) of saponin extract, when given orally to alloxan-induced diabetic rabbits, produced a significant reduction of plasma glucose concentration (2).

1. Nmila R, R Gross, H Rchid, M Roye, M Manteghetti, P Petit, M Tijane, G Ribes, Y Sauvaire; Insulinotropic effect of *Citrullus colocynthis* fruit extracts, *Planta Med* **66**(5), 418-23 (2000).

2. Abdel-Hassan IA, JA Abdel-Barry, S Tariq Mohammeda; The hypoglycaemic and anti-hyperglycaemic effect of *Citrullus colocynthis* fruit aqueous extract in normal and alloxan diabetic rabbits, *J Ethnopharmacol* **71**(1-2), 325-30 (2000).

Citrus paradisi Macfad. (Rutaceae)
(Grapefruit)

The grapefruit is a subtropical citrus tree grown for its edible fruit, which is yellow-skinned, largely oblate and ranges in diameter from 10-15 cm. The pulp is white, pink or red of varying sweetness. The effects of grapefruit on body weight and metabolic syndrome were studied in 91 obese patients in a randomized, placebo-controlled experiment. Half of a fresh grapefruit eaten before meals was associated with significant weight loss. Insulin resistance was improved with fresh grapefruit. Although the mechanism of this weight loss is unknown, it would appear reasonable to include grapefruit in a weight reduction diet.

Fujioka K, F Greenway, J Sheard, Y Ying; The effects of grapefruit on weight and insulin resistance: relationship to the metabolic syndrome, *J Med Food* **9**(1), 49-54 (2006)

Citrus sinensis (L) Osbeck (Rutaceae)
(Sweet orange, H. Santara)

Orange and apple were found to have lower glycaemic indices in comparison to white bread. Eight non-insulin-dependent diabetic subjects consumed apple (227 g), orange (280 g) or white bread (50 g) on three separate days. The mean postprandial blood glucose response area to white bread was significantly higher compared with orange and apple. The glycaemic indices of the fruits were nearly identical for orange and for apple. The low glycaemic response to orange and apple may be ascribed to the high content of fructose, which is rapidly cleared and metabolised by the liver, without elevating the blood glucose (1).

Insoluble fibre-rich fractions, isolated from the peel of *Citrus sinensis* cv. *Liucheng*, were found to effectively adsorb glucose, retard glucose diffusion, and inhibit the activity of *alpha*-amylase to different extents. These mechanisms were expected to create a concerted benefit in decreasing the rate of glucose absorption and eventually lower the concentration of postprandial serum glucose. The potential hypoglycaemic effects of these insoluble fibre-rich fractions suggested that they could be incorporated as low-calorie bulk ingredients in high-fibre foods to reduce calorie level and control blood glucose level. (2).

1. Gregersen S, O Rasmussen, S Larsen, K Hermansen; Glycaemic and insulinaemic responses to orange and apple compared with white bread in non-insulin-dependent diabetic subjects, *Eur J Clin Nutr* **46**(4), 301-03 (1992).
2. Chau CF, YL Huang, MH Lee; *In vitro* hypoglycaemic effects of different in-

soluble fibre-rich fractions prepared from the peel of *Citrus sinensis* L. cv. *Liucheng*, *J Agric Food Chem* **51**(22), 6623-26 (2003).

Clausena anisata (Willd) Hook f. ex Benth (Rutaceae) (Horsewood)

It is a small tree with leaves that are densely dotted with glands and have a strong scent when crushed. The hypoglycaemic effect of the methanol extract of *C. anisata* root was studied in normoglycaemic and streptozotocin-treated diabetic rats. By using graded doses of methanol extract of *C. anisata* root, a dose of 800 mg/kg of the extract was found to produce maximal hypoglycaemic effect in both fasted normal and diabetic rats The hypoglycaemic effect of this single dose of *C. anisata* root extract was compared with those of insulin (5 µU/kg s.c.) and glibenclamide (0.2 mg/kg p.o.) in both fasted normal and fasted diabetic rats. At the dose of 800 mg/kg p.o., the extract reduced the mean basal blood glucose concentrations of fasted normal and fasted diabetic rats by 57.52 and 51.30%, respectively. *C. anisata* contains a diverse group of chemical compounds. While it is possible that the hypoglycaemic effect of the plant extract may be due, at least in part, to its terpenoid and coumarin contents, the mechanism of its hypoglycaemic action remains largely speculative, and is unlikely to be due to the stimulation of pancreatic *beta*-cells and subsequent secretion of insulin.

Ojewole JA; Hypoglycaemic effect of *Clausena anisata* (Willd) Hook methanolic root extract in rats, *J Ethnopharmacol* **81**(2), 231-37 (2002).

Clausena lansium Skeels (Rutaceae) (Wampee))

Clausena lansium, also known as wampee, is a species of strongly scented evergreen trees with somewhat grapelike fruits, but the pulp is scant and the seeds are large. Wampee is native to south-east Asia. It is only occasionally grown in India and Sri Lanka. Oral administration of *Clausena* coumarin, isolated from the leaves *C. lansium,* was found to lower blood glucose level in normal and alloxan-induced diabetic mice at a dose of 200 mg/kg/d for three days. *Clausena* coumarin was also found to antagonise the elevation of blood glucose by injection of adrenaline to normal mice.

Shen ZP, QM Chen, HP Liu, MZ Xie; The hypoglycaemic effect of clausena coumarin, *Acta Pharm Sin* **24**(5), 391-92 (1989).

Cleistocalyx operculatus (Roxb) Merr and Perry (Myrtaceae)

Aqueous extracts of the flower buds of *C. operculatus* are commonly used as drink preparations in Vietnam. The anti-hyperglycaemic effects of this extract were studied *in vitro* and *in vivo*. The extract inhibited the rat-intestinal maltase and sucrase activities. Postprandial blood glucose testing of normal mice and streptozotocin-induced diabetic rats by maltose loading (2 g/kg b.w.) showed that the blood glucose reduction with the flower extract (500 mg/kg b.w.) was slightly less than that with acarbose (25 mg/kg bw). In an 8-week experiment, the blood glucose level of streptozotocin-induced diabetic rats, treated with this extract, was markedly lower than that of non-treated diabetic rats.

Mai TT, NV Chuyen; Anti-hyperglycaemic activity of an aqueous extract from flower buds of *Cleistocalyx operculatus* (Roxb.) Merr and Perry, *Biosci Biotechnol Biochem* **71**(1), 69-76 (2007)

Cleome felina Linn. (Cleomaceae / Capparaceae)

Oral administration of petroleum ether and benzene extracts of *C. felina* (300 mg/kg/day) to alloxan-induced diabetic rats for 30 days exhibited anti-diabetic and anti-hyperlipemic effects. A significant decrease in the activities of enzymes like alkaline phosphatase, acid phosphatase and HMG CoA reductase in the liver was also observed.

Nagarajan NS, N Murugesh, P Thirupathy Kumaresan, N Radha, A Murali; Anti-diabetic and anti-hyperlipemic effects of *Cleome felina*, *Fitoterapia* **76**(3-4), 310-15 (2005).

Cleome droserifolia (Forssk.) Delile (Cleomaceae)

The mechanism of the hypoglycaemic effect of *C. droserifolia* was studied in a group of albino rats, rendered glucose intolerant by tetracycline-induced fatty liver, and compared with normal control rats. The plant extract significantly suppressed the rise in peripheral blood glucose concentrations, both in the basal (fasting) state and after glucose intake. While the suppression of basal blood glucose indicated a lowering effect of the plant extract on hepatic glucose output, its postprandial hypoglycaemic effect without increasing insulin secretion indicated potentiation of peripheral and hepatic insulin sensitivity with diminished intestinal glucose absorption. This plant might prove to have a promising therapeutic value in the treatment of diabetes mellitus.

Nicola WG, KM Ibrahim, TH Mikhail, RB Girgis, ME Khadr; Role of the hypoglycaemic plant extract *Cleome droserifolia* in improving glucose and lipid metabolism and its relation to insulin resistance in fatty liver, *Boll Chim Farm* **135**(9), 507-17 (1996)

Clitoria ternatea Linn. (Fabaceae)
(Blue pea vine, H. Aparajita)

Clitoria ternatea is a vine native to tropical and equatorial Asia, but has been introduced to Africa, Australia and other parts of the world. It is grown as an ornamental plant and its flowers are used to colour food and drink. The ethanol extract of *C. ternatea* flowers significantly lowered the serum sugar level of alloxan-induced diabetic rats. It inhibited the enzymes β-galactosidase, α-glucosidase but not β-D-fructosidase.

Sharma AK, M Majumdar; Some observations on the effect of *Clitoria ternatea* Linn on changes in serum sugar level and small intestinal mucosal carbohydrases activities in alloxan diabetes, *Calcutta Med J* **87**(11-12), 168-71 (1990).

Clutia richardiana Linn. (Euphorbiaceae)

There are about 70 species of the plant genus *Clutia*, found in Africa and Arabia. *C. richardiana* is a traditional medicinal herb with demonstrated hypoglycaemic effects. Saudin, a novel diterpene isolated from the petroleum ether extract of *C. richardiana* leaves, showed hypoglycaemic activity. It caused marked hypoglycaemic effects in fasted mice at a dose of 80 mg/kg p.o. At a dose of 40 mg/kg ip, saudin exerted hypoglycaemic activity in non-alloxanized rather than in alloxanized fasted animals. In rats, saudin (40 mg/kg ip) was found to produce hypoglycaemic effect in fed but not fasted non-alloxanized animals. The hypoglycaemic effect of saudin was associated with a significant decrease in the plasma insulin activity in rats. The hypoglycaemic activity of saudin may involve a mechanism, not related to insulin secretion (1, 2).

An HPLC method was utilized to determine the levels of the major diterpenes of *C. richardiana* in extracts obtained by using solvents like methanol and acetonitrile as well as hot water. Organic solvent extracts are more efficient than aqueous extract but all the nine markers could be detected equally in all extracts. The aqueous extract was non-toxic against a number of human cell lines, which is a promising indication for its use as a safe and effective anti-diabetic herbal preparation (3).

1. Mossa JS, JM Cassady, MD Antoun, SR Byrn, AT McKenzie, JF Kozlowski, P Main; Saudin, a hypoglycaemic diterpenoid with a novel 6,7-secolabdane carbon skeleton, from *Cluytia richardiana, J Org Chem* **50**(6), 916-18 (1985).
2. Mossa JS, ES El-Denshary, R Hindawi, AM Ageel; The hypoglycaemic effect of saudin, *Int J Crude Drug Res* **26**(2), 81-87 (1988)
3. Abourashed EA, M Ganzera, LA Khan, S Khan, JS Mossa, FS El-Feraly; HPLC fingerprinting and estimation of the bioactive components of *Clutia richardiana* L. as a potential hypoglycaemic herbal tea, *Phytother Res* **17**(6), 657-60 (2003)

Cnidium officinale Mak. (Apiaceae Umbelliferae)

The effects of *C. officinale* on high glucose-stimulated extracellular matrix (ECM) protein accumulation and transforming growth factor-*beta* 1 (TGF-β 1) production were examined. The results of the study indicated that *C. officinale* inhibit the high glucose-induced glomerular mesangial cells (GMC) proliferation partially through suppression of the ECM accumulation and TGF-β 1 production and suggested that *C. officinale* might be a promising agent for treating the development and progression of diabetic glomerulopathy.

Jeong SL, DH Kwak, S Lee, YK Choo, WH Woo, KS Keum, BK Choi, KY Jung; Inhibitory effects of *Cnidium officinale* Makino and *Tabanus fulvus* Meigan on the high glucose-induced proliferation of glomerular mesangial cells, *Phytomedicine* **12**(9), 648-55 (2005)

Coccinia indica Wight and Arn (Cucurbitaceae)
(H. Kanduru, S. Bimba)

Coccinia indica is a creeper, which grows wildly in Bangladesh and in many parts of the Indian sub-continent. The plant has been used since ancient times as an anti-diabetic drug in the Ayurvedic system of medicine. *Coccinia indica* and *Cephalandra indica* are synonymous.

Brahmachari and Augusti (1) claimed the isolation of orally effective hypoglycaemic principles from *C. indica,* while Gupta and Variyar (2) studied the effect of this plant against the hyperglycaemic response of somatotropin and corticotropin hormones. Mukherjee *et al* (3) recognized the plant as a potential hypoglycaemic agent. Azad Khan and co-workers (4, 6) conducted a double blind controlled trial with a preparation from the leaves of the plant on uncontrolled, maturity onset diabetics. The trial lasted for six weeks for an individual patient. Ten out of 16 patients, who received the experimental preparations, showed marked improvement in their glucose tolerance. No such improvement was observed in any of the 16 patients in the dummy group.

The juice and decoction of leaves and stems of *C. indica* (20ml/kg) showed significant hypoglycaemic response in fasting rabbits. The decoction of the fruits of the plant also showed similar activity (5). The powdered stem of *C. indica* showed highly effective hypoglycaemic activity in human maturity onset diabetes mellitus cases. The drug was found to ameliorate clinical symptoms in the patients and was least toxic (7). Effect of *C. indica* in 6 patients of type II diabetes mellitus was tested. *C. indica* juice produced some hypoglycaemic action at 30, 60, 90 and 120 minutes and the area under the incremental glucose curve was significantly lower (8).

The blood sugar lowering effects of ethanol extracts of whole plant and root of *C. indica* were tested in different experimental models. While the plant extract reduced the blood sugar levels of fasted, glucose-loaded and streptozotocin-induced diabetic albino mice to different degrees, root extract reduced the blood sugar only of glucose-loaded animals (9). Effective and significant control of hyperglycaemia with highly significant elevation of serum insulin level was observed in streptozotocin-induced diabetic rats, treated with *C. indica* (11).

Rahman and co-workers (10, 12) studied the hypoglycaemic effect of alcoholic extract of *C. indica* leaves and observed that oral administration of the aqueous suspension of the residue, obtained from the extract, significantly lowered the blood glucose level of normal-fed, 48-hr starved as well as of streptozotocin-induced diabetic rats. Starvation-induced increase in the activity of glucose-6-phosphatase was depressed by extract feeding while basal activity of the enzyme in normal-fed rats remained unaffected. Similar result was also obtained by using 60% ethanol extract. Oral administration of the aqueous suspension of the residue (200 mg/kg b.w) obtained from the extract to normal fed and streptozotocin-induced male diabetic rats after 18 h of fasting resulted in lowering of blood sugar levels, depression of hepatic glucose-6-phosphatase and fructose-1,6-bisphosphatase activities and elevation of both the red-cell and hepatic glucose-6-phosphate dehydrogenase activities. From the results of detailed investigation, it was suggested that the observed hypoglycaemic effect of *C. indica* was partly due to the depression of the key gluconeogenic enzymes glucose-6-phosphatase and fructose-1,6-bisphosphatase and partly due to the enhancement of glucose oxidation by the shunt pathway through activation of its principal enzyme, glucose-6-phosphate dehydrogenase.

Alcoholic extract of *C. indica* proved to be a potent anti-diabetic agent. Thr hypoglycaemic activity and effectiveness on biochemical parameters of different fractions were found to be significant and comparable with the standard biguanide drug, phenformin (16).

Venkateswaran and Pari (14, 15, 17) studied the antioxidant effect of an ethanol extract of *C. indica* leaves in streptozotocin-induced diabetic rats. Oral administration of the extract (200 mg/kg b.w.) for 45 days resulted in a significant reduction in thiobarbituric acid reactive substances, hydroperoxides, vitamin E and ceruloplasmin. A significant increase in reduced glutathione, superoxide dismutase, catalase, glutathione peroxidase and glutathione-S-transferase in liver and kidney of streptozotocin induced diabetic rats was also observed. These authors also studied the effect of ethanol extract *C. indica* leaves on blood glucose, plasma insulin, cholesterol, triglycerides, free fatty acids and phospholipids and fatty acid composition of total lipids in liver, kidney and brain of normal and streptozotocin induced diabetic rats Oral administration of the extract (200 mg/kg body weight) for 45 days to diabetic rats decreased the concentrations of blood glucose, lipids and fatty acids, *viz.*, palmitic, stearic, and oleic acids whereas linolenic and arachidonic acids and plasma insulin were elevated. These effects were better than those of glibenclamide.

The fruits of *C. indica* were also found to be hypoglycaemic. Oral administration of the pectin, isolated from *C. indica* fruits, at a dose of 200 mg/100 g b.w./day showed a significant hypoglycaemic action in normal rats. The pectin administration resulted in a significant reduction in blood glucose and an increase in the liver glycogen. Glycogen synthetase activity was highly significant. Incorporation of labelled glucose into hepatic glycogen was also found to be higher. A significant reduction in phosphorylase activity was noted in the pectin-administered groups (13).

1. Brahmachari HD, KT Augusti; Orally effective hypoglycaemic principles from *Coccinia indica* Wight and Arn, *J Pharm Pharmacol* **15**(Jun), 411-12 (1963).
2. Gupta SS, MC Variyar; Experimental studies on pituitary diabetes IV. Effect of *Gymnema sylvestre* and *Coccinia indica* against the hyperglycaemic response of somatotropin and corticotropin hormones, *Indian J Med Res* **52** (Feb), 200-07 (1964).
3. Mukherjee K, NC Ghosh, T Datta; *Coccinia indica* Linn. as potential hypoglycaemic agent, *Indian J Exp Biol* **10**(5), 347-49 (1972)
4. Azad Khan AK, S Akhtar, H Mahtab; *Coccinia indica* in the treatment of patients with diabetes mellitus, *Bangladesh Med Res Counc Bull* **5**(2), 60-66 (1979)
5. Pillai NR, D Ghosh, R Uma, A Anandakumar; Hypoglycaemic activity of *Coccinia indica* W. & A., *Bull Med Ethnobot Res* **1**(2), 234-42 (1980)
6. Azad Khan AK, S Akhtar, H Mahtab; Treatment of diabetes mellitus with *Coccinia indica, Br Med J* **280**(6220), 1044 (1980)
7. Kuppurajan K, C Seshadri, R Revathi, S Venkataraghavan; Hypoglycaemic effect of *Ciccinia indica* in diabetes mellitus, *Nagarjun* **29**(5), 1-4 (1986).
8. Choudhury RR, M Mishra; *Coccinia indica* in type II diabetes mellitus, *Indian Med J* **81**(2), 31-32 (1987).
9. Mukherjee B, B Chandrasekar, SK Mukherjee; Blood sugar lowering effect of *Coccinia indica* root and whole plant in different experimental models, *Fitoterapia* **59**(3), 207-210 (1988).
10. Hossain MZ, BA Shibib, R Rahman; Hypoglycaemic effects of *Coccinia indica*: inhibition of key gluconeogenic enzyme, glucose-6-phosphatase, *Indian J Exp Biol* **30**(5), 418-20 (1992).
11. Basu DP, M Chatterjee, J Das; Evaluation of hypoglycaemic properties of *Coccinea indica* on streptozotocin-induced diabetes in rats, *Proc 25th Indian Pharmacol Soc Conf*, Muzaffarpur, Bihar, India, December 5-8, p.81, (1992).
12. Shibib BA, LA Khan, R Rahman; Hypoglycaemic activity of *Coccinia indica* and *Momordica charantia* in diabetic rats: depression of the hepatic gluconeogenic enzymes glucose-6-phosphatase and fructose-1,6-bisphosphatase and elevation of both liver and red-cell shunt enzyme glucose-6-phosphate dehydrogenase, *Biochem J* **292**(Pt.1), 267-70 (1993).
13. Kumar GP, S Sudheesh, NR Vijayalakshmi; Hypoglycaemic effect of *Coccinia indica*: mechanism of action, *Planta Med* **59**(4), 330-32 (1993)
14. Venkateswaran S, L Pari; Effect of *Coccinia indica* leaves on antioxidant status in streptozotocin- induced diabetic rats, *J Ethnopharmacol* **84**(2-3), 163-68 (2003)
15. Pari L, S Venkateswaran; Protective effect of *Coccinia indica* on changes in the

fatty acid composition in streptozotocin induced diabetic rats, *Pharmazie* **58**(6), 409-12 (2003)

16. Dhanabal SP, CK Kokate, MB Patil, K Elango, B Suresh; Hypoglycaemic effect of *Coccinia indica*: Influence on biochemical parameters, *National Conf of Indian Soc Pharmacognosy: Herb: The National Alternative* , p.A-01, Jan 17-18, 2003, Gandhinagar, Gujrat, India
17. Venkateswaran S, L Pari; Effect of *Coccinia indica* leaf extract on plasma anti-oxidants in streptozotocin- induced experimental diabetes in rats, *Phytother Res* **17**(6), 605-08 (2003)

Cocculus hirsutus (L) Diels (Menispermaceae)) (Jaljamini)

Cocculus hirsutus is a shrub, native to Tropical Africa, India and Nepal. Methanol extract of the roots of the plant exhibited significant hypoglycaemic activity in diabetic rats. Total alkaloid fraction, isolated from the extract, showed considerable hypoglycaemic activity in alloxan-induced diabetic rats (1). The aqueous extract of *C. hirsutus* leaves (250, 500, and 1000 mg/kg, p.o.) showed significant reduction of serum glucose level in alloxan-induced diabetic mice at 28th day. In oral glucose tolerance test, the extract increased the glucose tolerance. The significant anti-hyperglycaemic activity of *C. hirsutus* leaf extract was thus verified (2). The extract of aerial parts of the plant showed anti-diabetic activity in normal as well as in diabetic rats. The effect, however, was more pronounced in diabetic animals when the extract was administered for 15 days after streptozotocin-induced diabetes. The effect was comparable with that of glibenclamide. The findings suggested that *C. hirsutus* could be of benefit in diabetes mellitus in controlling blood sugar (3).

1. Satyanarayana K, V Mangathayaru, J Sreekanth, V Venkateswarlu, CK Kokate; Studies on hypoglycaemic and cardiotonic effects of roots of *Cocculus hirsutus*, *Indian J Pharm Sci* **56**(1), 30-35 (1994)
2. Badole S, N Patel, S Bodhankar, B Jain, S Bhardwaj; Anti-hyperglycaemic activity of aqueous extract of leaves of *Cocculus hirsutus* (L.) Diels in alloxan-induced diabetic mice, *Indian J Pharmacol* **38**(1), 49-53 (2006)
3. Sangameswaran B, B Jayakar; Anti-diabetic and spermatogenic activity of *Cocculus hirsutus* (L) Diels, *African J Biotechnol* **6**(10), 1212-16 (2007)

Cocos nucifera Linn. (Arecacea / Palmae) (Cocoanut palm, H. Nariyel)

Cocoanut is a pan-tropical species usually found in humid coastal areas. The origin of this plant is uncertain, but many experts believe it from the west Pacific and Indian Ocean islands. The effect of neutral detergent fibre (lignin, hemicellulose, and cellulose) from cocoanut kernel on the concentration of blood glucose, serum insulin and excretion of minerals was studied in rats. Increase in the intake of fibre resulted in significant decrease in the level of blood glucose and serum insulin and increase in the faecal excretion of metals like copper, chromium, manganese, magnesium, zinc and calcium. The results of the investigation suggest that inclusion of cocoanut fibre in the diet causes a significant hypoglycaemic action.

Sindurani JA, T Rajamohan; Effects of different levels of cocoanut fibre on blood glucose, serum insulin and minerals in rats, *Indian J Physiol Pharmacol* **44**(1), 97-100 (2000)

Cogniauxia podoleana Baillon (Cucurbitaceae)

The leaves of the plant are used in Congolese traditional medicine for the treatment of diabetes mellitus. The aqueous extract of leaves of the plant was sequentially extracted with benzene and diethyl ether. The diethyl ether fraction was found to contain the flavonoid constituents and oral administration of this fraction (100mg/kg) reduced the blood glucose levels of normal rats by 40.0% after 3h. Similar effect was also observed in alloxan-induced diabetic rats. The observations confirmed the anti-diabetic activity of the leaves of *C. podoleana,* used in Congolese traditional medicine for the treatment of diabetes mellitus.

Diatewa M, CB Samba, TC Assah, AA Abena; Hypoglycaemic and anti-hyperglycaemic effects of diethyl ether fraction isolated from the aqueous extract of the leaves of *Cogniauxia podoleana* Baillon in normal and alloxan-induced diabetic rats, *J Ethnopharmacol* **92**(2-3), 229-32 (2004).

Coix lachryma-jobi L. var. ***ma-yuen*** (Roman.) Stapf. (Poaceae)) (Coix seed, Chinese pearl barley, Adlay)

Coix lachryma-jobi var. *ma-yuen* (Adlay) is a cereal food for humans and has also been used as a functional food for traditional treatment of diabetes in China. The hypoglycaemic activity of the glycans (coixans A, B and C), isolated from the seeds of the herb was tested (1). The effect of dietary de-hulled adlay on plasma lipid and glucose concentrations was studied in diabetic rats. Streptozotocin-induced diabetic male Sprague-Dawley rats were fed a cholesterol-rich diet containing either corn starch or de-hulled adlay for four weeks. After completion of the experimental period, the abdominal adipose tissue and liver of rats were excised and weighed, and the plasma glucose, triglyceride, and lipoprotein cholesterol concentrations were assayed. Diabetic rats, fed a de-hulled adlay diet, exhibited a greater adipose tissue weight compared with animals, fed a corn starch diet. Significant decrease in the levels of plasma glucose, total cholesterol, LDL and VLDL-cholesterol and triglyceride was observed in rats fed the de-hulled adlay diet. A significant decrease in plasma thiobarbituric reactive substances was also observed in diabetic rats fed the de-hulled adlay diet. De-hulled adlay diet thus played an important role in the regulation of plasma lipid and glucose metabolisms in diabetic rats induced by streptozotocin (2).

1. Takahashi M, C Konno, H Hikino; Isolation and hypoglycaemic activity of coixans A, B and C, glycans of *Coix lachryma*-jobi var. *ma-yuen* seeds, *Planta Med* (1), 64-65 (1986)
2. Yeh PH, W Chiang, MT Chiang; Effects of dehulled adlay on plasma glucose and lipid concentrations in streptozotocin-induced diabetic rats fed a diet enriched in cholesterol, *Int J Vitam Nutr Res* **76**(5), 299-305 (2006)

Colchicum luteum Baker (Colchicaceae/ Liliaceae)

Colchicum luteum is native to sub-alpine North India, Afghanistan and SW China. It yields the highly poisonous pale-yellow alkaloid, colchicine, used for the treatment of rheumatic complaints and especially gout.

The drug administered in different forms (crude *C. luteum*, its ethanol extract and colchicines) showed a transitory hypoglycaemic effect. The crude drug and colchicines exhibited a highly significant lowering effect on total lipids and cholesterol. A significant but transitory increase in the activity of LDH, SGOT, SGPT and alkaline phosphatase was also observed. All the three forms of the drug caused a decrease in serum uric acid level.

Chaudry AR, M Alam, M Ahmad, FZ Khan, N Nomani; Studies on medicinal herbs: II. Effect of *Colchium luteum* on biochemical parameters of rabbit serum, *Fitoterapia* **64**(6), 510-15 (1993)

Commelina communis Linn. (Commelinaceae) (Asiatic dayflower)

Aqueous extract of *C. communis* is traditionally used for the treatment of diabetes in Korea. Extract of *C. communis* has been reported to decrease the blood glucose level in alloxan-induced diabetic rats and recover the loss of their body weight. The decrease in liver weight and the activity of glucose 6-phosphate dehydrogenase, caused by diabetes, were normalised by administration of the plant protein fraction. From the results of detailed investigation, it was suggested that glucose 6-phosphate dehydrogenase may be used as a marker enzyme to diagnose diabetes and that the hypoglycaemic activity of the extract is associated with the action of the enzyme on rat liver (1). Aqueous extract of the plant showed inhibitory activity of the *alpha*-glucosidase in a dose-dependent manner, *in vitro*. It also alleviated hyperglycaemia, caused by maltose or starch loading, in normal and streptozotocin-induced diabetic mice with better efficacy than that of acarbose. Prolonged administration of the extract tended to normalise hyperglycaemia in streptozotocin-induced diabetic mice. From the results of the investigation, it was inferred that the inhibitory activity of aqueous extract of *C. communis* on *alpha*-glucosidase might contribute to delay in carbohydrate digestion and glucose absorption. Thus, *C. communis* extract was considered to have the potential for use in the management of non-insulin-dependent diabetes (2).

1. Park SY, KH Cho; Effects of *Commelina communis* L. on the blood glucose level in alloxan-induced diabetic rat and the biochemical properties of glucose-6-phosphate dehydrogenase from the rat livers, *Korean J Pharmacogn* **25**(3), 238-48 (1994)
2. Youn JY, HY Park, KH Cho; Anti-hyperglycaemic activity of *Commelina communis* L.: inhibition of *alpha*-glucosidase, *Diabetes Res Clin Pract* **66**(Suppl. 1), S149-55 (2004).

Commiphora myrrha Arn (Burseraceae) (Myrrh)

Myrrh is a reddish-brown resinous material, the dried sap of *C. myrrha*, native to Yemen, Somalia and the eastern parts of Ethiopia. The scent of raw myrrh resin and of its essential oil is sharp, pleasant, and bitter.

The resin of *C. myrrha* was examined for its anti-hyperglycaemic compounds using *in vivo* bioactivity-guided fractionation. Furano-sesquiterpenes, isolated from the resin, exhibited anti-hyperglycaemic activity.

Ubillas RP, CD Mendez, SD Jolad, J Luo, SR King, TJ Carlson, DM Fort; Anti-hyperglycaemic furano-sesquiterpenes from *Commiphora myrrha*, *Planta Med* **65**(8), 778-79 (1999)

Coptis chinensis Franch (Ranunculaceae) (Chinese goldthread)

Coptis chinensis is a species native to China and is used in traditional Chinese medicine. It contains berberine and coptisine as the major alkaloids. Water extract of *C. chinensis* lowered serum glucose level in normal mice. The alkaloid, berberine also exhibited hypoglycaemic activity in mice (1).

The effect of the plant drug on lipid peroxidation and diabetes of rats, induced by alloxan, was studied. The malondialdehyde (MDA) product of both pancreas and liver homogenate in drug treated group was significantly lower than that in control and alloxan group. Superoxide dismutase activity in erythrocytes was the same in all groups. The blood catalase activity in alloxan group markedly decreased compared to the control group but no significant change was observed between the drug-treated and alloxan group. The experiment indicated that *C. chinensis* had a strong inhibitory effect on lipid peroxidation both *in vitro* and *in vivo*. The drug could protect rats from diabetes, induced by alloxan, and it was due to this fact that the drug was able to inhibit alloxan-induced free radicals (2). The increased levels of total and LDL-cholesterol of rats, fed a diet containing 1% cholesterol and 0.5% cholic acid, were reduced markedly in a dose dependent manner by oral administration of *Coptis* inflorescence extract at doses of 0.25, 0.5 g/kg.day for 4 weeks. The extract showed a significant blood sugar lowering activity at all experimented doses in alloxan-induced diabetic rats. The highest reduction (58%) of blood sugar was observed when the rats were given *Coptis* inflorescence extract orally at a dose of 0.5 g/kg day for 3 weeks. From the results of the investigation, the extract is considered to be effective in the prevention and management of coronary artery disease by lowering serum cholesterol and blood sugar (3).

1. Chen QM, MZ Xie; Studies on the hypoglycaemic effect of *Coptis chinensis* and berberine, *Acta Pharma Sin* **21**(6), 401-06 (1986)
2. Song LC, KZ Chen, JY Zhu; The effect of *Coptis chinensis* on lipid peroxidation and antioxidase activity of rats, *Chinese J Integr Trad & Western Med* **12**(7), 421-23 (1992)
3. Yuan L, D Tu, X Ye, J Wu; Hypoglycaemic and hypocholesterolemic effects of *Coptis chinensis* Franch inflorescence, *Plant Foods Hum Nutr* **61**(3), 139-44 (2006)

Coriandrum sativum Linn. (Apiaceae)
(Coriander, H. Dhania)

In a culinary context, the name 'coriander' may refer to either the seeds of the plant (used as a spice), or to its leaves (used as herb) but generally it refers to the seeds. Coriander has been documented as a traditional treatment of diabetes. Coriander incorporated into the diet (62.5 g/kg) and drinking water (2.5 g/l, prepared by 15 min decoction) was found to reduce hyperglycaemia of streptozotocin-diabetic mice. An aqueous extract of coriander (1 mg/ml) was found to increase transport of 2-deoxyglucose, oxidation of glucose and its incorporation into glycogen of isolated murine abdominal muscle. The effect is comparable with 10^{-8} M-insulin. In acute 20 min tests, 0.25-10 mg/ml aqueous extract of coriander evoked a stepwise stimulation of insulin secretion from a clonal B-cell line. Sequential extraction with solvents revealed insulin-releasing activity in hexane and water fractions indicating a possible cumulative effect of more than one insulin-releasing constituent in the extract. These results demonstrate the presence of anti-hyperglycaemic, insulin-releasing and insulin-like activity in *Coriandrum sativum.*

Gray AM, PR Flatt; Insulin-releasing and insulin-like activity of the traditional anti-diabetic plant *Coriandrum sativum* (coriander), *Br J Nutr* **81**(3), 203-09 (1999)

Cornus mas Linn. (Cornaceae)
(Cornelian cherry dogwood)

Cornus mas is native to southern Europe and southwest Asia. In North America, the plant is known by the common name of "Cornelian Cherry". Cornelian cherries are used in the preparation of beverages in Europe and also for the treatment of diabetes-related disorders in Asia. The anthocyanins and ursolic acid, isolated from *C. mas* fruits, were tested for their ability to ameliorate obesity and insulin resistance in C57BL/6 mice, fed a high-fat diet. Mice were initially fed a high-fat diet for 4 weeks and then switched to a high-fat diet containing anthocyanins (1 g/kg of high-fat diet) and ursolic acid (500 mg/kg of high-fat diet) for an additional 8 weeks. The high-fat diet-induced glucose intolerance was prevented by anthocyanins and ursolic acid. Anthocyanin and ursolic acid treated mice also exhibited extremely elevated insulin levels.

Jayaprakasam B, LK Olson, RE Schutzki, MH Tai, MG Nair; Amelioration of obesity and glucose intolerance in high-fat-fed C57BL/6 mice by anthocyanins and ursolic acid in Cornelian cherry (*Cornus mas*), *J Agric Food Chem* **54**(1), 243-48 (2006).

Cornus officinalis Sieb. et Zucc. (Cornaceae). (Dogwood)

Dogwoods are widely used in landscapes for their beautiful flowers, showy fruit, winter colour and attractive foliage. Dogwood fruit (Corni Fructus), a favourite food for birds, is also used in Chinese anti-diabetic prescription, 'Hachimi-Gan". Of the different components of this Chinese prescription, Corni Fructus was most important and its ether extract was found to be most effective towards diabetic rats. The extract yielded ursolic and oleanolic acids; the former showed anti-diabetic activity while the latter decreased the amount of water consumption and urine volume (1).

Administration of the alcoholic extract of the fruit pulp of *C. officinalis* (10 and 20 gm /kg, p.o.) for 7 days lowered the blood sugar and lipid levels of normal mice. The extract also significantly reduced the blood sugar levels of alloxan-induced diabetic mice. It also inhibited aggregation of platelets and decreased the viscosity of blood in rabbits (2).

Alcohol extract of *C. officinalis* was found to increase GLUT4 mRNA and its protein expression in NIDDM rats through promoting proliferation of islet and increasing postprandial secretion of insulin. The extract was, therefore, capable of accelerating glucose transport (3).

1. Yamahara J, H Mibu, T Sawada, H Fujimura, S Takino, M Yoshikawa, I Kitagawa; Biologically active principles of crude drugs: Anti-diabetic principles of corni fructus in experimental diabetes induced by streptozotocin, *Yakugaku Zasshi* **101**(1), 86- 90 (1981)
2. Liu Baoling, Zhu Danni,Yu Zhiling,Yan Yongqing, Effect of alcoholic extract of Fructus corni on blood glucose, lipid levels and platelets aggregation in experimental animals, *J China Pharmaceut Univ* **23**(1), 19-21 (1992)
3. Qian DS, YF Zhu, Q Zhu; Effect of alcohol extract of *Cornus officinalis* Sieb. et Zucc on GLUT4 expression in skeletal muscle in type 2 (non-insulin-dependent) diabetes mellitus rats, *Zhongguo Zhong Yao Za Zhi* **26**(12), 859-62 (2001)

Coronopus didymus (L.) Sm. (Brassicaceae) (Swinecress)

Oral administration of the aqueous extract of *C. didymus* showed significant antiallergic, antipyretic, hypoglycaemic and hepatoprotective activity in mice at 200 and 400 mg/kg doses. The plant extract acts as an antioxidant as evidenced by its ability to scavenge 2,2-diphenyl-1-picrylhydrazyl (DPPH) and superoxide radicals. The observed activities were considered to be due to the presence of flavonoids, saponins and tannins in the extract.

Mantena SK, S Mutalik, H Srinivasa, GS Subramanian, KR Prabhakar, KR Reddy, KK Srinivasan; Antiallergic, antipyretic, hypoglycaemic and hepatoprotective effects of aqueous extract of *Coronopus didymus* Linn., *Biol Pharm Bull* **28**(3), 468-72 (2005).

Coscinium fenestratum (Gaertn.) Colebr. (Menispermaceae) (Tree turmeric)

Coscinium fenestratum, is a medicinal plant indigenous to India and Sri Lanka and is used in Ayurveda and Siddha medicine for treating diabetes. Its root is used as a bitter tonic, in ulcers and dressing wounds.The anti-diabetic potential of the alcoholic extract of *C. fenestratum* stems was evaluated in the streptozotocin-nicotinamide-induced type-2 diabetic model. Significant reductions in fasting blood glucose levels were observed in the normal as well as in the treated diabetic animals when graded doses of the extract were administered to normal and experimental diabetic rats for 12 days. Serum insulin levels were not stimulated in the animals treated with the extract. The assessment of the changes in body weight, serum lipid profiles, thiobarbituric acid reactive substance levels, glycosylated hemoglobin and liver glycogen levels of the extract-treated diabetic rats in comparison with diabetic control and normal animals justifies the use of the plant for the treatment of diabetes mellitus in the indigenous system of medicine (1). Oral administration of the extract in graded doses caused a significant increase in enzymatic antioxidants such as catalase, superoxide dismutase, glutathione synthetase, and glutathione peroxidase and in the non-enzymatic antioxidants ascorbic acid, ceruloplasmin and tocopherol. A significant increase in the levels of glycolytic enzymes such as glucose-6-phosphate dehydrogenase, lactate dehydrogenase and hexokinase and a significant decrease in the levels of gluconeogenic enzyme, glucose-6-phosphatase and alanine aminotransferase were also observed in treated diabetic rats (2).

1. Shirwaikar A, K Rajendran, IS Punitha; Anti-diabetic activity of alcoholic stem extract of *Coscinium fenestratum* in streptozotocin-nicotinamide induced type-2 diabetic rats, *J Ethnopharmacol* **97**(2), 369-74 (2005)
2. Punitha ES, K Rajendran, A Shirwaikar, A Shirwaikar; Alcoholic stem extract of *Coscinium fenestratum* regulates carbohydrate metabolism and improves

antioxidant status in streptozotocin-nicotinamide induced diabetic rats, *Evid Based Compliment Alternat Med* **2**(3), 375-81 (2005)

Costus afer Ker Gawl (Costaceae / Zingiberaceae) (Spiral Ginger)

Costus afer is a rhizomitous herb, widespread in tropical Africa. The methanol extract of *C. afer* leaves exhibited a biphasic anti-hyperglycaemic activity. At 200 mg/kg b.w., p.o., it decreased the blood glucose level by 50% in streptozotocin-induced hyperglycaemia in male rats in 60 minutes post dosing. However, doses above 200 mg/kg b.w., p.o., caused increase in blood glucose level, potentiating the action of streptozotocin. At 10 mg/µl, the extract induced about 98% glucose uptake in differentiated 3T3-L1 adipocytes when compared with insulin. Brine shrimp lethality test showed that the extract was significantly cytotoxic.

Anaga AO, CJ Njoku, ES Ekejiuba, MN Esiaka, IU Asuzu; Investigations of the methanolic leaf extract of *Costus afer* Ker for pharmacological activities *in vitro* and *in vivo, Phytomedicine* **11**(2-3), 242-48 (2004).

Crataegus laevigata (Poir.) DC (Rosaceae) (English Hawthorn)

Hawthorn leaves, flowers and berries are used by herbal practitioners in the UK to treat hypertension in conjunction with prescribed drugs. Patients with type-2 diabetes were randomised to daily 1200 mg hawthorn extract or placebo for 16 weeks. A randomised controlled trial demonstrated a hypotensive effect of hawthorn in patients with diabetes taking medication.

Walker AF, G Marakis, E Simpson, JL Hope, PA Robinson, M Hassanein, HC Simpson; Hypotensive effects of hawthorn for patients with diabetes taking prescription drugs: a randomised controlled trial, *Br J Gen Pract* **56**(527), 437-43 (2006)

Croton cajucara Benth. (Euphorbiaceae)

Trans-Dehydrocrotonin, a 19-nor-clerodane diterpene isolated from the bark of *C. cajucara*, demonstrated a significant hypoglycaemic activity in alloxan-induced diabetic rats but not in normal rats, at oral doses of 25 and 50 mg/kg body weight. The drug also effectively lowered the blood sugar levels in glucose fed normal rats. It also significantly reduced streptozotocin-induced increases in blood glucose levels as well as ethanol-induced increases in blood triglycerides. The hypoglycaemic effect of the diterpene was almost comparable to that produced by glibenclamide. The results suggest that *trans*-dehydrocrotonin has an anti-diabetic potential that warrants further research on its mechanism and clinical significance (1, 2).

1. Farias RA, VS Rao, GS Viana, ER Silveira, MA Maciel, AC Pinto; Hypoglycaemic effect of *trans*-dehydrocrotonin, a nor-clerodane diterpene from *Croton cajucara, Planta Med* **63**(6), 558-60 (1997).

2. Silva RM, FA Santos, VS Rao, MA Maciel, AC Pinto; Blood glucose- and triglyceride-lowering effect of trans-dehydrocrotonin, a diterpene from *Croton cajucara* Benth., in rats, *Diabetes Obes Metab* **3**(6), 452-56 (2001).

Cryptolepis sanguinolenta (Lindl.) Schlecter (Asclepiadaceae / Periplocaceae)

The root of the plant is used in traditional African medicine to treat a variety of diseases. The compounds isolated from the plant material showed anti-bacterial, anti-hyperglycaemic, anti-inflammatory, anti-malarial, and anti-viral effects. Using an ethnobotanical approach in combination with a bioactivity-guided fractionation led to the isolation of cryptolepine, an indoloquinoline alkaloid, as an anti-hyperglycaemic component of *C. sanguinolenta*. The hydroiodide, hydrochloride, and hydrotrifluoromethanesulfonate salts of cryptolepine were prepared and a comparison of their *in vitro* activities in a 3T3-L1 glucose transport assay was made. Cryptolepine and its salts were found to lower blood glucose levels in rodent models of type-2 diabetes. The anti-hyperglycaemic effect of cryptolepine leads to a significant decline in plasma insulin concentration, associated with evidence of an enhancement in insulin-mediated glucose disposal. It also increases glucose uptake by 3T3-L1 cells. A series of substituted and hetero-substituted cryptolepine analogues were also synthesized and their anti-hyperglycaemic activity was measured *in vitro* and in an NIDDM mouse model to generate the first structure-bioactivity study about the cryptolepine nucleus (1-3).

1. Bierer DE, DM Fort, CD Mendez, J Luo, PA Imbach, LG Dubenko, SD Jolad, RF Gerber, J Litvak, Q Lu, P Zhang, MJ Reed, N Waldeck, RC Bruening, BK Noamesi, RF Hector, TJ Carlson, SR King; Ethnobotanical-directed discovery of the anti-hyperglycaemic properties of cryptolepine: its isolation from *Cryptolepis sanguinolenta*, synthesis, and *in vitro* and *in vivo* activities, *J Med Chem* 41(6), 894-901 (1998).

2. Bierer DE, GM Reaven; *Cryptolepis sanguinolenta*: an ethnobotanical approach to drug discovery and the isolation of a potentially useful new anti-hyperglycaemic agent, *Diabet Med* **15**(5), 367-74 (1998).

3. Bierer DE, LG Dubenko, P Zhang, Q Lu, PA Imbach, AW Garofalo, PW Phuan, DM Fort, J Litvak, RE Gerber, B Sloan, J Luo, R Cooper, GM Reaven; Anti-hyperglycaemic activities of cryptolepine analogues: an ethnobotanical lead structure isolated from *Cryptolepis sanguinolenta, J Med Chem* **41**(15), 2754-64 (1998).

Cucurbita ficifolia Bouche (Cucurbitaceae) (Malabar squash)

Cucurbita ficifolia is an annual vine grown for its edible seeds, fruit, and greens. Native to Mexico, it is now grown in many parts of Eurasia, from France to India to Japan. It shows considerable biochemical difference from other members of its genus.

Oral administration of a raw extract of *C. ficifolia* to type-2 diabetic patients with moderate hyperglycaemia was followed by a significant decrease in blood glucose levels after 3 h and 5 h. The hypoglycaemic action of the plant extract agrees with its effects previously observed in laboratory animals (1).

Acute hypoglycaemic effects of freeze-dried juice of *C. ficifolia* fruits were studied in healthy and alloxan-induced diabetic mice. *C. ficifolia* fruit juice, administered by intra-peritoneal route, produced a significant decrease of glycaemia in healthy mice in a dose-dependent manner. Administration of *C. ficifolia* fruit juice by oral route also caused significant reductions of blood glucose levels in healthy mice but the effect was minor. The juice administered by intra-peritoneal route showed an acute hypoglycaemic effect in alloxan-diabetic mice. Freeze- dried juice caused acute toxicity when administered intra-peritoneally and also when it was administered daily by the oral route (2, 3).

Oral administration of *C. ficifolia* fruit extract (300 and 600 mg/kg body weight/ day) for 30 days resulted in a significant reduction in blood glucose, glycosylated haemoglobin, and an increase in plasma insulin and total haemoglobin (4).

1. Acosta-Patino JL, E Jimenez-Balderas, MA Juarez-Oropeza, JC Diaz-Zagoya; Hypoglycaemic action of *Cucurbita ficifolia* on Type-2 diabetic patients with moderately high blood glucose levels, *J Ethnopharmacol* 77(1), 99-101 (2001).
2. Alarcon-Aguilar FJ, E HernandezGalicia, AE Campos-Sepulveda, S Xolalpa-Molina, JF Rivas-Vilchis, LI Vazquez-Carrillo, R Roman-Ramos; Evaluation of the hypoglycaemic effect of *Cucurbita ficifolia* Bouche (Cucurbitaceae) in different experimental models, *J Ethnopharmacol* **82**(2-3), 185-89 (2002)
3. Hernandez-Galicia E, AE Campos-Sepulveda, FJ Alarcon-Aguilar, LI Vazquez-Carrillo, JL Flores-Saenz, R Roman-Ramos; Acute toxicological study of *Cucurbita ficifolia* juice in mice, *Proc West Pharmacol Soc* **45**,42-43 (2002)
4. Xia T, Q Wang; Anti-hyperglycaemic effect of *Cucurbita ficifolia* fruit extract in streptozotocin-induced diabetic rats, *Fitoterapia* 77(7-8), 530-33 (2006)

Cucurbita moschata Duchesne ex poir (Cucurbitaceae) (Pumpkin/Squash)

A protein-bound polysaccharide was isolated from the water-soluble fraction of pumpkin fruits by an activity-guided search. The hypoglycaemic activity and the effect on serum insulin levels of this protein-bound polysaccharide were studied in alloxan-induced diabetic rats using different doses. Administration of different doses of this protein bound polysaccharide to diabetic rats reduced the blood glucose level, improved glucose tolerance and increased insulin levels in a dose dependent manner. The effect of a high dose (1000 mg/kg body weight) excelled that of a low dose (500 mg/kg body weight).

Quanhong L, F Caili, R Yukui, H Guanghui, C Tongyi; Effects of protein-bound polysaccharide isolated from pumpkin on insulin in diabetic rats, *Plant Foods Hum Nutr* **60**(1), 13-16 (2005).

Cudrania tricuspidata (Carrière) Bureau ex Lavallée (Moraceae) (Cudrang, Chinese mulberry)

Cudrania tricuspidata is a tree, occasionally grown for its fruits, somewhat similar to that of mulberry. Methanol extract of *C. tricuspidata* root bark, at a dose of 1000 mg/kg, showed significant blood glucose lowering effect in alloxan-induced hyperglycaemic rats. It also showed potent inhibitory effect on bovine lens aldose reductase.

Park WY, JS Ro, KS Lee; Hypoglycaemic effect of *Cudrania tricuspidata* root bark, *Korean J Pharmacogn* **32**(3), 248-52 (2001)

Cuminum cyminum Linn. (Apiaceae) (Cumin seed, H. Jeera, S. Jeerak)

It is an annual herb, native from the Mediterranean to India. The seed-like fruit of this plant is used for seasoning, as in curry. Orally administered seed powder of *C. cyminum* lowered the blood glucose levels in hyperglycaemic rabbits (1).

The hypoglycaemic activity of cumin oil, the steam volatile fraction of petroleum ether (60-80°) extract of cumin seeds, and of cuminaldehyde, isolated from cumin oil, were studied in normal, glucose-induced hyperglycaemic, and streptozotocin-induced diabetic rats. Both the oil and cuminaldehyde lowered the fasting plasma glucose levels with corresponding increase in circulating insulin levels. However, the blood glucose lowering response was not significant in streptozotocin-induced diabetic rats. Cuminaldehyde also improved glucose tolerance test by increasing insulin secretory response. From the results of investigation, it was suggested that cuminaldehyde is a potential anti-diabetic compound, which might be acting by increasing insulin secretion from the islet of Langerhans, particularly in patients with NIDDM. The compound was found to be more potent than tolbutamide (2).

Cuminaldehyde, derived from *C. cyminum* seed oil, was found to be a potent inhibitor of aldose reductase and *alpha*-glucosidase. The inhibitory activities were compared with quercitrin, an aldose reductase inhibitor and acarbose, an *alpha*-glucosidase inhibitor. The study showed that cuminaldehyde was about 1.8 times less active than acarbose and 1.6 times less active than quercitrin (3).

1. Jain SC, M Purohit, R Jain; Pharmacological evaluation of *Cuminum cyminum*, *Fitoterapia* **63**(4), 291-94 (1992)
2. Kalia AN, Harbans Lal; Hypoglycaemic and insulin release effects of cuminaldehyde: A new hypoglycaemic natural compound from cumin oil, *J Sci Pharm* **6**(2), 45-47 (1995)
3. Lee HS; Cuminaldehyde: Aldose reductase and *alpha*-glucosidase inhibitor derived from *Cuminum cyminum* L. seeds, *J Agric Food Chem* **53**(7), 2446-50 (2005)

Cuminum nigrum Linn. (Apiaceae)

The effects of oral administration of various doses of *C. nigrum* seeds and their extracts on blood glucose and total lipid levels were studied in normal and alloxan-treated diabetic rabbits. Oral administration of 1, 2, 3 and 4 g/kg of seeds was found to produce a significant hypoglycaemic effect in normal as well as in diabetic rabbits. The aqueous and methanol extracts of seeds showed similar activity. However, the total blood lipids were not influenced by *C. nigrum* seeds or extracts in either normal or diabetic rabbits (1). The total flavonoids of *C. nigrum* seeds caused a hypoglycaemic effect at a dose range of 0.5 to 1.5 g/kg, both in normal and alloxan-diabetic rabbits. The hypoglycaemic effect started 2 h after drug administration, reached a maximum within 4-8 h and the blood glucose levels returned close to normal within 24 h of drug administration. The alkaloid fraction, isolated from *C. nigrum* seeds, however, failed to exert any significant hypoglycaemic effect in either normal or diabetic rabbits (2).

1. Akhtar MS, MR Ali; Study of hypoglycaemic activity of *Cuminum nigrum* seeds in normal and alloxan diabetic rabbits, *Planta Med* (2), 81-85 (1985)
2. Ahmad M, MS Akhtar, T Malik, AH Gilani; Hypoglycaemic action of the flavonoid fraction of *Cuminum nigrum* seeds, *Phytother Res* **14**(2), 103-06 (2000)

Curcuma longa Linn. (Zingiberaceae) (Turmeric, H. Haldi, S. Haridra)

Turmeric (*C. longa*) is a rhizomatous perennial plant of the ginger family, which is native to tropical South Asia. The rhizome of turmeric has long been used in traditional Asian medicine to treat a variety of ailments. Sangli, a town in Maharashtra, India, is the largest and most important trading centre for turmeric in Asia or perhaps in the entire world.

Adminstration (ip) of an aqueous alcoholic extract of *C. longa* (10 mg) decreased the blood glucose level of normal mice and more significantly of streptozotocin-induced diabetic mice (1). The extract also showed blood glucose lowering activity in alloxan-induced diabetic rats (2).

The lower rate of weight gain by diabetic rats in comparison to non-diabetic ones was normalised by oral administration of aqueous extract of turmeric (1g/kg b.w.) or its active constituent, curcumin (0.08g/kg b.w.) for a period of 3 weeks. Treatment of diabetic rats with turmeric extract or curcumin drastically reduced glucose-6-phosphatase and increased the activity of liver and serum hexokinase, lactate dehydrogenase and glucose-6-phosphate dehydrogenase. A decrease in the cellular leakage of acid phosphatase, alkaline phosphatase and lactate dehydrogenase into the serum of diabetic animals was also observed. Curcumin was obviously more effective than turmeric extract (3).

The effects of turmeric and of its active principle, curcumin on alloxan-induced diabetic rats were studied. Administration of turmeric or curcumin to diabetic rats reduced the blood sugar, haemoglobin and glycosylated haemoglobin levels significantly. Turmeric and curcumin also reduced the oxidative stress encountered by diabetic rats, as was evident from lower levels of TBARS (thiobarbituric acid reactive substances). This effect is surmised to be due to the decreased influx of glucose into the polyol pathway leading to an increased NADPH/NADP ratio and increased activity of the potent antioxidant enzyme, glutathione peroxidase. Also, the activity of sorbitol dehydrogenase, which catalyses the conversion of sorbitol to fructose, was significantly lowered by treatment with turmeric or curcumin (4).

Turmeric has a wide range of effect on human health. Curcuminoids and sesquiterpenoids, present in turmeric, are known to have anti-oxidative, anti-carcinogenic, and anti-inflammatory activities. The effects of different turmeric extracts on blood glucose levels were studied in 6 weeks old type-2 diabetic KK-A(y) mice. Both curcuminoids and sesquiterpenoids in turmeric were found to exhibit hypoglycaemic effects *via* peroxisome proliferator-activated receptor (PPAR)-*gamma* activation as one of the mechanisms. Ethanol extract containing both curcuminoids and sesquiterpenoids showed additive or synergistic effects of both components (5). Ethanol extract of turmeric, which contains curcumin, demethoxycurcumin, bisdemethoxycurcumin, and ar-turmerone as its main constituents, significantly suppressed an increase in blood glucose level in type-2 diabetic KK-A(y) mice. In an *in vitro* evaluation, the extract stimulated human adipocyte differentiation in a dose-dependent manner and showed human peroxisome proliferator-activated receptor (PPAR)-*gamma* ligand-binding activity in a GAL4-PPAR-*gamma* chimera assay. The major constituents of the extract mainly contribute to the effects *via* PPAR-*gamma* activation (6).

The effect of turmeric and curcumin on streptozotocin-induced diabetic cataract was studied in rats and it was observed that these supplements delayed the progression and maturation of cataract. The study also revealed that curcumin and turmeric treatment countered the hyperglycaemia-induced oxidative stress, as was manifest from a reversal of changes with respect to lipid peroxidation, reduced glutathione, protein carbonyl content and activities of antioxidant enzymes in a significant manner (7).

Turmeric oleoresin, an extract of turmeric, contains both curcuminoids and turmeric essential oil. The effect of turmeric oleoresin on hepatic gene expression was comprehensively assessed in obese diabetic KK-Ay mice using DNA microarray analysis and quantitative real-time polymerase chain reaction (PCR). Ingestion of turmeric oleoresin inhibited the development of increased blood glucose and abdominal fat mass, while curcuminoids only inhibited the increase in blood glucose. DNA microarray analysis indicated that turmeric oleoresin ingestion up-regulated the expression of genes related to glycolysis, *beta*-oxidation, and cholesterol metabolism in the liver of KK-Ay mice, while expression of gluconeogenesis-related genes was down-regulated. These changes in gene expression were considered to be the mechanism by which the turmeric oleoresin affected the control of both blood glucose levels and abdominal adipose tissue masses (8).

Tetrahydrocurcumin is a major colourless metabolite of curcumin and it also possesses anti-diabetic, anti-inflammatory and antioxidant activity. Oral administration of tetrahydrocurcumin to diabetic rats showed a decrease in the level of blood glucose and plasma glycoproteins. The levels of plasma insulin and tissue sialic acid were increased whereas the levels of tissue hexose, hexosamine and fucose were near normal in diabetic rats treated with tetrahydrocurcumin. The study indicates that tetrahydrocurcumin possesses a significant beneficial effect on glycoprotein moiety in addition to its anti-diabetic effect (9).

1. Tank R, N Sharma, VP Dixit; Hypoglycaemic .activity of *Curcuma longa* (50% EtOH) extract on streptozotocin induced diabetic mice, *Indian Zoologist* **12**(3-4), 321-22 (1988).

2. Tank R, N Sharma, T Sharma, VP Dixit; Anti-diabetic activity of *Curcuma longa* (50 per cent EtOH Extr.) in alloxan-induced diabetic rats, *Indian Drugs,* **27**(11), 587-89 (1990).

3. NarayannasamyA, N Namasivayam, K Radha; Effect of turmeric on the enzymes of glucose metabolism in diabetic rats, *J Herbs, Spices, Med Plants* **10**(1), 75-84 (2002)

4. Arun N, N Nalini; Efficacy of turmeric on blood sugar and polyol pathway in diabetic albino rats, *Plant Foods Hum Nutr* **57**(1), 141-50 (2002)

5. Nishiyama T, T Mac, H Kishida, M Tsukagawa, Y Mimaki, M Kuroda, Y Sashida, K Takahashi, T Kawada, K Nakagawa, M Kitahara; Curcuminoids and sesquiterpenoids in turmeric (*Curcuma longa* L.) suppress an increase in blood glucose level in type-2 diabetic KK-Ay mice, *J Agric Food Chem* **53**(4), 959-63 (2005).

6. Kuroda M, Y Mimaki, T Nishiyama, T Mae, H Kishida, M Tsukagawa, K Takahashi, T Kawada, K Nakagawa, M Kitahara; Hypoglycaemic effects of

turmeric (*Curcuma longa* L. rhizomes) on genetically diabetic KK-Ay mice, *Biol Pharm Bull* **28**(5), 937-39 (2005)

7. Suryanarayana P, M Saraswat, T Mrudula, TP Krishna, K Krishnaswamy, GB Reddy; Curcumin and turmeric delay streptozotocin-induced diabetic cataract in rats, *Invest Ophthalmol Vis Sci* **46**(6), 2092-99 (2005)
8. Honda S, F Aoki, H Tanaka, H Kishida, T Nishiyama, S Okada, I Matsumoto, K Abe, T Mae; Effects of ingested turmeric oleoresin on glucose and lipid metabolisms in obese diabetic mice: a DNA microarray study, *J Agric Food Chem* **54**(24), 9055-62 (2006)
9. Pari L, P Murugan; Changes in glycoprotein components in streptozotocin–nicotinamide induced type-2 diabetes: influence of tetrahydrocurcumin from *Curcuma longa, Plant Foods Hum Nutr* **62**(1), 25-29 (2007)

Cyamopsis tetragonoloba (L.) Taub. (Fabaceae)
(Cluster bean, Guar, H. Gowar, Babachi)

The guar plant grows primarily in Pakistan and the northern regions of India, where it is grown principally for its green fodder and for the pods that are used for food and feed. It is known as "cluster bean" because of the manner in which its pods are clustered together. The primary importance of guar is the commercial value of its seed gum (galactomannan gum), which has a wide variety of food and medicinal uses. Guar gum can best be described as a natural food thickener, similar to corn starch or tapioca flour.

The hypoglycaemic effect of an aqueous extract of fruits and seeds of *C. tetragonoloba* was tested in healthy fasting, glucose fed, and alloxan-induced diabetic rabbits, the extract being administered by gastric intubation. The extract showed significant hypoglycaemic effect in normal rabbits. It also exhibited an activity similar to tolbutamide in glucose tolerance test. It showed hypoglycaemic effect in alloxan-induced diabetic rabbits only at a higher dose. The involvement of an extra-pancreatic site rather than pancreatic *beta*-cell stimulation has been considered to be the mechanism of action (1). The effect of feeding an aqueous extract of beans of *C. tetragonoloba* was investigated on fasting blood glucose levels in glucose-loaded, normal and alloxan-induced diabetic rats and compared with gliclazide. The aqueous extract of beans at 250 mg/kg body weight significantly lowered blood glucose levels in alloxan-induced diabetic rats within 3 hr of administration. Continued administration of the extract at the same dose daily for 10 days produced statistically significant reduction in the blood glucose levels while marginal activity was seen in normal and glucose-loaded rats (16). Rats fed on whole seed of *C. tetragonoloba* (Guar) showed significant reduction in the serum cholesterol and blood sugar levels. While petroleum ether extract of guar was found to increase blood sugar levels, defatted seed meal was both hypocholesterolemic and hypoglycaemic (2). When normal and alloxan-induced diabetic guinea pigs were kept on the whole seed diet of 'Guar' for four weeks, blood sugar and total lipid levels were found to be decreased significantly in normal as well as in diabetic animals. Free and esterified cholesterol levels were also observed to be lowered significantly in normal animals, whereas esterified fraction alone was found to be lowered in diabetics. Significant fall in the levels of triglycerides, phospholipids and total lipids was also noticed (7). Exposure of normal rats to fructose-containing drinking water represents a current model of insulin resistance. The effect of diet supplementation with guar upon the metabolic consequences of exposure to exogenous fructose was assessed. For this purpose, the changes in body weight, plasma D-glucose and insulin concentrations, and D-glucose infusion rate during a hyperinsulinemic-euglycaemic clamp were measured after 65 days exposure to exogenous fructose and guar-enriched diet. The results of the detailed investigation indicated that guar opposed the effect of exogenous fructose on glucose homeostasis (18).

In order to study the effect of guar granules on glycaemic control and lipid levels, 20 diabetic patients (12 non-insulin treated and 8 insulin-treated) were given guar granules (10 g daily) for two months. The treatment significantly lowered the level of glycosylated haemoglobin (HbA1c) without any significant change in the levels of lipid, fasting blood glucose, 1 h postprandial blood glucose after a test meal and 24 h urinary glucose excretion (6). The effects of guar granules (Guarem, Rybar Laboratories, Amersham, Bucks) sprinkled over food on carbohydrate and lipid metabolism were studied in a double blind crossover trial in 18 patients with non-insulin-dependent diabetes mellitus without changing diabetic treatment during the study. Guar ingestion reduced postprandial insulin and significantly reduced enteroglucagon responses. The treatment had, however, no apparent effect on gastric inhibitory polypeptide, pancreatic glucagon, gastrin, and pancreatic polypeptide (9)

The activity of guar seeds is considered to be due to its gum, which contains about 75% soluble fibre. Statistically significant and sustained reductions in the levels of blood sugar and glycosylated haemoglobin (HbA1) were observed in diabetic patients (both IDDM and NIDDM), receiving a single daily dose (5g) of guar gum for 32 weeks (8). Guar gum, obtained from the endosperm of *C. tetragonoloba* was found to exhibit hypoglycaemic and hypocholesteolaemic activity. Botany, chemistry, pharmacology and toxicology of guar gum have been reviewed (10)

Administration of petroleum ether extract of guar gum (200 mg/kg, p.o.) reduced hyperglycaemia, induced by a single i.v. injection of streptozotocin (65 mg/kg) in male albino rats. The extract also exhibited hypocholesterolaemic activity (11, 14). The effects of guar gum on food intake, levels of serum cholesterol, triacylglycerols, glucose and LDL and HDL-cholesterol were studied. Diets containing 0%, 10% and 20% (w/w) guar gum or 10% and 20% cellulose powder (reference) were fed to normal rats for 60 days. The rats fed the guar gum diets showed significantly lower levels of serum cholesterol, triacylglycerols, reduced food intake and body weight gain. A concomitant increase in HDL-cholesterol with a substantial elevation of the HDL/LDL cholesterol ratio was also noted. Guar gum decreased blood serum glucose only during the first month of the experiment (13).

Postprandial hypotension occurs frequently in diabetes; the fall in blood pressure is greatest after ingestion of carbohydrate, particularly glucose. Investigation was carried out to determine whether slowing of gastric emptying by guar gum reduces the fall in blood pressure after oral glucose in patients with type-2 diabetes. From the results of the investigation, it was concluded that guar gum attenuates the fall in blood pressure after oral glucose in patients with type-2 diabetes mellitus, presumably by slowing glucose absorption (15). The short-term and long-term effects of guar gum on plasma insulin and glucagon-like peptide 1 concentration were studied in healthy rats. In the short-term experiments, concomitant intragastric administration of glucose and guar reduced the early increment in plasma glucose, insulin and glucagon-like peptide 1 concentration otherwise induced by glucose alone. Long term intake of guar gum was found to improve glucose tolerance and insulin response to glucose absorption, without improving insulin sensitivity, in healthy rats (17).

A new guar gum-containing wheat-flake product was developed and its effect on carbohydrate tolerance was assessed in healthy subjects having normal-weight. The extruded wheat-flake breakfast cereals containing 0 (control) or approximately 90 g guar gum/kg wheat-flake product were fed to ten fasting, healthy subjects using a repeated measures design. The meals were similar in energy, available carbohydrate, protein and fat content. Significant reductions in postprandial glucose and insulin responses were seen following the guar wheat-flake meal compared with the control meal. The study revealed that the use of a severe method of heat extrusion to produce guar wheat-flakes does not diminish the physiological activity of the guar gum (12).

Even the guar by-product, the fraction left after removal of guar gum, was found to possess hypoglycaemic properties. A de-gummed fraction of *C. tetragonoloba*, fed to normal and induced diabetic rats, showed significant hypoglycaemic activity in both cases (3). One percent guar by-product suspensions, administered immediately before a glucose challenge (1 g/kg body weight), caused a 31% reduction in the integrated plasma glucose response area during a 180 min test. Ten percent guar by-product caused a similar reduction in plasma glucose during a 360-minute test. Ten percent oat bran and 10% soy bran had no effect upon plasma glucose responses. The study demonstrated the ability of guar by-product suspensions to significantly reduce plasma glucose after carbohydrate challenge. Because of the different chemical characteristics of these two guar bean fractions, it seems that their hypoglycaemic properties are probably due to different mechanisms (4, 5).

1. Pillai NR, C Seshadri, G Santhakumari; Hypoglycaemic effect of *Cyamopsis tetragonoloba, Indian J Med Res* **72**(July), 128-31 (1980)

2. Joshi LD, PC Singhal, RK Gupta; Change in serum cholesterol and blood sugar levels on feeding with *Cyamopsis tetragonoloba* (Guar) and its solvent extracts, *Curr Sci* **51**(21), 1037-39 (1982)
3. Joshi LD, PC Singhal, RK Gupta; Effect of de-gummed fraction of *Cyamopsis tetragonoloba* (Guar) on blood sugar, *Indian J Pharm Sci* **44**(5), 115-16 (1982).
4. Chiu SS, NS Track; Guar by-product improves carbohydrate tolerance in rats, *Metabolism* **34**(5), 481-85 (1985)
5. Track NS, VW Lai, SS Chiu; Guar by-product improves carbohydrate tolerance in healthy human subjects, *Diabetes Res Clin Pract* **1**(2), 115-19 (1985)
6. Jones DB, S Lousley, R Jelfs, P Slaughter, RD Carter JI Mann; Low-dose guar improves diabetic control, *J Royal Soc Med* **78**(7), 546-48 (1985).
7. Srivastava A, GS Longia, SP Singh, LD Joshi; Hypoglycaemic and hypolipaemic effects of *Cyamopsis tetragonoloba* (guar) in normal and diabetic guinea pigs, *Indian J Physiol Pharmacol* **31**(2), 77-83 (1987).
8. Gupta A, V Singh; Diabetic glucose control on long term guar gum therapy, *J Diabetic Assoc India* **29**(2), 58-62 (1989)
9. Fuessl HS, G Williams, TF Adrian, SR Bloom; Guar sprinkled on food: Effect on glycaemic control, plasma lipids and gut hormones in non-insulin dependent diabetic patients, *Diabet Med* **4**(5), 463-68 (1987)
10. Guar gum: A monograph, *Lawrence Review of Natural Products,* **November,** 1-2 (1990)
11. Bhandari U, JN Sharma; Comparison of hypolipidaemic and hypoglycaemic activities of *Cyamopsis tetragonoloba* (Guar gum) and *Zingiber officinale* (ginger) in experimental animals, *Int Conf Curr Prog Med Aromat Pl Res* p.133, Dec 30, 1994—Jan 1, 1995, Calcutta, India
12. Fairchild RM, PR Ellis, AJ Byrne, SD Luzio, MA Mir; A new breakfast cereal containing guar gum reduces postprandial plasma glucose and insulin concentrations in normal-weight human subjects, *Br J Nutr* **76**(1), 63-73 (1996)
13. Frias AC, VC Sgarbieri; Guar gum effects on food intake, blood serum lipids, and glucose levels of Wister rats, *Plant Foods Hum Nutr* **53**(1), 15-28 (1998)
14. Bhandari U, JN Sharma; Effect of petroleum ether extract of guar gum in streptozotocin-induced hyperglycaemic rats, *Pharmaceut Biol* **37**(3), 248-50 (1999)
15. Russo A, JE Stevens, T Wilson, F Wells, A Tonkin, M Horowitz, KL Jones; Guar attenuates fall in postprandial blood pressure and slows gastric emptying of oral glucose in type-2 diabetes, *Dig Dis Sci* **48**(7), 1221-29 (2003).
16. Mukhtar HM, SH Ansari, M Ali, ZA Bhat, T Naved; Effect of aqueous extract of *Cyamopsis tetragonoloba* Linn. beans on blood glucose level in normal and alloxan-induced diabetic rats, *Indian J Exp Biol* **42**(12), 1212-15 (2004)
17. Prieto PG, J Cancelas, ML Villanueva-Penacarrillo, WJ Malaisse, I Valverde;

Short-term and long-term effects of guar on postprandial plasma glucose, insulin and glucagon-like peptide 1 concentration in healthy rats, *Horm Metab Res* **38**(6), 397-404 (2006)

18. Prieto PG, J Cancelas, P Moreno, ML Villanueva-Penacarrillo, WJ Malaisse, I Valverde; Effects of diet supplementation with olive oil and guar upon fructose-induced insulin resistance in normal rats, *Endocrine* **31**(3), 294-99 (2007)

Cyclocarya paliurus (Batalin) Iljinsk. (Juglandaceae) (Wheel Wingnut)

Cyclocarya is a genus in the walnut family and its fruits have a circular wing around. It is native to eastern and central China. *Cyclocarya paliurus* is rich in a polysaccharide complex. This polysaccharide complex was found to have obvious blood sugar reducing activity with the capability of improving glucose tolerance in diabetic mice (1).

The blood glucose levels of sucrose-loaded animals were found to be significantly lower in the *C. paliurus* extract-treated group than in the control group. This difference was, however, not observed following the administration of glucose. The chronological change in the level of blood glucose in genetically hyperglycaemic obese KK-Ay mice was significantly lower when *C. paliurus* extract was administered daily for three weeks. An *in vitro* study showed that *C. paliurus* inhibits *alpha*-glucosidase, a disaccharide-degrading enzyme in the small intestinal mucosa, leading to a decrease in the absorption of glucose into the blood and a subsequent lowering of the blood glucose level (2)

1. Li L, M Xie, X Yi; Study on reducing blood sugar of polysaccharide from *Cyclocarya paliurus* (Batal) Iljins, *Zhong Yao Cai* **25**(1), 39-41 (2002) [Article in Chinese].
2. Kurihara H, H Fukami, A Kusumoto, Y Toyoda, H Shibata, Y Matsui, S Asami, T Tanaka; Hypoglycaemic action of *Cyclocarya paliurus* (Batal.) Iljinskaja in normal and diabetic mice, *Biosci Biotechnol Biochem* **67**(4), 877-80 (2003).

Cyperus rotundus L. (Cyperaceae) (Coco-grass)

Cyperus rotundus is a perennial plant that is often known by "nut grass" and "nut sedge". This is because of its tubers, which somewhat resemble nuts. Oral administration of an aqueous alcoholic extract of *Cyperus rotundus* (500 mg/kg, once a day for seven consecutive days) significantly lowered the blood glucose levels of alloxan-induced diabetic rats. This anti-hyperglycaemic activity can be attributed to its antioxidant activity as it showed a strong radical scavenging action *in vitro.*

Rant NA, NJ Gaikwad; Anti-diabetic activity of hydro-ethanolic extract of *Cyperus rotundus* in alloxan induced diabetes in rats, *Fitoterapia* **77**(7-8), 585-88 (2006)

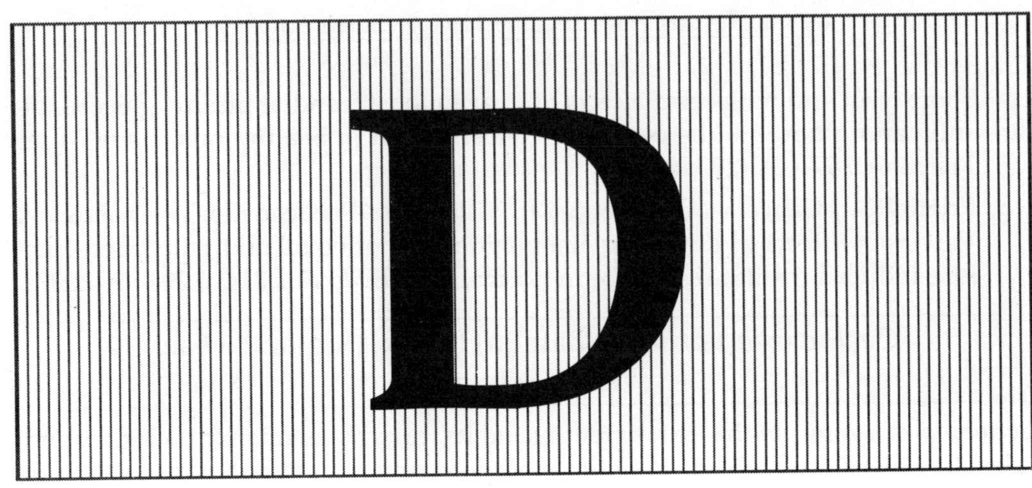

Daemia extensa (Jacq.) R.Br. (Asclepiadaceae)
(H. Sagovani, S. Karambha)

D. extensa is commonly used as a substitute for the potent anti-diabetic herb, *Gymnema sylvestre* by the folks of Sheveroy hills of Tamilnadu, India. It was, therefore, felt necessary to evaluate the anti-diabetic efficacy of this plant and preliminary investigation on alloxanised albino rats confirmed anti-diabetic activity of its ethanol extract (1). The anti-diabetic activity of alcoholic and aqueous extracts of *Daemia extensa* was evaluated using alloxan-induced diabetic rats. Administration of a single dose of alcoholic extract to diabetic rats caused a significant reduction of the blood glucose level after one hour and this level was maintained up to three hours. Its chronic administration for one week also resulted in a fall in the blood sugar level, the maximum effect being on second day. Reduction in blood sugar levels was comparable to a reference drug, chlorpropamide (2).

1. Ravi J, AK Wahi; Anti-diabetic studies of *Daemia extensa, Int Seminar on Recent Trends in Pharmaceutical Sciences,* Ootacamund, India, Abstr. No **E38,** February 18-20, 1995
2. Wahi AK, J Ravi, S Hemalatha, PN Singh; Anti-diabetic activity of *Daemia extensa* R.Br, *J Nat Remedies,* **2**(1), 80- 83(2002).

Datura metel Linn. (Solanaceae)
(Thorn-apple, H. Dhatura)

Datura metel is a shrub-like annual herb with large flowers. Native to China, India and South East Asia, it is now used in landscaping and gardening even in North America. The plant may be toxic, if ingested in any quantity, and tropane alkaloids are principal toxic elements. It is one of the 50 fundamental herbs used in traditional Chinese medicine,

Graded doses (25, 50 and 75 mg/kg, p.o.) of the seed powder of *D. metel*, given to both normal and alloxan-induced diabetic rats, produced significant reduction in blood glucose at the 8 h. The effect was found to be dose dependent.

Krishna Murthy B, S Nammi, MK Kota, RV Krishna Rao, N Koteswara Rao, A Annapurna; Evaluation of hypoglycaemic and anti-hyperglycaemic effects of *Datura metel* (Linn.) seeds in normal and alloxan-induced diabetic rats, *J Ethnopharmacol* **91**(1), 95-98 (2004).

Dendrobium candidum Wall. Ex Lindl (Orchidaceae / Ericaceae)

The anti-hyperglycaemic effect of *D. candidum* was studied and its mechanism of action was postulated. The plant drug failed to decrease the serum glucose concentration in normal mice but could increase serum insulin levels and decrease serum glucagon concentrations in streptozotocin-induced diabetic rats. The results of immunohistochemical study demonstrated that the number of islet *beta*-cells was increased and that of islet *alpha*-cells was decreased in streptozotocin-induced diabetic rats. The plant drug was suggested to stimulate the secretion of insulin from *beta*-cells and inhibit the secretion of glucagons from *alpha*-cells.

Wu HS, JH Xu, LZ Chen, JJ Sun; Studies on anti-hyperglycaemic effect of *Dendrobium candidum* and its mechanism *Zhongguo Zhong Yao Za Zhi* **29**(2), 160-63 (2004) [Article in Chinese].

Dioscorea dumetorum (Kunth) Pax (Dioscoreaceae) (Bitter yam)

Dioscorea is a genus of hundreds of species of flowering plants, native throughout the tropical and warm temperate regions of the world. Most of these species are tuberous herbaceous perennial woody vines. Yam is the common name for some of these species, which are cultivated for the consumption of their starchy tubers in Africa, Asia, Latin America and Ocenia. Yams are not sweet potatoes, but are used in a fashion similar to potatoes and sweet potatoes.

The aqueous alcoholic extract of the tubers of *D. dumetorum* was fractionated and the alkaloid-containing fraction was found to be hyperglycaemic in fasting normal mice but the whole extract and the fractions containing steroidal derivatives evinced significant hypoglycaemic activities in fasting normal mice or rabbits and in fasting alloxan-diabetic rabbits. The hypoglycaemic action of the glycosidic portion, in particular, was prompt and potent, in normal as well as in alloxan-diabetic rabbits (1). Dioscoretine, isolated from the aqueous fraction of the methanol extract of *D. dumetorum* tubers, was found to produce significant hypoglycaemic effects at a dose of 20 mg/kg when administered intraperitoneally to normal and alloxan-induced diabetic rabbits. The fasting blood sugar in normoglycaemic rabbits was reduced after 4 hours. In alloxan diabetic rabbits, the blood sugar was lowered at the same time interval. The acute toxicity studies gave LD_{50} values of 1.4 g/kg for the aqueous extract and 0.58 g/kg for dioscoretine when tested on mice. The hypoglycaemic effects were compared to those of tolbutamide (2, 3).

1. Undie AS, PI Akubue; Pharmacological evaluation of *Dioscorea dumetorum* tuber used in traditional anti-diabetic therapy, *J Ethnopharmacol* **15**(2), 135-44 (1986).
2. Iwu MM, CO Okunji, P Akah, MS Tempesta, D Corley; Dioscoretine: the hypoglycaemic principle of *Dioscorea dumetorum*, *Planta Med* 56(1), 119-20 (1990).
3. Iwu MM, CO Okunji, GO Ohiaeri, P Akah, D Corley, MS Tempesta; Hypoglycaemic activity of dioscoretine from tubers of *Dioscorea dumetorum* in normal and alloxan diabetic rabbits, *Planta Med* 56(3), 264-67 (1990).

Dioscorea japonica Thunb (Dioscoreaceae) (Japanese Yam)

See glycans in Appendix: Hikino *et al*; *Planta Med* No. 3, 168-71 (1986)

Dioscorea opposita Thunb (Dioscoreaceae) (Chinese wild yam)

D. opposita extract reduced significantly the blood insulin and glucose levels in dexamethasone-induced diabetic rats. *In vitro*, the extract significantly enhanced insulin-stimulated glucose uptake in 3T3-L1 adipocytes. It also increased the mRNA expression of GLUT-4 in 3T3-L1 adipocytes.

Gao X, B Li, H Jiang, F Liu, D Xu, Z Liu; *Dioscorea opposita* reverses dexamethasone induced insulin resistance, *Fitoterapia* **78**(1), 12-15 (2007)

Dolichos biflorus (Linn.) (Fabaceae / Leguminosae) (Horse gram, S. Kulattha)

Dolichos biflorus seed diets showed blood sugar and total cholesterol lowering effect in normal fasting albino rats (1). A high fat diet is known to induce oxidative stress in the cells by producing reactive oxygen species. Elevated levels of TBARS in liver, heart, and aorta in high fat diet-fed rabbits are a clear manifestation of excessive formation of free radical and activation of lipid peroxidation. The significant decline in the level of TBARS, in rabbits administered with *D.biflorus* (200 and 400 mg/kg b.w.) unveils the antioxidant potential of the plant extract. From the results of detailed investigation it was concluded that administration of *D .biflorus* manifests a protective action against high fat diet-induced oxidative stress in different tissues in rabbits (2).

1. Pant MC, I Uddin, UR Bhardwaj, RD Tewari; Blood sugar and total cholesterol lowering effect of *Glycine soja* (Sieb and Zucc.), *Mucuna pruriens* (D.C.) and *Dolichos biflorus* (Linn.) seed diets in normal fasting albino rats, *Indian J Med Res.* **56**(12):1808-12 (1968)

2. Kottai Muthu A, S. Sethupathy, R. Manavalan, P.K. Karar, Antioxidant potential of methanolic extract of *Dolichos biflorus* Linn. In high fat diet fed rats, *Indian J Pharmacol* **38** (2), 131-32 (2006)

Dorstenia psilurus Welw. (Moraceae / Cyperaceae)

Dorstenia psilurus is common in Central Africa, and is found in Angola, Cameroon, Tanzania and Uganda, growing in well drained peat. The effects of methanol/ methylene chloride extract of *D. psilurus* (100 and 200 mg/kg/day for 3 weeks) on systolic blood pressure, plasma glucose, insulin, cholesterol, triglycerides and creatinine were studied in male Wistar rats with fructose-rich diet induced hypertension. Treatment with *D. psilurus*-extract lowered systolic blood pressure of rats, raised by fructose-diet. Plasma insulin, cholesterol and triglycerides were higher in the fructose-rich diet fed rats compared with the controls, receiving standard chow. However, plasma insulin and cholesterol levels were lowered by treatment with *D. psilurus*-extract. These results suggested that treatment with *D. psilurus*-extract could prevent and reverse high blood pressure, induced by a diet rich in fructose, probably by improvement of plasma insulin levels (1). Antiradical activity (2) and antioxidant potential (3) of the plant extract have also been reported.

1. Dimo T, A Rakotonirina, PV Tan, E Dongo, AB Dongmo, P Kamtchouing, J Azay, BM Abegaz, G Cros, TB Nagadjui; Anti-hypertensive effects of *Dorstenia psilurus* extract in fructose-fed hyperinsulinemic, hypertensive rats, *Phytomedicine* **8**(2), 101-06 (2001)
2. Kansci, G., E. Dongo, C. Genot, 2,2-Diphenyl-1-picrylhydrazyl (DPPH*) test demonstrates antiradical activity of *Dorstenia psilurus* and *Dorstenia ciliata* plant extracts. *Nahrung* **47**(6), 434-37 (2003)
3. Atawodi SE, Antioxidant potential of African medicinal plants, *African J Biotech* **4**(2), 128-33 (2005)

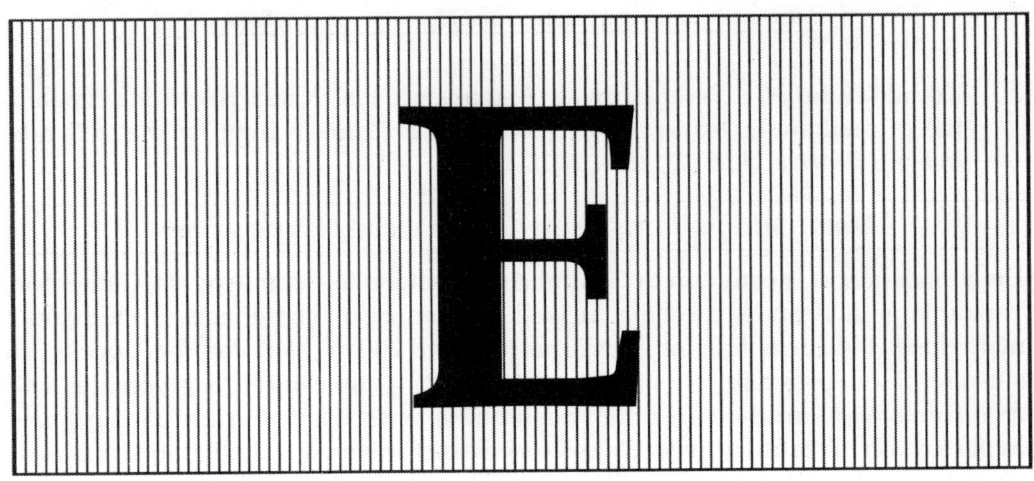

Eclipta alba (L) Hassk. (Asteraceae)
(False Daisy, H. Bhringraj)

Eclipta alba is widely distributed throughout India, China, Thailand, and Brazil. The plant finds various uses in Ayurveda. *Eclipta alba* has a folk reputation in rural South India as a hypoglycaemic agent. Oral administration of a leaf suspension of *E. alba* (2 and 4 g/kg b.w.) to alloxan-induced diabetic rats for 60 days resulted in a significant reduction in blood glucose, glycosylated haemoglobin, a decrease in the activities of glucose-6 phosphatase and fructose 1,6-bisphosphatase, and an increase in the activity of liver hexokinase. A lower dose (2 gm/kg b.w.) was found to be relatively more effective than a higher dose (4 g/kg b.w.) in decreasing blood sugar levels. Oral administration of *E. alba* was thus proved to possess potent anti-hyperglycaemic activity.

Ananthi J, A Prakasam, KV Pugalendi; Anti-hyperglycaemic activity of *Eclipta alba* leaf on alloxan-induced diabetic rats, *Yale J Biol Med* **76**(3), 97-102 (2003).

Elaeodendron glaucum Pers. (Celastraceae)

The bark powder of *E. glaucum* as well as its alcoholic extract exhibited significant hypoglycaemic activity in both normal and alloxan-induced diabetic rats (1, 2)

1. Jain VC, PS Gandhi, DR Shah; Evaluation of bark of *Elaeodendron glaucum* Pers, for hypoglycaemic activity, *National convention on Current Trends in Herbal Drugs & Annual Conference of Indian Soc Pharmacogn, Herb: The National Alternative* , Gandhinagar, Gujrat,, India, **A04**, January 17-18, 2003
2. Prajapati A, AK Singhal, VK Dixit; Investigation of hypoglycaemic activity of bark of *Elaeodendron glaucum* Pers, *National convention on Current Trends in Herbal Drugs & Annual Conference of Indian Soc Pharmacogn , Herb: The National Alternative* , Gandhinagar, Gujrat,, India **A06**, January 17-18, 2003

Elaeophorbia drupifera Thonn. Stapf (Euphorbiaceae)

E. drupifera is dioecious, that is, it has male and female plants. The latex of this species is dangerous. It has been used to remove warts, and can cause blindness, if it reaches the eyes.

Administration of crude leaf extract of *E, drupifera* (20 mg/kg p.o.), two hours before giving glucose or adrenaline, significantly reduced the blood sugar levels by 34% and 35%, respectively. However, when the extract was given 24 hrs after glucose or adrenaline administration the blood sugar levels decreased by 52% and 29%, respectively. The extract was found to be comparatively more effective in lowering blood sugar levels than glibenclamide.

Enoa E, EH Itam; Hypoglycaemic agent(s) in leaves of *Elaeophorbia drupifera, Phyther Res* **10**(8), 680-82 (1996)

Eleusine coracana Linn. (Poaceae)
(Finger millet, African millet, H. Ragi)

Finger millet, originally native to the Ethiopian highlands, was introduced into India approximately 4000 years ago. It is very adaptable to higher elevations and is grown in the Himalayas up to 2300 metres altitude. Incorporation of four commonly available millets [*Eleusine coracana* (Ragi), *Panicum miliare* (Samai), *Sorghum vulgare* (Jowar) and *Zea mays* (Maize)] in the breakfast, fed to non-insulin dependent diabetics for one month, lowered their blood sugar levels. Of these millets, *E. coracana* (Ragi) caused maximum reduction of blood sugar level. It was suggested that Ragi might be added to the diet of diabetic patients.

Geetha C, PP Easwaran; Hypoglycaemic effects of millet incorporated breakfast items on selected non-insulin dependent diabetic patients, *Indian J Nutr Dietet* **27**(11), 316-20 (1990).

Eleutherococcus senticosus Rupr. & Maxim (Araliaceae)
Syn. *Acanthopanax senticosus* (Siberian ginseng)

Eleutherococcus senticosus was formerly known as *Acanthopanax senticosus.* It is a species of small, woody shrub and its native habitat is East Asia, China, Japan and Russia. It is commonly called 'eleuthero", and was previously marketed in the United States as Siberian ginseng because of its herbal properties similar to those of *Panax* ginseng.

Hypoglycaemic effect and toxicity of *E. senticosus* following acute and chronic administration in mice have been studied.

For further reports, see *Acanthopanax senticosus* and also Hypoglycaemic glycans in Appendix.

Medon PJ, EB Thompson, NR Farnsworth; Hypoglycaemic effect and toxicity of *Eleutherococcus senticosus* following acute and chronic administration in mice, *Zhongguo Yao Li Xue Bao* **2**(4), 281-85 (1981).

Embelia keniensis R.E. Fries (Myrsinaceae)

The toluene-soluble fraction of the methanol extract of *E. keniensis* showed hypoglycaemic and lipid-lowering activity 7 hours after intra-peritoneal administration of the drug at a dose of 100 mg/kg. It also significantly decreased the blood glucose level in epinephrine-induced hyperglycaemic mice. The effects were different from those of the methanol extract of *Embelia schiperi.*

Kato A, T Miura, Y Nishiyama, Y Tachibana, Y Ohnishi, SG Mathenge, R Albert; A comparative study of *Embelia schiperi* and *Embelia keniensis* on blood glucose and triglycerides in normal and epinephrine-induced hyperglycaemic mice, *Am J Chin Med* **27**(3-4), 365-70 (1999).

Embelia ribes Burm (Myrsinaceae) (Flase Pepper, S. Vidanga, H. Baiberang)

This climbing shrub is present throughout India. Berries, leaves and root-bark of *Embelia ribes* are used in traditional medicine for a variety of ailments. In Ayurveda, vidanga, the berries, have been described as anthelmintic, alterative and tonic and recommended its use along with liqorice root for the purpose of strengthening the body and preventing the effects of ageing.

Oral feeding of an ethanol extract of *E. ribes* (200 mg/kg) to streptozotocin-induced diabetic rats for 20 days resulted in significant decrease in blood glucose, serum total cholesterol, and triglycerides and increase in HDL-cholesterol levels in comparison to diabetic rats. The extract also lowered the liver and pancreas thiobarbituric acid reactive substances in comparison to those of diabetic rats. The results of this plant drug were found to be comparable to gliclazide (25 mg/kg, p.o.), a standard anti-hyperglycaemic agent. The findings provided evidence of the potential of *E. ribes* in diabetic dyslipidemia.

Bhandari U, R Kanojia, KK Pillai; Effect of ethanolic extract of *Embelia ribes* on dyslipidemia in diabetic rats, *Int J Exp Diabetes Res* **3**(3), 159-62 (2002).

Embelia schimperi Vatke (Myrsinaceae)

Intra-peritoneal administration of methanol extract of *Embelia schimperi* to normal mice caused a significant decrease in blood glucose and a significant increase in triglycerides 4 hours after administration at 100 mg/kg. Unlike *E. keiensis,* which tended to decrease the blood triglycerides in epinephrine-induced diabetic mice, *E. schimperi* tended to increase these. The activities on blood glucose and triglycerides in normal and epinephrine-induced hyperglycaemic mice of the two species (*E.*

keiensis and *E. schimperi*) were different.

Kato A, T Miura, Y Nishiyama, Y Tachibana, Y Ohnishi, SG Mathenge, R Albert; A comparative study of *Embelia schmiperi* and *Embelia keniensis* on blood glucose and triglycerides in normal and epinephrine-induced hyperglycaemic mice, *Am J Chin Med* **27**(3-4), 365-70 (1999).

Enicostemma littorale Blume (Gentianaceae) (H. Chhota chirayata)

E. littorale is a perennial herb, found throughout India up to a height of 1500 feet. The plant is reported to contain bitter principles in addition to alkaloids. Gupta and co-workers (1, 3-4) studied the anti-diabetic effect of an aqueous extract of the whole plant on normoglycemic, hyperglycaemic, and alloxan-induced diabetic rats but the blood glucose lowering effect of *E. littorale* was observed only in alloxan-induced diabetic rats with no change in normoglycaemic control rats. However, the fall of blood sugar in diabetic rats after 30 days treatment with the extract was found to be significant. The decrease in the plasma glucose level was accompanied with a decrease in the level of glycosylated haemoglobin and glucose-6-phosphatase activity in liver. A single dose of aqueous extract of *E. littorale* (15 g dry plant equivalent extract per kg) had shown significant increase in the serum insulin levels in alloxan-induced diabetic rats at 8 h. This extract enhanced the glucose induced insulin release from isolated rat pancreatic islets and partially reversed the effect of diazoxide. Incubation with Ca^{2+} chelator (EGTA) and Ca^{2+} channel blocker did not affect the augmentation of insulin release by the extract. The hypoglycaemic effect of this drug was attributed to augmentation of glucose induced insulin release through K^+ ATP channel dependent pathway without Ca^{2+} influx. The effective dose was found to be 1.5 g dry plant equivalent extract/100 g body wt. This effective dose caused significant decrease in glycosylated haemoglobin, liver glucose-6-phosphatase activity and significant increase in serum insulin levels of the diabetic rats. No significant changes were observed in the toxicity parameters of extract treated diabetic rats.

The effect of oral administration of an aqueous extract of *E. littorale* whole plant on some key enzymes, meant for carbohydrate metabolism and antioxidant defence, was studied in alloxan-induced diabetes in rats. Oral administration of the extract for 45 days increased the activity of hexokinase and decreased the activities of glucose 6-phosphatase and fructose 1,6-bisphosphatase significantly in the serum, liver and kidney of diabetic rats. The extract significantly lowered the concentration of thiobarbituric acid reactive substances and lipid hydroperoxides in brain and increased it significantly in heart of diabetic rats. It also increased the concentration of reduced glutathione and the activity of glutathione peroxidase in diabetic rats. The activities of superoxide dismutase and catalase were also increased significantly. The results established the anti-diabetic activity of *E. littorale* aqueous extract (8).

The effect of oral administration of the aqueous extract of the plant (2 g/kg) daily for 6 weeks in neonatal non-insulin-dependent diabetes mellitus (NIDDM) rats was studied. Results of the oral glucose tolerance test showed a significant decrease in AUC (glucose) and AUC (insulin) values in NIDDM treated group. Insulin sensitivity index of NIDDM control was significantly increased after treatment with *E. littorale*. The extract also decreased the elevated cholesterol, triglyceride and creatinine levels observed in NIDDM rats (2).

Aqueous extract of the whole plant of *E. littorale* was reported to exhibit effective anti-diabetic activity in experimental animals as well as clinically. The extract was found to contain triterpenoids, flavonoids, alkaloids, phenolics and tannins (6).

Methanol extract of the plant also resulted in significant lowering of blood sugar levels of alloxan-induced diabetic rats after treatment for 20 days at a dose 2.5 g/kg. This extract also raised the serum insulin levels and improved the antioxidant status of diabetic rats (5).

Administration of pills, prepared from *E. littorale,* to patients with type-2 diabetes for three months reduced their blood glucose levels and prevented the progression of complications in diabetic patients. Significant improvement in kidney function, lipid profile and blood pressure was also observed (7).

1. Vijayvargia R, M Kumar, S Gupta; Hypoglycaemic effect of aqueous extract of *Enicostemma littorale* Blume (chhota chirayata) on alloxan induced diabetes mellitus in rats, *Indian J Exp Biol* **38**(8), 781-84 (2000)
2. Murali B, UM Upadhyaya, RK Goyal; Effect of chronic treatment with *Enicostemma littorale* in non-insulin-dependent diabetic (NIDDM) rats, *J Ethnopharmacol* **81**(2), 199-204 (2002).
3. Maroo J, VT Vasu, R Aalinkeel, S Gupta; Glucose lowering effect of aqueous extract of *Enicostemma littorale* Blume in diabetes: a possible mechanism of action, *J Ethnopharmacol* **81**(3), 317-20 (2002).
4. Maroo J, VT Vasu, S Gupta; Dose dependent hypoglycaemic effect of aqueous extract of *Enicostemma littorale* Blume in alloxan induced diabetic rats, *Phytomedicine* **10**(2-3), 196-99 (2003).
5. Maroo J, A Ghosh, R Mathur, VT Vasu, S Gupta, Anti-diabetic efficacy of *Enicostemma littorale* methanol extract in alloxan induced diabetic rats, *Pharmaceut Biol* **41**(5), 388-91 (2003)
6. Upadhyay UM, MN Ravishanker, M Rajani, H Padh, RK Goyal; *National convention on Current Trends in Herbal Drugs & Annual Conference of Indian Soc Pharmaconosyg* , Herb: The National Alternative , Gandhinagar, Gujrat,, India, p. **D04**, January 17-18, 2003
7. Upadhyay UM, RK Goyal; Efficacy of *Enicostemma littorale* in Type 2 diabetic patients, *Phytother Res* **18**(3), 233-35 (2004).

8. Srinivasan M, M Padmanabhan, PS Prince; Effect of aqueous *Enicostemma littorale* Blume extract on key carbohydrate metabolic enzymes, lipid peroxides and antioxidants in alloxan-induced diabetic rats, *J Pharm Pharmacol* **57**(4), 497-503 (2005)

Ephedra distachya Linn. (Ephedraceae) (Syn. *E. vulgaris*)

Ephedra distachya is a shrub that grows in southern Europe and parts of western and central Asia. It is sometimes identified with the legendary drug, "Soma", as described in the Rig-Veda, the ancient sacred text of Hindu faiths. Ephedrine, the major alkaloid of the plant, is a stimulant and often used to control asthma.

See Hypoglycaemic Glycans in Appendix: (Hikino *et al, Planta Med* **(2)**, 162-63 (1985)

Ephedrae sinica **stapf.** (Ephedraceae)

Ephedrae herba consists of the dried stem or aerial part of *Ephedra sinica* Stapf or other ephedrine-containing *Ephedra* species. The hypoglycaemic effects of crude *Ephedrae herba*, its alkaloid fraction and its major alkaloid component, l-ephedrine were studied in streptozotocin-induced diabetic mice. Only the alkaloid fraction and 1-ephedrine were found to suppress hyperglycaemia significantly. The suppression of hyperglycaemia by *Ephedrae herba* was, therefore, considered to be due to l-ephedrine. It was further observed that the crude drug, its alkaloid fraction and 1-ephedrine promoted the regeneration of pancreas islets following atrophy induced by streptozotocin. It was, therefore, suggested that *Ephedrae herba* might regenerate atrophied pancreatic islets, restore the secretion of insulin, and thus correct hyperglycaemia.

Xiu LM, AB Miura, K Yamamoto, T Kobayashi, QH Song, H Kitamura, JC Cyong; Pancreatic islet regeneration by ephedrine in mice with streptozotocin-induced diabetes, *Am J Chin Med* **29**(3-4), 493-500 (2001).

Equisetum myriochaetum Schlecht and Cham (Equisetaceae) (Mexican Giant Horsetail)

Equisetum is a genus of vascular plants that reproduce by spores rather than seeds. These are plants with jointed stems, with distinct nodes and small whorled leaves, fused into sheaths. *E. myriochaetum* is found in Nicaragua, Costa Rica, Colombia, Venezuela, Ecuador, Peru and Mexico. Water as well as butanol extracts of the aerial parts of *E. myriochaetum* were examined for their hypoglycaemic activity on streptozotocin-induced diabetic rats. Oral administration of water extract (7 and 13 mg/kg) and butanol extract (8 and 16 mg/kg) significantly lowered the plasma glucose levels in diabetic rats after three hours. The hypoglycaemic effects of the extracts were comparable to that of glibenclamide. Three kaempferol glucosides and one caffeoyl glucoside were the main constituents in the extracts (1). A single dose of aqueous extract of the aerial parts of *E. myriochaetum* (0.33g/kg) to type-2 diabetes mellitus patients significantly decreased the blood glucose levels within 90, 120 and 180 minutes. However, no significant change was noted in insulin levels (2).

1. Andrade-Cetto A, H Wiedenfeld, MC Revilla, IA Sergio; Hypoglycaemic effect of *Equisetum myriochaetum* aerial parts on streptozotocin diabetic rats, *J Ethnopharmacol* **72**(1-2), 129-33 (2000).
2. Revilla MC, A Andrade-Cetto, S Islas, H Wiedenfeld; Hypoglycaemic effect of *Equisetum myriochaetum* aerial parts on type 2 diabetic patients, *J Ethnopharmacol* **81**(1), 117-20 (2002)

Eriobotrya japonica (Thunb) Lindl (Rosaceae) (Loquat)

E. japonica is a fruit tree, indigenous to south-eastern China. It was introduced into Japan and became naturalised there in very early times. It has also become naturalised in India and many other countries. Eaten in quantity, loquats are reported to induce gentle but noticeable sedative effect.

The effects of *Eriobotrya japonica* on blood sugar levels of normal and alloxan-induced diabetic rabbits were studied by Wadood and co-workers (1, 2).

De-Tommasi and co-workers studied the effects of the terpenoid constituents of the plant in genetically diabetic mice (C57BL/KS-db/db/Ola). A sesquiterpene glycoside and two polyhydroxy tritrpenoids, isolated from the methanol extract *E. japonica,* produced a marked inhibition of glycosuria. The triterpenoids were also able to reduce blood glucose levels in normoglycaemic rats (3).

1. Wadood N, A Wadood, HH Khan, SA Shah; Effect of *Eriobotrya japonica* on blood glucose levels of normal and alloxan diabetic rabbits, *J Pak Med Assoc* **38**(4), 108-13 (1988).
2. Noreen W, A Wadood, HK Hidayat, SA Wahid; Effect of *Eriobotrya japonica* on blood glucose levels of normal and alloxan-diabetic rabbits, *Planta Med* **54**(3), 196-99 (1988).
3. De-Tommasi N, F De-Simone, G Cirino, C Cicala, C Pizza; Hypoglycaemic effects of sesquiterpene glycosides and polyhydroxylated triterpenoids of *Eriobotrya japonica, Planta Med* **57**(5), 414-16 (1991).

Eriosema kraussianum (N. E. Br.) Meisn. (Fabaceae) (Zulu name. "uBangalala")

Zulu traditional health practitioners use the roots of *E. kraussianum* for the treatment of erectile dysfunction and/or impotence. The present study was undertaken to investigate the hypoglycaemic and vasodilatory properties of the two main bioactive pyrano-isoflavones (K1 and K2), obtained from the roots of the plant, in experimental rat models. The compounds (20-80 mg/kg p.o.) caused dose-dependent and significant hypoglycaemia in rats. The hypoglycaemic activity of compounds was confirmed.

Ojewole JA, SE Drewes, F Khan; Vasodilatory and hypoglycaemic effects of two pyrano-isoflavone extractives from *Eriosema kraussianum* N. E. Br. [Fabaceae] rootstock in experimental rat models, *Phytochemistry* **67**(6), 610-17 (2006)

Eruca sativa Mill (Brassicaceae / Cruciferae) (Garden Rocket)

Eruca sativa is a leafy vegetable, available throughout the world but cultivated mainly in Italy. It has a rich, peppery taste, and used mainly in salads but also used as cooked vegetable.

Oil of *E. sativa* seeds has been found to be useful for prevention and treatment of diabetes mellitus, induced experimentally by alloxan injection. Oral administration of *E. sativa* oil to alloxan-induced diabetic rats (daily for 2 weeks) ameliorated hyperglycaemia, improved lipid profile, and reduced oxidative stress. The oil also showed preventive effect.

El-Missiry MA, AM El-Gindy; Amelioration of alloxan-induced diabetes mellitus and oxidative stress in rats by oil of *Eruca sativa* seeds, *Ann Nutr Metab* 44(3), 97-100 (2000)

Eucalyptus globulus Labill. (Myrtaceae) (Eucalyptus)

Eucalyptus (*E, globulus*) is traditionally used for the treatment of diabetes. An incorporation of eucalyptus in the diet (62.5 g/kg) and drinking water (2.5 g/l) reduced hyperglycaemia and associated weight loss of streptozotocin-treated mice. An aqueous extract of eucalyptus (0.5 g/l) enhanced transport of 2-deoxy-glucose, glucose oxidation and incorporation of glucose into glycogen in mouse abdominal muscle. In acute, 20 min incubations, the aqueous extract (0.25-0.5 g/l) evoked a stepwise 70-160% enhancement of insulin secretion from the clonal pancreatic *beta*-cell line (BRIN-BD11). Sequential extraction with solvents revealed that the activity resides in both methanol and water soluble fractions, indicating the presence of more than one biologically active constituent in the plant. *E, globulus* was considered by the authors to be an effective anti-hyperglycaemic dietary adjunct for the treatment of diabetes.

Gray AM, PR Flatt; Anti-hyperglycaemic actions of *Eucalyptus globulus* (Eucalyptus) are associated with pancreatic and extra- effects in mice, *J Nutr* **128**(12), 2319-23 (1998).

Eucommia ulmoides **Oliv. (Eucommiaceae)**
(Chinese rubber tree)

Eucommia ulmoides is a small tree, native to China, where it is widely cultivated for its bark. The bark of the plant is highly valued in Traditional Chinese medicine. The plant is used for the treatment of diabetes in Korea. In alloxan and streptozotocin-induced diabetic rats, anti-hyperglycaemic activity of methanol extracts of different parts of *E. ulmoides* was evaluated. Cortex and leaf extracts significantly lowered blood glucose levels along with an increase in the serum insulin levels. These extracts markedly increased the body weight of diabetic animals. An improvement in glucose tolerance test was also observed in treated diabetic rats (1). Quercetin 3-O-α-L-arabinopyranosyl-(1→2)-β-D-glucopyranoside, kaempferol 3-O-β-D-glucopyranoside (astragalin) and quercetin 3-O-β-D-glucopyranoside (isoquercitrin), isolated from the leaves of *E. ulmoides*, exhibited glycation inhibitory activity comparable to that of aminoguanidine, a known glycation inhibitor. The anti-diabetic action of *E. ulmoides* leaves is considered to be due to the glycation inhibitory activity of flavonol glycosides (2)

The anti-hyperglycaemic activity of the plant was studied in streptozotocin-induced diabetic rats. Male Sprague-Dawley rats were divided into four groups; a non-diabetic group, a diabetic group, a diabetic group supplemented with powdered *E. ulmoides* leaves and a diabetic group supplemented with water extract of the powdered *E. ulmoides* leaves. The plant drugs were added to a standard diet based on 1% dried *E. ulmoides* leaves (1 g powdered leaves/100 g diet and 0.187 g water extract/100 g diet, respectively). The blood glucose levels were significantly lower in the diabetic groups receiving plant drug in either forms. The plasma insulin and C-peptide levels were significantly higher in the plant drug supplemented groups than in the diabetic group. *E. ulmoides* leaves supplement seemed to be helpful in preserving the normal histological appearance of pancreatic islets as well as the insulin-positive *beta*-cells but it did not reverse the effect of streptozotocin to a great extent (3). The anti-diabetic efficacy of water extract of *E. ulmoides* leaves was investigated in type-2 diabetic animals. Dietary supplement based on 1% dried leaves of *E. ulmoides,* given to C57BL/KsJ-db/db mice for 6 weeks, lowered the blood glucose level and enhanced the glucose disposal in an intra-peritoneal glucose tolerance test. The plasma insulin and C-peptide levels were significantly higher in the dietary supplement group than in the control group, while the glucagon level was lower. The hepatic glucokinase activity was significantly higher in the group receiving dietary supplement, but the glucose-6-phosphatase and phosphoenolpyruvate carboxykinase activities were significantly lower. From the results of detailed investigation, it was inferred that dietary supplementation with water extract of *E. ulmoides* leaves (0.187 g extract/100 g standard diet) partly ameliorate hyperglycaemia and hyperlipidemia with type-2 diabetes through increasing glycolysis, suppressing gluconeogenesis and the biosynthesis of fatty acid and cholesterol in the liver (4).

1. Hong ND, YS Rho, DH Won, NJ Kim, BS Cho, Studies on the anti-diabetic activity of *Eucommia ulmoides* Oliver, *Korean J Pharmacogn* 18(2), 112-17 (1987)
2. Kim HY, BH Moon, HJ Lee, DH Choi; Flavonol glycosides from the leaves of *Eucommia ulmoides* with glycation inhibitory activity, *J Ethnopharmacol* **93**(2-3), 227-30 (2004).
3. Lee MK, MJ Kim, SY Cho, SA Park, KK Park,UJ Jung, HM Park, MS Choi; Hypoglycaemic effect of Du-zhong (*Eucommia ulmoides* Oliv.) leaves in streptozotocin-induced diabetic rats, *Diabetes Res Clin Pract* **67**(1), 22-28 (2005).
4. Park SA, MS Choi, MJ Kim, UJ Jung, HJ Kim, KK Park, HJ Noh, HM Park, YB Park, JS Lee, MK Lee; Hypoglycaemic and hypolipidaemic action of Du-zhong (*Eucommia ulmoides* Oliver) leaves water extract in C57BL/KsJ-db/db mice, *J Ethnopharmacol* **107**(3), 412-17 (2006)

Eugenia jambolana Lam. (Myrtaceae)
Syn. ***Syzygium cumini*** (L.) Skeels
(Black plum. Java Plum, H. Jamun, S. Jambu)

Eugenia jambolana (Syn. *Syzigium cumin* (L) Skeels, *Syzygium jambolana* DC, *Syzygium jambolanum* DC), is native to India, Pakistan and Indonesia but grown in other areas of southern and south-eastern Asia, particularly for its fruits. It is commonly known as 'jamun' in India and widely used in Indian folk medicine for the treatment of diabetes mellitus. Considerable work has been done on the hypoglycaemic activity of different parts of the plant, particularly on its seeds and seed kernels. Ratsimamanga and coworkers reported the isolation of an active principle from the young bark of the plant and studied its hypoglycaemic and anti-diabetic activity. The activity of the active principle was compared with that of NN-methyldimethyl biguanide and glybutamide on induced hyperglycaemia in rats and rabbits (1-3). Botanical characters, varieties, phytochemistry, therapeutics and anti-diabetic properties of *Eugenia jambolana* have been reviewed (9). A recent study shows that *Syzygium cumini* bark possesses a significant beneficial effect on glycoproteins in addition to its anti-diabetic action (39).

Oral administration of *E jambolana* has been reported to exhibit significant hypoglycaemic effect in both normal and streptozotocin-induced diabetic rats (14). The effect of varying doses of alcoholic and aqueous extracts of *E jambolana* on body weight, serum glucose, insulin and triglyceride was investigated in fructose fed rats. Serum glucose and insulin levels were significantly increased following feeding of fructose for 15 days. Administration of aqueous extract of *E jambolana* (400 mg/day) markedly prevented high fructose diet induced hyperglycaemia and hyperinsulinemia (24). The effects of daily oral feeding *E. jambolana* extract (200 mg/kg) for 40 days on blood glucose concentrations and kidney functions were studied in streptozotocin-induced diabetic rats. Plasma glucose concentrations in streptozotocin-diabetic mice were reduced by 20.84 per cent after the administration of the extract. Urine volume was significantly higher in diabetic controls but treatment with *E. jambolana* extract prevented polyuria. Treatment with the extract also significantly prevented the rise in urinary albumin levels. Renal hypertrophy was significantly higher in diabetic controls as compared to non-diabetic controls but treatment with the extract partially but significantly prevented renal hypertrophy as compared to diabetic controls (25).

Ethanol extract (20 and 40 mg/kg), chloroform extract (40 and 80 mg/kg) and aqueous extract (40 mg/kg) of *E. jambolana* leaves exhibited significant hypoglycaemic activity in normal and hyperglycaemic rabbits. A significant reduction (20-30%) of blood sugar levels was observed in two diabetic volunteers, who consumed a decoction of 6 or 12 g of leaves. (11). Administration of a decoction of *E. jambolana* leaves (15% w/v) as a substitute for drinking water to stroptozotocin-induced diabetic rats did not affect the blood sugar, cholesterol, HDL-cholesterol and triglyceride levels. The angiotensin converting enzyme also remained unaffected in treated diabetic rats. It was suggested that in this particular experimental model, *E. jambolana* did not elicit any anti-diabetic effect (23).

Effects of oral administration of *E. jambolana* seeds and chloropropamide on blood glucose level and pancreatic cathepsin B were studied in rats (4). Oral administration of *E. jambolana* seeds in caesein diet (1 g/kg) to streptozotocin-induced diabetic animals significantly lowered the elevated post-meal values of blood sugar, cholesterol, free fatty acids and triglycerides down to levels comparable to that obtained by phenformin. Like phenformin, *E. jambolana* seeds also failed to control glycogenolysis in streptozotocin-induced diabetes (5). In an experiment carried out on 28 diabetic patients, treatment with *Syzygium cumini* seed powder (4-24 g, tds) showed significant fall of fasting and postprandial blood sugar level in 20 cases (6). Administration of *E. jambolana* seed extract to alloxan-induced diabetic rats for 14 days reduced blood sugar, blood urea, serum cholesterol and triglyceride levels significantly. Continuation of treatment for another 15 days further decreased blood sugar, cholesterol and triglyceride levels (7). The effect of an aqueous extract of *E. jambolana* seeds on blood glucose levels was studied in normal fasting, alloxan-induced diabetic and glucose fed rabbits. The extract showed hypoglycaemic effect, the magnitude of which showed time related variation (29). Administration of an aqueous suspension of seed kernel of *S. cumini* (4g/kg) exhibited significant lowering of blood sugar levels in alloxan-induced diabetic rats after 3 hours. The results were comparable with those produced by tolbutamide. It was suggested that like tolbutamide, *S. cumini* might stimulate the endogenous insulin release (10). Administration of aqueous, alcoholic and acetone extracts of *S. cumini* to alloxan-induced diabetic rats for 2 to 5 weeks caused significant lowering of blood sugar levels. Interestingly, the blood glucose levels remained lower even after 15 days of discontinuation of the treatment. (12, 13). Seed powder of *E. jambolana*, given to patients of non-insulin dependent diabetes mellitus for 3 months, provided marked symptomatic relief, which increased progressively with the duration of therapy (16). Diabetics in Porto Alegre, Brazil are reported to use a tea, prepared from leaves and seeds of *S. cumini*, for their treatment. However, administration of such tea at different concentration levels (2-64 g/l), to normal and streptozotocin-induced diabetic rats failed to exhibit any detectable anti-hyperglycaemic effect either in normal or in diabetic rats. Similar observations were made also in a randomised, parallel, placebo controlled trial on 30 non-diabetic young volunteers. While the results of the investigation do not rule out hypoglycaemic effects in patients with type-2 diabetes mellitus, the authors are of the opinion that *S. cumini* cannot be recommended as an anti-hyperglycaemic agent (17, 21). Intra-peritoneal administration of 50% alcoholic extract of *S. cumini* seeds (20 mg) significantly decreased blood sugar levels in both normal and alloxan induced diabetic mice after 3 and 6 hours. However, lowering of blood sugar levels was more marked in diabetic mice compared to normal animals. The results were comparable to insulin administration. The hypoglycaemic effect of *S. cumini* seeds was attributed to its direct effect on tissue and/or on insulin secretion (20). Administration of ethanol extract of *E. jambolana* seed (100 mg/kg) to sub-diabetic rabbits for one day and to alloxan-induced mild and severely diabetic rabbits respectively, for 7 and 15 days led to a significant fall in fasting blood sugar levels at 90 min. Daily treatment with the extract for 15 days also produced significant fall in fasting blood sugar and glycosylated haemoglobin along with an increase in insulin levels in mild and severely diabetic animals. The treated diabetic animals also exhibited a significant lowering of total serum cholesterol, LDL-cholesterol and HMG-CoA reductase activity. Almost normal morphological appearance was noted in the pancreas, liver and aorta of treated diabetic rats (27). The quantitative determination showed that *S. cumini* seeds contained 40% water-soluble gummy fibre and 15% water-insoluble neutral detergent fibre. The effect of feeding diets supplemented with different fractions of *S. cumini* seeds was tested on fasting blood glucose and glucose tolerance in normal and alloxan-induced diabetic rats. The study revealed that the hypoglycaemic effect of *S. cumini* seeds was due to water-soluble gummy fibre and that water-insoluble neutral detergent fibre and other constituents of the seeds had no significant hypoglycaemic effects (26). Oral administration of an alcoholic extract of *S. cumini* seeds to alloxan-induced diabetic rats, at a dose of 100 mg/kg body weight, resulted in a significant reduction in blood glucose, urine sugar, and serum and tissue lipids of experimental animals. The extract also increased total haemoglobin and brought back all the parameters to normal levels. The effect of this alcoholic extract was similar to that of insulin (32). In order to ascertain which part of *E. jambolana* seeds is responsible for its hypoglycaemic activity, the effects of whole seeds, seed kernels, and seed coat were investigated using streptozotocin-induced diabetic rats. The ethanol extract of kernel, at a concentration of 100 mg/kg of body weight, significantly decreased the levels of blood glucose, blood urea, and cholesterol, increased glucose tolerance and levels of total proteins and liver glycogen, and decreased the activities of glutamate oxaloacetate transaminase and glutamate pyruvate transaminase in experimental diabetic rats. However, only moderate hypoglycaemic activity was observed following the administration of whole seed kernel, while the seed coat failed to show any hypoglycaemic activity (31).

Aqueous extract of *Syzygium cumini* seeds (2.5g/kg) increased the hexokinase activity along with a lowering of glucose-6-phosphatase activity in the liver of alloxan-induced diabetic rats. A decrease in serum acid and alkaline phosphatase and lacatate dehydrogenase activity was also observed in these animals. Such an effect of this extract was more marked than glibenclamide (18). In alloxan-induced diabetic rats, oral administration of aqueous extract of the seeds of *S. cumini* (2.5 and 5.0 g/kg/b.w.) for 6 weeks led to a significant reduction of blood glucose along with an increase in the haemoglobin level but this effect was not significant at a dose of 7.5 g/kg body weight. The aqueous extract also resulted in decreased free radical formation in tissues studied. The decrease in thiobarbituric acid reactive substances and increase in reduced glutathione, superoxide dismutase and catalase clearly showed the antioxidant property of the extract, the effect being most prominent at a dose of 5.0 g/kg body weight (19).

The anti-diabetic effects of aqueous and alcoholic extracts and lyophilized powder of *E. jambolana* seed kernel were studied in mild, moderate and severe diabetic animals. Mice having mild diabetes exhibited maximum reduction in blood sugar levels following administration of lyophilized powder of *E. jambolana* seed kernel (200 mg/kg/day for 3 wks). However, the percent reduction of blood sugar levels decreased in moderately and severely diabetic animals, treated with this lyophilized powder. The alterations in hepatic and skeletal muscle glycogen content and hepatic glucokinase, hexokinase, glucose-6-phosphate and phosphofructokinase levels in diabetic mice were partially restored by this treatment. The mechanism of action has been discussed (22). The antioxidant effect of oral administration of ethanol extract of *E. jambolana* seed kernel was evaluated. Administration of seed kernel to streptozotocin-induced diabetic rats significantly decreased the levels of blood glucose, glycosylated haemoglobin, and increased body weight gain, plasma insulin and haemoglobin. The diabetic rats showed low activities of superoxide dismutase, catalase, glutathione peroxidase and reduced glutathione content in liver and kidney, which were restored to near normal levels by treatment with the seed kernel extract. The increased levels of lipid peroxidation and hydroperoxides in diabetic rats were reverted back to near normal levels after the treatment with seed kernel extract (33). A significant increase in the levels of plasma glucose, vitamin-E, ceruloplasmin, lipid peroxides and a concomitant decrease in the levels of vitamin-C, reduced glutathione, observed in diabetic rats, were reverted back to near normal levels after the treatment with ethanol extract of *E. jambolana* seed kernel. Histopathological studies also revealed the protective effect of *E. jambolana* seed kernel on pancreatic *beta*-cells (34). Abnormalities in lipid profile are one of the most common complications in diabetes mellitus and *E. jambolana* seed kernel was found to rectify these abnormalities. Streptozotocin-induced diabetic rats showed significant increase in the levels of cholesterol, phospholipids, triglycerides, and free fatty acids, which were considerably restored to near normal levels in *E. jambolana* seed-kernel or glibenclamide treated animals (37).

Oral administration of *E. jambolana* seed powder (500 or 1000 mg/kg) to streptozotocin-induced diabetic rats showed an increase in body weight on day 20 in relation to day 5. It also showed a decrease in fasting blood glucose, a difference in post-treatment fasting and peak blood glucose and a difference in liver glycogen. The best results were obtained with an oral dose of 500 mg/kg. These findings on the anti-diabetic effect of *E. jambolana* seed powder are considered adequate for approval of phase 2 clinical trials to evaluate this seed powder as complementary therapy in type-2 and type-1 diabetes (36).

Oral administration of F-IIc, an active compound isolated from *E. jambolana,* to steptozotocin-induced diabetic rats at a dose of 7 mg/kg body weight, caused a fall (23%) in fasting blood glucose level after 90 minute. It also showed a fall (34%) in peak blood glucose during glucose tolerance test. In alloxan-induced diabetic rabbits prolonged (7days) treatment with F-IIc resulted a fall (42%) in fasting blood glucose level and 60% fall in peak blood glucose during glucose tolerance test. Plasma insulin levels were also significantly increased in both alloxan and streptozotocin-induced diabetic animals. Determination of the activity of key enzymes of glycolysis and gluconeogenesis in experimental animals revealed both pancreatic as well as extra-pancreatic action of F-IIc. (28).

The chromium contents of *Eugenia jambolana* and of five other herbs, widely used for the treatment of diabetes mellitus, were determined using Atomic absorption technique. All these plants contained chromium in varying amounts ranging from 1.25 to 15 μg/g dry plant material. These observations perhaps confirm the therapeutic value of chromium in diabetes (8). The inorganic trace elements present in *E. jambolana* seeds were analysed and the hypoglycaemic activity of inorganic part of the seeds was determined using streptozotocin-induced diabetic rats. The *E. jambolana* seed ash contained elements such as zinc, chromium, vanadium, potassium and sodium. Administration of seed ash to diabetic rats significantly reduced the blood sugar levels and improved the glucose tolerance. It was suggested that the inorganic constituents might play an important role in the anti-diabetic activity of *E. jambolana* (30).

The extract of fruit pulp of *Eugenia jambolana* showed hypoglycaemic activity. The effect of pulp was seen in 30 min, while the seeds of the same fruit required 24 hr. The incubation of isolated islets of Langerhans from normal as well as from diabetic animals with the pulp extract stimulated insulin secretion. The extract inhibited insulinase activity from liver and kidney (15). The fruit pulp of Brazilian *E. jambolana,* however, failed to show any anti-diabetic potential. This lack of anti-diabetic effect of *E. jambolana* fruits of Brazilian origin could be attributed to regional ecosystem from where the fruits were collected and/or the severity of experimental diabetes (35). The oral anti-hyperglycaemic effect of the water and ethanol extracts of the fruit-pulp of *E. jambolana* was studied in alloxan-induced diabetic as well as severely diabetic rabbits. Water extract was found to be more effective than the ethanol extract in reducing fasting blood glucose and improving blood glucose in glucose tolerance test. Chromatographic purification of the water extract yielded not only two hypoglycaemic fractions (F-III and F-IV) but also two hyperglycaemic compounds (F-I and F-II). A significant fall in fasting blood glucose level was observed in diabetic (21% fall) and severely diabetic (24% fall) rabbits by treatment with F-III once daily with 25mg/kg body weight. The mechanism of action of FIII fraction appears to be both pancreatic by stimulating release of insulin and extra pancreatic by directly acting on the tissues (38).

1. Sigogneau-Jagodzinski M, P Bibal-Prot, M Chanez, P Boiteau, AR Ratsimamanga; Contribution to the study of the hypoglycaemic and anti-diabetic activity of a principle extracted from the Madagascar myrtle (*Eugenia jambolana* Lamarck), *C R Acad Sci Hebd Seances Acad Sci D* **264**(8), 1119-23 (1967) [Article in French]
2. Ratsimamanga AR, C Lefournier-Contensou, P Bibal-Prot; Comparative study of the effect of a principle extracted from *Eugenia jambolana* bark with NN-methyldimethyl biguanide and glybutamide on induced hyperglycaemia in normal rats, *C R Acad Sci Hebd Seances Acad Sci D* **275**(8), 913-15 (1972) [Article in French]
3. Ratsimamanga AR, A Loiseau, S Ratsimamanga-Urverg, P Bibal-Prot; Action of a hypoglycaemic agent found in the young bark of *Eugenia jambolania* (Myrtaceae) on induced hyperglycaemia of the rabbit and continuation of its purification, *CR Acad Sci Hebd Seances acad Sci D* **277**(20), :2219-22 (1973) [Article in French]
4. Bansal R, N Ahmad, JR Kidwai; Effects of oral administration of *Eugenia jambolana* seeds & chloropropamide on blood glucose level & pancreatic cathepsin B in rat, *Indian J Biochem Biophys* **18**(5), 377 (1983)
5. Kedar P, CH Chakrabarti; Effects of jambolan seed treatment on blood sugar, lipids and urea in streptozotocin induced diabetes in rabbits, *Indian J Physiol Pharmacol* **27**(2), 135-40 (1983)
6. Srivastava Y, HV Bhatt, OP Gupta, SP Gupta; Hypoglycaemia induced by *Syzygium cumini* Linn. seeds in diabetes mellitus, *Asian Med J* **26**(7), 489-491 (1983).
7. Giri J, TK Sakthidevi, N Dushyanthy; Effect of Jamun seed extract on alloxan induced diabetes in rats, *J Diab. Assoc. India* **25** (4), 115-19 (1985)
8. Jasmal H, H Raza, KM Januja, MK Bhatty; Effect of minor minerals containing chromium on human health, Part I, Diabetic control with herbs, *Pak J Sci Ind*

Res, **29** (1), 45- 47 (1986)

9. Kohli KR, RH Singh; *Eugenia jambolana*: a plant drug with potential anti-diabetic property (a review), *J Sci Res Pl Med*, **6**(1-4), 21-28 (1986)
10. Nair RB, G Shanthakumari; Anti-diabetic activity of the seed kernel of *Syzygim cumini* Linn. *Ancient Sci Life* **2**(Oct), 80-84 (1986)
11. Arbab AG, T Akhtar, F Rab; Hypoglycaemic activity of *Eugenia jambolana* (EJ) leaves, *Pakistan J Med Res* **28**(3), 165-68 (1989)
12. Singh N, SD Tyagi, V Garg, S Joneja, SC Agarwal, SC Asthana; Effect of long term feeding of different extracts of *Syzygium cumini* seeds on alloxan induced diabetes in albino rats. *Agr Biol Res* **6**(2), 80- 88 (1990)
13. Singh N, SD Tyagi, SC Agarwal; Anti-diabetic effect of ethanolic extract of *Sygygium cumini* seeds powder, *Biosphere* **3**(1), 26- 36 (1991)
14. Al-Zaid, Hassan MAM, N Badir, KA Gumma; Evaluation of blood glucose lowering activity of three plant diet additives. *Int J Pharmacogn* **29** (2), 81-88 (1991)
15. Achrekar S, GS Kaklij, MS Pote, SM Kelkar; Hypoglycaemic activity of *Eugenia jambolana* and *Ficus bengalensis*: mechanism of action, *In Vivo* **5**(2),:143-47 (1991)
16. Kohli KR, RH Singh, A clinical trial of Jambu (*Eugenia jambolana*) in non insulin dependent diabetes mellitus, *Jour Res Ay Siddha* **14**(3-4), 89-97 (1993)
17. Teixeira CC, LP Pinto, FH Kessler, L Knijnik, CP Pinto, GJ Gastaldo, FD Fuchs; The effect of *Syzygium cumini* (L.) Skeels on post-prandial blood glucose levels in non-diabetic rats and rats with streptozotocin-induced diabetes mellitus, *J Ethnopharmacol* **56**(3), 209-13 (1997)
18. Prince PSM, VP Menon, L Pari; Effect of *Syzygium cumini* extract on hepatic hexokinase and glucose-6-phophatase in experimental diabetes, *Phytother Res* **11**(7), 529-31(1997)
19. Prince PS, VP Menon, L Pari; Hypoglycaemic activity of *Syzigium cumini* seeds: effect on lipid peroxidation in alloxan diabetic rats, *J Ethnopharmacol* **61**(1), 1-7 (1998)
20. Purohit A, HMM Daradka, Anti-diabetic activity of *Syzgium cumini* seeds extract in alloxan induced diabetic mice. *Hamdard Medicus* 43(4), 33-34 (2000)
21. Teixeira CC, CA Rava, P Mallman da Silva, R Melchior, R Argenta, F Anselmi, CR Almeida, FD Fuchs; Absence of anti-hyperglycaemic effect of jambolan in experimental and clinical models, *J Ethnopharmacol* **71**(1-2), 343-47 (2000)
22. Grover JK, V Vats, SS Rathi; Anti-hyperglycaemic effect of *Eugenia jambolana* and *Tinospora cordifolia* in experimental diabetes and their effects on key metabolic enzymes involved in carbohydrate metabolism, *J Ethnopharmacol* **73**(3), 461-70 ((2000)
23. Pepato MT, VB Folgado, IC Kettlehut, IL Brunetti, Lack of anti-diabetic effect

of a *Eugenia jambolana* leaf decoction on rat streptozotocin diabetes, *Braz J Med Biol Res* **34**(3), 389-95 (2000)

24. Vikrant V, JK Grover, N Tandon, SS Rathi, N Gupta; Treatment with extracts of *Momordica charantia* and *Eugenia jambolana* prevents hyperglycaemia and hyperinsulinemia in fructose fed rats, *J Ethnopharmacol* **76**(2):, 39-43 (2001)
25. Grover JK, V Vats, SS Rathi, R Dawar; Traditional Indian anti-diabetic plants attenuate progression of renal damage in streptozotocin induced diabetic mice, *J Ethnopharmacol* **76**(3), 233-38 (2001)
26. Pandey M, A Khan; Hypoglycaemic effect of defatted seeds and water soluble fibre from the seeds of *Syzygium cumini* (Linn.) Skeels in alloxan diabetic rats, *Indian J Exp Biol* **40**(10), 1178-82 (2002)
27. Sharma SB, A Nasir, KM Prabhu, PS Murthy, G Dev; Hypoglycaemic and hypolipidaemic effect of ethanolic extract of seeds of *Eugenia jambolana* in alloxan-induced diabetic rabbits, *J Ethnopharmacol* **85**(2-3), 201-06 (2003)
28. Sharma SB, A Nasir, PS Murthy, KM Prabhu; Novel herbal anti- diabetic drug from *Eugenia jambolana, IUPAC International Conference in Biodiversiy and Natural Products Chemistry and Medical Applications,* New Delhi, India, p. OP-27, January 26-31, 2004
29. Jasmine R, P Daisy; Comparative effect of plant extracts on the blood glucose level of alloxan diabetic rabbits, *J Exp Biol* **7**(2), 337-40 (2004)
30. Ravi K, DS Sekar, S Subramanian; Hypoglycaemic activity of inorganic constituents in *Eugenia jambolana* seed on streptozotocin-induced diabetes in rats, *Biol Trace Elem Res* **99**(1-3), 145-55 (2004)
31. Ravi K, K Sivagnanam, S Subramanian; Anti-diabetic activity of *Eugenia jambolana* seed kernels on streptozotocin-induced diabetic rats, *J Med Food* **7**(2), 187-91 (2004)
32. Prince PS, N Kamalakkannan, VP Menon; Anti-diabetic and anti-hyperlipidaemic effect of alcoholic *Syzigium cumini* seeds in alloxan induced diabetic albino rats, *J Ethnopharmacol* **91**(2-3), 209-13 (2004)
33. Ravi K, B Ramachandran, S Subramanian; Protective effect of *Eugenia jambolana* seed kernel on tissue antioxidants in streptozotocin-induced diabetic rats, *Biol Pharm Bull* **27**(8), 1212-17 (2004)
34. Ravi K, B Ramachandran, S Subramanian; Effect of *Eugenia jambolana* seed kernel on antioxidant defense system in streptozotocin-induced diabetes in rats, *Life Sci* **75**(22), 2717-31 (2004)
35. Pepato MT, DM Mori, AM Baviera, JB Harami, RC Vendramini, IL Brunetti; Fruit of the jambolan tree (*Eugenia jambolana* Lam.) and experimental diabetes, *J Ethnopharmacol* **96**(1-2), 43-48 (2005)
36. Sridhar SB, UD Sheetal, MR Pai, MS Shastri; Preclinical evaluation of the antidiabetic effect of *Eugenia jambolana* seed powder in streptozotocin-diabetic rats,

Braz J Med Biol Res **38**(3), 463-68 (2005)

37. Ravi K, S Rajasekaran, S Subramanian; Anti-hyperlipidaemic effect of *Eugenia jambolana* seed kernel on streptozotocin-induced diabetes in rats, *Food Chem Toxicol* **43**(9), 1433-39. (2005)
38. Sharma SB, A Nasir, KM Prabhu, PS Murthy; Anti-hyperglycaemic effect of the fruit-pulp of *Eugenia jambolana* in experimental diabetes mellitus, *J Ethnopharmacol* **104**(3), 367-73 (2006)
39. Saravanan G, L Pari; Effect of *Syzygium cumini* bark extract on plasma and tissue glycoproteins in streptozotocin-induced diabetic rats, *J Cell Tissue Res* 7(1), 881-87 (2007)

Eugenia uniflora Linn. (Myrtaceae)
(Surinam cherry, Pitanga)

The leaves of *E. uniflora* are used in Paraguayan natural medicine as an anti-diabetic agent. The water-soluble extract of *E. uniflora* leaves was found to inhibit the increase of plasma glucose level in sucrose tolerance test, conducted with mice. The extract was found to inhibit *alpha*-glucosidases. The structures of uniflorines A and B, isolated from the active fraction, were elucidated.

Matsumura T, M Kasai, T Hayashi, M Arisawa, Y Momose, I Arai, S Amagaya, Y Komatsu; *Alpha*-glucosidase inhibitors from Paraguayan natural medicine, Nangapiry, the leaves of *Eugenia uniflora*, *Pharmaceut Biol* **34** (4), 302-07 (2000).

Euonymus alatus (Thunb.) Siebold (Celastraceae)
(Burning Bush, Chinese. Gui Jeon Wu)

Euonymus alatus is native to eastern Asia; in central and northern China, Japan, and Korea. It is a popular ornamental plant in gardens and parks due to its bright pink or orange fruit and attractive fall colour. The common name "burning bush" comes from its bright red fall colour. The plant is used as a folk medicine for regulating blood circulation, relieving pain, eliminating blood clot, and treating dysmenorrhea in Asian countries. The effect of treatment of high-fat diet-induced hyperglycaemic and hyperlipidemic ICR mice with a 50% ethanol extract of the plant for a 10-week period was studied. The extract not only reduced body weight in a dose dependent manner but also corrected associated hyperinsulinemia and hyperlipidemia. The extract exerted beneficial effects on glucose and lipid homeostasis in diabetes. A marked improvement in obesity-related diabetes and non-alcoholic fatty liver disease was also observed.

Park SH, SK Ko, SH Chung; *Euonymus alatus* prevents the hyperglycaemia and hyperlipidaemia induced by high-fat diet in ICR mice, *J Ethnopharmacol* **102**(3), 326-35 (2005)

Euphorbia prostrata Aiton (Euphorbiaceae)

In normal rabbits a significant hypoglycaemic effect was observed following oral administration of the methanol extract of *Euphorbia prostrata*. The extract of *E. prostrata* caused lowering of blood glucose.

Akhtar MS, QM Khan, T Khaliq; Effects of *Euphorbia prostrata* and *Fumaria parviflora* in normoglycaemic and alloxan-treated hyperglycaemic rabbits, *Planta Med* **50**(2), 138-42 (1984)

Euphrasia officinalis (Linn.) (Scrophulariaceae) (Eyebright)

It is an elegant little plant, that flowers from July to September, with deeply-cut leaves and numerous, small, white or purplish flowers. *E. officinalis* has been used for centuries for various eye problems.

The treatment of alloxan-induced diabetic rats with an aqueous extract of *Euphrasia officinale* leaves brought down the raised glucose levels. The extract was, however, not effective in lowering the blood glucose level of normal rats.

Porchezhian E, SH Ansari, NK Shreedharan; Anti-hyperglycaemic activity of *Euphrasia officinale* leaves, *Fitoterapia* **71**(5), 522-26 (2000)

Eurycoma longifolia Jack. (Simaroubaceae)

E. longifolia is a flowering plant, native to Indonesia and Malaysia. The blood glucose lowering effect of an aqueous extract of *E. longifolia* was studied in normoglycaemic and streptozotocin-induced hyperglycaemic rats. A positive result in hyperglycaemic rats was obtained only at a dose of 150 mg/kg body weight.

Husen R, AH Pihie, M Nallappan; Screening for anti-hyperglycaemic activity in several local herbs of Malaysia, *J Ethnopharmacol* **95** (2-3), 205-08 (2004)

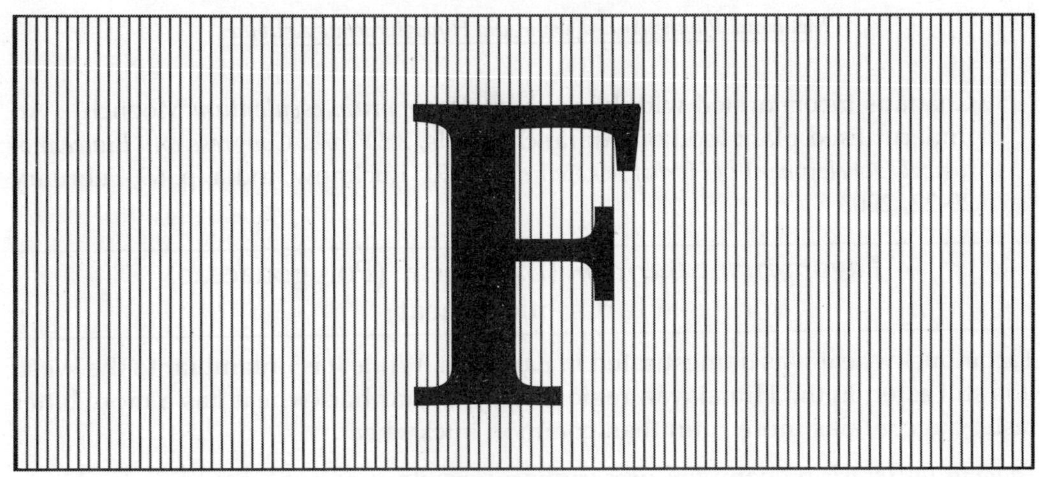

Fagopyrum esculentum Moench (Polygonaceae)
(Common buckwheat, H. Kotu)

F. esculentum is classed as a pseudocereal, as it is used in the same way as cereals but is not a member of the grass family. Consumption of diet, supplemented with whole buckwheat (*F. esculentum*) for 12 and 14 weeks, resulted in lowering of fasting blood glucose levels along with an improvement in glucose tolerance test. The volunteers consuming this supplemented diet also showed a significant increase in HDL-cholesterol/total cholesterol ratio with a significant fall in triglyceride levels (1).

The anti-hyperglycaemic effects of synthetic d-*chiro*-inositol, a component of an insulin mediator, have been demonstrated in rats. Buckwheat, a rich source of d-*chiro*-inositol, is obviously expected to reduce serum glucose concentrations in diabetics. The effects of a buckwheat concentrate on hyperglycaemia and glucose tolerance was studied in streptozotocin-induced diabetic rats. Buckwheat concentrates, containing 10 and 20 mg of d-*chiro*-inositol/kg of body weight, were effective in lowering serum glucose concentrations in streptozotocin-induced diabetic rats at 90 and 120 min after administration. Buckwheat concentrate may, therefore, be useful in the treatment of diabetes (2). A study, undertaken to evaluate the nutritional composition and glycaemic indices of different varieties of buckwheat grains, showed that in addition to promising values of nutritional composition, buckwheat has lower glycaemic index properties and can be suitably used to design foods for diabetic patients (3).

1. Bijlani RL, BM Gandhi, MC Gupta, S Manocha, BN Tandon; Effect of whole buckwheat (*Fagopyrum esculantum*) flour supplemention on lipid profile and glucose tolerance, *Indian J Med Res* **81**(2), 162-68 (1985)
2. Kawa JM, CG Taylor, R Przybylski; Buckwheat concentrate reduces serum glucose in streptozotocin-diabetic rats, *J Agric Food Chem* **51**(25), 7287-91 (2003)
3. Raghuvanshi RS, M Verma; Nutritional evaluation and glycaemic response of

Chapatis incorporated with buckwheat (*Fagopyrum esculentum* Moench) : An underutilised plant food of Uttaranchal hills, 2nd *World Congress on "Biotechnological Development of Herbal Medicine"*, NBRI, Lucknow, India, p. 69, February 20-22, 2003

Fagopyrum tataricum (L.) Gaertn. (Polygonaceae) (Tartar buckwheat)

Tartar buckwheat was domesticated in East Asia. While it is unfamiliar to the West, it is still eaten in the Himalayan region today. Tartar buckwheat has a more bitter taste, but contains more rutin than common buckwheat.

Fagopyrum tataricum complex prescription was close or superior to glyburide in decreasing blood glucose level, improving insulin-sensitivity and preventing obesity. It could also prevent chronic complication of diabetes.

Gao T, Q You; The study of *Fagopyrum tataricum* complex prescription on type-II diabetes rats, *Zhong Yao Cai* **24**(6), 424-26 (2001) [Article in Chinese]

Ficus bengalensis Linn. (Moraceae) (Bengal fig, Banyan tree, H. Bargad)

Banyan tree is endemic to Bangladesh, India and Sri Lanka. It can grow into a giant tree covering several hectares. *Ficus bengalensis* is a medicinal plant reputed for its anti-diabetic properties in Ayurvedic and other traditional systems of medicine of India.

Early experimental and clinical studies revealed hypoglycaemic activity in the bark of *F, bengalensis* (1, 3, 5, 6, 9). There are also some reports of the isolation of hypoglycaemic principles from this plant (2, 4). The extract of stem bark of *F, bengalensis* significantly decreased the blood sugar levels after three hours, the hypoglycaemic response being more marked than tolbutamide. The magnitude of hypoglycaemic effect of the extract varied with dosage and storage time (10). Oral administration of hot water extract of the plant bark (50 mg/kg/day) for 3 days and its repetition after a gap of 5 days resulted in a fall (55.8%) of fasting blood glucose level in mildly diabetic rabbits with improvement of glucose tolerance test. A more significant fall in fasting blood glucose level was observed in severely diabetic rabbits. The treatment, however, failed to exhibit any significant change in fasting blood glucose level or in glucose tolerance test in normal rabbits. Treatment of alloxan-induced diabetic rabbits with the extract (50 mg/kg/day) for three months brought down serum lipid values close to those in healthy controls (22, 23), Administration of a partially purified aqueous extract of bark of the plant to alloxanised rabbits was found to exhibit hypoglycaemic and hypocholesterolemic activity. Chronic toxicity studies, using three doses of aqueous extract (50, 100 and 150 mg/kg) for three months, did not reveal any adverse effect (27). Oral administration of the extract (25mg/kg b.w.) once daily for one month to streptozotocin-induced diabetic rats resulted in a fall in the levels of fasting blood glucose, glycosylated haemoglobin, triacylglycerol, and LDL+VLDL-cholesterol (28).

The extract of *F. bengalensis* bark caused reduction in blood sugar level in streptozotocin-induced diabetic animals. Oral administration of the extract resulted in enhancement in serum insulin levels in normoglycaemic and diabetic rats. The incubation of isolated islets of Langerhans from normal as well as from diabetic animals with the plant extract stimulated insulin secretion. The extract inhibited insulinase activity from liver and kidney (15). In addition to significant hypoglycaemic activity in alloxan-induced diabetic rats, the extract also lowered the serum cholesterol and blood urea levels in these animals (16).

Bengalenoside, an uncharacterised flavone glycoside isolated from the ethanol extract of the bark of *F. bengalensis*, produced a fall in fasting blood glucose level in normal and alloxan-induced diabetic rabbits. The glucoside was found to be more active than the crude extract and half as potent as tolbutamide (7). An acetone-soluble highly active hypoglycaemic principle was isolated from the ethanol extract of the bark, which was found to be more potent than tolbutamide (11, 12).

The effects of the flavonols, morin and quercetin and of their corresponding glycosides quercitrin and rutin were studied on the blood glucose levels of rats. Quercetin and quercitrin caused hypoglycaemia in rats, while rutin and morin showed almost no difference. Quercetin, which showed 50% pronounced hypoglycaemic effect, reduced significantly the blood glucose level of alloxan diabetic rats (13)

Several anthocyanidine derivatives were isolated from the ethanol extract of the bark of the plant and fully characterized (8). Oral administration of a dimethoxy derivative of leucocyanidin 3-O-β-D-galactosyl cellobioside, isolated from the bark of *F. bengalensis*, significantly lowered the blood glucose levels and increased serum insulin levels at a dose of 250 mg/kg in normal and moderately diabetic rats. Treatment for one month at a dose of 100 mg/kg significantly decreased blood and urine sugar levels, certain lipid components and hepatic glucose-6-phosphatase activity. This compound also increased the body weight and activities of hexokinase and HMG-CoA reductase in tissues (14). The insulin sparing action of the compound has also been reported (19, 20).

In moderately diabetic rats the acute and chronic hypoglycaemic effects of dimethoxy derivative of pelargonidin-3-O-α-L-rhamnoside, isolated from the bark of *F. bengalensis* were evaluated and compared with those of glibenclamide. Administration of a single dose the glycoside (250 mg /kg) caused lowering of fasting blood sugar levels by 29 %. This hypoglycaemic effect of the glycoside was comparatively more marked than glibenclamide. Following 30 days of the treatment, the blood sugar levels were reduced by 50 % of pretreatment level. The glycoside also raised the serum insulin levels in these animals very much like glibenclamide but while the glycoside significantly increased the faecal excretion of sterols and bile acids, glibenclamide did not exert such activity. In normal and alloxan induced diabetic dogs, the dimethoxy ether of leucopelargonidin -3-O-α-L-rhamnoside (100 mg/kg p.o.) produced significant hypoglycaemic effect along with an increase of serum insulin level after 2 hours of administration. Such an effect of the glycoside was similar to that of known drugs, which stimulates insulin secretion. Acute (0.2-1.8 g/kg) or chronic (100, 250 and 500 mg/kg) administration of the glycoside for one month did not produce any side effect (17, 18, 21, 25).

A leucodelphinidin derivative, also isolated from the bark of *F. bengalensis*, demonstrated hypoglycaemic action at a dosage of 250 mg/kg given both in normal and alloxan-induced diabetic rats. Its action was similar to that of an effective dose of glibenclamide (2 mg/kg) tested under the same conditions. However, after a glucose load, the plant product was just significantly active but not as effective as sulphonylurea (24).

An ethanol extract of the fruits of *F. bengalensis*, at a dosage of 120 mg/kg body weight, was found to exert a more pronounced anti-diabetic activity than the ethanol extract of the root or bark (29).

1. Shrotri DS, R Aiman; The relationship of the post absorptive state to the hypoglycaemic action studies on *Ficus bengalensis*, *Indian J Med Res* **48,** 162-63 (1960)
2. Deshmukh VK. DS Shrotri, R Aiman; Isolation of hypoglycaemic principle from the bark of *Ficus bengalensis*: A preliminary note, *Indian J Physiol Pharmcol* **4**, 182-85 (1960)
3. Joglekar GV, DS Shrotri, R Aiman, JH Balwani; A study on *Ficus bengalensis* Linn., *J Indian Med Assoc* **40,** 11 (1963)
4. Brahmachari HD, KT Augusti; Isolation of orally effective hypoglycaemic compounds from *Ficus bengalensis*, Linn, *Indian J Physiol Pharmacol* **8,** 60-64 (1964)
5. Vad BG, Joglekar GV, Mutalik GS, Balwani JH; Clinical experience with *Ficus bengalensis* Linn, *Indian Med J* **59,** 94-95 (1965)
6. Vohra SB, GC Parasar; Anti-diabetic studies on *Ficus bengalensis* Linn., *Indian J Pharmacy* **32,** 68-69 (1970)
7. Augusti KT; Hypoglycaemic action of bengalenoside, a glucoside isolated from *Ficus bengalensis* Linn, in normal and alloxan diabetic rabbits, *Indian J Physiol Pharmacol* **19**(4), 218-20 (1975)
8. Prema MS, GS Misra; Chemical Constituents of *Ficus bengalensis*, *Indian J Chem* **15**, 762-63 (1977)
9. Ikram M; Biologically active medicinal plants, *Hamdard Med* **27**(3), 73-85 (1984)

10. Fernando MR, MI Thabrew, EH Karunanayake; Oral hypoglycaemic activity of the stem bark of *Ficus bengalensis*, *Ceylon J Med Sci* **30**(2), 73-81 (1987)
11. Venkanna Babu B, KM Prabhu, PS Murthy; Studies on the hypoglycaemic activity of the bark of *Ficus bengalensis* employing alloxan recovered rabbits. *Diabetes Bulletin* **7,** 105-08 (1987)
12. Venkanna Babu B, Radha Moorti, S Pugazenthi, KM Prabhu, PS Murthy; Alloxan recovered rabbits as animal model for screening for hypoglycaemic activity of compounds, *Indian J Biochem Biophys* **25**, 714-18 (1988);
13. Nagwa M, Ammar, SY Al-Okhi; Effect of four flavonoids on blood glucose of rats, *Arch Pharm Res* **11**(2), 166-68 (1988)
14. Vinod Kumar R, KT Augusti; Anti-diabetic effect of a leucocyandin derivative isolated from the bark of *Ficus bengalensis* Linn., *Indian J Biochem Biophys* **26**(6), 400-04 (1989)
15. Achrekar S, GS Kaklij, MS Pote, SM Kelkar; Hypoglycaemic activity of *Eugenia jambolana* and *Ficus bengalensis*: mechanism of action, *In Vivo* **5**(2), 143-47 (1991)
16. Neera Singh, SD Tyagi, SC Agarwal; Study of anti-diabetic effect of alcoholic extract of *Ficus bengalensis* (Linn.) on alloxan diabetic albino rats, *Jour Res Ayur Siddha***13**(1-2), 56-62 (1992)
17. Cherian S, RV Kumar, KT Augusti, JR Kidwai; Anti-diabetic effect of a glycoside of pelargonidin isolated from the bark of *Ficus bengalensis* Linn, *Indian J Biochem Biophys* **29**(4), 380-82 (1992)
18. Cherian S, KT Augusti; Anti-diabetic effects of a glycoside of leucopelargonidine isolated from *Ficus bengalensis* Linn. *Indian J Exp Biol* **31**(1), 26-29 (1993)
19. Vinod Kumar R, KT Augusti; Insulin sparing action of a leucocyanidin derivative, isolated from *Ficus bengalensis* Linn,, *Amala Res Bull* **13**(Aug), 32-36 (1993)
20. Kumar RV, KT Augusti; Insulin sparing action of a leucocyanidin derivative isolated from *Ficus bengalensis* Linn, *Indian J Biochem Biophys* **31**(1), 73-76 (1994)
21. Augusti KT, RS Daniel, S Cherian, CG Sheela, CR Sudhakaran Nair, Effect of leucopelargonidine derivative from *Ficus bengalensis* Linn. in diabetic dogs, *Indian J Med Res* **99**(2), 82-86 (1994)
22. Rimi Shukla, Kiran Anand, KM Prabhu, P Suryanarayana Murthy; Hypoglycaemic effect of the water extract of *Ficus bengalensis* in alloxan recovered, mildly diabetic and severely diabetic rabbits, *Int J Diab Dev Countries* **14,** 78 (1994)
23. Rimi Shukla, Kiran Anand, KM Prabhu, P Suryanarayana Murthy; Hypolipidemic effect of water extract of *Ficus bengalensis* in alloxan induced diabetes mellitus in rabbits, *Indian J Clin Biochem* **10**(2), 119-21 (1995)

24. Geetha BS, BC Mathew, KT Augusti; Hypoglycaemic effects of leucodelphinidin derivative isolated from *Ficus bengalensis* (Linn), *Indian J Physiol Pharmacol* **38**(3), 220-22 (1994)

25. Cherian S, KT Augusti; Insulin sparing action of leucopelargonin derivative from *Ficus bengalensis* Linn., *Indian J Exp Biol* **33**(8), 608-11 (1995)

26. Shukla R, SB Sharma, D Puri, KM.Prabhu, PS Murthy; Medicinal plants for treatment of diabetes mellitus, *Indian J Clin Biochem* **15**(Suppl. 1), 169-77 (2000)

27. Gupta S, P. Shukla, KM Prabhu, S Agrawal, V Rusia, PS Murthy; Acute and chronic toxicity studies on partially purified hypoglycaemic preparation from water extract of bark of *Ficus bengalensis*, *Ind J Clin Biochem* **17**(1), 58-63 (2002)

28. Gupta S, R Shukla, PS Murthy, KM Prabhu; Hypoglycaemic effect of aqueous extract of the bark of *Ficus bengalensis* in streptozotocin-induced diabetic rats, *IUPAC International Conference on Biodiversity and Natural Product Chemistry and Medical Applications,* New Delhi, p.P-101, January 26-31, 2004

29. Sharma S, M Chaturvedi, E Edwin, S Shukla, H Sagrawat; Evaluation of the phytochemicals and anti-diabetic activity of *Ficus bengalensis*, *Int J Diab Dev Ctries* **27**(2), 56-59 (2007)

Ficus carica Linn. (Moraceae)
(The common fig tree,)

Hypoglycaemic effect of aqueous extract of *F. carica* leaves was evaluated using streptozotocin-induced diabetic rats. Oral or intra-peritoneal administration of the extract produced significant reduction of blood sugar levels. It also prevented body weight loss and improved the survival index of diabetic rats (1). The effect of a decoction of fig leaves, as a supplement to breakfast, on diabetes control was studied in insulin-dependent diabetes mellitus (IDDM) patients. From the results of the investigation, it was inferred that the addition of fig leaf decoction to diet could be of help to control postprandial glycaemia of IDDM patients (2). Aqueous extract of fig leaves significantly lowered the blood sugar levels of diabetic rats without affecting the glucose levels in normal rats. In non-diabetic rats, the extract also decreased the plasma insulin levels (4). An aqueous decoction of fig leaves was acidified with hydrochloric acid, centrifuged, and the supernatant was neutralized with sodium hydroxide and extracted with chloroform. Administration of this solvent extract to streptozotocin-induced diabetic rats led to a decline in the levels of total cholesterol and a decrease in the total cholesterol/HDL cholesterol ratio (with respect to the control group), together with a reduction of the hyperglycaemia (3).

1. Perez C, E Dominguez, JM Ramiro, A Romero, JE Campillo, MD Torres; A study on the glycaemic balance in streptozotocin diabetic rats with an aqueous extract of *Ficus carica* (Fig tree) leaves, *Phytother Res* **10**(1), 82-83 (1996)

2. Serraclara A, F Hawkins, C Perez, E Dominguez, JE Campillo, MD Torres; Hypoglycaemic action of an oral fig-leaf decoction in type-I diabetic patients, *Diabetes Res Clin Pract* **39**(1), 19-22 (1998)

3. Canal JR, MD Torres, A Romero, C Perez; A chloroform extract obtained from a decoction of *Ficus carica* leaves improves the cholesterolaemic status of rats with streptozotocin-induced diabetes, *Acta Physiol Hung* **87**(1), 71-76 (2000)

4. Perez C, E Dominguez, JR Canal, JE Campillo, MD Torres; Hypoglycaemic activity of an aqueous extract from *Ficus carica* (Fig tree) leaves in streptozotocine diabetic rats . *Pharmaceut Biol* **38**(3), 181-86 (2000)

Ficus glomerata Roxb. (Moraceae) Syn. *Ficus racemosa* (Cluster Fig Tree, H. Gular, S. Udumbara)

Administration of an alcoholic extract of the bark of *F racemosa* (75 mg /100 g b.w.) to alloxan-induced diabetic rats for 15 days significantly reduced the levels of blood sugar, urea and cholesterol. Further, no increase in blood sugar level was observed even after 15 days of discontinuation of the drug (1). The petroleum ether extract of the stem bark of the plant reduced the blood sugar level significantly. The extract completely inhibited the enzymes glucose-6-phosphatase and arginase and activated the enzyme glucose-6-phosphate dehydrogenase from rat liver. A number of components were isolated from this extract and characterized (2). Administration of petroleum ether extract of *F. racemosa* leaves (200 and 400 mg /kg, p.o.) to streptozotocin-induced diabetic rats caused lowering of blood sugar levels by 29.8% and 34.6%, respectively at the end of nine days. The hypoglycaemic activity of the extract was comparable to glibenclamide (3). The methanol extract of the stem bark of *F. racemosa* (200 and 400 mg/kg p.o.) exhibited significant hypoglycaemic activity both in normal and alloxan-induced diabetic rats, when compared with the control group. The activity was also comparable to that of glibenclamide (10 mg/kg). The findings provided pharmacological evidence in support of its folklore use as an anti-diabetic agent (4).

1. Singh N, SD Tyagi, SC Agarwal; Anti-diabetic activity of Gular, *J Natl Integr Med Assoc* **32**(2), 9-12 (1991)

2. Rahman NN, M Khan, R Hasan; Bioactive components from *Ficus glomerata*, *Pure & Appl. Chem* **66**(10), 2287-90 (1994)

3. Mandal SC, Muckerjee PK, Saha K, Das J. Pal M, Saha BP, Hypoglycaemic activity of *Ficus racemosus* L. (Moraceae) leaves in streptozotocine induced diabetic rats, *Nat Prod Sci* 3 (1) 38-41 (1997)

4. Bhaskara Rao R, T Murugesan, S Sinha, BP Saha, M Pal, SC Mandal; Glucose lowering efficacy of *Ficus racemosa* bark extract in normal and alloxan diabetic rats, *Phytother Res* **16**(6), 590-92 (2002)

Ficus racemosa Linn. (Moraecae)
(H. Gular; S. Udumbara)

See *Ficus glomerata* Roxb above

Ficus religiosa Linn. (Moraceae)
(Sacred Fig, S. Ashvatha, H. Pipal)

This plant is considered sacred by the followers of Hinduism, Jainism and Buddhism, and hence the name 'Sacred Fig' was given to it. It is native to Sri Lanka, Nepal and India, and also found in southwest China to Vietnam. The extract of *F. religiosa* (200, 250 and 300 mg/kg b.w.) exerted a significant hypoglycaemic effect in normal rabbits, which was however short lived. The hypoglycaemic effect was not significant in alloxan-treated rabbits. It has been inferred that the extract acts by initiating the release of insulin by pancreatic *beta* cells of normal rabbits.

Wadood N, A Wadood, M Nisar; Effect of *Ficus relegiosa* on blood glucose and total lipid levels of normal and alloxan diabetic rabbits, *J Ayub Med Coll Abbottabad* **15**(4), 40-42 (2003)

Fraxinus excelsior Linn. (Oleaceae)
(European Ash)

European Ash is native to most of the European countries. It is also found in northern Turkey and in Alburz mountain range in northern Iran. It is readily distinguished from other species of ash in that it has black buds, unlike the brown or grey buds of most other ashes.

Hypoglycaemic/anti-hyperglycaemic effect of an aqueous extract of *F. excelsior* seeds was evaluated in normal and streptozotocin-induced diabetic rats. Oral administration of the extract (20 mg/kg single dose or 15 daily doses) significantly lowered the blood glucose levels in normal and diabetic rats. The extract did not affect the basal plasma insulin level in either normal or diabetic rats. It was suggested that the seed extract of the plant reduced blood sugar level in normal and diabetic rats without affecting plasma insulin levels (1). The mechanism of action of hypoglycaemic activity of the aqueous extract of *F. excelsior* was investigated in normal and streptozotocin-induced diabetic rats. Intravenous administration of the extract (10 mg/kg/h) to normal and diabetic rats significantly decreased the blood sugar levels. The decrease in the levels was more marked in the diabetic rats than in normal ones. Since the basal insulin levels remained unchanged following the treatment, it was suggested that the hypoglycaemic effect of the extract could be due to some extra pancreatic action. In both normal and diabetic animals, the extract also significantly increased glycosuria. It was inferred that the plant extract induced inhibition of glucose re-absorption, which could at least be one of the mechanisms of hypoglycaemic activity of this plant (2).

1. Maghrani M, NA Zeggwagh, A Lemhadri, M El-Amraoui, JB Michel, M Eddouks; Study of the hypoglycaemic activity of *Fraxinus excelsior* and *Silybum marianum* in an animal model of type 1 diabetes mellitus, *J Ethnopharmacol* **91**(2-3), 309-16 (2004)
2. Eddouks M, M Maghrani; Phlorizin-like effect of *Fraxinus excelsior* in normal and diabetic rats, *J Ethnopharmacol* **94**(1), 149-54 (2004)

Fumaria parviflora Lam. (Fumariaceae) (Indian fumitory, H. Pitpapra)

Fumaria parviflora is native to Europe, Asia, and Africa, but widely distributed in many other parts of the world.

In normal rabbits, a significant hypoglycaemic effect was observed following oral administration of *F. parviflora.* However, methanol extract of the plant drug failed to decrease the blood glucose level of rabbits.

Akhtar MS, QM Khan, T Khaliq; Effects of *Euphorbia prostrata* and *Fumaria parviflora* in normoglycaemic and alloxan-treated hyperglycaemic rabbits, *Planta Med* **50**(2), 138-42 (1984).

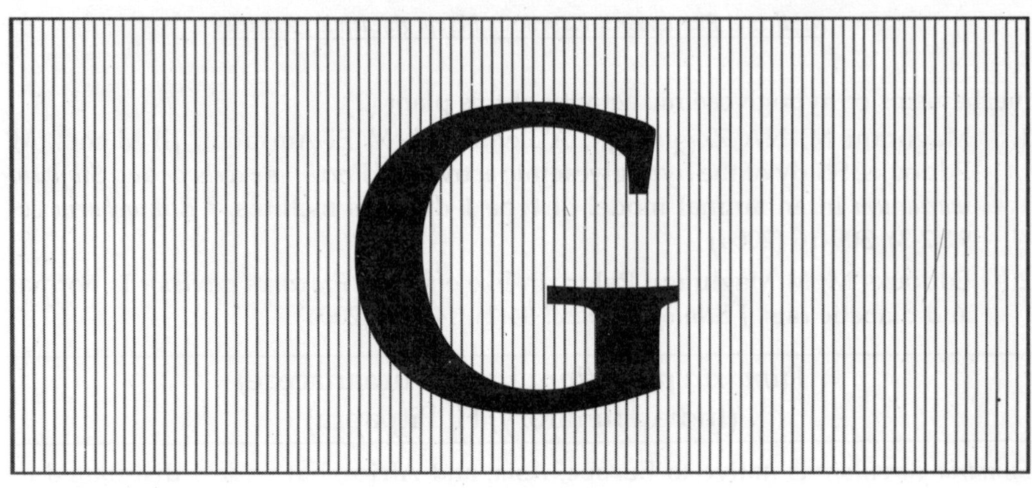

Galega officinalis Linn. (Fabaceae)
(Goat's rue)

G. officinalis, an herbaceous plant, is native to the Middle East, but it has been naturalised in Europe, western Asia, and western Pakistan. The plant has been used as a galactogogue in small domestic animals and it is for this reason that it is known as "Goat's rue". The plant has been known for relieving the symptoms of diabetes mellitus. The plant contains guanidine derivative, which is considered to be responsible for its anti-diabetic activity.

A method for the extraction and spectrophotometeric determination of galegine in *G. officinalis* and its dry extracts has been described. Gastric administration of dry extract (1.1 g) and galegine sulphate (30 mg/kg) reduced blood sugar in alloxan-induced diabetic rats (1).

Crude extracts of fresh and dry herbs of *G. officinalis* failed to exhibit any hypoglycaemic activity in normal or diabetic mice after acute administration. Repeated treatment of normal mice with alcoholic extract for 4 days also showed no hypoglycaemic activity. The alcoholic extract showed the presence of galegine and hydroxygalegine (2).

In addition to established hypoglycaemic effects, *G. officinalis* has a novel weight reducing action in normal mice, independent of a reduction in food intake. The mechanism of the weight reducing action of galega is unclear but involves loss of body fat. *G. officinalis* is a constituent of an anti-diabetic formulation, which is a powdered mixture of equal proportions of *G. officinalis, Cressa cretica, Mangifera indica* and *Syzygium jambolanum* (3).

1. Patricic J, Z Kalodera; Galegine in the goat's rue herb: Its toxicity, anti-diabetic activity and content determination, *Acta Pharm Jugosl* **32**(3), 219-23 (1982)

2. Pundarikakshudu K, AI Gray, BI Purman; Studies on the hypoglycaemic activity of *Galega officinalis* (goat's rue), *Fitoterapia* **65**(5), 423-26 (1994)

3. Palit P, Furman BL, Gray AI, Novel weight-reducing activity of *Galega officinalis* in mice, *J Pharm Pharmacol* **51**(11), 1313-19 (1999)

Garcinia cambogia (Linn.) Desr. (Clusiaceae) (Gambooge, S. Vrikshamla)

Garcinia cambogia is a shrub native to India and South-East Asia. It is regarded as an ideal plant for slimming, as it not only helps reduce storage of fatty tissue, but also activates their elimination.

The effects of 3.3% *G. cambogia* extract on 10% sucrose loading in mice for 4 weeks were studied. The treatment was found to have no effect on body weight or serum glucose level. Detailed investigation, however, showed that *G. cambogia* extract efficiently improved glucose metabolism and displayed leptin-like activity.

Hayamizu K, H Hirakawa, D Oikawa, T Nakanishi, T Takagi, T Tachibana, M Furuse; Effect of *Garcinia cambogia* extract on serum leptin and insulin in mice, *Fitoterapia* **74**(3), 267-73 (2003).

Garcinia kola Heckel.(Clusiaceae / Guttiferae) (Bitter-kola)

The natural habitat of *G. kola* is subtropical or tropical moist lowland forests. It is native to west and south tropical Africa. *G. kola* seeds are considered to be poison antidote in Africa.

Kolaviron, a defatted ethanol extract from the seeds of *Garcinia kola*, is a mixture of three compounds - Garcinia biflavonoid GB1, GB2 and Kola flavanone in ratio 2:2:1. Kolaviron was found to produce significant hypoglycaemic effects when administered intraperitoneally to normal and alloxan diabetic rabbits at a dose of 100 mg/kg. The blood sugar levels of fasting normoglycaemic and alloxan-induced diabetic rabbits were significantly reduced after 4 h and 12 h, respectively. The hypoglycaemic effects were compared with those of tolbutamide. Kolaviron was found to inhibit rat lens aldose reductase activity. The significance of these findings in the potential use of kolaviron as an anti-diabetic agent was discussed (1).

Kolaviron, a biflavonoid complex from *G. kola* seed, was separated by thin-layer chromatography into three fractions, F-1, F-2 and F-3. Kolaviron, F-1 and F-2, administered at a dose of 100mg/kg b.w., elicited significant hypoglycaemic activity within 4 h of oral administration. In streptozotocin-induced diabetic rats, these fractions also significantly reduced blood sugar levels within 4 h of oral administration. Kolaviron alone produced a significant anti-diabetic effect from day 3 to day 7 of oral intubation of streptozotocin-induced diabetic rats. It also showed favourable effect on the plasma lipid profile and decreased significantly the streptozotocin-induced increase in the activity of microsomal glucose-6-phosphatase and lipid peroxidation products. This study confirmsed the anti-diabetic and hypolipidaemic effects of kolaviron in streptozotocin-induced-diabetic rats. The observed effects of kolaviron were attributed to fractions, F-1 and F-2 (2).

1. Iwu MM, OA Igboko, CO Okunji, MS Tempesta; Anti-diabetic and aldose reductase activities of biflavanones of *Garcinia kola*, *J Pharm Pharmacol* **42**(4), 290-92 (1990);
2. Adaramoye OA, EO Adeyemi; Hypoglycaemic and hypolipidaemic effects of fractions from kolaviron, a biflavonoid complex from *Garcinia Kola* in streptozotocin-induced diabetes mellitus rats, *J Pharm Pharmacol* **58**(1), 121-28 (2006).

Gardenia jasminoides Ellis (Rubiaceae) Syn. *G. grandiflora* (Cape Jasmine)

It is a fragrant flower producing plant growing in Vietnam, Southern China, Taiwan and Japan. The name "Cape Jasmine" comes from the earlier belief that the flower originated in the Cape of Good Hope, South Africa.

Of the four iridoidal glycosides isolated from *G. jasminoides* leaves, only deacetylasperulosidic acid methyl ester was found to lower the blood glucose level in normal mice but the others did not affect the blood glucose level. The importance of stereochemical requirement for the desired activity was discussed (1). Crocetin is a natural product isolated from *G. jasminoides*. The beneficial effects of crocetin on the state of insulin resistance, induced by dexamethasone in a rat model, were studied. Male Wistar rats treated with subcutaneous dexamethasone (0.08 mg/kg/d) for 6 weeks exhibited reduced insulin sensitivity and impaired glucose tolerance. In the dexamethasone-treated group, serum insulin, free fatty acids, triglyceride and tumor necrosis factor *alpha* levels were significantly increased and the hepatic glycogen content was reduced. Treatment with crocetin (40 mg/kg/d) significantly attenuated all the described effects of dexamethasone (2).

1. Miura T, Y Nishiyama, M Ichimaru, M Moriyasu, A Kato; Hypoglycaemic activity and structure-activity relationship of iridoidal glycosides, *Biol Pharm Bull* **19**(1), 160-61 (1996).
2. Xi L, Z Qian, X Shen, N Wen, Y Zhang; Crocetin prevents dexamethasone-induced insulin resistance in rats, *Planta Med* **71**(10), 917-22 (2005).

Garuga pinnata Roxb. (Burseraceae) (Garuga)

Members of *Garuga* genus are shrubs, found in Asia and America. The anti-hyperglycaemic activity of an aqueous extract of the bark of *G. pinnata* was studied using normal and streptozotocin-nicotinamide induced type-2 diabetic rats. Treatment with the extract at two dose levels showed a significant increase in the liver glycogen and serum insulin level and a significant decrease in fasting blood glucose and glycated hemoglobin levels. The extract also reduced serum cholesterol and triglyceride levels and increased the level of HDL-cholesterol.

Shirwaikar A,, K Rajendran, R Barik, Effect of aqueous bark extract of *Garuga pinnata* Roxb. in streptozotocin-nicotinamide induced type-2 diabetes mellitus, *J Ethnopharmacol* **107**(2), 285-90 (2006)

Genista tenera (Jacq. ex Murray) Kuntze (Fabaceae)

Genista tenera is endemic to the Portuguese island of Madeira, where an infusion of the aerial parts of the plant is used in folk medicine as an anti-diabetic agent. *G. tenera* is a rich source of quinolizidine alkaloids and a number of alkaloids were isolated from the aerial parts of the plant and fully identified. Of the major alkaloids isolated from this source, N-methylcytisine and lupanine are known for their hypoglycaemic activity. Capillary electrophoresis-mass spectrometric analysis led to the characterisation of many more secondary metabolites from this anti-hyperglycaemic plant (1, 2)

1. Martins A, M Wink, A Tei, M Brum-Bousquet, F Tillequin, AP Rauter; A phytochemical study of the quinolizidine alkaloids from *Genista tenera* by gas chromatography-mass spectrometry, *Phytochem Anal* **16**(4), 264-66 (2005).
2. Edwards EL, JA Rodrigues, J Ferreira, DM Goodall, AP Rauter, J Justino, J Thomas-Oates; Capillary electrophoresis-mass spectrometry characterisation of secondary metabolites from the anti-hyperglycaemic plant *Genista tenera*, *Electrophoresis* **27**(11), 2164-70 (2006)

Gentiana olivieri Griseb. (Gentianaceae) (S. Trayamana)

Isoorientin, a known C-glycosylflavone isolated from *Gentiana olivieri* through an *in vivo* bioassay-guided fractionation procedure, exhibited significant hypoglycaemic and anti-hyperlipidaemic effects at a dose of 15mg/kg b.w.

Sezik E, M Aslam, E Yesilada, S Ito; Hypoglycaemic activity of *Gentiana olivieri* and isolation of the active constituent through bioassay-directed fractionation techniques, *Life Sci* **76**(11), 1223-38 (2005).

Gentianella nitida (Griseb.) Fabris (Gentianaceae)

Administration of an aqueous extract of *G. nitida* 60 min before a glucose load significantly reduced (40%) the level of blood glucose in alloxan-induced diabetic rats. Methanol and dichloromethane extracts of the plant showed similar but less significant effect. Three of the isolated phytochemicals showed similar effect in strptozotocin-induced diabetic mice at a dose of 10 mg/kg (1).

The ethyl acetate-soluble fraction of ethanol extract of *G. nitida* showed strong free radical scavenging activity (2)

1. Callo N, CM Alvarez, H Jurupe, UO Lock De, K Hostettmann; Chemistry and hypoglycaemic activity of *Gentianella nitida* and *Gentianella tristricha, International Joint Symposium: Chemistry, Biological and Pharmacological Properties of Medicinal Plants from the Americas,* Panama, Republic of Panama, B-25, February 23-26, 1997.
2. Rojas R, V Doroteo, B Bustamante, J Bauer, O Lock; Antimicrobial and free radical scavenging activity of *Gentianella nitida, Fitoterapia* **75**(7-8), 754-57 (2004)

Gentianella tristricha (Gilg) J. Pringle (Gentianaceae)

The hypoglycaemic activity of *Gentianella tristricha* extracts (water, methanol and dichloromethane) were tested in alloxan and streptozotocin-induced diabetic animals. The effects were similar but slightly weaker than those of *Gentianella nitida*.

Callo N, CM Alvarez, H Jurupe, UO Lock De, K Hostettmann; Chemistry and hypoglycaemic activity of *Gentianella nitida* and *Gentianella tristricha, International Joint Symposium: Chemistry, Biological and Pharmacological Properties of Medicinal Plants from the Americas,* Panama, Republic of Panama, B-25, February 23-26, 1997.

Ginkgo biloba Linn. (Ginkgoaceae)
(Maidenhair Tree)

Ginkgos are very large trees, reaching a height upto 164 feet. Ginkgo has long been cultivated in China; some planted trees at temples are believed to be over 1,500 years old. The extract of the Ginkgo leaves has many alleged nootropic properties, and is mainly used as memory and concentration enhancer. Chronic use of *G. biloba* extract is claimed to enhance mental focus and improve cognitive function in the elderly.

Kudolo (1, 2) studied the effect of 3-month ingestion of *Ginkgo biloba* extract on glucose-stimulated pancreatic *beta*-cell function in normal glucose-tolerant individuals as well as in those with non-insulin dependent diabetes mellitus. Twenty individuals underwent a 2-hour 75 g oral glucose tolerance test before and after ingestion of *G. biloba* extract (120 mg/day at bed time) for 3 months. The ingestion of the extract caused a decrease in systolic and diastolic blood pressure and a significant increase in pancreatic *beta*-cell insulin and C-peptide response. A follow-up study was later designed to determine the effect of the same *G. biloba* treatment on glucose-stimulated pancreatic *beta*-cell function in non-insulin-dependent diabetes mellitus (NIDDM) subjects. In diet-controlled subjects ingestion of *G. biloba* produced no significant effect on the insulin but in hyperinsulinaemic NIDDM subjects taking oral hypoglycaemic medications ingestion of *G. biloba* caused blunted plasma insulin levels from 30 to 120 minutes during oral glucose tolerance test leading to a reduction of the insulin. The C-peptide levels increased creating a dissimilar insulin/C-peptide ratio indicative of an enhanced hepatic extraction of insulin relative to C-peptide. Thus, in pancreatic *beta*-cells that are already maximally stimulated, ingestion of *G. biloba* may cause a reduction in plasma insulin levels. Only in NIDDM subjects with pancreatic exhaustion, who also took oral hypoglycaemic agents, did *Ginkgo biloba* ingestion significantly increase pancreatic *beta*-cell function in response to glucose loading paralleled by a C-peptide but this increased pancreatic *beta*-cell activity failed to cause a reduction of blood glucose during the oral glucose tolerance test. From these observations, it was concluded that ingestion of *G. biloba* extract by an NIDDM subject might increase the hepatic metabolic clearance rate of not only insulin but also the hypoglycaemic agents resulting in reduced insulin-mediated glucose metabolism.

The hepatic cytochrome P450-mediated interactions between *Ginkgo biloba* extract and tolbutamide, an oral anti-diabetic agent, were studied in aged and young rats. The study showed that simultaneous and continuous intake of ginkgo extract significantly affects the hypoglycaemic action of tolbutamide, possibly *via* a hepatic cytochrome P450 enzyme-mediated mechanism, particularly in the aged rats (3).

From a randomised double blind placebo-controlled crossover study, Kundolo and co-workers inferred that a short-term ingestion of *Ginkgo biloba* extract does not alter whole body insulin sensitivity in non-diabetic, pre-diabetic and type-2 diabetic subjects (4). *Ginkgo biloba* extract has been shown to ameliorate some defects associated with the insulin resistance syndrome and, therefore, patients with type-2 diabetes mellitus may be inclined to co-ingest the herb with their medications, such as metformin. It was observed that co-ingestion of *Ginkgo biloba* extract (120 mg) with metformin (500 mg) did not significantly affect the pharmacokinetic properties of metformin (5). It has, however, been suggested that patients, particularly elderly ones, should be cautious in using a combination of *Ginkgo biloba* extract with drugs like tolbutamide or midazolam because of potential interactions (6).

1. Kudolo GB, The effect of 3-month ingestion of *Ginkgo biloba* extract on pancreatic *beta*-cell function in response to glucose loading in normal glucose tolerant individuals, *J Clin Pharmacol* **40**(6), 647-54 (2000).
2. Kudolo GB, The effect of 3-month ingestion of *Ginkgo biloba* extract (EGb 761) on pancreatic *beta*-cell function in response to glucose loading in individuals with non-insulin-dependent diabetes mellitus, *J Clin Pharmacol* **41**(6), 600-11 (2001).
3. . Sugiyama T, Y Kubota, K Shinozuka, S Yamada, J Wu, K Umegaki; *Ginkgo biloba* extract modifies hypoglycaemic action of tolbutamide *via* hepatic cytochrome P450 mediated mechanism in aged rats, *Life Sci* **75**(9), 1113-22 (2004).
4. Kudolo GB, W Wang, R Elrod J Barrientos, A Hasse, J Blodgett; Short term

ingestion of *Ginkgo biloba* extract does not alter whole body insulin sensitivity in non-diabetic, pre-diabetic, or type-2 diabetic subjects—a randomised double-blind placebo controlled crossover study, *Clin Nutr* **25**(1), 123-34 (2006)

5. Kudolo GB, W Wang, M Javors, J Blodgett; The effect of the ingestion of *Ginkgo biloba* extract (EGb 761) on the pharmacokinetics of metformin in non-diabetic and type-2 diabetic subjects—a double blind placebo controlled, crossover study, *Clin Nutr* **25**(4), 606-16 (2006)
6. Uchida S, H Yamada, XD Li, S Maruyama, Y Ohmori, T Oki, H Watanabe, K Umegaki, K Ohashi, S Yamada; Effects of *Ginkgo biloba* extract on pharmacokinetics and pharmacodynamics of tolbutamide and midazolam in healthy volunteers, *J Clin Pharmacol* **46**(11), 1290-98 (2006).

Gleditsia macracantha Desf. (Fabaceae / Leguminosae)

Gleditsia macracantha is an alkaloid-bearing plant that grows along the streamsides and open countrysides in East Asian region. Galactomannan, a non-toxic polysaccharide isolated from the seed coats of the plant, was found to prevent development of alloxan-induced hyperglycaemia and diabetes in rats.

Rakhmanberdyeva RK, DA Rakhimov, AA Vakhabov, ZA Khushbaktova, VN Synov; Galactomannan from *Gleditsia macracantha* seeds and its biological activity, *Chemistry of Natural Compounds* **41**(1), 11-13 (2005)

Globularia alypum Linn. (Plantaginaceae / Globulariaceae)

Globularia alypum is a small shrub, growing on the European shores of the Mediterranean, Oral and intra-peritoneal administration of an infusion of *G. alypum* (0.7 g/kg) produced a significant hypoglycaemic effect in normal as well as in hyperglycaemic rats. The infusion significantly increased plasma insulin levels in normal rats. The hypoglycaemic activity of the plant is probably mediated through enhancement of peripheral metabolism of glucose and an increase in insulin release (1).

The effect of oral administration of an aqueous extract of *G. alypum* leaves on blood glucose levels in normal and in streptozotocin-induced diabetic rats was studied. In normal rats, single and repeated oral administration of *G. alypum* treatment did not change blood glucose level but in streptozotocin-induced diabetic rats it produced significant decrease of blood glucose level. The treatment did not affect insulin secretion both in normal and streptozotocin-induced diabetic rats, indicating that mechanism by which the plant decreases blood glucose levels is extra-pancreatic at least, for the doses used. The plant represents a potential source for discovery of new orally active component(s) for future therapy (2)

1. Skim F, HB Lazek, A Kaaya, H el-Amri, M Jana; Pharmacological studies of two anti-diabetic plants: *Globularia alypum* and *Zygophyllum gaetulum*, *Therapie* **54**(6), 711-15 (1999).

2. Jouad H, M Maghrani, M Eddouks; Hypoglycaemic effect of *Rubus fructicosis* L. and *Globularia alypum* L. in normal and streptozotocin-induced diabetic rats, *J Ethnopharmacol* **81**(3), 351-56 (2002).

Glossostemon bruguieri Desf (Sterculiaceae) (Moghat)

Glossostemon bruguieri is a shrub with thick long tapering dark coloured roots. The root mucilages of *G. bruguieri* showed remarkable hypoglycaemic activity, decreasing the blood glucose level in diabetic rats by 54.5% within 15 days. Galactose constituted 33.7 to 34.5% of the root mucilage, while rhamnose, xylose, mannose and galacturonic acid were the other sugars present in root mucilage.

Ibrahim N, W el-eraky, S el-Gengaihi, AS Shalaby; Chemical and biological evaluation of proteins and mucilages from roots and seeds of *Glossostemon bruguieri* Desf. (Moghat), *Plant Foods Hum Nutr* **50**(1), 55-61 (1997)

Glycine max (L) Merr.(Fabaceae / Leguminosae) (Soya bean, Soybean)

Soya bean (*Glycine max*) is a species of legume native to East Asia. The pods, stems, and leaves of Soya bean are covered with fine brown or grey hairs. The leaves of the plant fall before the seeds are mature. The pods grow in clusters and each pod contains 2-4 seeds. Seeds furnish one of the world's most important sources of oil and protein.

Supplementation of soy polysaccharide was found to result in an increase in wet faecal content and improvement in glucose tolerance response (1). The effect of soy polysaccharide on postprandial plasma glucose levels was examined in a crossover experiment involving seven obese non-insulin dependent maturity-onset diabetic patients. The patients were fed a standard meal without or with 10 g of this fibre source. Supplementation of soy polysaccharide significantly enhanced return of serum glucose levels towards fasting level during the latter half of the meal test. Addition of soy polysaccharide had no effect on plasma insulin levels but appeared to lessen postprandial increases in glucagon and pancreatic polypeptide levels, while it raised somatostatin levels. The changes in plasma glucagon, pancreatic polypeptide, and somatostatin levels may have been instrumental in reducing the postprandial glucose (2).

Incorporation of defatted soy flour to other cereals (Ragi, wheat or rava) in 1:4 ratio has been found to have a beneficial effect in the dietary management of non-insulin dependent diabetes mellitus (3).

The effect on serum glucose and insulin of a preprandial ingestion of 7 g of soy fibres or of an equal amount of purified cellulose on eight non-insulin-dependent (type-2) diabetic patients was studied. From the result of detailed investigation it was concluded that soy fibre compared with purified cellulose has a favourable effect on the rise of postprandial glycaemia in type-2 diabetic patients. Further, the use of soy fibres did not carry any untoward side effect (4).

Though rats fed a lipid-enriched diet have shown an impairment of insulin secretion, a significant increase of insulin secretion and glucose oxidation without any alteration of the ionic movements were detected in pancreatic islets from rats fed a soybean oil enriched diet (5)

Soya bean contains certain isoflavones, which are known as phytoestrogens. The isoflavone-containing extract of soybean showed antioxidant and potential anti-diabetic properties (6). Dietary phytoestrogens play a beneficial role in obesity and diabetes. In animal models of obesity and diabetes, soy protein associated with isoflavones has been shown to reduce serum insulin and insulin resistance. In studies of human subjects with or without diabetes, soy protein also appears to moderate hyperglycaemia and reduce body weight, hyperlipidaemia, and hyperinsulinaemia, supporting its beneficial effects on obesity and diabetes. However, to evaluate the long-term effects of phytoestrogens on obesity and diabetes further investigation was considered essential (11). Soy isoflavones were proved to exert anti-diabetic and hypolipidaemic effects through the PPAR pathways in obese Zucker rats and it was hypothesised that the isoflavones improve lipid and glucose metabolism by acting as an anti-diabetic PPAR agonist. Using obese Zucker rats as a model of type-2 diabetes, it was observed that a high isoflavone soy protein diet displayed improvements in lipid metabolism consistent with results in humans treated with anti-diabetic PPAR agonists such as the fibrates or glitazones (12). Soybean and its isoflavones have been shown to have beneficial effects on carbohydrate and lipid metabolism and on renal function. It was assumed that probiotics might potentiate the beneficial effects of isoflavones by converting the inactive isoflavone glycoside to active aglycones, and thereby producing a synergistic effect. It was with this assumption that the effects of soybean isoflavones in the presence and absence of probiotics were studied on glucose and triglyceride metabolism and the peptide hormones involved in their metabolism. Isoflavones given alone lowered plasma glucose in both lean and obese SHR/N-cp rats, while triglyceride was decreased only in lean animals. Isoflavones had significant effect on plasma insulin, leptin and glucagon in lean rats but not in obese rats. From the results of investigation it was inferred that isoflavones have hypoglycaemic and hypolipidaemic effects and the effect is mediated by changes in peptide hormones. Isoflavones fail to lower plasma triglyceride levels when triglyceride levels are high as in obese rats. Probiotics do not appear to enhance the effect of isoflavones (15).

Certain dietary components are known to suppress the initiation of experimental insulin-dependent diabetes mellitus (IDDM) in animal models. Dietary soybean prevents induction of experimental hyperglycaemia by retaining *beta*-cell activity.

In rats fed raw soybean, expression of insulin mRNA in pancreatic *beta* cells was significantly increased compared to those fed with normal diet. Injection of streptozotocin to these raw soybean fed rats caused death of only few *beta* cells but most of them demonstrated active viability with enhanced mRNA expression and insulin content and as a result blood glucose level was normalised after a transitory hyperglycaemic state. Dietary soybean was thus found to prevent *beta*-cell injury by streptozotocin. Although, this protective effect was not observed in the rats that were fed with heated soybean, some *beta*-cells were found to retain their cell organelles for insulin secretion indicating that some heat-stable components of soybean might prevent the cytotoxic insult. Dietary soybean was thus shown to protect the streptozotocin-induced *beta*-cell damage and restrain the development of hyperglycaemia in rats (7).

Water-soluble extracts of soybean, optimized for phenolic content *via* sprouting or bio-processing by dietary fungus (*Rhizopus oligosporus*, *Lentinus edodes*), were investigated for their inhibitory activity against porcine pancreatic *alpha*-amylase, yeast *alpha*-glucosidase, and rabbit lung hypertension-linked angiotensin I-converting enzyme *in vitro*. All soybean extracts possessed marked anti-amylase activity, but only slight anti-glucosidase activity. Again, the anti-amylase activity of each extract seemed to be associated with its antioxidant activity and the strongest inhibitory activity was shown by soybean bio-processed by *R. oligosporus*. The results suggest that sprouting and dietary fungal bioprocessing of soybean improve the anti-diabetic potential of soybean extracts (13)

Touchi is a traditional Chinese food, derived by fermentation of soybean. Water-extracted Touchi- exerts a potent inhibitory activity against rat intestinal *alpha*-glucosidase and elicits anti-hyperglycaemic effects in rats and humans after a single oral administration. A long-term ingestion of a fermented soybean-derived Touchi-extract with *alpha*-glucosidase inhibitory activity was found to be safe and effective in humans with borderline and mild type-2 diabetes (8-10).

The effects of soybean-derived D-pinitol (3-O-methyl-D-*chiro*-inositol) on glycaemic control and cardiovascular risk factors in Korean patients with type-2 diabetes mellitus were assessed. A total of 30 patients with type-2 diabetes received an oral dose of 600 mg soybean-derived pinitol or placebo twice daily for 13 weeks. Pinitol significantly decreased mean fasting plasma glucose, insulin, fructosamine, HbA1c, and the homeostatic model assessment insulin resistance index. Pinitol significantly decreased total cholesterol, LDL-cholesterol, the LDL/HDL-cholesterol ratio, and systolic and diastolic blood pressure and increased HDL-cholesterol. The soybean-derived pinitol was considered beneficial in controlling postprandial increases in blood glucose and reducing cardiovascular risk in patients with type-2 diabetes (14, 16).

1. Tsai AC, EL Mott, GM Owen, MR Bennick, GS Lo, PH Steinke; Effects of soy polysaccharide on gastrointestinal functions, nutrient balance, steroid

excretions, glucose tolerance, serum lipids and other parameters in humans, *Am J Clin Nutr* **38**(4), 504-11 (1983).

2. Tsai AC, AI Vinik, A Lasichak, GS Lo; Effects of soy polysaccharide on postprandial plasma glucose, insulin, glucagon, pancreatic polypeptide, somatostatin, and triglyceride in obese diabetic patients, *Am J Clin Nutr* **45**(3), 596-601 (1987).
3. Subbulakshmi G, LD Bolaki ; Glycaemic response of diabetics and non-diabetics to different soy supplemented food mixes, *J Diabet Assoc India* **31**(1), 15-18 (1991)
4. Librenti MC, M Cocchi, E Orsi, G Pozza P Micossi; Effect of soya and cellulose fibres on postprandial glycaemic response in type II diabetic patients, *Diabetes Care* **15**(1), 111-13 (1992).
5. Picinato MC, R Curi, UF Machado, AR Carpinelli; Soybean- and olive-oils-enriched diets increase insulin secretion to glucose stimulus in isolated pancreatic rat islets, *Physiol Behav* **65**(2):289-94 (1998)
6. Vedavanam K, S Srijayanta, J O'Reilly, A Raman, H Wiseman; Antioxidant action and potential anti-diabetic properties of an isoflavonoid-containing soya bean phytochemical extract (SPE), *Phytother Res* **13**(7), 601-08 (1999)
7. Lee SH, IS Park; Effects of soybean diet on the *beta* cells in the streptozotocin treated rats for induction of diabetes, *Diabetes Res Clin Pract* **47**(1), 1-13 (2000).
8. Fujita H, T Yamaguchi, K Ohshima; Fermented soybean-derived water-soluble Touchi extract inhibits *alpha*-glucosidase and is anti-glycaemic in rats and humans after single oral treatments, *J Nutr* **131**(4), 1211-13 (2001)
9. Fujita H, T Yamaguchi, K Ohshima; Long-term ingestion of a fermented soybean-derived Touchi-extract with *alpha*-glucosidase inhibitory activity is safe and effective in humans with borderline and mild type-2 diabetes, *J Nutr* **131**(8), 2105-8 (2001)
10. Fujita H, T Yamaguchi; Fermented soybean-derived Touchi extract with anti-diabetic effect *via alpha* -glucosidase inhibitory action in a long-term administration study with KKAy mice, *Life Sci* **70**(2), 219-27 (2001).
11. Bhathena SJ, MT Velasquez; Beneficial role of dietary phytoestrogens in obesity and diabetes, *Am J Clin Nutr***76**(6), 1191-201 (2002)
12. Mezei O, WJ Banz, RW Steger, MR Peluso, TA Winters, N Shay; Soy isoflavones exert anti-diabetic and hypolipidemic effects through the PPAR pathways in obese Zucker rats and murine RAW 264.7 cells, *J Nutr* **133**(5), 1238-43 (2003).
13. McCue P, YI Kwon, K Shetty; Anti-diabetic and anti-hypertensive potential of sprouted and solid-state bio-processed soybean, *Asia Pac J Clin Nutr* **14**(2), 145-52 (2005).
14. Kim JI, JC Kim, MJ Kang, MS Lee, JJ Kim, U Cha; Effects of pinitol isolated from soybeans on glycaemic control and cardiovascular risk factors in Korean

patients with type II diabetes mellitus: a randomized controlled study, *Eur J Clin Nutr* **59**(3), 456-58 (2005).

15. Ali AA, MT Valasquez, CT Hansen, AL Mohamed, SJ Bhathena; Modulation of carbohydrate metabolism and peptide hormones by soybean isoflavones and probiotics in obesity and diabetes, *J Nutr Biochem***16**(11, 693-99 (2005)
16. Kang MJ, JI Kim, SY Yoon, JC Kim, IJ Cha; Pinitol from soybeans reduces postprandial blood glucose in patients with type 2 diabetes mellitus, *J Med Food* **9**(2), 182-86 (2006)

Glycine soja Siebold.& Zucc. (Fabaceae / Leguminosae) (Wild Soya bean)

Glycine soja is native to China, India and Turkey. The seeds are rich in protein and used like Soya bean. Blood sugar and total cholesterol lowering effect of *Glycine soja* was studied.

Pant MC, I Uddin, UR Bhardwaj, RD Tewari; Blood sugar and total cholesterol lowering effect of *Glycine soja* (Sieb and Zucc.), *Mucuna pruriens* (D.C.) and *Dolichos biflorus* (Linn.) seed diets in normal fasting albino rats, *Indian J Med Res* **56**(12), 1808-12 (1968).

Glycyrrhiza glabra Linn. (Fabaceae) (Liquorice, Licorice, S. Yashti Madhu, H. Mulhathi)

Glycyrrhiza glabra is native to southern Europe and parts of Asia. Liquorice stick is the sweet, flavoured underground stem of the plant, which can be chewed to impart its sweet flavour.

The effects of hydrophobic flavonoids from *G. glabra* on abdominal fat accumulation and blood glucose level were studied in obese diabetic KK-A(y) mice. Liquorice flavonoid oil rich in hydrophobic flavonoids (with 1.25% concentration of, glabridin, the major flavonoid of liquorice), was found to have abdominal fat-lowering and hypoglycaemic effects, possibly mediated *via* activation of peroxisome proliferator-activated receptor-*gamma* (PPAR-*gamma*).

Nakagawa K, H Kishida, N Arai, T Nishiyama, T Mae; Licorice flavonoids suppress abdominal fat accumulation and increase in blood glucose level in obese diabetic KK-A(y) mice, *Biol Pharm Bull* **27**(11), 1775-78 (2004).

Glycyrrhiza uralensis Fisch. (Fabaceae) (Chinese liquorice)

G. uralensis is a flowering plant native to Asia. It is known to be one of the fundamental herbs used in traditional Chinese medicine.

The ethyl acetate extract of *G. uralensis* roots exhibited considerable PPAR-*gamma* ligand-binding activity. The ingredients of the plant (four isoflavonoids and three arylcoumarins) that exhibited PPAR- *gamma* ligand-binding activity were isolated by a bioassay-guided fractionation of the extract. The structural requirements for PPAR- *gamma* ligand-binding activity of the isolated compounds were established. Glycyrin, one of the main PPAR- *gamma* ligands of *G. uralensis*, significantly decreased the blood glucose levels of genetically diabetic KK-A(y) mice.

Kiroda M, Y Mimaki, Y Sashida, T Mac, H Kishida, T Nishiyama, M Tsukagawa, E Konishi, K Takahashi, T Kawada, K Nakagawa, M Kitahara; Phenolics with PPAR-*gamma* ligand-binding activity obtained from licorice (*Glycyrrhiza uralensis* roots) and ameliorative effects of glycyrin on genetically diabetic KK-A(y) mice, *Bioorg Med Chem Lett* **13**(24), 4267-72 (2003).

Gmelina asiatica Linn. (Verbanaceae / Lamiaceae) (Asian bushbeech, S. Gopalbhadra)

The hypoglycaemic and anti-hyperglycaemic effect of alcoholic extract of *G. asiatica* roots was investigated in normal and in alloxan induced diabetic rats. The extract showed significant dose dependent reduction of blood glucose in normal and diabetic rats at 6 h after treatment. The anti-hyperglycaemic effect of *G. asiatica* was compared with the reference standard drug tolbutamide.

Kasiviswanath R, A Ramesh, KE Kumar; Hypoglycaemic and anti-hyperglycaemic effect of *Gmelina asiatica* Linn. in normal and in alloxan induced diabetic rats, *Biol Pharm Bull* **28**(4), 729-32 (2005).

Gongronema latifolium Benth. (Asclepiadaceae)

Gongronema latifolium, commonly called 'utazi' in Nigeria, is a tropical rainforest plant, used in traditional folk medicine for the management of diabetes. Oral administration of aqueous and ethanol extracts of *G. latifolium* leaves for 2 weeks to streptozotocin-induced diabetic rats significantly increased the activity of superoxide dismutase and the level of reduced glutathione. The extracts were proved to exert their anti-diabetic activities through their antioxidant properties (1). Ethanol extract of *G. latifolium* leaves also significantly decreased triglyceride levels and normalised total cholesterol concentration (2). The anti-hyperglycaemic potency of the ethanol extract of *G. latifolium* leaves is thought to be mediated through the activation of hepatic hexokinase, phosphofructokinase, glucose-6-phosphate dehydrogenase and inhibition of glucokinase in the liver (3).

The ethanol extract normalised catalase activity, increased glutathione peroxidase activity, and reduced reactive oxygen species concentrations. It also non-significantly normalised superoxide dismutase activity, increased GSH/GSSG ratio and reduced malondialdehyde concentrations in diabetic kidney. The aqueous extract had no effect on the superoxide dismutase activity in the diabetic animals and caused a non-significant increase in catalase activity. Ethanol extract appeared to be more effective in reducing oxidative stress, lipid peroxidation, and increasing the GSH/GSSG ratio, thus ameliorating the oxidative stress found in diabetics and indicating its possible use in lessening morbidity in affected individuals (4). The anti-lipid peroxidative effects of aqueous extract of *G. latifolium* leaves were studied in non-diabetic and streptozotocin-induced diabetic rats. The oxidative stress in untreated diabetic rats, is indicated by significantly low level of their antioxidant enzyme, superoxide dismutase and high level of plasma lipid peroxidation product, malondialdehyde in comparison to non-diabetic rats. The aqueous extract of *G. latifolium* leaves reversed this situation by significantly increasing the activity of superoxide dismutase and decreasing the levels of plasma malondialdehyde. The results suggested hypoglycaemic as well as anti-lipid peroxidative properties of the aqueous extract of *G. latifolium* leaves (5).

1. Ugochukwu NH, NE Babady; Antioxidant effects of *Gongronema latifolium* in hepatocytes of rat models of non-insulin dependent diabetes mellitus, *Fitoterapia* **73**(7-8), 612-18 (2002)
2. Ugochukwu NH, NE Babady, M Cobourne, SR Gasset; The effect of *Gongronema latifolium* extracts on serum lipid profile and oxidative stress in hepatocytes of diabetic rats, *J Biosci* **28**(1), 1–5 (2003)
3. Ugochukwu NH, NE Babady; Anti-hyperglycaemic effect of aqueous and ethanolic extracts of *Gongronema latifolium* leaves on glucose and glycogen metabolism in livers of normal and streptozotocin-induced diabetic rats, *Life Sci* **73**(15), 1925-38 (2003)
4. Ugochukwu NH, K M Cobourne, Modification of renal oxidative stress and lipid peroxidation in streptozotocin-induced diabetic rats treated with extracts from *Gongronema latifolium* leaves, *Clin Chim Acta* **336**, 73–81 (2003)
5. Nwanjo HU, MC Okafor, GO Oze; Antilipid peroxidative activity of *Gongronema latifolium* in streptozotocin-induced diabetic rats, *Nigerian J Physiol Sci* 21(1-2), 61-65 (2006)

Gymnema montanum (Roxb.) Hook (Asclepiadaceae)

Gymnema montanum, an endangered plant endemic to India, is reported to be used in ancient medicine for the treatment for various ailments. Ananthan and co-workers published a series of papers (1-6) reporting the efficacy of the plant in the treatment of diabetes and associated complications.

Oral administration of the alcoholic extract (200 mg/kg b.w.) of *G. montanum* leaves in alloxan-induced diabetic rats for 3 weeks resulted in a significant reduction in blood glucose and an increase in plasma insulin. The anti-diabetic efficacy of the extract was better than that of glibenclamide (1). In addition to the suppression of elevated level of blood glucose, the treatment also suppressed elevated lipid levels in diabetic rats (2). The extract also resulted in decreased free radical formation in plasma of diabetic rats. *G. montanum* leaf extract was thus proved to possess anti-hyperglycaemic and anti-peroxidative effect. The antioxidant properties of the extract were manifest from the decrease in lipid peroxides and increase in reduced glutathione, ascorbic acid and *alpha*-tocopherol (3). Liver and kidney from diabetic animals exhibited disturbances in antioxidant defence when compared with normal rats. *G. montanum* leaf extract at a dose of 200 mg/kg of body weight exhibited a significant antioxidant defence level. In light of evidence that some complications of diabetes mellitus may be caused or exacerbated by oxidative damage, the effect of *G. montanum* leaf extract on tissue antioxidant defence systems in alloxan-induced diabetes in rats was studied. The antioxidant responsiveness mediated by *G. montanum* may be anticipated to have biological significance in eliminating reactive free radicals that may otherwise affect normal cell functioning and provide a scientific rationale for the use of *G. montanum* as an anti-diabetic plant. These effects were comparable with glibenclamide, a reference drug (4). The effects of leaf extract were also examined on brain lipid peroxidation in experimental diabetic rats. The changes in blood glucose, plasma insulin, and lipid peroxidation markers such as thiobarbituric acid-reactive substances, hydroperoxides, and levels of antioxidants, namely, superoxide dismutase, catalase, glutathione peroxidase, reduced glutathione, and glutathione-S-transferase, were examined in the brain of alloxan-induced diabetic rats after oral administration of the extract (50, 100, and 200 mg/kg bw) for 3 weeks. A significant increase in the activities of antioxidants was observed in brain on treatment with *G. montanum* leaf extract and glibenclamide for 3 weeks. The findings indicate that *G. montanum* leaf extract possesses anti-peroxidative and antioxidant effects in addition to its anti-diabetic activity (5). Hyperglycaemia significantly enhances TBARS levels in brain and retinal tissue and decreases acetylcholinesterase and butyrylcholinesterase activity. Treatment with *G. montanum* leaf extract significantly reversed the impairment in enzymatic activity in addition to reducing the level of TBARS, suggesting that the extract protects against the adverse effect of lipid peroxidation on brain and retinal cholinesterases (6).

1. Ananthan R, M Latha, L Pari, KM Ramkumar; CG Baskar, VN Bai; Effect of *Gymnema montanum* on blood glucose, plasma insulin, and carbohydrate metabolic enzymes in alloxan-induced diabetic rats, *J Med Food* **6**(1), 43-49 (2003).
2. Ananthan R, M Latha, KM Ramkumar, L Pari, C Baskar, V Narmatha Bai; Effect of *Gymnema montanum* leaves on serum and tissue lipids in alloxan diabetic rats, *Experimental Diabesity Research* **4(3)**, 183-89 (2003)
3. Ananthan R, C Baskar, V Narmatha Bai, M Latha, KM Ramkumar; Anti-diabetic effect of *Gymnema montanum* leaves: effect on lipid peroxidation-induced oxidative stress in experimental diabetes, *Pharmacol Res* **48**(6), 551-56 (2003).
4. Ananthan R, M Latha, KM Ramkumar; L Pari, C Baskar, V Narmatha Bai; Modulatory effects of *Gymnema montanum* leaf extract on alloxan-induced

oxidative stress in Wistar rats, *Nutrition* **20**(3), 280-85 (2004).

5. Ramkumar KM; M Latha, S Venkateswaran, L Pari, R Ananthan, VN Bai; Modulatory effect of *Gymnema montanum* leaf extract on brain antioxidant status and lipid peroxidation in diabetic rats, *J Med Food* **7**(3), 366-71 (2004).
6. Ramkumar KM; M Latha, N Ashokkumar, L Pari, R Ananthan; Modulation of impaired cholinesterase activity in experimental diabetes: effect of *Gymnema montanum* leaf extract, *J Basic Clin Physiol Pharmacol* **16**(1), 17-35 (2005)

Gymnema sylvestre R.Br. (Asclepiadaceae)
(H. Gurmar, S. Meshasringi, Madhunaashini)

Gymnema sylvestre is a large climber, native to the tropical forests of southern and central India. It has been used extensively in the Ayurvedic system of medicine for the treatment diabetes for centuries. It reduces the taste of sugar when it is placed in the mouth, thus some use it to fight sugar cravings. Gurmarin, the chemical constituent of the plant responsible for blocking sweet taste in humans, was recognised to be a polypeptide. While the effects of the herb are not entirely known, it has been shown to reduce blood sugar levels, particularly when used for an extended period of time. Several early publications, reporting different aspects of hypoglycaemic activity of *G. sylvestre* appeared during 1963-1988 (1-9). These include the effect of *Gymnema sylvestre* on glucose tolerance in albino rats (1), the insulinotropic activity of *G. sylvestre* (3), the hypoglycaemic activity of *G. sylvestre* in normal and diabetic persons (5) and the hypoglycaemic and life-prolonging properties of *G. sylvestre* leaf extract in diabetic rats (6). Srivastava and co-workers reported that oral administration of an aqueous suspension of dry leaves of the plant (0.2 g/2 ml) exhibited hypoglycaemic activity in moderately diabetic rats and that the effect persisted beyond a period of two months even after discontinuation of the treatment. The drug, however, failed to show reduction of blood sugar levels in severely diabetic animals but was able to enhance their longevity (2, 7). Rathi *et al* reported that the elevated levels of some protein-bound polysaccharides and glycosaminoglycans in serum and tissues (brain, kidney, heart and liver) in alloxan-induced diabetic rats were brought down to the normal levels by treatment with *G. sylvestre* for one month. The levels of chondroitin sulphates, which showed a decrease in diabetic animals, were restored to normal levels by treatment with *G. sylvestre* (4). In addition to the effective control of hyperglycaemia, the lipid abnormalities observed in alloxan-induced diabetic rabbits were restored to near normal levels by treatment with *G. sylvestre* (8). An isolate from *Gymnema sylvestre* is claimed to control diabetes mellitus and the associated pathological changes (9). A hypoglycaemic action of *G. sylvestre* has been discussed in animal models and NIDDM patients (21).

Okabayashi *et al* studied the effect of *G. sylvestre* (GS4) on glucose homeostasis in rats. Administration of GS4 (1 g/kg b.w.) to 18-h fasted non-diabetic rats significantly attenuated the serum glucose response to oral administration of glucose (1 g/kg). The immunoreactive insulin response in GS4-administered rats was lower than that in control rats. In mildly diabetic rats, a 60 min increment in serum glucose concentrations was significantly reduced by GS4 administration. In another set of experiments, the chronic effect of GS4 was examined in mildly diabetic rats. Two weeks after the induction of diabetes, the rats were divided into two groups that had similar impairment of glucose tolerance, assessed by an oral glucose-loading test. The rats were fed for 32-35 days with either a control diet or a diet supplemented with GS4. After 4 weeks, GS4 showed a tendency to reduce the serum glucose concentrations in the fed state and to improve the glucose tolerance. Gain in body weight, food intake, pancreas weight and the pancreatic contents of immunoreactive insulin response, protein, amylase and trypsinogen were unaltered in the GS4-treated group compared with the control. These results suggested the usefulness of *G. sylvestre* in the treatment of certain classes of non-insulin-dependent diabetes mellitus (10).

GS3 and GS4, two water soluble extracts of *G. sylvestre* leaves, were tested in streptozotocin treated rats for their effects on blood glucose homeostasis and pancreatic endocrine tissue. Oral administration of GS3 to diabetic rats for 60 days brought down fasting blood glucose to normal levels. The same effect was achieved by GS4 within 20 days. GS3 and GS4 therapy led to a rise in serum insulin to levels closer to normal fasting levels. In diabetic rat pancreas, both GS3 and GS4 were able to double the islet number and *beta* cell number. This herbal therapy appears to bring about blood glucose homeostasis through increased serum insulin levels provided by repair/regeneration of the endocrine pancreas (11). It is, however, not clear whether GS4 of Okabayashi group (10) corresponds with that of Shanmugasundaram group. Administration of GS4 (400 mg/day) to patients with insulin-dependent diabetes mellitus on insulin therapy brought down the requirement of insulin together with a fall in fasting blood glucose and glycosylated haemoglobin (HbA1c) and glycosylated plasma protein levels. GS4 therapy appears to enhance endogenous insulin, possibly by regeneration/revitalisation of the residual *beta* cells in IDDM patents (12). The effectiveness of GS4 in controlling hyperglycaemia was investigated in 22 type-2 diabetic patients on conventional oral anti-hyperglycaemic agents. GS4 (400 mg/day) was administered for 18-20 months as a supplement to the conventional oral drugs. During GS4 supplementation, the patients showed a significant reduction in blood glucose, glycosylated haemoglobin and glycosylated plasma proteins. Five of the 22 diabetic patients were able to discontinue their conventional drug and maintain their blood glucose homeostasis with GS4 alone. While these observations suggested that the *beta* cells might be regenerated / repaired in type-2 diabetic patients on GS4 supplementation, the appearance of raised insulin levels in the serum of patients after GS4 supplementation supported the suggestion (13). The effects of an alcoholic extract of *G. sylvestre* (GS4) on insulin secretion from rat islets of Langerhans and several pancreatic *beta*-cell lines were examined. The results of this investigation confirmed the stimulatory effects of *G. sylvestre* on insulin release, but indicated that GS4 acted by increasing cell permeability, rather than by stimulating exocytosis by regulated pathways (23).

The hypoglycaemic effect observed on administration of *G. sylvestre* leaf powder (10g per day) to normal subjects and mild diabetics indicated it to be comparable to tolbutamide (15).

G. sylvestre leaf extract was found to exhibit hypoglycaemic and anti-hyperglycaemic effects in rats. The leaf extract, by itself, failed to alter the hepatic glycogen content in normal rats but lowered the glycogen content of the tissue significantly in glucose fed rats. The glycogen content was further lowered when both exogenous insulin and leaf extract were administered. The results have been discussed (18, 22).

Gastric inhibitory peptide release into the portal vein in response to duodenal infusion of D-glucose was studied in the presence of a leaf extract of *G. sylvestre* and gymnemic acid, a pure constituent of the plant. The increase in the portal immunoreactive gastric inhibitory peptide induced by glucose was significantly depressed by concomitant infusion of leaf extract of *G. sylvestre* and gymnemic acids. These results suggest that the glucose receptor interacts with the leaf extract of *Gymnema sylvestre* and purified gymnemic acid (14).

The hypoglycaemic and anti-hyperglycaemic activities of gymnemasins A-D, the four new triterpenoid saponins, isolated from the hot aqueous extract of dried leaves of *G. sylvestre,* have been discussed. The non-sugar part of these saponins was recognised as 3β, 16β, 22α, 23, 28-pentahydroxyolean-12-ene with or without tigloyl group at 22-position (16). Major saponin constituents were isolated from "gymnemic acid", a crude saponin fraction of *G. sylvestre.* Gymnemoside-b and gymnemic acid V were recognised as the active principles (20).

The anti-hyperglycaemic action of a crude saponin fraction and five triterpene glycosides (gymnemic acids I-IV and gymnemasaponin V) derived from the methanol extract of *G. sylvestre* leaves was studied in streptozotocin-induced diabetic mice. While the saponin fraction (60 mg/kg) reduced blood glucose levels 2-4h after the intra-peritoneal administration, gymnemic acid IV, at doses of 3.4-13.4 mg/kg, reduced the blood glucose levels by 13.5-60.0% 6h after the administration. This activity is comparable to the potency of glibenclamide. Gymnemic acid IV increased plasma insulin levels in streptozotocin diabetic mice at a dose of 13.4 mg/kg and did not inhibit *alpha*-glycosidase activity in the brush border membrane vesicles of normal rat small intestines. The results indicate that insulin-releasing action of gymnemic acid IV possibly contributes to the anti-hyperglycaemic effect by the leaves of *G. sylvestre* (24).

Administration of *G. sylvestre* extract decreased serum glucose concentration in dexamethasone induced hyperglycaemic animals. The effects were comparable to the standard corticosteroid-inhibiting drug, ketoconazole (26).

The effects of OSA, a virgin isolate of *G. sylvestre*, on pancreatic β-cell function was determined. OSA ($\geq$0.125 mg/ml) caused a dose-dependent and a statistically significant increase in insulin secretion from MIN6 insulin-secreting cells at both 2mM and 20mM glucose. The stimulatory effects of OSA on insulin secretion were significantly reduced in the absence of extracellular Ca^{2+}, indicating that at least part of the effect of OSA was dependent on Ca^{2+} influx.. OSA significantly stimulated insulin secretion from isolated human islets of Langerhans in perifusion experiments.(27).

Oral administration of conduritol-A, a polyol isolated from the leaves of *G, sylvestre*, to fasting rats at a dose level of 1 mg/kg body weight with every 1g of glucose inhibited increase of blood sugar level. Conduritol and its derivatives are used as hypoglycaemic agents (17). Further, administration of conduritol-A to streptozotocin-induced diabetic rats prevented them from getting cataracts. This was due to its ability to inhibit aldose reductase, an enzyme capable of reducing aldoses to sugar alcohols. In an *in vitro* assay, lens aldose reductase was most effectively inhibited by conduritol A when β-D-glucose was used as a substrate. This finding suggests that the inhibition of lens aldose reductase by conduritol-A may be responsible for its cataract-suppressing effect (19).

Gymnema sylvestre, a plant with potent anti diabetic properties, is also used for controlling obesity in the form of Gymnema tea. The active compound of the plant is a group of acids termed as gymnemic acids. A possible link between obesity, gymnemic acids and diabetes has been visualised. This review attempts to put forth an overall idea about the plant and presents a molecular perspective linking the common medicine to the most common metabolic disorders (28). Across the globe, an estimated 150 million people are suffering from diabetes mellitus and associated complications resulting in a reduction in quality of life and an increase in individual morbidity and mortality. One treatment that is emerging as a potential panacea for the management of diabetes is *Gymnema sylvestre*, which, however, needs a systematic review of the literature describing its effects (29). Advances in the study on hypoglycaemic constituents of *Gymnema sylvestre* have also been reviewed (25).

1. Gupta SS; Effect of *Gymnema sylvestre* and *Pterocarpus marsupium* on glucose tolerance in albino rats, *Indian J Med Res* **17**, 501-05 (1963)
2. Srivastava Y, CI Jhala, SK Nigam, Ashok Kumar, H Venkatakrishna-Bhatt, Experimental evaluation of hypoglycaemic effect of *Gymnema sylvestre* R. Br. in alloxan diabetic Charles Foster rats, *J Diabetic Assoc India* **21**(4), 139-42 (1981)
3. Shanmugasundaram KR, C Panneerselvam, P Samudram, ER Shanmugasundaram; The insulinotropic activity of *Gymnema sylvestre*, R. Br. An Indian medical herb used in controlling diabetes mellitus, *Pharmacol Res Commun* **13**(5), 475-86 (1981).

4. Rathi AN, A Visvanathan, KR Shanmugasundaram; Studies on protein-bound polysaccharide components and glycosaminoglycans in experimental diabetes:-Effect of *Gymnema sylvestre* R. Br., *J Indian Exp Biol* **19**(8), j715-21 (1981)
5. Khare AK, RN Tondon, JP Tewari; Hypoglycaemic activity of an indigenous drug (*Gymnema sylvestre*, 'Gurmar') in normal and diabetic persons, *Indian J Physiol Pharmacol* **27**(3), 257-58 (1983).
6. Srivastava Y, SK Nigam, HV Bhatt, Y Verma, AS Prem; Hypoglycaemic and life-prolonging properties of *Gymnema sylvestre* leaf extract in diabetic rats, *Isr J Med Sci* **21**(6), 540-42 (1985).
7. Srivastava Y, H Venkatakrishna-Bhatt, CI Jhala, SK Nigam, Ashok Kumar, Y Verma, Oral *Gymnema sylvestre* R. Br. leaf extracts inducing protracted longevity and hypoglycaemia in alloxan diabetic rats: review and experimental study, *Int J Crude Drug Res* **24**(4), 171-76 (1986)
8. Rathi NA, KR Shanmugasundaram; Glycaemic control in the development of vascular disease in diabetes mellitus: effect of *Gymnema sylvestre* R.Br., *Biomedicine* **7**(2), 39-44 (1987)
9. Shanmugasundaram ER, M Venkatasubrahmanyam, N Vijendran, KR Shanmugasundaram, Effect of an isolate from *Gymnema sylvestre* R. Br. in the control of diabetes mellitus and the associated pathological changes, *Ancient Science of Life* **7**, 183-94 (1988)
10. Okabayyashi Y, S Tani, T Fujisawa, M Koide, H Hasegawa, T Nakamura, M Fujii, M Otsuki; Effect of *Gymnema sylvestre*, R.Br. on glucose homeostasis in rats, *Diabetes Res Clin Pract* **9**(2), 143-48 (1990).
11. Shanmugasundaram ER, KL Gopinath, KR Shanmugasundaram, VM Rajendran; Possible regeneration of the islets of Langerhans in streptozotocin-diabetic rats given *Gymnema sylvestre* leaf extracts, *J Ethnopharmacol* **30**(3), 265-79 (1990).
12. Shanmugasundaram ER, G Rajendran, K Baskaran, BR Tajesh Kumar, KR Shanmugasundaram, B Kizar Ahmath; Use of *Gymnema sylvestre* leaf extract in the control of blood glucose in insulin-dependent diabetes mellitus, *J Ethnopharmacol* **30**(3), 281-94 (1990).
13. Baskaran K, B Kizar Ahamath, KR Shanmugasundaram, ER Shanmugasundaram; Anti-diabetic effect of a leaf extract from *Gymnema sylvestre* in non-insulin-dependent diabetes mellitus patients, *J Ethnopharmacol* **30**(3), 295-300 (1990).
14. Fushiki T, A Kojima, T Imoto, K Inoue, E Sugimoto; An extract of *Gymnema sylvestre* leaves and purified gymnemic acid inhibits glucose-stimulated gastric inhibitory peptide secretion in rats, *J Nutr* **122**(12), 2367-73 (1992).
15. Balasubramaniam KB, V Arasaratnam, A Nageswaran, S Anushiyanthan, N Mugunthan; Studies on the effect of *Gymnema sylvestre* on diabetics, *J Nat Sci*

Counc Sri Lanka **20**(1), 81-89 (1992).

16. Mahato SB, NP Sahu, SK Sarkar, G Podder; New hypoglycaemic and anti-hyperglycaemic principles from *Gymnema sylvestre, Int Seminar Trad Med,* Calcutta November 7-9, p. 128 (1992).
17. Ituo K, Y Fumiio, N Toshikazu, F Tadashi, N Yoshihisa, T Hideki; Use of conduritol to inhibit increase of blood sugar level , *Eur Pat Appl Ep474,358* (CLA61K31/10), 1992, 9pp.
18. Chattopadhyay RR, C Medda, S Das, TK Basu, G Poddar; Hypoglycaemic and anti-hyperglycaemic effect of *Gymnema sylvestre* leaf extract in rats, *Fitoterapia* **64**(5), 450-54 (1993)
19. Miyatake K, Kensho G, Fujimoto T, Noguchi E, Shinohara M, Takenaka S, Taira T, Upadhaya PS, Ichimoto I, Nakano Y; Effect of conduritol A, a polyol from *Gymnema sylvestre*, on the development of diabetic cataracts in streptozotocin-treated rats and on aldose reductase, *Biosci Biotechnol Biochem* **58**(4), 756-57 (1994)
20. Murakami N, T Murakami, M Kadoya, H Matsuda, J Yamahara, M Yoshikawa; New hypoglycaemic constituents in "gymnemic acid" from *Gymnema sylvestre, Chem Pharm Bull* (Tokyo) **44**(2), 469-71 (1996).
21. Bhandari U, JK Grover; A reappraisal of clinical studies on the comparative influences of three indigenous plant drugs in diabetes mellitus, *Hamdard Medicus* **41**(2), 9-15 (1998)
22. Chattopadhyay RR, Possible mechanism of anti-hyperglycaemic effect of *Gymnema sylvestre* leaf extract, part I, *Gen Pharmacol* **31**(3), 495-96 (1998).
23. Persaud SJ, H Al-Majed, A Raman, PM Jones; *Gymnema sylvestre* stimulates insulin release *in vitro* by increased membrane permeability, *J Endocrinol* **163**(2), 207-12 (1999).
24. Sugihara Y, H Nojima, H Matsuda, T Murakami, M Yoshikawa, I Kimura; Anti-hyperglycaemic effects of gymnemic acid IV, a compound derived from *Gymnema sylvestre* leaves in streptozotocin-diabetic mice, *J Asian Nat Prod Res* **2**(4), 321-27 (2000).
25. Jiang H; Advances in the study on hypoglycaemic constituents of *Gymnema sylvestre* (Retz.) Schult, *Zhong Yao Cai* **26**(4), 305-07 (2003) [Article in Chinese]
26. Gholap S, A Kar; Efficacy of some plant extracts in regulating corticosteroid-induced hyperglycaemia in mice, *Pharmaceut Biol* **41**(5), 315-18 (2003)
27. Asare-Anane H, GC Huang, SA Amiel, PM Jones, SJ Persaud; Stimulation of insulin secretion by an aqueous extract of *Gymnema sylvestre*: role of intracellular calcium, *Endocrine Abstracts* **10,** DP1 (2005) (Annual Meeting, 2005, Society for Endocrinology, November 7-9, London, U.K., 2005,
28. Kanetkar P, R Singhal, M Kamat; *Gymnema sylvestre*: A Memoir, *J Clin Biochem Nutr* 41(2), 77-81 (2007)

29. Leach MJ; *Gymnema sylvestre* for diabetes mellitus: a systematic review, *J Altern Compliment Med* **13**(9), 977-83 (2007)

Gymnema yunnanense Tsiang (Asclepiadaceae)

The anti-hyperglycaemic effect and body weight reduction activity of *G. yunnanense* extract in obese ob/ob and diabetic db/db mice were examined by intra-peritoneal injections of the extract (100 mg/kg for 12 days). On Day 5, the extract-treated ob/ob mice had significantly lower fasting blood glucose levels, which became normal on Day 12, compared to vehicle-treated animals. Glucose tolerance improved significantly and in addition, the extract-treated ob/ob mice lost weight significantly in comparison to the vehicle treated group. In db/db mice, after treatment with the same dose of the extract, fasting blood glucose levels also decreased significantly from Day 0 to Day 12. After 12 days of treatment with the extract, body weight in db/db mice also reduced. The results support an *in vivo* anti-hyperglycaemic and body weight reduction activity of *G. yunnanense* extract.

Xie JT, A Wang, S Mehendale, J Wu, HH Aung, L Dey, S Qiu, CS Yuan; Anti-diabetic effects of *Gymnema yunnanense* extract, *Pharmacol Res* **47**(4), 323-29 (2003).

Gynandropsis gynandra (L.) Briq. (Capparidaceae) (African spiderflower)

The roots of the plant are used in folk medicine for a variety of ailments. Alcoholic extract of *G. gynandra* roots exhibited significant hypoglycaemic activity in a dose dependent manner.

Rao PR, MR Babu, RV Krishna Rao, GV Mohan Babu; Studies on antipyretic, analgesic, and hypoglycaemic activities of root of *Gynandropsis gynandra* Linn., *Indian Drugs* **34**(12), 690-94 (1997)

Gynostemma pentaphyllum (Thunb) Makino (Cucurbitaceae) (Jiaogulan)

Jiaogulan is a hardy vine indigenous to Southeast Asia. It is known as an adaptogen and antioxidant and often consumed as herbal tea.

Phanoside, a dammarane-type saponin and its four inter-convertible stereoisomers, isolated from the ethanol extract of *G. pentaphyllum,* were found to stimulate insulin release from isolated rat pancreatic islets. Phanoside at 500 μM stimulates insulin release *in vitro*. Phanoside improved glucose tolerance and enhanced plasma insulin levels in hyperglycaemic situations (1). The possible mechanisms by which phanoside stimulates insulin secretion from rat islets have been investigated (3).

The anti-hyperlipidaemic and hypoglycaemic effectiveness of *G. pentaphyllum* was studied in the obese Zucker fatty diabetic rat model. Treatment with *G. pentaphyllum*

(250 mg/kg) for 4 days reduced triglyceride, total cholesterol, and low density lipoprotein cholesterol levels. These effects were dose-dependent and maintained for at least 5 weeks. Chronic treatment for 3-5 weeks also reduced post-prandial hypertriglyceridaemia induced by olive oil in the Zucker fatty rats but had no significant effect in lowering sucrose-induced hyperglycaemia in Sprague-Dawley rats. *G. pentaphyllum* improved glucose tolerance at 120 min in obese Zucker fatty rats but not in lean rats. It is suggested that the drug improves insulin receptor sensitivity (2)

1. Norberg A, NK Hoa, E Liepinsh, D Van-Phan, ND Thuan, H Jornvall, R Sillard, CG Ostenson; A novel insulin-releasing substance, phanoside, from the plant *Gynostemma pentaphyllum*, *J Biol Chem* **279**(40), 41361-67 (2004).
2. Megalli S, NM Davies, BD Roufogalis; Anti-hyperlipidemic and hypoglycaemic effects of *Gynostemma pentaphyllum* in the Zucker fatty rat, *J Pharm Pharm Sci* **9**(3), 281-91 (2006)
3. Hoa NK, A Norberg, R Sillard, D Van Phan, ND Thuan, DT Dzung, H Jornvall, CG Ostenson; The possible mechanisms by which phanoside stimulates insulin secretion from rat islets, *J Endocrinol* **192**(2), 389-94 (2007)

Gynura procumbens (Lour.) Merr. (Asteraceae)

Oral administration of an ethanol extract of *G. procumbens* leaves (150 mg/kg) significantly suppressed the elevated serum glucose levels in streptozotocin-induced diabetic rats but the effect was not significant in normal rats. When the optimum dose (150 mg/kg) was given to diabetic rats for 7 days, the extract significantly reduced serum cholesterol and triglyceride levels in these rats. These results indicated a biguanide-like activity in the leaves of *G. procumbens.*

Zhang XF, BK Tan; Effects of an ethanolic extract of *Gynura procumbens* on serum glucose, cholesterol and triglyceride levels in normal and streptozotocin-induced diabetic rats, *Singapore Med J* **41**(1), 9-13 (2000).

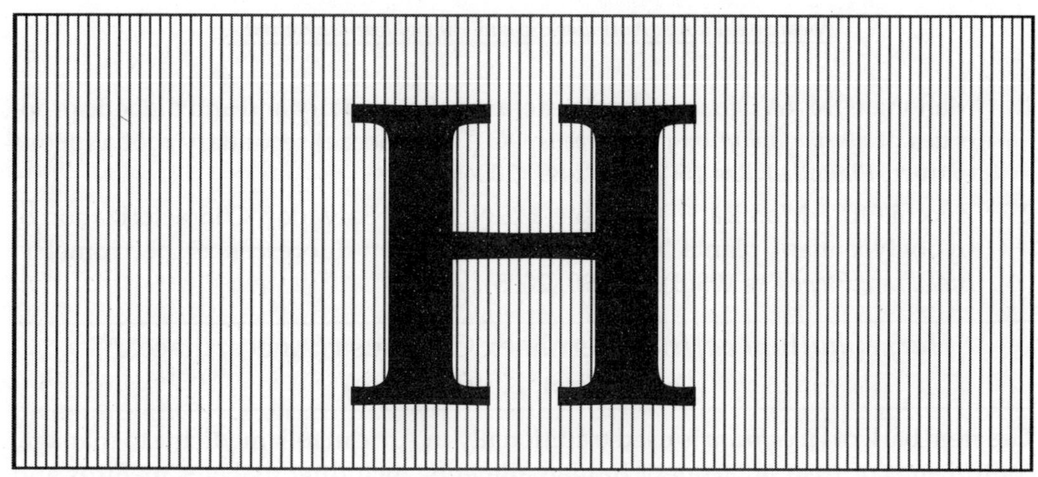

Hammada salicornica (Moq) Iljin. (Chenopodiaceae)

Ethanol extract of *Hammada salicornica* has been reported to exhibit anti-diabetic activity in mice without adverse effects.

Ajabnoor MA, ML Al-Yahya, M Tariq, AA Jayyab; Anti-diabetic activity of *Hammada salicornica, Fitoterapia* **55**(2), 107-09 (1984).

Hamiltonia suaveolens Roxb. (Rubiaceae)

Oral administration of an alcoholic extract of *H. suaveolens* roots (500 mg/kg) effected a fall of 45% and 37% in blood sugar levels in normal and alloxan-induced diabetic rats, respectively after 5h.

Desai AC, MB Bhide; Hypoglycaemic activity of *Hamiltonia suaveolens, Indian J Med Res* **81**, 86-91 (1985)

Harpagophytum procumbens DC (Pedaliaceae) (Devil's claw, Wood spider)

H. procumbens is found in the eastern and south eastern parts of Namibia, Southern Botswana and the Kalahari region of South Africa. The plant's large tuberous roots are widely used in South African traditional medicine for the treatment and management of a variety of human ailments including diabetes.

The aqueous extract of *H. procumbens* roots (50-800 mg/kg ip) produced dose-dependent, significant reductions in the blood glucose concentrations of both fasted normal and fasted diabetic rats. The results of this experimental animal study lent support to folklore uses of *H. procumbens* roots in the management and control of type-2 diabetes mellitus (1).

The elements P, K, Ca, Ti, Mn, Fe, Cu, Zn, Rb, and Sr were detected in the plant by use of synchrotron radiation total reflection X-ray fluorescence spectrometry (2).

1. Mahomed JM, JA Ojewole; Analgesic, antiinflammatory and anti diabetic properties of *Harpagophytum procumbens* DC (Pedaliaceae) secondary root aqueous extract, *Phytother Res* **16**(12), 982-89 (2004).
2. Zucchi OL, S Moreira, FF de-Jesus, HS Neto, MJ Salvador; Characterization of hypoglycemiant plants by total reflection X-ray fluorescence spectrometry, *Biol Trace Elem Res* **103**(3), 277-90 (2005).

Harpephyllum caffrum Bernh. ex C. Krauss (Anacardiaceae) (Wild plum, Kaffir-plum)

The stem bark of *H. caffrum* is used traditionally in African folk medicine to manage, control and/or treat an array of human ailments, including diabetes mellitus and hypertension. Acute oral administrations of an aqueous extract of the stem bark of the plant (50-800 mg/kg) caused a dose-related, significant hypoglycaemia in normal and streptozotocin-treated diabetic rats. The numerous polyphenolic compounds and flavonoids present in the plant are speculated to account for the observed hypoglycaemic and hypotensive effects of the extract. The findings validate the folkloric, and ethnomedical uses of the plant in the management and/or control of adult-onset type-2 diabetes mellitus and hypertension in some rural communities of southern Africa.

Ojewole JA; Hypoglycaemic and hypotensive effects of *Harpephyllum caffrum* Bernh ex CF Krauss (Anacardiaceae) stem-bark aqueous extract in rats, *Cardiovasc J S Afr* **17**(2), 67-72 (2006)

Helianthus tuberosus Linn. (Asteraceae) (Jerusalem artichoke, Sunchoke)

It is a species of sunflower, native to North America. It is also cultivated widely across the temperate world for its tuber, which is used as a root vegetable.

The influence of fructans, isolated from *H. tuberosus,* on blood glucose, insulin, and C-peptide responses was studied in eight healthy subjects and compared with those for fructose ingestion. The blood glucose and insulin increments were very low after fructan ingestion, lower than after fructose ingestion, whereas breath-hydrogen production was much higher. Areas under blood glucose curves tended to be smaller when 10 g fructans was added to a 50-g wheat-starch meal, but there was no apparent interference with starch absorption.

Rumessen JJ, S Bode, O Hamberg, E Gudmand-Hoyer; Fructans of Jerusalem artichokes: intestinal transport, absorption, fermentation, and influence on blood glucose, insulin, and C-peptide responses in healthy subjects, *Am J Clin Nutr* **52**(4), 675-81 (1990).

Helichrysum plicatum DC. ssp. ***plicatum*** (Asteraceae)

Helichrysum species are widely found in Anatolia. Decoctions prepared from the flower heads (capitulums) of *H. plicatum* ssp. *plicatum* are used to alleviate the symptoms of diabetes mellitus in folk medicine. The hypoglycaemic and antioxidant potential of the plant was evaluated in normal and streptozotocin-induced-diabetic rats. Water and ethanol extracts of the plant capitulums (500mg/kg b.w.) demonstrated significant anti-hyperglycaemic and antioxidant activity in streptozotocin-induced rats which confirmed its folkloric utilization. Polyphenolic components, present in the extracts, are considered responsible for the observed activity.

Aslam M, D Deliorman-Orhan, N Orhan, F Sezik, E Yesilada; *In vivo* anti-diabetic and antioxidant potential of *Helichrysum plicatum* ssp. *plicatum* capitulums in streptozotocin-induced-diabetic rats, *J Ethnopharmacol* **109**(1), 54-59 (2007)

Helicteres isora Linn. (Sterculiaceae)
(East Indian Screw Tree)

It is an East Indian shrub, often cultivated for its hairy leaves and orange-red flowers. The roots and stem barks of the plant are used medicinally for a variety of ailments. The root juice of the plant is known to be used for the treatment of diabetes by several ethnic groups in different parts of India. Ethanol extract of *H. isora* root (300 mg/kg) caused a significant reduction in plasma glucose, triglyceride and insulin levels after 9 days of administration to insulin resistant and diabetic C57BL/KsJdb/db mice. In normoglycaemic and mildly hypertriglyceridaemic Swiss albino mice, the extract also showed significant reduction in plasma triglyceride and insulin levels, without affecting plasma glucose level. The activity of the extract was distinctly different from glibenclamide and acarbose but similar to troglitazone in these models. The study suggested insulin-sensitizing and hypolipidaemic activity of the extract and recognized its potential for use in the treatment of type-2 diabetes (1). Of the different solvent extracts of *Helicteres isora* roots tested, butanol extract (250 mg/kg) showed maximum anti-hyperglycaemic activity in alloxan-induced and also on glucose loaded rats and the effect was comparable to that of glibenclamide (2, 3).

The bark extract significantly reduced blood glucose levels of normal, glucose-loaded and streptozotocin-induced diabetic rats (4). Oral administration of an aqueous extract of *H. isora* bark (100, 200 mg/kg) in steptozotocin-induced diabetic rats caused a significant increase in body weight, hepatic hexokinase activity and significant decrease in hepatic glucose-6-phosphatase, serum acid phosphatase, alkaline phosphatase and lactate dehydrogenase. The plant extract was thus found to ameliorate biochemical damage in streptozotocin-induced diabetic rats and possess hypoglycaemic and hepatoprotective activity (5).

1. Chakrabarti R, RK Vikramadithyam, R Mullangi, VM Sharma, H Jagadheshan, YN Rao, P Sairam, R Rajagopalan; Anti-diabetic and hypolipidaemic activity of *Helicteres isora* in animal models, *J Ethnopharmacol* **81**(3), 343-49 (2002).
2. Venkatesh S, GD Reddy, BM Reddy; Anti-hyperglycaemic activity of *Helicteres isora* roots in alloxan-induced diabetic rats, *Pharmaceut Biol* **41**(5), 347-50 (2003)
3. Venkatesh S, G Dayanand Reddy, YS Reddy; Effect of *Helicteres isora* root extracts on glucose tolerance in glucose-induced hyperglycaemic rats, *Fitoterapia* **75**(3-4), 364-67 (2004).
4. Kumar G, GS Banu, AG Murugesan, MR Pandian; Hypoglycaemic effect of *Helicteres isora* bark extract in rats, *J Ethnopharmacol* **107**(2), 304-07 (2006)
5. Kumar G, AG Murugesan, M Rajasekara Pandian; Effect of *Helicteres isora* bark extract on blood glucose and hepatic enzymes in experimental diabetes, *Pharmazie* **61**(4), 353-55 (2006)

Heliotropium zeylanicum (Burm. f.) Lam. (Boraginaceae)

Oral administration of a methanol extract of *Heliotropium zeylanicum* (150 and 300 mg/kg/d) for 14 days significantly decreased the blood glucose level and considerably increased the body weight, food intake, and liquid intake of streptozotocin-induced diabetic rats. The extract significantly decreased thiobarbituric acid reactive substances and significantly increased reduced glutathione, superoxide dismutase and catalase in streptozotocin-induced diabetic rats at the end of 14 days of treatment.

Murugesh K, V Yeligar, DK Dash, P Sengupta, BC Maiti, TK Maity; Anti-diabetic, antioxidant and anti-hyperlipidaemic status of *Heliotropium zeylanicum* extract on streptozotocin-induced diabetes in rats, *Biol Pharm Bull* **29**(11), 2202-05 (2006)

Hematoxylon campechianum Linn. (Fabaceae / Caesalpiniaceae) (Bloodwood, Campeche)

Campeche is a fast growing ornamental tree that can reach a height up to 50 feet. A black to blue dye, also called logwood extract, is obtained from the heartwood. Campeche is native to Guatemala and Mexico but it has been naturalised in many South American countries as well. In Brazilian herbal medicine, the bark is used internally for a variety of ailments.

Hydroxybrazilin, a phenolic constituent of *H. campechianum* significantly inhibited phospholipase A2 activity in normal and streptozotocin-induced diabetic rats.

Moon CH, DS Lim, TS Cho, JY Kim; Inhibitory effects of hydroxybrazilin on the platelet phospholipase A2 activities in normal and streptozotocin-induced diabetic rats, *Yakhak Hoeji* **38**(1), 97-101 (1994)

Hemionitis arifolia (Burm. f.) T. Moore (Pteridaceae) (Heart Fern)

It is an attractive and unusual dwarf fern with dark green heart shaped fronds, which grow on blackish stems. In Asian folklore, *Hermionitis arifolia* is used to treat diabetes. Of different extracts tested, ethanol and, to some extent, water extracts were found to lower the levels of blood glucose in glucose fed rats. While the ethanol extract showed optimum activity at 200 mg/kg, its ethyl acetate-soluble fraction exhibited this activity at 50 mg/kg. This fraction containing steroids and coumarins showed anti-diabetic activity in alloxan diabetic rats as judged from serum glucose levels, liver glycogen content and body weight.

Ajikumaran Nair S, BS Shyleash, B Gopakumar, A Subramoniam; Anti-diabetes and hypoglycaemic properties of *Hemionitis arifolia* (Burm.) Moore in rats, *J Ethnopharmacol* **106**(2), 192-97 (2006)

Hexachlamys edulis (O. Berg) Kausel & D. Legrand (Myrtaceae) (Yvahai)

The hypoglycaemic activity of an ethanol (70%) extract of the crude drug was assessed in normoglycaemic and alloxan-induced diabetic rats. The glycaemia in normal and diabetic rats was significantly reduced during glucose tolerance test after 7 days of oral treatment with the extract (100 mg/kg b.w.). The maximum effect was discernible between 1.5 and 2.5 h after glucose administration in normoglycaemic rats and after 1 h in diabetic animals. A single oral dose of the extract (500 mg/kg) administered to normoglycaemic rats 1 h before glucose loading elicited significant reduction in the increase of glycaemia compared to untreated animals. The effect was comparable to tolbutamide.

Rodriguez CJ, J Loyola, G Schmeda-Hirschmann; Hypoglycaemic activity of *Hexachlamys edulis* (Yvahai) extract in rats, *Phytother Res* **6**(1), 47-49 (1992).

Hibiscus esculenta Linn. (Malvaceae) (Lady's finger, Okra, H. Bhindi)

Hypoglycaemic activities of *Hibiscus esculenta* (okra) and hibiscus mucilages were studied (1). The effects of hot water, cold water and ethanol (80%) extracts of roasted seeds of the plant, respectively, in doses of 435 mg/kg, 230 mg/kg and 210 mg/kg were studied in normoglycaemic, glucose loaded hyperglycaemic, and streptozotocin-induced diabetic rats. The extracts were ineffective in normoglycaemic rats, prevented the rise in blood glucose level in glucose loaded animals but showed pronounced and significant effect in streptozotocin-induced diabetic animals (2).

1. Tomoda M, N Shimizu, R Gonda, M Kanari, H Yamada, H Hikino; Anti-complementary and hypoglycaemic activity of okra and hibiscus mucilages,

Carbohydr Res **190**(2), 323-28 (1989).

2. Aslam M, E Sezik, E Yesilada; Effect of *Hibiscus esculenta* L. seeds on blood glucose levels in normoglycaemic, glucose-hyperglycaemic and streptozotocin-induced diabetic rats, *J Faculty of Pharmacy, Gazi Univ* **20**(1), 1-7 (2003)

Hibiscus rosa sinensis Linn. (Malvaceae) (China rose, H. Gurhal, S. Japapushpam)

The hypoglycaemic activity of an ethanol extract of *H. rosa-sinensis* was studied in glucose loaded rats. After repeated administration of the extract (once a day for seven consecutive days) a statistically significant reduction in blood glucose levels was observed at 30, 90 and 120 min after glucose loading. At a dose of 250 mg/kg, the efficacy of the extract was found to be 84% of tolbutamide (100 mg/kg). The mechanism of action may be a stimulation of pancreatic *beta* cells to produce more insulin or an increase of the glycogen deposition in liver The mechanism of action could be attributed partly to increased utilization of glucose, either by direct stimulation of glucose uptake or *via* the mediation of enhanced insulin secretion (1-2).

Repeated administration of an aqueous extract of the drug plant (once a day for seven consecutive days), at an oral dose equivalent to 250 mg/kg significantly improved glucose tolerance in rats. The peak blood glucose level was obtained at 30 min of glucose load (2 g/kg), thereafter a decreasing trend was recorded up to 120 min. In streptozotocin-induced diabetic rats, no significant effect was observed with the extract, while glibenclamide significantly lowered the glucose level up to 7 hr. The data suggest that hypoglycaemic activity of *H. rosa sinensis* leaf extract is comparable to tolbutamide and not to glibenclamide treatment (3).

The effect of oral administration of an ethanol extract of the flowers of *H. rosa sinensis* on blood glucose and total lipid levels was determined in streptozotocin-induced diabetic rats. The hypoglycaemic effect obtained after 7 and 21 days of oral administration of the extract was comparable to that of glibenclamide. The extract also lowered the levels of total cholesterol and serum triglycerides and increased the level of HDL-cholesterol. The hypoglycaemic activity of the extract, though comparable with that of glibenclamide, is not mediated through insulin release (4).

1. Sachdewa A, LD Khemani; A preliminary investigation of the possible hypoglycaemic activity of *Hibiscus rosa-sinensis*, *Biomed Environ Sci* **12**(3), 222-26 (1999).
2. Sachdewa A, D Rama, AK Srivastava, LD Khemani; Effect of *Aegle marmelos* and *Hibiscus rosa sinensis* leaf extract on glucose tolerance in glucose induced hyperglycaemic rats (Charles foster), *J Environ Biol* **22**(1), 53-57 (2001).
3. Sachdewa A, R Nigam, LD Khemani; Hypoglycaemic effect of *Hibiscus rosa sinensis* L. leaf extract in glucose and streptozotocin induced hyperglycaemic

rats, *Indian J Exp Biol* **39**(3), 284-86 (2001).

4. Sachdewa A, LD Khemani; Effect of *Hibiscus rosa sinensis* Linn. ethanol flower extract on blood glucose and lipid profile in streptozotocin induced diabetes in rats, *J Ethnopharmacol* **89**(1), 61-66 (2003)

Hibiscus vitifolius Linn. (Malvaceae) (Tropical rose mallow)

A new flavonol glycoside (3′,4′, 6, 8-tetrahydroxyflavonol-5′-methyl ether 7-O-neohesperidoside), isolated from the flowers of the plant, exhibited hypoglycaemic activity in albino rats.

Ragunathan V, N Sulochana; A new flavonol bioside from the flowers of *Hibiscus vitifolius* Linn. and its hypoglycaemic activity, *J Indian Chem Soc* **71**(11), 705-06 (1994)

Himanthalia elongata (Linn.) S.F. Gray (Himanthaliaceae) (Thongweed)

Polysaccharides and proteins from *Himanthalia elongata*, a sea-weed, caused a significant reduction in blood glucose 8 h after intravenous administration. Crude polysaccharides of *H. elongata* (5 mg/kg) were found to lower glycaemia in normal and alloxan-induced diabetic rabbits by about 18 and 50 per cent, respectively. The protein solution lowered glycaemia in diabetic animals by about 30 per cent.

Lamela M, J Anca, R Villar, J Otero, JM Calleja; Hypoglycaemic activity of several seaweed extracts, *J Ethnopharmacol* **27**(1-2), 35-43 (1989)

Hintonia latiflora (DC) Bullock (Rubiaceae) (Copalchi)

The hypoglycaemic effect of Copalchi extract (Sucontral) was tested in 60 adult Wistar rats (both sexes) in a randomised, placebo-controlled, parallel-comparative animal study and a distinctly significant blood glucose-lowering effect of the extract was demonstrated. The onset of action of the Copalchi extract was observed between day 1 and day 3 of the treatment. A 20-25% decrease in the blood glucose concentration was achieved between the 7th and 15th day of treatment and remained at that level, thereafter (1). Intragastric administration of coutareagenin, a neoflavonoid isolated from Copalchi extract, demonstrated a statistically significant blood sugar-lowering effect in streptozotocin-induced diabetic animals suggesting the isolated compound to be one of the active constituents of Copalchi bark (2).

1. Pinto A, A Capasso, L Sorrentino; Experimental animal studies on the hypoglycaemic effects of a Copalchi extract, *Arzneimittel-Forschung* **47**(7), 829-33 (1997)

2. Korec R, K Heinz-Sensch, T Zoukas; Effects of the neoflavonoid coutareagenin, one of the anti-diabetic active substances of *Hintonia latiflora*, on streptozotocin-induced diabetes mellitus in rats, *Arzneimittel-Forschung* **50**(2), 122-28 (2000)

Hintonia standleyana Benth (Rubiaceae)

An extract (100 mg/kg) of the stem bark of *H. standleyana* caused a significant decrease in blood glucose levels in both normal and streptozotocin-induced diabetic rats when compared with vehicle-treated groups. The cucurbitacin glycoside 3-O-β D-glucopyranosyl-23,24-dihydrocucurbitacin F and the coumarin 5-O-[β-D-apiofuranosyl-(1→6)-β-D-glucopyranosyl]-7-methoxy-3',4'-dihydroxy-4-phenylcoumarin, isolated from the active extract, failed to decrease blood glucose levels in normal rats but in two different long-term sub-acute experiments, using animals with a developing diabetes condition and with streptozotocin-induced diabetes, both compounds induced a significant anti-hyperglycaemic activity. The phenylcoumarin also restored normal blood glucose levels in streptozotocin-induced diabetic rats.

Guerrero-Analco JA, P Hersch-Martinez, J Pedraza-Chaverri, A Navarrete, R Mata; Anti-hyperglycaemic effect of constituents from *Hintonia standleyana* in streptozotocin-induced diabetic rats, *Planta Med* **71**(12), 1099-105 (2005).

Holarrhena antidysenterica (Linn.) Wall. (Apocynaceae) (Connessi tree, S. Kutaja, H. Kurchi)

The connessi tree is a valuable medicinal plant of India. It grows throughout India up to an altitude of 4,000 ft. It is especially abundant in the sub-Himalayan tract. A significant fall in blood glucose level was observed both in normal and diabetic rats, treated with aqueous and alcoholic extracts of the seeds of the plant (1). Aqueous as well as ethanol, butanol, chloroform and butanone extracts of *H. antidysenterica* bark (250 mg/kg, b.w.) showed significant anti-diabetic activity both in acute and chronic study on alloxan-induced diabetic rats. Ethanol extract was found to be most active in reducing blood glucose level after a single dose (2).

1. Gopal V, MG Chauhan; *Holarrhena antidysenterica*: a novel herbal anti-diabetic seed drug, *Indian J Pharmaceut Sci* **56**(4), 156 (1994)
2. Jalapure SS, S Bamne, MB Patil, B Shah, M Salahuddin; Anti-diabetic activity of *Holarrhena antidysenterica* (Linn.) Wall. bark on alloxan-induced diabetic rats, *J Nat Remedies* **6**(1), 26-30 (2006)

Hordeum vulgare Linn. (Poaceae) (Barley)

Barley is of major commercial importance as a cereal grain, which is also used as fodder crop and for malting in beer and whiskey production. It is native throughout the temperate Northern hemisphere, temperate South America, and also South Africa. Barley grains have been found to exhibit hypoglycaemic and hypocholesterolemic activity (1).

Investigation showed that barley bread containing lactic acid, eaten at breakfast, has the potential to improve second-meal glucose tolerance at a high glycaemic index lunch meal 4 h later (2). Experiment with horses showed that the glycaemic index of barley was slightly more than half of that of glucose (3). Malted barley extract was shown to alleviate many of the symptoms of diabetes in genetically obese mice. It, therefore, offers promise as a therapeutic supplement for the normalization of blood glucose levels in humans with hyperglycaemia and has the beneficial effects in patients with non-insulin-dependent diabetes mellitus (4). High amounts of soluble *beta*-glucan in barley products have been shown to exert beneficial effects on glucose tolerance and blood lipids. Products prepared from barley flour enriched with *beta*-glucan exhibit favourable responses on glucose metabolism, and particularly on insulinemic responses (5).

1. Olin BR, C Dombek, D Rubber, L Liberti; Barley: a monograph, *Lawrence Review of Natural Products* p.1-2, Nov. (1994)
2. Ostman EM, HG Liljeberg Elmstahl, IM Bjorck; Barley bread containing lactic acid improves glucose tolerance at a subsequent meal in healthy men and women, *J Nutr* **132**(6), 1173-75 (2002)
3. Jose-Cunilleras E, LE Taylor, KW Hinchcliff; Glycaemic index of cracked corn, oat groats and rolled barley in horses, *J Anim Sci* **82**(9), 2623-29(2004)
4. Hong H, W Jai Maeng; Effects of malted barley extract and banaba extract on blood glucose levels in genetically diabetic mice, *J Med Food* **7**(4), 487-90 (2004)
5. Casiraghi MC, M Garsetti, G Testolin, F Brighenti; Post-prandial responses to cereal products enriched with barley *beta*-glucan, *J Am Coll Nutr* **25**(4), 313-20 (2006)

Hovenia dulcis Thunb (Rhamnaceae)
(Japanese Raisin Tree)

Hovenia dulcis is a hardy tree that occurs in Japan, eastern China, Korea and to the Himalayas, The sweet and fragrant fruits of the plant are edible in raw or cooked state. In dried condition, they look and taste like raisins.

The effects of *H. dulcis* on blood sugar and hepatic glycogen were studied in alloxan-induced diabetic mice and compared with that of glibenclamide. The blood sugar levels of mice treated with the plant drug and glibenclamide were significantly lowered, while the hepatic glycogen levels were significantly increased. *Hovenia dulcis* may become an effective anti-diabetic herb.

Ji Y, S Chen, K Zhang, W Wang; Effects of *Hovenia dulcis* Thunb on blood sugar and hepatic glycogen in diabetic mice, *Zhong Yao Cai* **25**(3), 190-91 (2002) [Article in Chinese].

Humulus lupulus Linn. (Cannabaceae) (Hops)

Humulus lupulus is a small genus of flowering plants, native to the temperate Northern hemisphere. Its female flowers, commonly called hops, are used for flavouring and as stabilisers during beer brewing. Hop fruit powder and extracts were clinically tested and found effective in the treatment of diabetes (1).

Oral administration of the bitters of hop, humulone and lupulone (200 mg/kg) to streptozotocin-induced diabetic rats decreased the blood sugar level by more than 50% within a period of 6 hour (2). Peroxisome proliferator-activated receptors (PPARs) are dietary lipid sensors that regulate fatty acid and carbohydrate metabolism. Isohumulones, the bitter compounds derived from hops that are present in beer, were found to activate PPARs. Among the three major isohumulone homolouegs, isohumulone and isocohumulone were found to activate PPAR *alpha* and *gamma*. Diabetic KK-Ay mice that were treated with these humulones showed reduced plasma glucose, triglyceride, and free fatty acid levels similar to the thiazolidinedione drug, pioglitazone. A double blind, placebo-controlled pilot study for studying the effect of isohumulones on diabetes suggested that isohumulones significantly decreased blood glucose and haemoglobin A1c levels after 8 weeks. These results suggest that isohumulones can improve insulin sensitivity in high fat diet-fed mice with insulin resistance and in patients with type-2 diabetes (3).

Xanthohumol is a chalcone of beer hops and xanthohumol-fed KK-A(y) mice exhibited lowered levels of plasma glucose, plasma, and hepatic triglycerides. They also showed decreased amounts of water intake, lowered weights of white adipose tissue and exhibited increased levels of plasma adiponectin, indicating that xanthohumol attenuated diabetes in KK-A(y) mice (4).

1. Tokutaro M; Hop fruit extracts for treatment of diabetes, *Patent/Japan Kokai Tokkyo Koho JP* 58,09,084 (Cl.A61,K35/78), 1983
2. Aigo Nutritive Chemicals Ltd., Humulone and lupulone as anti-diabetics from hops, *Japan Kakai Tokkyo Koho* JP 59, 59, 623, (Cl. A61. K35/78, 4 pp 1984).
3. Yajima H, E Ikeshima, M Shiraki, T Kanaya, D Fujiwara, H Odai, N Tsuboyama-Kasaoka, O Ezaki, S Oikawa, K Kondo; Isohumulones, bitter acids derived from hops, activate both peroxisome proliferator-activated receptor *alpha* and *gamma* and reduce insulin resistance, *J Biol Chem* **279**(32), 33456-62 (2004)
4. Nozawa H; Xanthohumol, the chalcone from beer hops (*Humulus lupulus* L.), is the ligand for farnesoid X receptor and ameliorates lipid and glucose metabolism in KK-A(y) mice, *Biochem Biophys Res'Commun* **336**(3), 754-61 (2005)

Hydnocarpus wightiana Blume (Flacourtiaceae) (Chaulmoogra)

Chaulmoogra is the Bengali name for an evergreen tree of the Indian subcontinent. This leathery-leaved tree bearing round fruits with brown densely-hairy rind is the source of well known Chaulmoogra oil.

Hydnocarpus wightiana is advocated in traditional Indian medicine to possess strong anti-diabetic activity. Investigation revealed that acetone extract of the seed hulls of *H. wightiana* possesses strong free radicals (DPPH and ABTS) scavenging, a-glucosidase and N-acetyl-b-D-glucosaminidase inhibitory activities. Fractionation of the extract led to the isolation of hydnocarpin, luteolin and isohydnocarpin, which showed varying degrees of antioxidant and enzyme inhibitory activities. These properties of the isolated phytochemicals and of the acetone extract of *H. wightiana* justify the use of the plant for the treatment of diabetes in traditional medicine.

Reddy SV, AK Tiwari, US Kumar, RJ Rao, JM Rao; Free radical scavenging, enzyme inhibitory constituents from anti-diabetic Ayurvedic medicinal plant *Hydnocarpus wightiana* Blume, *Phytother Res* **19**(4), 277-81 (2005).

Hygrophila auriculata (Schumach.) Heine.(Acanthaceae) (Waterleaf, H. Talmakhana)

Hygrophila auriculata is a wild herb widely used in 'Ayurveda' as a 'Rasayana' drug for treatment of various disorders. Treatment of diabetic rats with an extract of its aerial parts (100 and 250 mg/kg b.w.) for 3 weeks showed significant reduction in blood glucose, thiobarbituric acid reactive substances and hydroperoxide in both liver and kidney. The treatment significantly increased the glutathione, glutathione peroxidase, glutathione S-transferase and catalase. Significant anti-diabetic activity with potent antioxidant potential of the plant extract was revealed by the study.

Vijayakumar M, R Govindarajan, GM Rao, ChV Rao, A Shirwaikar, S Mehrotra, P Pushpangadam; Action of *Hygrophila auriculata* against streptozotocin-induced oxidative stress, *J Ethnopharmacol* **104**(3), 356-61 (2006)

Hygrophila longifolia (Mart) Nees (Acanthaceae)

It is an aquatic plant. Administration of an aqueous extract of this plant prior to glucose loading resulted in a significant increase in the glycogen content of liver and muscle along with a significant increase in triacylglycerol content of adipose tissue in comparison with control rats. The plant has been suggested to exert hypoglycaemic action by mechanisms similar to those of sulphonylureas.

Fernando MR, SMDN Vickramasinghe, MI Thabrew; Extra-pancreatic action of *Hygrophila longifolia, Pharmaceut Biol* **36**(5), 352-56 (1998)

Hypoxis hemerocallidea Fisch. Mey. & Ave-Lall (Hypoxidaceae) (African potato)

Hypoxis hemerocallidea is a medicinal plant native to South Africa.

The hypoglycaemic effect of aqueous extract of the corms of *H. hemerocallidea* was studied in normoglycaemic and streptozotocin-induced diabetic rats. In a pilot experiment, graded doses of the aqueous extract of African potato (100-800 mg/kg p.o.) were administered to 12-h fasted normal and diabetic rats, and a dose-dependent, significant reduction in the blood glucose concentrations of fasted normal and diabetic rats was observed. While the exact mechanism of the hypoglycaemic action of the extract is still obscure, the phytosterols present in the extract might play a role. Anyway, the suggested folkloric use of African potato extract in the control and/or management of adult-onset, type-2 diabetes mellitus in some communities of South Africa is well justified (1,2).

1. Mahomed IM, JA Ojewole; Hypoglycaemic effect of *Hypoxis hemerocallidea* corm (African potato) aqueous extract in rats, *Methods Find Exp Clin Pharmacol* **25**(8), 617-23 (2003).
2. Ojewole JA; Anti-nociceptive, anti-inflammatory and anti-diabetic properties of *Hypoxis hemerocallidea* Fisch. & C.A. Mey. (Hypoxidaceae) corm ['African Potato'] aqueous extract in mice and rats, *J Ethnopharmacol* **103**(1), 126-34 (2006)

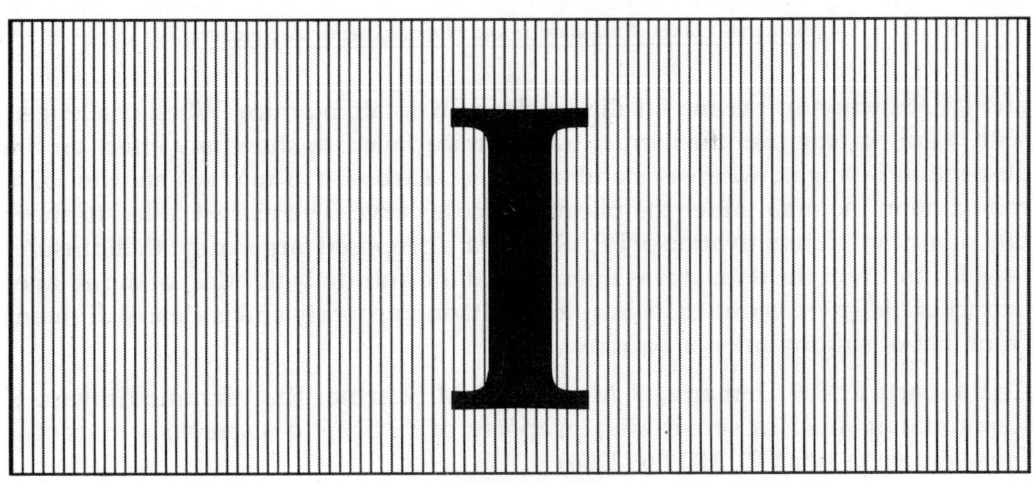

Ibervillea sonorae Greene (Cucurbitaceae) (Wareque)

This rare plant is native to northwestern Mexico. For centuries, the roots of the plant have been used in the preparation of medicines used to treat diabetes.

The effects produced by acute and chronic administration of various extracts of *I. sonorae* were investigated. Both aqueous decoction and juice of *I. sonorae* roots resulted in significant reductions of glycaemia in healthy mice after intra-peritoneal administration at a dose of 600 mg/kg. The dichloromethane extract of roots also induced a reduction of glycaemia in healthy and alloxan-induced diabetic mice but it caused a severe hypoglycaemia that produced lethality in all the treated animals when administered intra-peritoneally at doses of 300 and 600 mg/kg b.w. Daily administration of the extract per os to alloxan-induced diabetic rats at a dose of 300 mg/kg/day, showed improvement in glycaemia, body weight, triglycerides, and GPT in comparison with the diabetic control group after 41 days.

Alarcon-Aguilar FJ, F Calzada-Bermejo, E Hernandez-Galicia, C Ruiz-Angeles, R Roman-Ramos; Acute and chronic hypoglycaemic effect of *Ibervillea sonorae* root extracts-II, *J Ethnopharmacol* **97**(3), 447-52 (2005).

Indigofera mysorensis DC (Fabaccae Indigofereae) (Mysore Panicled Indigo)

Indigofera mysorensis is a shrub used for its anti-diabetic activity in rural India. Administration of an ethanol extract of the whole shrub of *I. mysorensis* (300 mg/kg for 10 days) produced a 63% reduction in plasma glucose, 41% reduction in plasma triglycerides and 77% reduction in plasma insulin levels in insulin resistant db/db mice. Unlike sulphonylureas, the plant extract failed to show any acute hypoglycaemic effect in normoglycaemic Swiss albino mice. Like insulin sensitizers, the extract (300 mg/kg, for 10 days) showed no effect on plasma glucose, but caused an 81% reduction in plasma insulin levels in Swiss albino mice. When challenged with 3 gm/kg sucrose, the extract treated mice failed to show any effect on the absorption of sugar, whereas standard drug, acarbose (10 mg/kg) showed 52% reduction in the area under the plasma glucose curve. The extract failed to show any significant transactivation of PPAR *gamma*, a proposed target of synthetic insulin sensitizers. From the data, it was inferred that the anti-diabetic effect of the ethanol extract of *Indigofera* is due to its insulin sensitizing property and is clearly different from that of sulfonylurea or acarbose.

Chakrabarti R, RK Damaria, R Mullangi, VM Sharma, RK Vikramadithyan, R Rajagopalan; Insulin sensitizing property of *Indigofera mysorensis* extract, *J Ethnopharmacol* **105**(1-2), 102-06 (2006)

Inula britannica L. subsp. ***japonica*** Kitam. (Asteraceae)

The effects of flower extract of the plant on autoimmune diabetes, induced by multiple low doses of streptozotocin (40 mg/kg/day for 5 daily doses, ip), were studied in C57BL/KsJ mice. The treatment with the flower extract (500 mg/ kg/ day) starting 7 days before the first streptozotocin injection significantly suppressed the increase of blood glucose levels. Histological analysis of the pancreas showed that the degree of insulitis and destruction of β-cells were reduced by the treatment. The results of the investigation suggest that the flower extract of *I. britannica* subsp. *japonica* has a preventative effect on autoimmune diabetes by regulating cytokine production.

Kobayashi T, QH Song, T Hong, H Kitamura, JC Cyong; Preventative effects of the flowers of *Inula britannica* on autoimmune diabetes in C57BL/KsJ mice induced by multiple low doses of streptozotocin, *Phytother Res* **16**(4), 377-82 (2002).

Inula japonica Regel (Asteraceae)
(Japanese inula)

The anti-diabetic and hypolipidaemic effects of aqueous extract of *I. japonica* flowers and its two fractions (IJR and IJP) were investigated in alloxan-induced diabetic mice. Significant reduction of blood glucose levels in diabetic mice was observed by oral administration of the aqueous extract (1000 mg/kg). Similar effects were obtained by IJR (500 mg/kg) and IJP (250 mg/kg). The aqueous extract and IJP also markedly decreased serum triglyceride concentrations in diabetic mice. The aqueous extract of the plant was thus shown to have both anti-diabetic and hypolipidemic effects.

Shan JJ, M Yang, JW Ren; Anti-diabetic and hypolipidaemic effects of aqueous extract from the flower of *Inula japonica* in alloxan-induced diabetic mice, *Biol Pharm Bull* **29**(3), 455-59 (2006)

Inula racemosa (Hook.f) (Asteraceae)
(H & S. Pushkarmool)

Inula racemosa grows in the temperate and alpine western Himalayas, and it is common in Kashmir. The roots are widely used locally in indigenous medicine. Of the different Indian drugs tested for their hypoglycaemic activity in normal and glucose induced hyperglycaemic rabbits, *Inula racemosa* proved to be the most effective one (1). The petroleum ether extract of *I. racemosa* roots lowered plasma insulin and glucose levels within 75 min of oral administration to albino rats and it significantly counteracted adrenaline-induced hyperglycaemia in rats. Alcoholic extract of the root of *I. racemosa* was found to lower blood glucose and enhance liver glycogen without increasing plasma insulin in rats. No increase in degree of de-granulation of the *beta* cells of pancreas was observed. It appears that hypoglycaemic response of *I. racemosa* is not due to enhanced secretion/synthesis of insulin; but may be due to potentiation of insulin sensitivity (2-3). Like *G. sylvestre*, *I. racemosa* extract also decreased serum glucose concentration in dexamethasone-induced hyperglycaemic animals. The effects were comparable to the standard corticosteroid-inhibiting drug, ketoconazole (4).

1. Tripathi SN, CM Tiwari, BN Upadhyay, RS Singh; Screening og hypoglycaemic action in certain indigenous drugs, *J Res Indian Med Yoga Homeopath* **14**(3-4), 159-69 (1979)
2. Tripathi YB, P Tripathi, BN Upadhyay, Assessment of the adrenergic *beta*-blocking activity of *Inula racemosa, J Ethnopharmacol* **23**(1), 3-9 (1988).
3. Tripathi YB, P Chaturvedi; Assessment of endocrine response of *Inula racemosa* in relation to glucose homeostasis in rats, *Indian J Exp Biol* **33**(9), 686-89 (1995).
4. Gholap S, A Kar; Efficacy of some plant extracts in regulating corticosteroid-induced hyperglycaemia in mice, *Pharmaceut Biol* **41**(5), 315-18 (2003)

Ipomoea aquatica Forssk. (Convolvulaceae)
(Water spinach, Water morning-glory)

Ipomoea aquatica is a semi-aquatic tropical plant, commonly consumed as green leafy vegetable in Sri Lanka, Bangladesh and some eastern States of India. The plant is supposed to possess an insulin-like activity (1). Malalavidhane and co-workers studied the oral hypoglycaemic activity of single and multiple doses of *I. aquatica* extract in healthy, male Wistar rats after a glucose challenge and observed a significant reduction in the serum glucose concentrations with both single and multiple doses. The optimum dose was 3.4 g/kg while the optimum activity was observed 2 h after the administration of the extract (2). A comparison of the oral hypoglycaemic activity of an aqueous extract of this green leafy vegetable (dose equivalent to 3.3 g starting material /kg b.w.) with that of the known oral hypoglycaemic drug tolbutamide (15 mg/kg b.w.) in glucose challenged Wistar rats (3 g/kg b.w. given 30 min after the administration of plant drug or tolbutamide) revealed that the plant drug was as effective as tolbutamide in reducing the blood glucose levels of glucose-challenged Wistar rats (3). The results of the oral hypoglycaemic activity of *I. aquatica* extract in streptozotocin induced diabetic Wistar rats, and type-2 diabetic patients were also promising. Consumption of the shredded, fresh, edible portion of the vegetable (3.4 g/kg) for one week effectively reduced the fasting blood sugar level of streptozotocin-induced diabetic rats. When subjected to a glucose challenge, type-2 diabetic subjects, treated with the plant extract, showed a significant reduction in the serum glucose concentration 2 h after the glucose load (4).

1. Jayaweera, D.M.A., Medicinal Plants (Indigenous and Exotic) Used in Ceylon. Part 11. National Science Council, Colombo, Sri Lanka, pp. 99 (1982).
2. Malalavidhane TS, SM Wickramasinghe, ER Jansz; Oral hypoglycaemic activity of *Ipomoea aquatica, J Ethnopharmacol* **72**(1-2), 293-98 (2000)'
3. Malalavidhane TS, SM Wickramasinghe, ER Jansz; An aqueous extract of the green leafy vegetable *Ipomoea aquatica* is as effective as the oral hypoglycaemic drug tolbutamide in reducing the blood sugar levels of Wistar rats, *Phytother Res* **15**(7), 635-37 (2001).
4. Malalavidhane TS, SM Wickramasinghe, MS Perera, ER Jansz; Oral hypoglycaemic activity of *Ipomoea aquatica* in streptozotocin-induced, diabetic wistar rats and Type II diabetics, *Phytother Res* **17**(9), 1098-100 (2003).

Ipomoea batatas (L) Lam. (Convolvulaceae)
(Sweet potato)

I. batatas is a crop plant whose large, starchy, sweet tasting tuberous roots are an important root vegetable. Of the different varieties of sweet potatoes, it is the white skinned variety that has drawn the attention of researchers for the management of diabetes. Hyperinsulinaemia in Zucker fatty rats was reduced significantly by oral administration of white skinned sweet potato (WSSP) and about 50% reduction was observed 8 weeks after starting its oral administration; the effect being comparable to troglitazone, an insulin sensitizer. In the glucose tolerance test after 7 weeks of treatment with WSSP, increases in blood glucose levels after glucose loading were inhibited. Histological examinations of the pancreas of Zucker fatty rats revealed remarkable re-granulation of pancreatic islet *beta* cells in the sweet potato and troglitazone treated groups after 8 weeks of treatment. White skinned sweet potato showed remarkable anti-diabetic activity and improved the abnormality of glucose and lipid metabolism by reducing insulin resistance (1). WSSP showed anti-diabetic activity in streptozotocin-induced diabetic rats and genetically diabetic models (yellow KK, db/db mice and Zucker fatty rats). The anti-diabetic component of WSSP was isolated and it was found to be present in its cortex. The active component was presumed to be an acidic glycoprotein (M.W.

22,000) because it contained protein and sugar and was adsorbed onto the anion exchange QA column at neutral pH (2). Ludvik *et al* studied the beneficial effects of the nutraceutical Caiapo, the extract of white-skinned sweet potato, on fasting plasma glucose, as well as on total and low-density lipoprotein cholesterol (LDL-c) in type-2 diabetic patients. Efforts were made to understand the underlying mechanism responsible for the improvement in metabolic control following administration of Caiapo in type-2 diabetic subjects. From the results of the investigation it was concluded that a short-term treatment with 4 g/d of Caiapo consistently improved metabolic control in type-2 diabetic patients by decreasing insulin resistance without affecting body weight, glucose effectiveness, or insulin dynamics (3, 5). The effect of Caiapo in reducing fasting blood glucose and insulin resistance in type-2 diabetic patients required 2-4 weeks after its single administration. A combination therapy of Caiapo with a mulberry leaf powder, which inhibits α-glucosidase, or with a loquat leaf (Folium *Eriobotrya japonica*) extract, which shows an insulin-like effect, shortened the time necessary for the inhibition of increasing blood glucose levels (6). Effects on immune response by white-skinned sweet potato were studied and it was proved to be a beneficial food not only due to its anti-diabetic effects but also for its ability to increase immune activity (8).

The diacylated anthocyanin, peonidin {3-O-[2-O-(6-O-*E*-feruloyl-β-D-glucopyranosyl)-6-O-*E*-caffeoyl-β-D-glucopyranoside]-5-O-β-D-glucopyranoside}, isolated from storage roots of the purple sweet potato (*Ipomoea batatas* cv. Ayamurasaki), showed a potent maltase inhibitory activity. When the diacylated anthocyanin (100 mg/kg) was administered following maltose (2 g/kg), a maximal blood glucose level at 30 min was significantly decreased compared to vehicle. A reduction of serum insulin level was also observed corresponding to the decrease in blood glucose level. No significant change in blood glucose level was, however, observed when sucrose or glucose was ingested, suggesting that the anti-hyperglycaemic effect of the anthocyanin was achieved by maltase inhibition, not by sucrase or glucose transport inhibition at the intestinal membrane (4). The anti-hyperglycaemic function of 6-O-caffeoylsophorose, obtained from red vinegar by fermented purple-fleshed sweet potato, was investigated. Like diacylated anthocyanin, the administration of caffeoylsophorose (100 mg/kg) following maltose (2 g/kg) to Sprague-Dawley rats resulted in the maximal blood glucose level after 30 min but this level was significantly lower compared to the control. A reduction in the serum insulin secretion was also observed in parallel to the decrease in blood glucose level. No blood glucose change was apparent when sucrose or glucose was ingested, suggesting that the anti-hyperglycaemic effect of caffeoylsophorose was achieved by maltase inhibition, rather than by sucrase or glucose transport inhibition (7).

1. Kusano S, H Abe; Anti-diabetic activity of white skinned sweet potato (*Ipomoea batatas* L.) in obese Zucker fatty rats, *Biol Pharm Bull* **23**(1), 23-26 (2000).

2. Kusano S, H Abe, H Tamura; Isolation of anti-diabetic components from white-skinned sweet potato (*Ipomoea batatas* L.), *Biosci Biotechnol Biochem* **65**(1), 109-14 (2001).
3. Ludvik BH, K Mahdjoobian, W Waldhaeusl, A Hofer, R Prager, A Kautzky-Willer, G Pacini; The effect of *Ipomoea batatas* (Caiapo) on glucose metabolism and serum cholesterol in patients with type 2 diabetes: a randomized study, *Diabetes Care* **25**(1), 239-40 (2002).
4. Matsui T, S Ebuchi, M Kobayashi, K Fukui, K Sugita, N Terahara, K Matsumoto; Anti-hyperglycaemic effect of diacylated anthocyanin derived from *Ipomoea batatas* cultivar Ayamurasaki can be achieved through the *alpha*-glucosidase inhibitory action, *J Agric Food Chem* **50**(25), 7244-48 (2002).
5. Ludvik B, W Waldhausl, R Prager, A Kautzky-Willer, G Pacini; Mode of action of *Ipomoea batatas* (Caiapo) in type 2 diabetic patients, *Metabolism* **52**(7), 875-80 (2003).
6. Sakuramata Y, H Oe, S Kusano, O Aki; Effects of combination of Caiapo with other plant-derived substance on anti-diabetic efficacy in KK-Ay mice, *Biofactors* **22**(1-4), 149-52 (2004).
7. Matsui T, S Ebuchi, K Fukui, K Matsugano, N Terahara, K Matsumoto; Caffeoylsophorose, a new natural *alpha*-glucosidase inhibitor, from red vinegar by fermented purple-fleshed sweet potato, *Biosci Biotechnol Biochem* **68**(11), 2239-46 (2004).
8. Miyazaki Y, S Kusano, H Doi, O Aki; Effects on immune response of anti-diabetic ingredients from white-skinned sweet potato (*Ipomoea batatas* L.), *Nutrition* **21**(3), 358-62 (2005).

Ipomoea pes-caprae (L.) R. Brown (Convolvulaceae) (Beach morning glory)

Ipomoea pes-caprae, which produces purple or pink funnel-shaped flowers, is commonly known as beach morning glory. Alcoholic extract of the leaves of this vine was found to stimulate release of insulin from islets of Langerhans *in vitro* and the effect was dose dependent. Oral administration of the extract (250 mg/kg) to normal rats for 7 days caused significant lowering of blood glucose with concomitant increase in serum insulin and liver glycogen levels and decrease in the activity of glucose 6-phosphatase. Significant improvement in glucose tolerance was also observed.

Khan MM, F Ahmad, AK Rastogi, JR Kidwai; Insulinogenic and hypoglycaemic activities of *Ipomoea pes-caprae, Fitoterapia* **65**(3), 231-37 (1994)

Irvingia gabonensis (Aubry-Lecomte ex O'Rorke) Baill. (Irvingiaceae)

Irvingia is a genus of African and Southeast Asian trees, known by the common name, wild mango. They bear edible mango-like fruits, and are especially valued for their fat and protein-rich nuts, known as dikanuts. The high content of mucilage in dikanuts enables them to be used as thickening agents for dishes such as ogbono soup. The effects of dikanut in the diet of eleven type-2 diabetics were studied. The dikanut supplement elicited hypolipidaemic activity primarily due to a decrease in LDL + VLDL-cholesterol and triglycerides levels. It also increased HDL-cholesterol levels. Consumption of dikanut supplement for 4 weeks by diabetics significantly increased three ATPases of the erythrocyte membrane, which correlated well with significant reduction of plasma glucose levels. Desirable biochemical effects mediated by ingestion of a naturally-occurring dietary fibre were accompanied by improved clinical states.

Okafor C, A Abu-Bakare; A supplement of Dikanut (*Irvingia gabonensis*) improves treatment of type II diabetics, *West Afr J Med* **9**(2), 108-15 (1990)

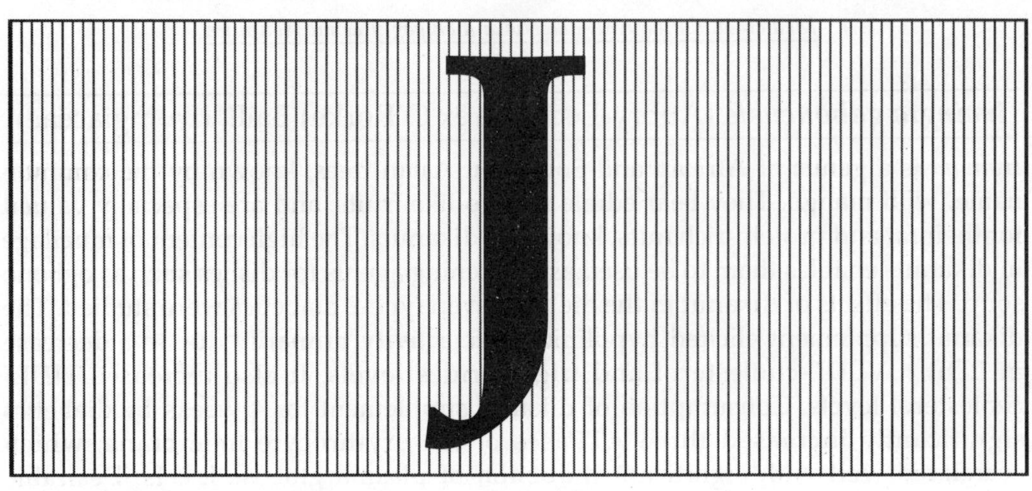

Jasonia montana (Vahl.) Botsch (Asteraceae)

Of the different extracts of the plant that were screened for their putative hypoglycaemic and anti-diabetic activities, only the petroleum ether and ethanol extracts exhibited the desired activity. The plant yielded three new diterpenes (jasonins-A, B and C) and a known flavone (centaureidin).

Al-Howiriny TA, AL Al-Rehaily, JR Polsc, JR Porter, JS Mossa, B Ahmed; Three new diterpenes and the biological activity of different extracts of *Jasonia montana, Nat Prod Res* **19**(3), 253-65 (2005).

Juniperus communis Linn. (Cupressaceae) (Common Juniper)

Common Juniper grows throughout the cool temperate Northern hemisphere in North America, Europe and Asia. The hypoglycaemic activity of a decoction from juniper "berries" (*J. communis*) was studied both in normoglycaemic and in streptozotocin-induced diabetic animals. The decoction was found to decrease glycaemic levels in normoglycaemic rats at a dose of 250 mg/kg. The administration of the decoction (125 mg /kg) to streptozotocin-induced diabetic rats for 24 days resulted in a significant reduction both in blood glucose levels and in the mortality index. The treatment also prevented the loss of body weight. This effect appears to be mediated by an increase of peripheral glucose consumption.

Sanchez de Medina F, MJ Gamez, I Jimenez. J Jimenez, H Osuna, A Zarzuelo; Hypoglycaemic activity of juniper "berries", *Planta Med* **60**(3), 197-200 (1994).

Juniperus procera Hoechst ex Endl. (Cupressaceae)

The essential oil of *Juniperus procera* was examined for its potential radical scavenging activities. The ability of the volatile oil to act as non-specific donor for hydrogen atoms or electrons was checked in the diphenylpicrylhydrazyl assay and it showed positive results. The oil of *J. procera* was also found to be effective hydroxyl radical scavenging agent when assessed in the deoxyribose degradation assay. In the *in vitro* assay for non-enzymatic lipid peroxidation in liposomes, the oil of *J. procera* also displayed antioxidant potential. The compounds that contribute to the radical scavenging activities of *J. procera* were also identified.

Burits M, K Asres, F Bucar; The antioxidant activity of the essential oils of *Artemisia afra, Artemisia abyssinica* and *Juniperus procera, Phytother Res* **15**(2), 103-08 (2001)

Jussiaea suffruticosa Linn. (Onagraceae)

The effect of methanol extract of the plant on the blood glucose levels of normal and alloxan-induced diabetic rats was studied. The extract (200 and 400 mg/kg, p.o.) produced significant reduction in normal and alloxan-induced blood glucose levels, the maximum effect being observed in rats at 4.5 hours at a dose of 400 mg/kg. The effect was comparable to that of glibenclamide. The potent hypoglycaemic activity elicited by the extract is considered to be due to the flavonoids and steroids present in the extract.

Marugesan T, PK Mukherjee, M Pal, BP Saha; Hypoglycaemic potential of *Jussiaea suffruticosa* extract in rats, *Phytomedicine* 7(Suppl. II), 68 (2000)

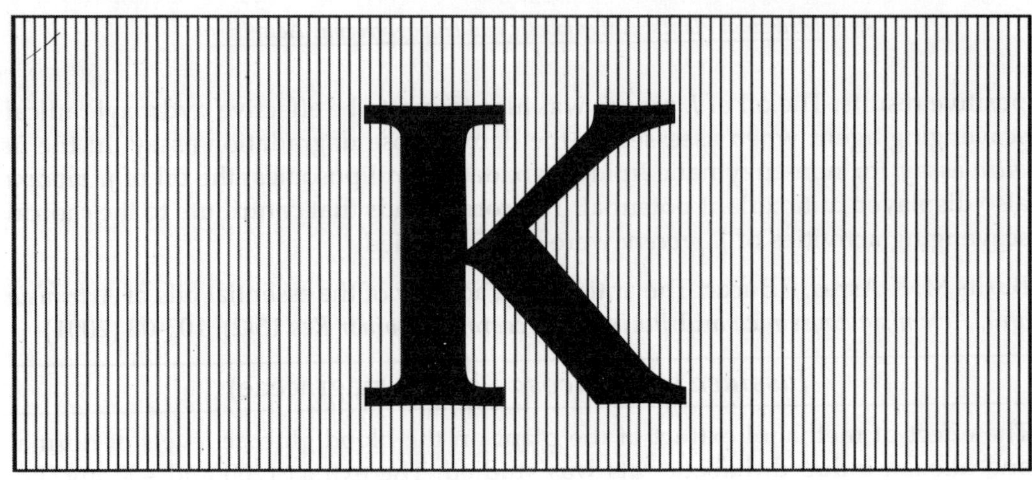

Kalopanax pictus (Thunb.)Nakai (Araliaceae) (Prickly Castor-oil Tree, Kalopanax)

It is the sole species in the genus *Kalopanax,* native to northeastern Asia, from Sakhalin and Japan to south-western China. Of the different phytochemicals isolated from the plant, kalopanax saponin a hedragenin glycoside exhibited a potent anti-diabetic activity in contrast to a mild activity of hederagenin, when tested in the streptozotocin-induced diabetic rats. Both the compounds exhibited significant hypocholesterolaemic and hypolipidaemic activities. The structure-activity relationship of kalopanaxsaponin A was also investigated in the present work.

Park HJ, DH Kim, JW Choi, JH Park, YN Han; A potent anti-diabetic agent from *Kalopanax pictus, Arch Pharm Res* **21**(1), 24-29 (1998).

Kochia scoparia (L.) Schrad (Amaranthaceae) (Fireweed)

K. scoparia, also known as fireweed for its bright red foliage in autumn, is a drought-resistant forage crop. The methanol extract of the fruits of Japanese *K. scoparia* was found to inhibit the increase in serum glucose in glucose-loaded rats. Through bioassay-guided separation, momordin 1c and its 2'-O-β-D-glucopyranoside (principal saponin constituents of this plant) were isolated as the active principles from this medicinal foodstuff. These were found to potently inhibit glucose and ethanol absorption in rats (2). The inhibitory effects of oleanolic acid glycosides on the increase of serum glucose in oral glucose-loaded rats were evaluated and their mechanism of action was examined using momordin and oleanolic acid 3-O-glucuronide. Both the compounds inhibited the increase in serum glucose concentration in oral glucose loaded rats but failed to do so in normal rats, intra-peritoneally glucose loaded rats and in alloxan-induced diabetic mice. These glycosides were found to suppress gastric emptying in rats, and also inhibit glucose uptake in rat small intestine *in vitro*. The findings led to suggest that these glycosides, given orally, have neither insulin-like nor insulin-releasing activity. The hypoglycaemic activity of the compounds is due to suppression of the transfer of glucose from the stomach to small intestine and due to inhibition of glucose transport at the brush border of small intestine (3).

Rankins *et al*, however, reported that livestock grazing on *K. scoparia*, sometimes experience body weight loss, hyperbilirubinaemia, photosensitization, and polyuria. Animals fed kochia hay may fail to utilize nutrients efficiently and exhibit mild or negligible signs of toxicosis (1).

1. Rankins DL Jr, GS Smith, DM Hallford; Altered metabolic hormones, impaired nitrogen retention, and hepatotoxicosis in lambs fed *Kochia scoparia* hay, *J Animal Sci* **69**(7), 2932-40 (1991)
2. Yoshikawa M, H Shimada, T Morikawa, S Yoshizumi, N Matsumura, T Murakami, H Matsuda, K Hori, J Yamahara; Medicinal foodstuffs. VII. On the saponin constituents with glucose and alcohol absorption-inhibitory activity from a food garnish "Tonburi", the fruit of Japanese *Kochia scoparia* (L.) Schrad.: structures of scoparianosides A, B, and C, *Chem Pharm Bull* (Tokyo), **45**(8), 1300-05 (1997).
3. Matsuda H, Y Li, T Murakami, N Matsumura, J Yamahara, M Yoshikawa; Anti-diabetic principles of natural medicines. III. Structure-related inhibitory activity and action mode of oleanolic acid glycosides on hypoglycaemic activity, *Chem Pharm Bull* **46**(9), 1399-1403 (1998)

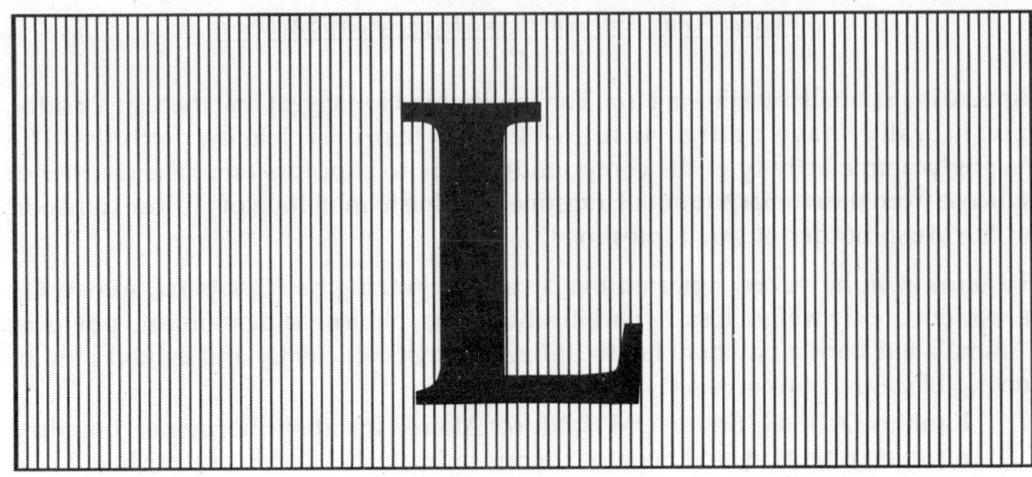

Lactuca indica Linn. (Asteraceae)
(Indian lettuce)

Lactuca, commonly known as lettuce, is a genus of flowering plants in the Sunflower family. Of the different phytochemicals isolated from the plant, the sesquiterpene lactone, lactucain C and a new furofuran lignan, lactucaside showed significant anti-diabetic activity (1). Chemical components of *Lactuca* and their bioactivities have also been discussed (2).

1. Hou CC, SJ Lin, JT Cheng, FL Hsu; Anti-diabetic dimeric guianolides and a lignan glycoside from *Lactuca indica, J Nat Prod* **66**(5), 625-29 (2003).
2. Ren Yu-lin, Ya-wei Zhou, Yun-hua Ye; Chemical components of *Lactuca* and their bioactivities, *Acta Pharmaceutica sinica* **39**(11), 954-60 (2004).

Lagerstroemia speciosa (L.) Pers. (Lythraceae)
(Pride of India, Banabá Plant, H. & Bengali. Jarul)

Lagerstroemia speciosa is native to tropical southern Asia and known by the name of banaba in the Phillipines. Spray-dried leaf extract of *L. speciosa* in the powder form showed significant hypoglycaemic and anti-diabetic activities in mice. Tannin-free leaf extract also showed similar activities (1). In addition to tannins and lipids, sixteen amino acids were isolated from the leaves of the plant. Preliminary biological studies indicated the presence of active constituents in both the crude and tannin-free spray dried extract that were responsible for the blood sugar lowering activity.The study established that the amino acids constitute the insulin-like principle responsible for hypoglycaemic activity (2).

The hypoglycaemic effects of hot-water extract of *L. speciosa* leaves and its two different fractions (HPWE and HPME) were studied using hereditary diabetic mice (Type II, KK-AY/Ta Jcl). The mice were fed a test diet containing either 5% of the hot-water extract from banaba leaves or 3% of HPWE or 2% or HPME for a period of 5 weeks. The elevation of blood plasma glucose level in non-insulin dependent diabetic mice, fed cellulose as the control diet, was almost entirely suppressed by hot water extract of the leaves of the plant or HPME. The extract or HPME also lowered the level of serum insulin, urinary glucose and plasma total cholesterol in mice. From the results of the investigation, it is suggested that hot water extract of *L. speciosa* leaves and especially the fraction, HPME. have beneficial effects in the control of plasma glucose level in non-insulin dependent diabetes mellitus (3). The effects of *L. speciosa* extracts on glucose transport and adipocyte differentiation in 3T3-L1 cells were studied. The hot water extract and a chromatographic fraction (BME) stimulated glucose uptake in 3T3-L1 adipocytes with an induction time and a dose-dependent response similar to those of insulin. There were no additive or synergistic effects found between water extract and insulin on glucose uptake, and the glucose uptake activity of insulin could be reduced to basal levels by adding increasing amounts of the extract. From the results of the investigation it was suggested that *L. speciosa* leaf extract may be useful for prevention and treatment of hyperglycaemia and obesity in type-2 diabetics (4). Three active ellagitannins (lagerstroemin, flosin B and reginin A), isolated by bioassay-guided fractionation of aqueous acetone extract of the leaves of the plant, were found to increase glucose uptake by rat adipocytes. These ellagitannins are considered to be responsible for lowering blood glucose level. Further, lagerstroemin was found to exhibit insulin-like actions by a mechanism different from that of insulin (5, 7).

Corosolic acid is an ingredient of the leaves of *Lagerstroemia speciosa*. The anti-diabetic activity of an extract from the leaves of *L. speciosa*, standardized to 1% corosolic acid (Glucosol), has been demonstrated in a randomized clinical trial involving Type-2 diabetics. Subjects receiving Glucosol, at daily dosages of 32 and 48 mg for 2 weeks, showed a significant reduction in the blood glucose levels. Glucosol in a soft gel capsule formulation showed a better bioavailability than a dry-powder formulation (6). Miura *et al* reported that corosolic acid (10 mg/kg) reduced the blood glucose level of KK-Ay mice (animal model of type-2 diabetes) 4h after a single oral administration but it did not change the plasma insulin level. From the results of investigation it was inferred that the hypoglycaemic effect of corosolic acid is derived, at least in part, from an increase in GLUT4 translocation in muscle (8). In a later publication, this group of authors reported that corosolic acid, at a dose of 2 mg/kg, reduced the blood glucose level of KK-Ay mice 2 weeks after a single oral dose and also lowered plasma insulin levels. The decrease in blood glucose level of these mice was also observed in insulin tolerance test. The results support the hypothesis that corosolic acid improves glucose metabolism by reducing insulin resistance. It may, therefore, be useful for the treatment of type 2 diabetes (9).

1. Vito-de-vera FE, JB Manalo, S Bonifacio, FD Unalivia, VP Arida; Development of an anti-diabetic drug from *Lagerstroemia speciosa* (Banaba) , Biological studies, *ASOMPS VII, Manila*, February 2-7, (1992).

2. Manalo JB, FV Vera, TS Bonifacio, FD Unalivia, VP Arida; Phytochemical investigation of *Lagerstroemia speciosa* leaves, *Philippine J Sci* **122**(1), 15-31 (1993)

3. Kakuda T, I Sakane, T Takihara, Y Ozaki, H Takeuchi, M Kuroyanagi; Hypoglycaemic effect of extracts from *Lagerstroemia speciosa* L. leaves in genetically diabetic KK-AY mice, *Biosci Biotechnol Biochem* **60**(2), 204-08 (1996).

4. Liu F, J Kim, Y Li, X Liu, J Li, X Chen; An extract of *Lagerstroemia speciosa* L. has insulin-like glucose uptake-stimulatory and adipocyte differentiation-inhibitory activities in 3T3-L1 cells, *J Nutr* **131**(9), 2242-47 (2001).

5. Hayashi T, H Maruyama, R Kasai, K Hatxxx, S Takasuga, O Hazeki, K Yamasaki, X Tanaka; Ellagitannins from *Lagerstroemia speciosa* on activators of glucose transport in fat cells, *Planta Med* **68**(2), 173-75 (2002)

6. Judy WV, SP Hari, WW Stogsdill, JS Judy, YM Naguib, R Passwater; Anti-diabetic activity of a standardized extract (Glucosol) from *Lagerstroemia speciosa* leaves in Type II diabetics: A dose-dependence study, *J Ethnopharmacol* **87**(1), 115-17 (2003).

7. Hattori K, N Sukenobu, T Sasaki, S Takasuga, T Hayashi, R Kasai, K Yamasaki, O Hazeki; Activation of insulin receptors by lagerstroemin, *J Pharmacol Sci* **93**(1), 69-73 (2003).

8. Miura T, Y Itoh, T Kaneko, N Ueda, T Ishida, M Fukushima, F Matsuyama, Y Seino; Corosolic acid induces GLUT4 translocation in genetically type-2 diabetic mice, *Biol Pharmaceut Bull* **27**(7), 1103-05 (2004)

9. Miura T, N Ueda, K Yamada, M Fukushima, T Ishida, T Kaneko, F Matsuyama, Y Seino; Anti-diabetic effects of corosolic acid in KK-Ay diabetic mice, *Biol Pharmaceut Bull* **29**(3), 585-87 (2006)

Laportea ovalifolia (Schum and Thonn) Chew (Urticaceae)

The leaves of *Laportea ovalifolia* is widely used in Cameroon for the treatment of several diseases including diabetes mellitus. The anti-diabetic and hypolipidaemic effects of a methanol-methylene chloride extract of the aerial parts of *L. ovalifolia* were investigated in normal and alloxan-induced diabetic rats. Intra-gastric treatment of diabetic rats with *L. ovalifolia* extract for 2 weeks caused a significant reduction in the fasting serum glucose concentrations, a lowering of the serum concentrations of total cholesterol, triglycerides, LDL-cholesterol and the ratio of total cholesterol to HDL-cholesterol.

Momo CE, JE Oben, D Tazoo, E Dongo; Anti-diabetic and hypolipidaemic effects of a methanol-methylene chloride extract of *Laportea ovalifolia* (Urticaceae), measured in rats with alloxan-induced diabetes, *Ann Trop Med Parasitol* **100**(1), 69-74 (2006).

Larrea tridentata (DC.) Coville (Zygophyllaceae) (Creosote bush, Chaparral)

Larrea tridentata is an important flowering plant in the deserts of western North America. It is closely related to the South American *Larrea divaricata* and was formerly treated as the same species. The ability of masoprocol (nordihydroguaiaretic acid), isolated from *L. tridentata* to lower plasma glucose concentration was studied in two mouse models of type-2 diabetes. Oral administration of masoprocol, a well-known lipoxygenase inhibitor, significantly lowered the plasma glucose concentration in male C57BL/ks-db/db or C57BL/6J-ob/ob mice. The decline in plasma glucose concentration was achieved without any change in plasma insulin concentration. Masoprocol also improved oral glucose tolerance and accentuated the ability of insulin to lower plasma glucose concentrations in treated db/db mice. The lipoxygenase inhibitors like masoprocol, represent a new approach to the pharmacological treatment of type-2 diabetes.

Luo J, T Chuang, J Cheung, J Quan, C Sullivan, RF Hector, MJ Reed, K Meszaros, SR King, TJ Carlson, GM Reaven; Masoprocol (nordihydroguaiaretic acid): a new anti-hyperglycaemic agent isolated from the creosote bush (*Larrea tridentata*), *Eur J Pharmacol* **346**(1), 77-79 (1998).

Lathyrus sativus Linn. (Fabaceae)) (Grass pea, H. Khesari)

Lathyrus sativus, is a legume commonly grown for human consumption and livestock feed in Asia and East Africa. It is an important crop in areas that are prone to drought. *L. sativus* seed protein contains variable amounts of a neurotoxic amino acid that is known to be responsible for a neurodegenerative disease, neurolathyrism.

The glycolipid glycosyl-phosphatidylinositol (GPI), isolated from grass pea seeds, showed similarities to GPI previously isolated from other sources such as rat liver. Inositol phosphoglycan was generated from *L. sativus* seed GPI by hydrolysis with a GPI-specific phospholipase D. Water-soluble inositol phosphoglycan from *L. sativus* seed possesses insulin-mimetic activities. This explains why *L. sativus* seeds are used in some traditional medicines to ameliorate diabetic symptoms.

Paneda C, AV Villar, A Alonso, FM Goni, F Varela, U Brodbeck, Y Leon, I Varela-Nieto, DR Jones; Purification and characterization of insulin-mimetic inositol phosphoglycan-like molecules from grass pea (*Lathyrus sativus*) seeds, *Mol Med* 7(7), 454-60 (2001).

Laurus nobilis Linn. (Lauraceae)
(Sweet Bay)

Laurus nobilis is known commonly as Sweet Bay. It is distributed across the Mediterranean region from Spain to Greece. Oral administration of an ethanol extract (200 and 600 mg/kg) produced a significant decrease in blood glucose levels in diabetic rabbits.

Yanardag R, S Can; Effect of *Laurus nobilis* L. leaves on blood glucose levels in normal and alloxan-diabetic rabbits. *Chimica Acta Turcica* **22**(2), 169-75 (1994)

Lavandula species (Lamiaceae)
(Lavender)

The Lavenders *Lavandula* are a genus of about 25-30 species of flowering plants in the mint family, native to the Mediterranean region, tropical Africa and to the southeast regions of India. Gamez and coworkers (1, 2) studied the hypoglycaemic activities of *Lavandula dentata, Lavandula latifolia, Lavandula multifida* and *Lavandula stoechas*. Oral administration of water suspension of *L. dentata* (10%) exhibited marked hypoglycaemic activity in normoglycaemic rats. *L. dentata* suspension was active at all doses (0.5, 1.0 and 2 g/kg) assayed but the activity was maintained only at a dose of 2 g/kg. *L. latifolia* also showed activity at this dose. Suspension of *L. dentata* was effective even in glucose loaded hyperglycaemia in rats but ineffective in alloxan-induced hyperglycaemic rats.

1. Gamez MJ, J Jimenez, S Risco, A Zarzuelo; Hypoglycaemic activity in various species of the genus *Lavandula* Part 1: *Lavandula stoechas* L. and *Lavandula multifida* L, *Pharmazie* **42**(10), 706-07 (1987)
2. Gamez MJ, A Zarzuelo, S Risco, P Utrilla, J Jimenez; Hypoglycaemic activity in various species of the genus *Lavandula* Part 2: *Lavandula dentata* and *Lavandula latifolia, Pharmazie* **43**(6), 441-42 (1988).

Lemna gibba G3 Linn. (Araceae)
(Gibbous Duckweed)

Lemna is a genus of free-floating aquatic plant from the duckweed family. From this plant source, a material, very similar to mammalian insulin, was isolated by solvent extraction and extensive chromatographic resolution of the extract. The protein nature of the material was suggested by its destruction by pronase but not by the inactivated enzyme. On TSK chromatography it eluted in a position similar to that of insulin, i.e. equivalent to a protein of 6000 daltons.This plant-derived insulin-like material was found to bind to insulin receptors on IM-9 lymphocytes and stimulate glucose oxidation and lipogenesis in isolated adipocytes from young rats. The bioactivity was neutralized in the presence of anti-insulin antibodies, but not in the presence of normal guinea pig IgG.

Collier E, A Watkinson, CF Cleland, J Roth; Partial purification and characterization of an insulin-like material from spinach and *Lemna gibba* G3, *J Biol Chem* **262**(13), 6238-47 (1987)

Leonotis leonurus (L.) R. Br. (Lamiaceae) (Lion's Tail)

The plant *Leonotis leonurus* is a member of the mint family and native to southern Africa. The anti-diabetic activity of the aqueous extract of *L. leonurus* leaf powder, obtained by Soxhlet extraction with distilled water, was evaluated using streptozotocin-induced diabetic rats and chlorpropamide as reference compound. The aqueous extract of *L. leonurus* leaves (50-800 mg/kg ip) caused significant hypoglycaemic effects in rats. The different flavonoids, diterpenoids, polyphenolics, and other chemical constituents present in the plant might be involved in the anti-diabetic effects of the plant extract.

Ojewole JA; Antinociceptive, antiinflammatory and anti-diabetic effects of *Leonotis leonurus* (L.) R. BR. [Lamiaceae] leaf aqueous extract in mice and rats, *Methods Find Exp Clin Pharmacol* **27**(4), 257-64 (2005).

Lepechinia caulescens (Ortega) Epling (Lamiaceae)

The traditional preparation as well as different solvent extracts of the flowers of *Lepechinia caulescens* were administered to fasting healthy mice. The results of investigation showed that only the traditional preparation and the water extract significantly reduced blood glucose level after intra-peritoneal administration. The water extract, which showed blood sugar lowering activity in a dose-dependent manner, yielded a precipitate (F1 fraction) on maceration with methanol. This fraction F1 showed significant hypoglycaemic activity in healthy and mild alloxan-induced diabetic mice, but not in severe alloxan-diabetic mice.

Roman-Ramos R, C.C. Contreras-Weber, G. Nohpal-Grajeda, J.L. Flores-Saenz, F.J. Alarcon-Aguilar; Blood glucose level decrease caused by extracts and fractions from *Lepechinia caulescens* in healthy and alloxan-diabetic mice, *Pharmaceut Biol* **39**(4), 317-21 (2001)

Lepidium sativum Linn. (Brassicaceae) (Garden cress)

Garden cress is a fast-growing, edible plant botanically related to mustard. Garden cress is found to contain significant amounts of iron, calcium and folic acid, in addition to vitamins A and C. Garden cress seeds, which showed 41% reduction in starch hydrolysis, were tested *in vivo* on 11 NIDDM subjects as well as on 14 normal healthy subjects. It was observed that for both controls and diabetics, garden cress seeds significantly lowered glycaemic response to meals. Further, diabetics showed higher reduction than the healthy subjects. (1). Hypoglycaemic effect of an aqueous extract of *L. sativum* seeds was investigated in normal and streptozotocin-induced diabetic rats. Oral administration of a single dose (20 mg/kg) of *L. sativum* extract produced a significant decrease in blood glucose levels in normal as well as in streptozotocin-induced diabetic rats and the blood glucose levels were normalized after daily repeated oral administration of aqueous extract (20 mg/kg) for 2 weeks. However, no changes were observed in basal plasma insulin concentrations after treatment either in normal or streptozotocin-induced diabetic rats indicating that the mechanism of this hypoglycaemic activity is independent of insulin secretion (2).

1. Patole AP, VV Agie, MC Phadnis; Effect of mucilaginous seeds on *in vitro* rate of starch hydrolysis and blood glucose levels of NIDDM subjects with special reference to garden cress seeds, *J Med Arom Plant Sci* **20**(4), 1005-08 (1998)
2. Eddouks M, M Maghrani, NA Zeggwagh, JB Michel; Study of the hypoglycaemic activity of *Lepidium sativum* L. aqueous extract in normal and diabetic rats, *J Ethnopharmacol* **97**(2), 391-95 (2005).

Leucaena leucocephala (Lam) de Wit (Fabaceae) (White popinac)

Leucaena leucocephala is a small tropical tree native to Mexico. It is used for a variety of purposes, such as firewood, fiber and livestock feed. In India it is known as 'Subabul'. Singhal and co-workers made a preliminary study on hypoglycaemic and hypocholesterolaemic activities of the plant (1). The total flavonoids of the plant significantly lowered the blood glucose levels in alloxan and adrenaline-induced diabetic mice as well as in hyperglycaemic mice but not in normal mice (2),

1. Singhal PC, RK Gupta, JB Singh, LD Joshi; Preliminary studies on hypoglycaemic and hypocholesterolemic activities of *Leucaena leucocephala* (Lam) de Wit, *Indian J Med Res* **78**(Suppl), 119-23 (1982).
2. Li XJ, JG Deng, ZL Qin, HB Huang; Experimental study on anti-diabetic effect of the total flavonoids in *Leucaena* seeds, *Zhonggno Zhong Yao Za Zhi* **30**(11),842-44 (2005) [Article in Chinese]

Leucas lavandulaefolia (Rees) J.E. Smith (Lamiaceae)

The anti-diabetic activity of *Leucas lavandulaefolia* extract on streptozotocin-induced diabetic rats was investigated. Administration of methanol extract of the plant (200 and 400 mg/kg) to streptozotocin-induced diabetic rats caused a significant reduction of blood glucose levels in comparison to control groups.

Saha K, PK Mukherjee , J Das, SC Mandal, M Pal, BP Saha; Hypoglycaemic activity of *Leucas lavandulaefolia* Rees. in streptozotocin-induced diabetic rats, *Phytother Res*

11(6):463-66 (1998)

Ligustrum lucidum W.T. Aiton (Oleaceae) (Chinese Privet)

Ligustrum lucidum, the largest species of the genus *Ligustrum* is native to the southern half of China. The berries of the plant are used in Chinese traditional medicine. Intra-gastric administration of a decoction of the fruits of the plant (15, 30 g/kg/d for 10 days) decreased the blood sugar level of normal mice. At a dose of 30g/kg it also reduced the blood sugar level alloxan-induced diabetic mice. The extract also antagonised the elevation of blood sugar level induced by adrenaline or glucose.

Hao Z. Hang B, Wang Y; Hypoglycaemic effect of the fruit of *Ligustrum lucidum, China J Chinese Materia Medica* **17**(7), 429-31(1992)

Liriope platyphylla Wang et Tang (Liliaceae) (Lily-turf)

Native to China and Japan, the plant is with ribbon-like foliage. The homoisoflavone-enriched fraction, isolated from the 70% methanol extract of the plant, worked as an insulin sensitizer. It was found to enhance insulin action using glucose uptake as an indicator. The fraction thus played an important role as an insulin sensitizer in adipocytes.

Choi SB, JD Wha, S Park; The insulin sensitizing effect of homoisoflavone-enriched fraction in *Liriope platyphylla* Wang et Tang via PI3-kinase pathway, *Life Sci* **75**(22), 2653-64 (2004).

Litchi chinensis Sonn. (Sapindaceae) (Lychee)

It is a tropical fruit tree, native to southern China, where it is known as lìzhî. The pharmacological mechanism of the aqueous extract of the seeds of *Litchi chinensis* (Semen Litchi) on enhancing insulin sensitivity in type-2 diabetic rats with insulin resistance was investigated. The extract was found to reduce the levels of tumor necrosis factor-*alpha*, hyper-leptinemia and hyperinsulinaemia, antagonize insulin resistance, fortify insulin sensitivity, readjust lipodystrophy and maladjustment of glycometabolism, enhance antioxidation, and improve functions of liver and kidney in type-2 diabetic rats with insulin resistance.

Guo J, L Li, J Pan, G Qiu, A Li, G Huang, L Xu; Pharmacological mechanism of Semen Litchi on antagonizing insulin resistance in rats with type 2 diabetes, *Zhong Yao Cai* **27**(6), 435-38 (2004). [Article in Chinese]

Lithospermum erythrorhizon Siebold &Zucc. (Boraginaceae)

See *Hypoglycaemic glycans* in Appendix

Konno C, T Mizuno, H Hikino; Isolation and hypoglycaemic activity of lithospermans A, B and C, glycans of *Lithospermum erythrorhizon* roots, *Planta Med* (2), 157-58 (1985)

Loranthus bengwensis Linn. (Loranthaceae) (African Mistletoe)

Mistletoe is a parasitic tree hugger and this African mistletoe, *Loranthus bengwensis* is known in folk medicine for its therapeutic values and it has been widely used in Nigerian folk medicine to treat diabetes mellitus. The aqueous extract or infusion (1.32 g/kg per day) of the leaves of this plant, parasitic on lemon, guava, and jatropha, were supplied *ad libitum* to separate groups of both non-diabetic and streptozotocin-induced diabetic rats, as their only source of fluid for a period of 28 days. The infusions of mistletoe, parasitic on both lemon and guava trees, significantly decreased serum glucose levels in non-diabetic and diabetic rats, whereas that prepared from mistletoe parasitic on jatropha did not. The observation indicates that the anti-diabetic activity of this mistletoe is highly dependent on the host plant species (1). The effect of an aqueous extract of *L. bengwensis* from two host plants (*Citrus limon* or *Vernonia amygdalina*) was studied in male Wistar rats, treated orally with either 1.32, 13.2 or 26.4 g/kg per day for 7 days. A significant dose-dependent reduction in the serum glucose and cholesterol was observed with both the extracts, accompanied by a reduction of urine flow rate and serum creatinine. Mistletoe extract, irrespective of source, appears to lower the blood sugar level offering the potential for clinical use of the ingredients of its extracts (2).

1. Obatomi DK, EO Bikomo, VJ Temple; Anti-diabetic properties of the African mistletoe in streptozotocin-induced diabetic rats, *J Ethnopharmacol* **43**(1), 13-17 (1994)
2. Obatomi DK, AAA Oye, ZN Jangber, VJ Temple; Metabolic and renal changes following the ingestion of African Mistletoe extract in rats, *Phytother Res* **11**(2), 171-73 (1997)

Loranthus micranthus Linn. (Loranthaceae) (Eastern Nigerian mistletoe)

This Nigerian mistletoe is parasitic on many species of trees but Osadebe and his colleagues focused their attention on those, parasitic on *Persea americana* (avocado), *Baphia nitida*, *Cola acuminata* (kola nut), *Pentaclethra macrophylla* (oil bean), and *Azadirachta indica* (neem), and evaluated hypoglycaemic and anti-hyperglycaemic activities of their dried leaves. The crude methanol extract of *L. micranthus* exhibited statistically significant hypoglycaemic and anti-hyperglycaemic activities in normoglycaemic and alloxan-induced diabetic albino rats. The hypoglycaemic effect was found to be dose-dependent. The strongest effect was seen with an extract from mistletoe with *P. americana* as the host plant. The maximum effect of the mistletoe extract (400 mg/kg) from *Persea americana* on alloxan-induced diabetic rats was found to be statistically comparable with that of glibenclamide at 24 h after administration. *L. micranthus* harvested from *Kola acuminata, Azadirchta indica* and *Baphia nitida* host trees also exhibited significant anti-hyperglycaemic activities.

Osadebe PO, GB Okide, IC Akabogu; Study on anti-diabetic activities of crude methanolic extracts of *Loranthus micranthus* (Linn.) sourced from five different host trees, *J Ethnopharmacol* **95**(2-3), 133-38 (2004).

Luffa aegyptiaca Mill (Cucurbitaceae) (Sponge gourd, H. Nenua)

Sponge gourd is a rampant, fast-growing annual vine that produces fruits that are edible when immature and used as back scrubbers or sponges when fully mature. It is grown throughout most of Asia for food. The effect of oral administration of an ethanol extract of the seeds of sponge gourd on blood glucose levels of normal as well as of streptozotocin-induced diabetic rats was studied. The extract significantly reduced the blood glucose levels in streptozotocin-induced diabetic rats during the first three hours of the treatment and its potency was similar to that of metformin. In normal rats, however, only an insignificant change in blood glucose level was observed.

El-Fiky FK, MA Abou Karam, EA Afify; Effect of *Luffa aegyptiaca* (seeds) and *Carissa edulis* (leaves) extracts on blood glucose level of normal and streptozotocin diabetic rats, *J Ethnopharmacol* **50**(1), 43-47 (1996)

Lupinus albus Linn.(Fabaceae) (White lupin)

The white lupin, an annual, pubescent plant, has a wide distribution in the Mediterranean region. It is an appreciated food crop and it is still cultivated in some Mediterranean countries, particularly Egypt. The hypoglycaemic fraction of lupin seed extract exhibited anti-hyperglycaemic activity only in animals having intact *beta*-pancreatic cells.

See also *Lupinus termis*.

Cabo J, J Jimenez, S Risco, A Zarzuelo; Hypoglycaemic activity of the seeds of lupin (*Lupinus albus*). IX. Anti-hyperglycaemic activity of the active fraction, *Plant Med Phytother* **18**(4), 237-42 (1984)

Lupinus species(Fabaceae)

The hypoglycaemic effect of lupin flour was tested in seven adult non-insulin dependent diabetic patients using the glucose tolerance test. Postprandial blood glucose concentration data was lower in individuals after a test meal of lupin marmalade compared to fructose marmalade. This result would allow diabetic people to eat foods such as marmalades, which are known to contain a large amount of carbohydrates (1). The effect of *Lupinus* alkaloids (lupanine, 13-α hydroxy lupanine, 17-oxo-lupanine and 2-thionosparteine) upon insulin secretion was studied. Isolated normal rat islets were incubated with different concentrations of glucose, in the presence or absence of different concentrations of the quinolizidine alkaloids from *Lupinus* species and insulin release was measured by radioimmunoassay. While 2-thionosparteine enhanced insulin secretion at all glucose concentrations, other alkaloids did so only at a higher concentration of glucose. Diazoxide (0.1 mM) decreased the effect of all alkaloids but did not suppress their effect completely. The fact that 13-α-hydroxy lupanine and 17-oxo-lupanine exert their secretagogue effect only at high glucose concentrations could be of additional value when considering their potential use in the treatment of type-2 diabetes (2).

Conglutin *gamma*, a lupin seed protein, was found to bind insulin *in vitro* and the interaction was specific, despite different origin of the two protein molecules. The effect of oral administration of conglutin *gamma* on the glycaemic levels of rats subjected to glucose overloading was studied. A statistically significant reduction in glycaemia comparable to that of metformin, a well-known glucose lowering drug, was observed (3).

1. Villarroel M, E Biolley E, G Larenas, E Wittig, V Diaz, Y Munoz; Chemical, sensory and clinical characterization of lupin marmalades, *Arch Latinoam Nutr* **46**(3), 234-37 (1996) [Article in Spanish].
2. Garcia Lopez PM, PG de la Mora, W Wysocka, B Maiztegui, ME Alzugaray, H Del-Zotto, MI Borelli; Quinolizidine alkaloids isolated from *Lupinus* species enhance insulin secretion, *Eur J Pharmacol* **504**(1-2), 139-42 (2004).
3. Magni C, F Sessa, E Accardo, M Vanoni, P Morazzoni, A Scarafoni, M Duranti; Conglutin *gamma*, a lupin seed protein, binds insulin *in vitro* and reduces plasma glucose levels of hyperglycaemic rats, *J Nutr Biochem* **15**(11), 646-50 (2004)

Lupinus termis Linn. (Fabaceae / Leguminosae) Syn: *Lupinus albus*

Hypoglycaemic and hypolipidaemic effects of diets supplemented with 20 % *Lupinus termis* seeds were studied in streptozotocin-induced diabetic rats. The rats, that were not pre-treated with supplemented diets and were given diets only after induction of diabetes, did not show any effect on blood sugar or lipid levels. Lupin seeds diet did not affect hyperglycaemia and hyperlipidaemia but reduced only the levels of triglycerides (1). It has, however, been reported by Al-Zaid and co-workers that oral administration of *Lupinus termis* exhibits significant hypoglycaemic effect in both normal and diabetic rats (2). The effects of *L. termis* on biochemical parameters in alloxan-induced diabetic rats were studied. The increased levels of plasma glucose, urea, creatinine and bilirubin of alloxan-induced diabetic rats were restored to their normal levels after 4 weeks of treatment with the aqueous suspension (1.5 ml /100 g b.w.) of the herb. The results of detailed investigation showed that the herb suspension exerted anti-hyperglycaemic effects and consequently might alleviate liver and renal damage caused by alloxan-induced diabetes (3).

1. Amin Riyad M, Abdul-Ghani, S Abdul-Salam, SM Suleman; Effect of Fenugreek and Lupin seeds on the development of experimental diabetes in rats, *Planta Medica* **54**(4), 286-90 (1988)

2. Al-Zaid, MAM Hassan, N Badir, KA Gumma; Evaluation of blood glucose lowering activity of three plant diet additives. *Int J Pharmacogn* **29**(2), 81-88 (1991).

3. Mansour HA, AS Newairy, MI Yousef, SA Sheweita; Biochemical study on the effects of some Egyptian herbs in alloxan-induced diabetic rats, *Toxicology* **170**(3), 221-28 (2002)

Lycium barbarum Linn. (Solanaceae)
(Wolfberry)

Wolfberry is the common name for the fruit of *Lycium barbarum* and wolfberry species are now grown around the world, primarily in China. Regardless of the plant's geographic origin, the names 'Tibetan goji' and 'Himalayan goji' are in common use in the health food market for products from this plant.

Aqueous decoction as well as the crude and purified polysaccharide fractions of *L. barbarum* fruits significantly reduced blood glucose, serum total cholesterol and triglyceride levels after 10 days of treatment in alloxan-induced diabetic or hyperlipidaemic rabbits. The treatment also enhanced high density lipoprotein cholesterol levels indicating substantial hypoglycaemic and hypolipidaemic effects of the drugs. Hypoglycaemic effect of purified polysaccharide fraction was more significant than those of water decoction and crude polysaccharide fraction. All three preparations from *L. barbarum* possessed antioxidant activity. However, purified polysaccharide fraction was a slightly weaker antioxidant than the others because crude extracts were rich in antioxidants (e.g., carotenoids, riboflavin, ascorbic acid, thiamine, nicotinic acid). *Lycium barbarum* polysaccharides, containing several monosaccharides and 17 amino acids, were major hypoglycaemic constituents of the plant.

Luo Q, Y Cai, J Yan, M Sun, H Corke; Hypoglycaemic and hypolipidemic effects and antioxidant activity of fruit extracts from *Lycium barbarum*, *Life Sci* **76**(2), 137-49 (2004).

Lycopodium species (Lycopodiaceae)

The members of the genus *Lycopodium* are flowerless, vascular, terrestrial or epiphytic plants, with widely-branched, erect, prostrate or creeping stems, with small, simple, needle-like or scale-like leaves that cover the stem and branches thickly. Extract of *Lycopodium* was found to act as a hypoglycaemic agent in *Lohita grandis* (Squash Bug). *Lycopodium* and insulin-injected insects showed a drop in the total carbohydrate content in haemolymph and a significant increase in the glycogen content level in the fat body. The dilute form of the extract in lower doses was more effective than the concentrate form in higher doses.

Mandal S, B Ghosh, D Choudhuri; Insulin and *Lycopodium* extract acting as a hypoglycaemic agent in *Lohita grandis* Gray (Heteroptera, Pyrrhococidae Insecta), *Curr Sci* **51**(1), 51-52 (1982).

Lygos raetam Forssk (Fabaceae)

Sixteen quinolizidine and dipiperidyl alkaloids were isolated from *Lygos raetam* and its different varieties (*L. raetam* var. *sarcocarpa* and *L. raetam* var. *bovei*) and fully characterized. Evaluation of hypoglycaemic effect of the different extracts and of the isolated alkaloids was performed. N-methylcytisine was proved to have a significant hypoglycaemic effect on the induced diabetic mice.

Abdel Halim OB, H Abdel Fattah, AF Halim, I Murakoshi; Comparative chemical and biological studies of the alkaloidal content of *Lygos* species and varieties growing in Egypt, *Acta Pharm Hung* **67**(6), 241-47 (1997).

Lythrum salicaria Linn. (Lythraceae) (Purple-loosestrife)

Purple-loosestrife is a flowering plant, native to Europe, Asia, northwest Africa and south-eastern Australia. Several extracts of *L. salicaria* were tested for their putative hypoglycaemic activity in normoglycaemic and hyperglycaemic rabbits. The variations in circulating insulin levels were also examined. The results of this preliminary study proved the hypoglycaemic activity of the plant (1). Of the different extracts of the plant tested, only ether extracts from stem or flowers, at a dose equivalent to 10 g of crude plant material/kg, caused a significant reduction in blood glucose level 4 h after oral administration and this effect was associated with an increase of circulating insulin (2). The extracts also exhibited significant hypoglycaemic activity in rats with glucose- and epinephrine-induced hyperglycaemia when the animals were given oral doses equivalent to 10 g/kg of starting material. These extracts were also found to be active in alloxan- and streptozotocin-induced diabetic rats and alloxan-induced diabetic mice. The elevated *gamma*-glutamyl transpeptidase activity, induced by streptozotocin in rats, was reduced by the extracts but the elevated lactic dehydrogenase activity was reduced only by the stem extract (3).

1. Torres IC, JC Suarex; A preliminary study of hypoglycaemic activity of *Lythrum salicaria, J Nat Prod* **43**(5), 559-63 (1980)
2. Lamela M, I Cadavid, A Gato, JM Calleja; Effects of *Lythrum salicaria* in normoglycaemic rats, *J Ethnopharmacol* **14**(1), 83-91 (1985).
3. Lamela M, I Cadavid, JM Calleja; Effects of *Lythrum salicaria* extracts on hyperglycaemic rats and mice, *J Ethnopharmacol* **15**(2), 153-60 (1986).

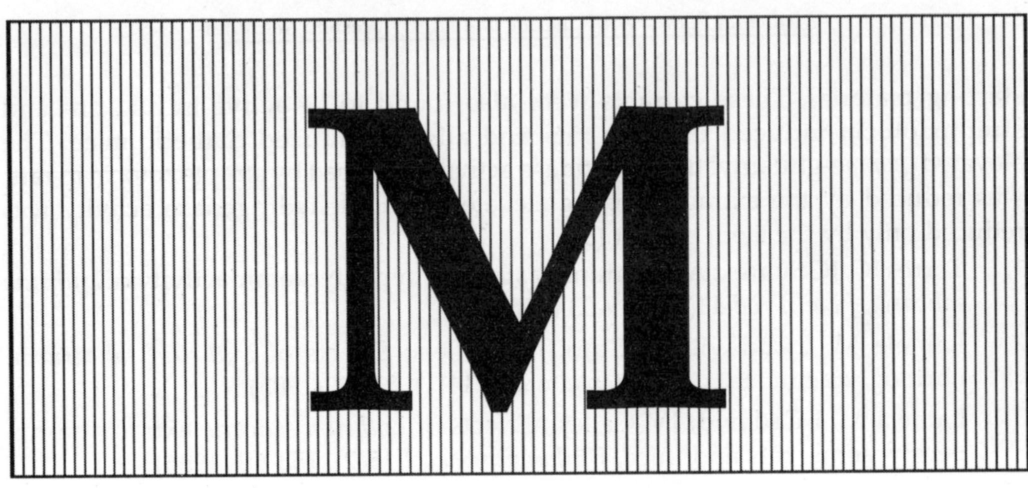

Malva verticillata Linn.(Malvaceae) (Cluster mallow)

Seven polysaccharides and peptidoglycans, obtained from the seeds of *M. verticillata*, were tested for anti-complementary and hypoglycaemic activities. The major neutral polysaccharide (MVS-I), the major peptidoglycan (MVS-V), and the polysaccharide-rich fraction were tested for hypoglycaemic activity. MVS-I especially showed remarkable activity, and the polysaccharide-rich fraction also exhibited significant activity. [See also glycans in the Appendix]

Tomoda M, N Shimizu, R Gonda, M Kanari, H Yamada, H Hikino; Anti-complementary and hypoglycaemic activities of the glycans from the seeds of *Malva verticillata, Planta Med* **56**(2), 168-70 (1990).

Mangifera indica Linn. (Anacardiaceae) (Mango, S. Aamraphal, H. Aam)

Mangifera indica retains special significance for its fruits (mango), which is considered to be divine fruit or the 'King of fruits' in India and other South Asian countries. Administration (per os) of a 50% ethanol extract of tender leaves of mango caused a decrease in plasma glucose levels of normal rats, the highest fall being noticed 8h after administration of a dose of 250 mg/kg. In diabetic rats, the extract (250 mg / kg, per os) produced a significant anti-hyperglycaemic effect within 3 days (1). The effect of the aqueous extract of the leaves of *M. indica* on blood glucose level was assessed in normoglycaemic, glucose-induced hyperglycaemic and streptozotocin-induced diabetic rats. Oral administration of the extract (1 g/kg) did not alter the blood glucose levels in either normoglycaemic or streptozotocin-induced diabetic rats. However, in glucose- induced hyperglycaemia, anti-diabetic activity was seen when the extract and glucose were administered simultaneously and also when the extract was given to the rats 60 min before the glucose. When the test was performed in mice, the extract produced a reduction of blood glucose level in normoglycaemic and glucose-induced hyperglycaemic animals but did not show any effect on streptozotocin-induced diabetic mice. The hypoglycaemic effect of the aqueous extract was comparable with that of an oral dose of chlorpropamide under the same conditions. From the results of the investigation, the hypoglycaemic activity of the aqueous extract of the leaves of *M. indica* was ascertained (2, 3).

Ethanol extract of *M. indica* bark exhibited significant *alpha*-glucosidase inhibitory activity (4). Aqueous extract of the stem bark of *M. indica* was prepared in a Soxhlett extractor using distilled water. The extract (50-800 mg/kg ip) caused significant hypoglycaemic effects in streptozotocin-induced diabetic rats. The chemical constituents of the plant, especially the polyphenolics, flavonoids, triterpenoids, mangiferin, etc., might be involved in the observed hypoglycaemic effects of the plant's extract (5).

1. Sharma SR, SK Dwivedi, D Swarup; Hypoglycaemic potential of *Mangifera indica* leaves in rats, *Int J Pharmacogn* **35**(2), 130-33 (1997)
2. Aderibigbe AO, TS Emudianughe, BA Lawal; Anti-hyperglycaemic effect of *Mangifera indica* in rat, *Phytother Res* **13**(6), 504-07 (1999).
3. Aderibigbe AO, TS Emudianughe, BA Lawal; Evaluation of the anti-diabetic action of *Mangifera indica* in mice, *Phytother Res* **15**(5), 456-58 (2001).
4. Prashanth D, A Amit, DS Samiulla, MK Asha, R Padmaja; *Alpha*-glucosidase inhibitory activity of *Mangifera indica* bark, *Fitoterapia* **72**(6), 686-88 (2001)
5. Ojewole JA; Antiinflammatory, analgesic and hypoglycaemic effects of *Mangifera indica* Linn. (Anacardiaceae) stem-bark aqueous extract, *Methods Find Exp Clin Pharmacol* **27**(8). 547-54 (2005).

Manihot esculenta Crantz (Euphorbiaceae) (Tapioca, Cassava)

The cassava, or tapioca is native to South America but it is extensively cultivated as an annual crop in tropical and subtropical regions of the world for its edible starchy tuberous root, a major source of carbohydrates. Cassava is the third largest source of carbohydrates for human food in the world, with Africa as the largest centre of its production. The extent of blood glucose increases, produced by products of cassava and wheat, were compared in experiments performed in cats and rats. In normal anaesthetised rats, a meal of 500 mg grated cassava preparation produced a mean maximum blood glucose increases, which is 200% less than the mean maximum blood glucose increases produced by a meal of 500 mg wheat flour preparation. In diabetic rats, a 20 g homogenous mixture consisting of 50% cassava bammy and 50% rat chow that was eaten within a 24 h period, produced a mean blood glucose increases which is 221% less than the blood glucose increase produced by a 20g homogenous mixture, consisting of 50% wheat flour bread and 50% rat chow eaten over a similar period of time.

Simon OR, R Gaskin; Supporting evidence for the use of Cassava (*Manihot esculenta*) products instead of wheat flour products in the diet of the diabetic, *West Indian Med J* **37**(2), 100-05 (1989)

Medicago sativa Linn. (Fabaceae) (Alfalfa, Lucerne)

Alfalfa (*Medicago sativa*), also known as Lucerne, is native to Iran and neighbouring regions. It is used for human consumption. Alfalfa sprouts are used as a salad ingredient in the United States, Australia and New Zealand.

Administration of *M. sativa* in the diet (62.5 g/kg) and drinking water (2.5 g/l) reduced the hyperglycaemia of streptozotocin-induced diabetic mice. An aqueous extract of lucerne (1 mg/ml) stimulated 2-deoxy-glucose transport, glucose oxidation, and incorporation of glucose into glycogen in mouse abdominal muscle.. In acute 20 min tests, 0.25-1 mg/ml of the extract evoked a stepwise stimulation of insulin secretion from the BRIN-BD11 pancreatic β-cell line. The results of detailed investigation demonstrated the presence of anti-hyperglycaemic, insulin-releasing and insulin-like activity in the traditional anti-diabetic plant, *Medicago sativa* (1).

Alfalfa has a long history of medicinal and nutritional uses. Hypoglycaemic and other important medicinal uses of alfalfa have been reviewed (2).

1. Gray AM, PR Flatt; Pancreatic and extra-pancreatic effects of the traditional anti-diabetic plant, *Medicago sativa* (lucerne), *Brit J Nutr* **78**(2), 325-34 (1997)
2. Basch E, C Ulbricht, M Harrison, D Sollars, M Smith, C Dennehy, P Szapary; Alfalfa (*Medicago sativa* L.): A clinical decision support tool, *J Herb Pharmacother* **3**(2), 69-90 (2003)

Melaleuca quinquenervia (Clav.) S. T. Blake (Myrtaceae) (Paper Bark Tea Tree)

Grandinin, the major ellagitannin isolated from the leaves of *M. quinquenervia*, showed radical scavenging properties by its reaction with 1,1-diphenyl-2-picrylhydrazyl (DPPH) radical. It exhibited a significant dose-dependent (35-70 mg/kg) hypoglycaemic effect by significantly reducing blood glucose level in basal condition and after heavy glucose load in normal mice. It also reduced the elevated blood glucose level in streptozotocin-induced diabetic mice.

Moharram FA, MS Marzouk, SA El-Toumy, AA Ahmed, EA Aboutabl; Polyphenols of *Melaleuca quinquenervia* leaves—pharmacological studies of grandinin, *Phytother Res* **17**(7), 767-73 (2003).

Memecylon umbellatum Burm.f. (Melastomataceae/Memecylaceae) (H. Anjan)

Memecylon umbellatum is native to Sri Lanka, India and Burma and it grows well in the dry lowlands and in intermediate forests. The plant has great ornamental value because of its blue beauty when in bloom.. Oral administration of an alcoholic extract of the leaves of *M. umbellatum* led to a significant lowering of serum glucose levels in normal and alloxan-induced diabetic mice. Though the mechanism of action could not be ascertained in this study, the plant has interesting possibilities as a source of oral hypoglycaemic agents.

Amalraj T, S Ignacimuthu; Evaluation of the hypoglycaemic effect of *Memecylon umbellatum* in normal and alloxan diabetic mice, *J Ethnopharmacol* **62** (3), 247-50 (1998)

Merremia mammosa (Lour.) Hallier f. (Convolvulaceae)

Merremosides, the resin glycosides isolated from the methanol extract of the roots of the plant, are reported to be useful in the treatment of diabetes.

Isao K (Eisal Company Limited, Japan), Merremosides for treatment of diabetes and tuberculosis, *Japan Kokai Tokkyo Koho JP 01, 139, 595* (C1C0711106), 1989, 6pp. (Jap, Eng)

Mimosa pudica Linn. (Fabaceae) (Sensitive plant, Touch me not)

Sensitive plant was first described from Brazil but today it has pan-tropical distribution. The compound leaves of the creeper fold inward and droop when touched, re-opening within minutes. Methanol extract of the plant exhibited good hypoglycaemic activity, when tested in albino rats.

Gopalkrishnan V, B Jaykar, T Balasaraswathi, VE Idachristy, B Parvathi, R Saraswathi; Pharmacognostical and pharmacological studies of *Mimosa pudica*, *International Seminar on Recent Trends in Pharmaceutical Science,* Ootacamund, India, Abst. No. A-8, February 18-20, 1995

Momordica charantia Linn. (Cucurbitaceae) (Bitter gourd, Bitter melon, H. Karela)

Of the different vegetables that are commonly consumed in India for their putative anti-diabetic potency, karela, the unripe fruits of *Momordica charantia,* is an important one (22, 38, 51). It is indigenous to South America and Asia and its hypoglycaemic activity is well known. A number of publications (1-6) reporting its anti-diabetic activity appeared between 1963 and 1980. Different parts of fruits and plant of *M. charantia* and their extracts have been tested for their potential anti-diabetic activity.

Wistar rats rendered hyperglycaemic by streptozotocin (50 mg/kg b.w., ip) were maintained on a semi-synthetic diet containing freeze dried bitter gourd powder at 0.5% level for 6 weeks. Analysis of plasma glucose, albumin, urea and cholesterol at the end of the experimental regime revealed that bitter gourd had no beneficial hypoglycaemic influence as evidenced by the blood glucose levels as well as the excretion of diabetes related metabolites (35). The effects of freeze-dried powder of bitter melon were studied in rats fed diets supplemented with and without cholesterol. Rats were fed the diets for 14 days containing bitter melon powder (0.5 - 3%) with or without an added dietary cholesterol. Dietary bitter melon resulted in a consistent decrease in serum glucose levels in rats fed cholesterol-free diets, but not in those fed cholesterol-enriched diets, although no dose-response was noted (41).

The effect of *M. charantia* on blood glucose level of normal and alloxan-diabetic rabbits was studied (8). Oral administration of a 50% methanol extract (30 mg/kg) of *M. charantia* decreased the blood glucose level by 25% at 3 h after administration. The n-butanol soluble fraction of the extract (30 mg/kg) was most effective and it lowered blood glucose level by 34%. In the oral and intra-peritoneal glucose tolerance test the n-butanol fraction of *M. charantia* inhibited the increase of blood glucose level significantly. The extract seems to act like insulin or *via* insulin secretion from the pancreas, like the action of sulfonylureas (27).

The effect of water-soluble extract of karela on glucose and insulin concentrations was studied in nine non-insulin-dependent diabetics and six non-diabetic laboratory rats. During a 50 g oral glucose tolerance test in the diabetics, a significant reduction of blood glucose concentrations was observed. Force-feeding in the rats also produced similar results. Fried karela fruits, consumed as a daily supplement to the diet, were also found to produce a small but significant improvement in glucose tolerance. Improvement in glucose tolerance was not associated with an increase in serum insulin responses (7). Experimental and clinical studies revealed anti-diabetic and adaptogenic properties of the aqueous extract of bitter gourd. The aqueous extract of the fruit was more effective in diabetes than the powder of the dried fruit (30). The effect of varying doses of alcoholic and aqueous extracts of *M. charantia* on body weight, serum glucose, insulin and triglycoside was investigated in fructose fed rats. Serum glucose and insulin levels were significantly increased following feeding of fructose for 15 days. Administration of an aqueous extract of *M. charantia* (400 mg/d) markedly prevented high fructose diet-induced hyperglycaemia and hyperinsulinaemia (44). The effects of daily oral feeding of an extract of *M. charantia* (200 mg/kg) for 40 days on blood glucose concentrations and kidney functions were studied in streptozotocin-induced diabetic rats. Plasma glucose levels, body weight, urine volume and urinary albumin levels were monitored on every 10th day over a 40-day period while plasma creatinine levels were assessed at the beginning and end of experiment. Renal hypertrophy was assessed as the ratio between the kidney weight and total body weight. Plasma glucose concentration in streptozotocin-induced diabetic animals was reduced by the administration of the extract by about 24.4%. The treatment prevented polyuria, the rise in urinary albumin levels and partially but significantly renal hypertrophy (46). The anti-diabetic activity of *M charantia* was investigated in KK-Ay mice, an animal model with type-2 diabetes with hyperinsulinaemia. The water extract of *M charantia* fruit reduced the blood glucose of KK-Ay mice 3 weeks after oral administration and also significantly lowered the serum insulin level. However, it did not affect the blood glucose in normal mice. The blood glucose level of the extract-treated KK-Ay mice decreased significantly in an insulin tolerance test. The glucose transporter isoform 4 (GLUT4) protein content in the plasma membrane fraction from muscle also significantly increased in the treated mice when compared with that of the controls. From this result it was inferred that the anti-diabetic activity *M charantia* fruit extract is derived, at least in part, from a decrease in insulin resistance because of the increase of GLUT4 protein content in the plasma membrane of the muscle (47). The effect of daily administration of karela extract (100g) for 2 weeks on fasting and postprandial blood and urine sugar levels was studied in 25 diabetics and 10 non-diabetics and no significant difference in blood sugar level was observed. The fasting and postprandial urine tests were negative for glycosurea throughout the 2 week period (10). The efficacy of bitter gourd as an oral hypoglycaemic agent was evaluated in a randomized controlled clinical trial (53).

Tongia and co-workers claimed the isolation of 15 chemical constituents (alkaloids, glycosides, aglycone, tannin, sterol, phenol and protein) from the methanol extract of *M. charantia* fruits. The active fraction (carbon tetrachloride-benzene extract of the semisolid form of *M. charantia* fruits) was used orally in a dose of 200 mg twice daily for pharmacological interactions with two diversely acting oral hypoglycaemic agents; metformin and glibenclamide, in 15 patients of NIDDM. It was observed that the active fraction plus half doses of metformin or glibenclamide or both in combination caused hypoglycaemia greater than that caused by full doses used in the study with 7 days treatment. It was concluded that the extract acts in synergism with oral hypoglycaemics and potentiates their hypoglycaemia in NIDDM (59). Cerasee, a wild variety of *Momordica charantia*, is traditionally prepared as a tea for the treatment of diabetes mellitus in the West Indies and Central America. Intra-peritoneal administration of a concentrated aqueous extract of cerasee improved glucose tolerance after 8 hr in normal mice, and in streptozotocin diabetic mice the level of hyperglycaemia was reduced by 50% after 5 hour. The cerasee extracts did not significantly alter plasma insulin concentrations, suggesting that cerasee may exert an extra-pancreatic effect to promote glucose disposal (14). The water extract of the fruit of *M. charantia* with exercise reduced the blood glucose of KK-Ay mice 5 weeks after oral administration and also significantly lowered the plasma insulin of KK-Ay mice under similar conditions. These results suggest that *M. charantia* extract with exercise is useful for cure of type-2 diabetes (57). The aqueous extract of *M. charantia* was found to inhibit primarily the uptake of glucose in a dose-dependent manner. Uptake of tyrosine was affected at high substrate concentrations only. The extract was also found to decrease the absorptive capacity of fluid across the small intestine and sodium ions. It is hypothesized that the effects of *Momordica* could involve a washout of glucose from the blood stream (56). Rodent studies suggest that the active components of extracts of the unripe fruit of *M. charantia* enhance the efficiency of postprandial glucose storage in muscle and liver, and diminish excessive hepatic glucose output, while often down-regulating serum insulin—effects comparable to those reported for metformin. The clinical efficacy of metformin has recently been traced to its ability to activate AMP-activated kinase and it would be of interest to determine whether bitter melon extracts contain activators of this enzyme. The fact that bitter melon has the potential to down-regulate insulin suggests that, beyond its likely utility in the management of diabetes, it may have preventive value with respect to a wide range of disorders in which hyperinsulinamia plays a pathogenic role (58). Ethanol (95%) extract of *Momordica charantia* lowered blood glucose by depressing its synthesis, on the one hand through depression of the key gluconeogenic enzymes glucose-6-phosphatase and fructose-1,6-bisphosphatase and on the other by enhancing glucose oxidation by the shunt pathway through activation of its principal enzyme glucose-6-phosphate dehydrogenase (29). It has been demonstrated by immunohistochemistry, that glutathione S-transferase (GST) isoenzymes are differentially expressed in the liver, kidney and testis of diabetic rats and that treatment with an extract of *M. charantia* modulates GST expression in diabetic rats and reverts them to the normal distribution as seen in the tissues of control rats. It has, therefore, been suggested that glutathione metabolism and GST distribution in the tissues of diabetic rats may play an important role in the etiology, pathology and prevention of diabetes (65).

Khanna and Jain (5) isolated a polypeptide (M.wt. 6553), from fruits, seeds and tissue culture of *M. charantia* and it showed hypoglycaemic action (i.v.) in desert rats, monkeys and human beings. The polypeptide was found to work very effectively in juvenile diabetes and its oral administration was equally effective. The active peptide, which was termed as 'plant insulin' is debatable. These workers later reported the isolation of a polypeptide p (M.wt. 11,000) from the same source and found it to be a very effective hypoglycaemic agent when administered subcutaneously to gerbils, langurs, and humans (9). The isolation of molecules with insulin-like bioactivity from fruits and seeds of the bitter gourd was also reported by Ng and co-workers. These authors extracted decorticated seeds of *M. charantia* by a method which was developed originally for the purification of insect and annelid insulins. Of the seven fractions collected, three fractions exhibited anti-lipolytic and lipogenic activities in isolated adipocytes and one fraction showed only lipogenic activity. The "p-fraction" exhibited anti-lipolytic activity in hamster adipocytes and stimulated ^{3}H-glucose incorporation into lipids. Chromatography of "p-fraction" led to the isolation of fractions F_1 and F_2. F_1, a saponin containing fraction, inhibited both lipolysis and incorporation of ^{3}H-glucose into lipids, while fraction F_2 enhanced ^{3}H-glucose incorporation into lipid. The presence of compounds with insulinomimetic activities in *M. charantia* fruits and seeds was thus validated (15, 19). Hypoglycaemic polypeptide, isolated from *M. charantia* seeds was judged as plant insulin on the basis of the analysis of its SDS-PAGE electrophoresis and its amino acid composition.(63).

The effects of the fruit pulp and seed extracts of *M. charantia* on glucose tolerance have been presented (43). Seeds of *M. charantia* (1.3g/day/rabbit) proved to be hypoglycaemic like glibenclamide and this activity was positively associated with lipogenesis. The seeds, however, failed to improve impaired renal functions caused by streptozotocin (11). Methanol and saline extracts of *M. charantia* seeds produced significant hypoglycaemia in starved rats and also prevented adrenaline-induced hyperglycaemia (20). The hypoglycaemic efficacy and antioxidant activities of the aqueous extract of the seeds of country and hybrid varieties of *M. charantia* were studied in streptozotocin-induced diabetic rats. Oral administration of both the seed extracts (150 mg/kg b.w.) for 30 days showed a significant decrease in fasting blood glucose, hepatic and renal thiobarbituric acid reactive substances and hydroperoxides. The treatment also resulted in a significant increase in reduced glutathione, superoxide dismutase, catalase, glutathione peroxidase and glutathione-S-transferase in the liver and kidney of diabetic rats. The results clearly indicate that the impaired antioxidant status in streptozotocin-induced-diabetes may be effectively normalised by *M. charantia* seed extract. The extract exerted rapid protective effects against lipid peroxidation by scavenging of free radicals and thereby reducing the risk of diabetic complications (66). The hypoglycaemic efficacy in aqueous extracts of the seeds of two varieties (country and hybrid variety) of *Momordica charantia* was evaluated in streptozotocin-induced diabetic rats. Treatment of diabetic rats with either of the extracts for a period of 30 days resulted in a significant reduction in blood glucose, glycosylated hemoglobin, lactate dehydrogenase, glucose-6-phosphatase, fructose-1,6-bisphosphatase and glycogen phosphorylase, and a concomitant increase in the levels of hemoglobin, glycogen and activities of hexokinase and glycogen synthase. Both the varieties showed significant hypoglycaemic effects, which were more pronounced in the country variety (67).

Considerable work has also been done on the fruit juice of *M. charantia*. It is reported to show significant hypoglycaemic activity and improvement in oral glucose tolerance in rats (13). The fruit juice of this plant caused an increased glucose uptake by tissues *in vitro* without concomitant increase of tissue respiration. Oral treatment with the juice prior to a glucose load was found to increase the glycogen content of liver and muscle. Pre-treatment of fasted rats with this fruit juice had no significant effect on the gluconeogenic capacity of kidney slices (16). In a clinical trial, however, the fruit juice of *M. charantia* was found to significantly improve the glucose tolerance of 73% of the patients investigated while the other 27% failed to respond (17). Karunanayake and co-workers, however, reported that oral administration of the juice (10 ml/kg for 30 days) to streptozotocin-induced diabetic rats did not show a significant effect, either acute or cumulative, on the ability to tolerate an external glucose load. Viable *beta*-cells capable of secreting insulin upon stimulation appear to be required for *M. charantia* to exert its oral hypoglycaemic activity (23). Oral administration of fruit juice, freeze-dried fruit juice and seed extract of *M. charantia* to healthy Sprague Dawley rats significantly improved their ability to tolerate an oral glucose load and the oral hypoglycaemic activity of these preparations were comparable (25). Fruit juice of *M. charantia* was found to be a scavenger of superoxide and hydroxyl radicals. Since oxygen radicals are implicated in the complications of diabetics, anti-diabetic activity of *M. charantia* has been suggested to be mediated through this mechanism (26). Hypoglycaemic efficacy of the fruit extract of *M. charantia* was found to be significantly improved when used in combination with the extracts of the fruits of *Emblica officinalis* and rhizomes of *Curcuma longa* (28). Pulp juice of *M. charantia* lowered fasting blood glucose levels in normal rats; the effect was more pronounced with the saponin-free methanol extract of the pulp juice. The pulp juice also had a significant hypoglycaemic effect in the glucose-fed normal rats when the extract was fed 45 minutes before the oral glucose load. In the IDDM model rats, the pulp juice had no significant effect on blood glucose levels either in fasting or postprandial states. In the NIDDM model rats, the saponin-free methanol extract of juice produced a significant hypoglycaemic effect both in fasting and in postprandial states. Methanol extracts of seed and of whole plant, and saponin-free methanol extract of whole plant produced no hypoglycaemic effects in normal or IDDM model rats either in fasting or in postprandial states (31). The residue left after centrifugation of the fruit juice of *M. charantia* was extracted with ethanol. The ethanol extract was concentrated and extracted with diethyl ether. Oral administration of this ether extract (0.75g/kg) to normal rabbits decreased the blood glucose level by 26 percent (34). Administration of the fruit juice of *M. charantia* (5 ml) to diabetic rabbits caused a significant fall in blood glucose (40). The effect of bitter melon on rats fed a hyperinsulinemic high fat diet was examined. In a dose-response study, oral glucose tolerance was improved in rats fed a high fat (30%) diet supplemented with freeze-dried bitter melon juice at a dose of 0.75% or higher. Rats switched to high fat plus bitter melon juice diet gained less weight and had less visceral fat than those fed high fat diet alone. Supplementation of high fat diet with bitter melon juice improved insulin resistance, lowered serum insulin and leptin but raised serum free fatty acid concentration. Bitter melon juice appears to have multiple influences on glucose and lipid metabolism that strongly counteract the untoward effects of a high fat diet (52). The anti-diabetic potential of *M. charantia* fruit juice was also found to restore impaired estrous cycle in alloxan-induced diabetic rats (69).

Intravenous administration of acidified water-chloroform extract of unripe fruits of *M. charantia* (10 and 20 mg/kg) to alloxan-induced diabetic rabbits caused a significant decrease in blood glucose level (18). Oral administration of the aqueous extract of *M. charantia* fruits reduced the fasting glucose levels of cyproheptadine-induced hyperglycaemic or normoglycaemic mice. The extract showed a hypoglycaemic activity without improving the tolerance to glucose in cyproheptadine-induced diabetic mice. On the other hand, oral glucose-loading of the cyproheptadine-induced hyperglycaemic animals reduced the fasting glucose levels significantly. The extract showed hypoglycaemic activity without improving the tolerance to glucose in cyproheptadine-induced diabetic mice (33). Aqueous extract of unripe fruits of *M. charantia* was also reported to be a potent stimulator of insulin release from *beta*-cell-rich pancreatic islets isolated from obese-hyperglycaemic mice. The stimulation of insulin release was partially reversible. It differed from that of D-glucose and other commonly employed insulin secretagogues in not being suppressed by L-epinephrine and in being potentiated even by the removal of Ca^{2+}. It has been suggested that the insulin-releasing action of the extract is the result of perturbations of membrane functions (12). The powder prepared from aqueous extract of fresh unripe whole fruits, at a dose of 20 mg/kg body weight, was found to reduce fasting blood glucose level by 48%, an effect comparable to that of glibenclamide. The extract did not show any sign of nephrotoxicity and hepatotoxicity, as judged by histological and biochemical parameters. The powder derived from the aqueous extract of *M. charantia* appeared to be a safe alternative for reduction of blood glucose (54). The influence of *M. charantia* fruit extract on the development of diabetic cataract was studied in alloxan-induced diabetic Charles Foster rats with greater than 150 mg% of blood sugar. While control group receiving 2 ml of 0.9% NaCl developed cataract in 90 to 100 days, the fruit extract treated diabetics showed cataract in 140 to 180 days (21). In normal mice, an aqueous extract of *M. charantia* fruit has been reported to lower the glycaemic response to both oral and intra-peritoneal glucose load, without altering the insulin response. This aqueous extract and the residue left after alkaline chloroform extraction reduced the hyperglycaemia in diabetic mice at 1 hour. Material recovered by acid water wash of the chloroform extract remaining after an alkaline water wash produced a more slowly generated hypoglycaemic effect. From the results it has been suggested that orally administered karela extracts lower glucose concentrations independently of intestinal glucose absorption and involve an extra-pancreatic effect. The presence of two types of hypoglycaemic substances with different time dependent effects was indicated. (24).

In order to ascertain the mechanism of action of the hypoglycaemic activity of the fruit juice of *M. charantia*, experiments (*in vitro* and *in vivo*) were carried out to study the role of bitter gourd juice on the diabetic status. The activity of this plant drug was tested in streptozotocin-treated RIN cells and isolated islets *in vitro*. The fruit juice markedly reduced streptozotocin-induced lipid peroxidation in pancreas of mice, RIN cells and islets. It also reduced streptozotocin-induced apoptosis in RIN cells indicating the mode of protection of the fruit juice on RIN cells, islets and pancreatic *beta*-cells. The study confirms hypoglycaemic effect of the fruit juice of *M. charantia* and defines its role for its potential use in treating diabetes (42). The beneficial effects of *M. charantia* juice in streptozotocin-induced diabetic rats and the mechanism of action were studied. The juice was found to exert marked beneficial effects in diabetic rats. Oral intake of *M. charantia* juice by streptozotocin-induced diabetic rats partially reversed all the diabetes-induced effects measured. Daily oral administration of *M. charantia* juice to these diabetic rats significantly reduced the Na^+- and K^+-dependent absorptions of glucose by the brush border membrane vesicles of the jejunum compared to the responses obtained in untreated streptozotocin-induced diabetic rats. It was also found to stimulate glucose uptake into skeletal muscle cells similar to the response obtained with insulin (60). In order to understand the mechanism of the hypoglycaemic action of *M. charantia, in vitro,* the effect of fruit juice on labeled 2-deoxyglucose or N-methyl-α-amino-isobutyric acid uptake in L6 rat muscle cells was investigated. Like insulin, fruit juice of *M. charantia* resulted in time-dependent increases in the uptakes of the above-mentioned labelled compounds with maximal uptakes taking place at 5 μg/ml. The results indicate that *M. charantia* fruit juice acts like insulin to exert its hypoglycaemic effect and moreover, it can stimulate amino acid uptake into skeletal muscle cells just like insulin (48, 61).

The effects of oral feeding of karela fruit juice on the hepatic cytochrome P450 and glutathione S-transferase drug-metabolizing enzymes in the streptozotocin induced diabetic rats were studied. The results of the investigation suggest that the changes in hepatic phase I and phase II drug-metabolizing enzyme activities in the streptozotocin-induced diabetic animals may be associated with the altered expression of different cytochrome P450 and glutathione S-transferase isozymes. It was also observed that karela does not always reverse the effects of drug-metabolizing enzymes in streptozotocin-induced diabetes (37). The effect of *Momordica charantia* fruit juice and seed extract on certain key hepatic enzymes was investigated using male Sprague-Dawley rats as the animal model. Oral administration of both the fruit juice and the seed extract (1 ml/100 g body weight for 30 days) significantly elevated the concentrations of serum *gamma*-glutamyl transferase and alkaline phosphatase. Though no significant histopathological changes in the liver was observed, the prevalence of dilatation and/or congestion of the central vein sinusoidal system appeared to be twice as high following fruit juice treatment. It was thus inferred that *M. charantia* may either contain hepatotoxins capable of causing cellular damage at the molecular level without causing significant histopathological changes or the plant may have an enzyme inducing effect (32). The chronic administration of an aqueous exract of *M. charantia* fruits (200 mg/kg/d) significantly decreased the plasma glucose levels in alloxanised rats and streptozotocin-induced diabetic mice. However, the reduction in the glucose level was more marked in alloxanised rats compared to streptozotocin-induced diabetic mice. Dibetes-induced changes in hepatic and skeletal muscle glycogen contents and hepatic glucokinase, hexokinase, glucose-6-phosphate and phosphofructokinase were also partially restored by *M. charantia* fruit extract (49).

The effects of long term feeding (10 weeks) of *M. charantia* fruit extract on blood plasma and tissue lipid profiles were studied in normal and streptozotocin-induced type-1 diabetic rats. A significant increase in plasma non-esterified cholesterol, triglycerides and phospholipids accompanied by a decrease in high-density lipoprotein-cholesterol and a moderate increase in plasma lipid peroxidation product, malonedialdehyde and about two-fold increase in kidney lipid peroxidation were observed in streptozotocin-induced diabetic rats. The treatment of these diabetic rats with *M. charantia* fruit extract over a 10-week period returned these levels close to normal. This extract also exhibited an inhibitory effect on membrane lipid peroxidation under *in vitro* conditions (45). The enzyme fraction, isolated from the unripe fruits of *M. charantia*, at doses of 25 and 50 mg/ml, showed significant anti-hyperglycaemic activity in alloxan-induced diabetic rats but not so significant effect in normal rats (50).

Sarkar and coworkers (36) demonstrated the hypoglycaemic action of *M. charantia* fruit extract in a validated animal model of diabetes. In the normal glucose primed rat model, *M. charantia* fruit extract (500 mg/kg), depressed the plasma glucose levels by 10-15% without any increase in insulin secretion at 1 h and its efficacy was 25-30% of tolbutamide. In streptozotocin-induced diabetes rats, it improved the oral glucose tolerance causing 26% reduction in plasma glucose at 3.5 h while metformin caused 40-50% reduction at 1, 2 and 3.5 h. The extract (500 mg/kg) caused a 4-5-fold increase in the rate of glycogen synthesis from U-^{14}C-glucose in the liver of normally fed rats. These data suggest that the mechanism of action of *M. charantia* could be partly attributed to increased glucose utilization in the liver rather than an insulin secretion effect.

Treatment of diabetic rats with fruit extract of *M. charantia* for 30 days showed a significant decrease in triglyceride, low density lipoprotein and a significant increase in high density lipoprotein level. A significant effect on oral glucose tolerance was also noted by chronic administration of the fruit extract (64)

Serious complications occur due to excess glucose in brain and other tissues in diabetic condition. In such situations, reversal of increased sugar levels becomes necessary for a good metabolic control. Insulin, trace metals and some plant extracts have been used to control diabetes and its complications in rats. Administration of vanadates, either alone or in combination with the extract of *M. charantia,* to diabetic animals almost completely reversed the metabolic changes in the activities of key enzymes and effectively controlled their blood glucose levels (39). Sodium orthovanadate is well known for its insulin mimetic and anti-diabetic activities.

The effects of treatment of *Momordica* fruit extract and sodium orthovanadate, separately and in combination, on serum and tissue lipid profile and on the activities of lipogenic enzymes were studied in alloxan induced diabetic rats. The treatment of alloxan diabetic rats with *Momordica* fruit extract and sodium orthovanadate prevented the alterations of lipid profile and activities of lipogenic enzymes and maintained all parameters near control values. Most effective prevention was however observed in a combined treatment of *Momordica* with a reduced dose of sodium orthovanadate (0.2%). The results suggest that *Momordica* fruit extract and sodium orthovanadate exhibit hypolipidaemic as well as hypoglycaemic effect in diabetic rats and their effect is pronounced when administered in combination (68).

Bioactivity guided fractionation of the methanol extract of dried bitter gourds led to the isolation and characterization of three new cucurbitane triterpenoids together with eight known compounds. In order to evaluate the contribution of the cucurbitane triterpenoids, the major compounds, 5β,19-epoxy-3β,25-dihydroxycucurbita-6,23(*E*)-diene and 3 β,7 β,25-trihydroxycucurbita-5,23(*E*)-dien-19-al were tested for their *in vivo* anti-diabetic effects. Both the compounds showed hypoglycaemic effects in the diabetes-induced male ddY mice strain at 400 mg/kg (70).

A modified *in vitro* procedure for identifying herbs possessing sulfonylurea-like activity has been developed. The collected data suggest that the hypoglycaemic properties of bitter melon are at least partially due to its sulfonylurea-like activity (62).

A significant decrease in malondialdehyde level and an increase in antioxidant activity were observed when *Momordica charantia* was administered to diabetic rats. Changes in metal ion status were also observed following administration of this herbal drug (55). The anti-diabetic properties of *M. charantia* (bitter gourd), a vegetable with pan tropical distribution is well established though some adverse effects have also been reported. It has been reported to contain substances with anti-diabetic properties as well as some non-specific bioactive components such as antioxidants. Metabolic and hypoglycaemic effects of bitter gourd extracts have been demonstrated in cell culture, animal, and human studies. Various mechanisms of action have been postulated but the exact one is still under debate. Nevertheless, bitter gourd has the potential to become a component of the diet or a dietary supplement for diabetic and pre-diabetic patients. Well-designed interdisciplinary research is needed before a dietary recommendation can be given and a product is brought to the market (71).

The cell reparative effects of the boiling water extract of *M. charantia* were studied on HIT-T15 Hamster pancreatic *beta*-cells. The extract at a relatively low concentration (0.02%, w/v) achieved the highest cell proliferation rate of 45.6% on alloxan-damaged HIT-T15 cells while the extract at a higher concentration (0.2%, w/v) increased the proliferation of the normal cells by 35.4%. The high molecular weight (M. wt. 3 kDa) fraction of the extract showed stronger effects in repairing alloxan damaged cells than that of the low molecular weight fraction (M. wt < or =3 kDa), while the latter showed a higher activity on increasing insulin secretion of normal or damaged cells. The extract (2%) and the low mol. wt. fraction showed the highest superoxide dismutase activities but failed to improve the proliferation rate of alloxan-damaged cells. These results indicated that the extract has significant repairing effects on HIT-T15 cells against superoxide anion radicals. It was hypothesized that the different fractions of the extract may make different contributions to its cell repairing activity and its ability of stimulating insulin secretion (72).

1. Chatterjee KP; On the presence of an anti-diabetic principle in *Momordica charantia, Indian Physiol Pharmacol* **52**, 240-44 (1963)
2. Aslam M, IH Stockley; Interaction between curry ingredient (karela) and drug (chlorpropamide), *Lancet* **1**(8116), 607 (1979).
3. Pitchumoni CS; Karela and blood sugar, *Lancet* **1**(8122), 924-25 (1979).
4. Shah K, E Hickman, Sr.; Karela and blood sugar, *Lancet* **1**(8122), 925 (1979).
5. Khanna P, JC Jain; A hypoglycaemic polypeptide from vegetable source with an alternate mode of action , *J Nat Prod (Lloydia)* **42**(6), 684 (1979)
6. Yakub M, MS Akhtar, MA Athar; Karela—anti diabetic agent, *J Pak Med Assoc* **30**(8), 181-84 (1980).
7. Leatherdale BA, RK Panesar, G Singh, TW Atkins, CJ Bailey, AH Bignell; Improvement in glucose tolerance due to *Momordica charantia* (karela), *Br Med J* (Clin Res Ed) **282**(6279), 1823-24 (1981).
8. Akhtar MS, MA Athar, M Yaqub; Effect of *Momordica charantia* on blood glucose level of normal and alloxan-diabetic rabbits, *Planta Med* **42**(3), 205-12 (1981).
9. Khanna P, SC Jain, A Panagariya, VP Dixit; Hypoglycaemic activity of polypeptide-p from a plant source, *J Nat Prod* **44**(6), 648-55 (1981).
10. Kirti S, Vinod Kumar, P Nigam, P Srivastava; Effect of *Momordica charantia* (karela) extract on blood and urine sugar in diabetes mellitus -Study from a diabetic clinic, *Clinician* **46**(1), 26-29 (1982)
11. Kedar P, CH Chakrabarti; Effects of bittergourd (*Momordica charantia*) seed & glibenclamide in streptozotocin induced diabetes mellitus, *Indian J Exp Biol* **20**(3), 232-35 (1982).
12. Welihinda J, G Arvidson, E Gylfe, B Hellman, E Karlsson; The insulin-releasing activity of the tropical plant *Momordica charantia, Acta Biol Med Ger* **41**(12), 1229-40 (1982).

13. Karunanayake ER, J Welihinda, SR Sirimanne, G Sinna dorai; Oral hypoglycaemic activity of some medicinal plants of Sri Lanka, *J Ethnopharmacol* **11**(2), 223-31 (1984)
14. Bailey CJ, C Day, SL Turner, BA Leatherdale; Cerasee, a traditional treatment for diabetes. Studies in normal and streptozotocin diabetic mice, *Diabetes Res* **2**(2), 81-84 (1985).
15. Ng TB, CM Wong, WW Li, HW Yeung; Insulin-like molecules in *Momordica charantia* seeds, *J Ethnopharmacol* **15**(1), 107-17 (1986).
16. Welihinda J, EH Karunanayake; Extra-pancreatic effects of *Momordica charantia* in rats, *J Ethnopharmacol* **17**(3), 247-55 (1986).
17. Welihinda J, EH Karunanayake, MH Sheriff, KS Jayasinghe; Effect of *Momordica charantia* on the glucose tolerance in maturity onset diabetes, *J Ethnopharmacol* **17**(3), 277-82 (1986).
18. Tiangda C, R Mekmance, K Praphapraditchote, M Ungsurungsie, C Paovalo; The hypoglycaemic activity of *Momordica charantia* Linn. in normal and alloxan-induced diabetic rabbits, *J Nat Res Council, Thailand* **19**(1), 1-11 (1987)
19. Ng TB, CM Wong, WW Li, HW Yeung; Acid-ethanol extractable compounds from fruits and seeds of the bitter gourd *Momordica charantia*: effects on lipid metabolism in isolated rat adipocytes, *Am J Chin Med* **15**(1-2), 31-42 (1987).
20. Dubey DK, AR Biswas, JS Bapna, SC Pradhan; Hypoglycaemic and anti-hyperglycaemic effects of *Momordica charantia* seed extracts in albino rats, *Fitoterapia* **58**(6), 387-90 (1987)
21. Srivastava Y, H Venkatakrishna-Bhatt, Y Verma; Effect of *Momordica charantia* Linn. pomous aqueous extract on cataractogenesis in murrin alloxan diabetics, *Pharmacol Res Commun* **20**(3), 201-09 (1988).
22. Jangle SN, MS Navthar; *Momordica charantia*: Plant having hypoglycaemic action, *Deerghayu International* **5**(20), 6-8 (1989)
23. Karunanayake EH, S Jeevathayaparan, KH Tennekoon; Effect of *Momordica charantia* fruit juice on streptozotocin-induced diabetes in rats, *J Ethnopharmacol* **30**(2), 199-204 (1990).
24. Day C, T Cartwright, J Provost, CJ Bailey; Hypoglycaemic effect of *Momordica charantia* extracts, *Planta Med* **56**(5), 426-29 (1990).
25. Jeevathayaparan S, KH Tennekoon, EH Karunanayake, SA Jayasinghe; Oral hypoglycaemic activity of different preparation of *Momordica charantia, J Natl Sci Council Sri Lanka* **19**(1), 19-24 (1991)
26. Sreejayan N, MNA Rao, Oxygen free radical scavenging activity of the juice of *Momordica charantia* fruits, *Fitoterapia* **62**(4), 344-46 (1991)
27. Higashino H, A Suzuki, Y Tanaka, K Pootakham; Hypoglycaemic effects of Siamese *Momordica charantia* and *Phyllanthus urinaria* extracts in streptozotocin-

induced diabetic rats (the 1st report), *Nippon Yakurigaku Zasshi* **100**(5), 415-21 (1992) [Article in Japanese]

28. Sankaranarayanan J, CJ Jolly; Phytochemical, antibacterial, and pharmacological investigations on *Momordica charantia* Linn., *Emblica officinalis* and *Curcuma longa* Linn. *Indian J Pharmaceut Sci* **55**(1), 6-13 (1993)
29. Shibib BA, LA Khan, R Rahman; Hypoglycaemic activity of *Coccinia indica* and *Momordica charantia* in diabetic rats: depression of the hepatic gluconeogenic enzymes glucose-6-phosphatase and fructose-1,6-bisphosphatase and elevation of both liver and red-cell shunt enzyme glucose-6-phosphate dehydrogenase, *Biochem J* **292**(Pt 1):267-70 (1993)
30. Srivastava Y, H Venkatakrishna-Bhatt, Y Verma, K Venkaiah, BH Raval; Antidiabetic and adaptogenic properties of *Momordica charantia* extract: An experimental and clinical evaluation, *Phytother Res* **7**(4), 285-89 (1993)
31. Ali L, AK Khan, ML Mamun, M Masihuzzaman, N Nahar, M Nur-e-Alam, B Rokeya; Studies on hypoglycaemic effects of fruit pulp, seed, and whole plant of *Momordica charantia* on normal and diabetic model rats, *Planta Med* **59**(5), 408-12 (1993).
32. Tennekoon KH, S Jeevathayaparan, P Angumawala, EH Karunanayake, KS Jayasinghe; Effect of *Momordica charantia* on key hepatic enzymes, *J Ethnopharmacol* **44**(2), 93-97 (1994).
33. Cakici I, C Hurmoglu, B Tunctan, N Abacioglu, I Kanzik, B Sener; Hypoglycaemic effect of *Momordica charantia* extracts in normoglycaemic or cyproheptadine-induced hyperglycaemic mice, *J Ethnopharmacol* **44**(2), 117-21 (1994).
34. Pugazhenthi S, PS Murthy; Partial purification of a hypoglycaemic fraction from the unripe fruits of *Momordica charantia* Linn. (bitter gourd), *Indian J Clin Biochem* **10**(1), 19-21 (1995)
35. Platel K, K Srinivasan; Effect of dietary intake of freeze dried bitter gourd (*Momordica charantia*) in streptozotocin induced diabetic rats, *Nahrung* **39**(4), 262-68 (1995).
36. Sarkar S, M Pranava, R Marita; Demonstration of the hypoglycaemic action of *Momordica charantia* in a validated animal model of diabetes, *Pharmacol Res* **33**(1), 1-4 (1996).
37. Raza H, I Ahmed, MS Lakhani, AK Sharma, D Pallot, W Montague; Effect of bitter melon (*Momordica charantia*) fruit juice on the hepatic cytochrome P450-dependent monooxygenases and glutathione S-transferases in streptozotocin-induced diabetic rats, *Biochem Pharmacol* **52**(10), 1639-42 (1996).
38. Platel K, K Srinivasan; Plant foods in the management of diabetes mellitus: vegetables as potential hypoglycaemic agents, *Nahrung* **41**(2), 68-74 (1997)
39. Baquer NJ, Glucose overutilization and underutilization in diabetes and effect of anti-diabetic compounds, *Anales de la Real Academia De Farmacia* **64**(1),

147–80 (1998)

40. Khan RA; A study of karela (*Momordica charantia* Linn.) on blood glucose, *Hamdard Medicus* **42**(2), 56-61 (1999)
41. Jayasooriya AP, M Sakono, C Yukizaki, M Kawano, K Yamamoto, N Fukuda; Effects of *Momordica charantia* powder on serum glucose levels and various lipid parameters in rats fed with cholesterol-free and cholesterol-enriched diets, *J Ethnopharmacol* **72**(1-2), 331-36 (2000).
42. Sitasawad SL, Y Shewade, R Bhonde; Role of bittergourd fruit juice in Stz-induced diabetic state *in vivo* and *in vitro, J Ethnopharmacol* **73**(1-2), 71-79 (2000).
43. Basnet P, T Namba, K Komatsu; *Momordica charantia*: What do we really know about its hypoglycaemic activity? *Phytomedicine* **7**(Suppl.II), 63 (2000)
44. Vikrant V, JK Grover, N Tandon, SS Rathi, N Gupta; Treatment with extracts of *Momordica charantia* and *Eugenia jambolana* prevents hyperglycaemia and hyperinsulinaemia in fructose fed rats, *J Ethnopharmacol* **76**(2), 139-43 (2001)
45. Ahmed I, MS Lakhani, M Gillett, A John, H Raza; Hypotriglyceridemic and hypocholesterolemic effects of anti-diabetic *Momordica charantia* (karela) fruit extract in streptozotocin-induced diabetic rats, *Diabetes Res Clin Pract* **51**(3), 155-61 (2001)
46. Grover JK, V Vats, SS Rathi, R Dawar; Traditional Indian anti-diabetic plants attenuate progression of renal damage in streptozotocin induced diabetic mice, *J Ethnopharmacol* **76**(3), 233-38 (2001).
47. Miura T, C Itoh, N Iwamoto, M Kato, M Kawai, SR Park, I Suzuki; Hypoglycaemic activity of the fruit of the *Momordica charantia* in type 2 diabetic mice, *J Nutr Sci Vitaminol* (Tokyo) **47**(5), 340-44 (2001).
48. Cummings EF, J Singh, H Wackerhage; Effect of insulin and *Momordica charantia* fruit extract on deoxyglucose uptake in L6 rat muscle cell line, *West Indian Med J* **50**(Suppl.2), 55 (2001)
49. Rathi SS, JK Grover, V Vats; The use of *Momordica charantia* and *Mucuna pruriens* in experimental diabetes and their effect on key metabolic enzymes invoved in carbohydrate metabolism, *Phytother Res* **16**(3), 236-43 (2002)
50. Bhuvaneswari S, P Chitra Devi, P Balamurugan, N Asish, MC Divakar; Studies on the anti-diabetic activity of the enzyme fraction of *Momordica charantia* fruits, *Antiseptic* **99**(12), 466-67 (2002)
51. Lu L, Y Zhao; Study on hypoglycaemic action and active constituents of *Momordica charantia* L. *Zhong Yao Cai* **25**(6), 449-51 (2002) [Article in Chinese]
52. Chen Q, LL Chan, ET Li; Bitter melon (*Momordica charantia*) reduces adiposity, lowers serum insulin and normalizes glucose tolerance in rats fed a high fat diet, *J Nutr* **133**(4), 1088-93 (2003).
53. John AJ, R Cherian, HS Subhash, AM Cherian; Evaluation of the efficacy of

bitter gourd (*Momordica charantia*) as an oral hypoglycaemic agent—a randomized controlled clinical trial, *Indian J Physiol Pharmacol* **47**(3), 363-65 (2003).

54. Virdi J, S Sivakami, S Shahani, AC Suthar, MM Banavalikar, MK Biyani; Anti-hyperglycaemic effects of three extracts from *Momordica charantia, J Ethnopharmacol* **88**(1), 107-11 (2003).
55. Chandra A, AA Mahdi, RK Singh, R El-hence, S Ahmad; Effect of herbal hypoglycaemic agents on antioxidative potential and metal ion status in STZ-induced diabetic rats, *National Symposium on Emerging Trends in Indian Medicinal Plants,* Lucknow, India, p. 57 (P-2), October 10-12, 2003
56. Mahomoodally MF, AG Fakim, AH Subratty; *Momordica charantia* extracts inhibit uptake of monosaccharide and amino acid across rat everted gut sacs *in vitro, Biol Pharm Bull* **27**(2), 216-18 (2004).
57. Miura T, Y Itoh, N Iwamoto, M Kato, T Ishida; Suppressive activity of the fruit of *Momordica charantia* with exercise on blood glucose in type 2 diabetic mice, *Biol Pharm Bull* **27**(2), 248-50 (2004).
58. McCarty MF; Does bitter melon contain an activator of AMP-activated kinase, *Med Hypotheses* **63**(2), 340-43 (2004).
59. Tongia A, SK Tongia, M Dave; Phytochemical determination and extraction of *Momordica charantia* fruit and its hypoglycaemic potentiation of oral hypoglycaemic drugs in diabetes mellitus (NIDDM), *Indian J Physiol Pharmacol* **48**(2), 241-44 (2004).
60. Ahmed I, E Adeghate, E Cummings, AK Sharma, J Singh; Beneficial effects and mechanism of action of *Momordica charantia* juice in the treatment of streptozotocin-induced diabetes mellitus in rat, *Mol Cell Biochem* **261**(1-2), 63-70 (2004).
61. Cummings E, HS Hundal, H Wackerhage, M Hope, M Belle, E Adeghate, J Singh; *Momordica charantia* fruit juice stimulates glucose and amino acid uptakes in L6 myotubes, *Mol Cell Biochem* **261**(1-2), 99-104 (2004).
62. Rotshteyn Y, SW Zito; Application of modified *in vitro* screening procedure for identifying herbals possessing sulfonylurea-like activity, *J Ethnopharmacol* **93**(2-3), 337-44 (2004).
63. Sheng Q, H Yao, H Xu, X Ling, T He; Isolation of plant insulin from *Momordica charantia* seeds by gel filtration and RP-HPLC, *Zhong Yao Cai* **27**(6), 414-16 (2004) [Article in Chinese].
64. Chaturvedi P, S George, M Milingamyo, YB Tripathi; Effect of *Momordica charantia* on lipid profile and oral glucose tolerance in diabetic rats, *Phytother Res* **18**(11), 954-56 (2004).
65. Raza H, I Ahmed, A John; Tissue specific expression and immunohistochemical localization of glutathione S-transferase in streptozotocin induced diabetic

rats: modulation by *Momordica charantia* (karela) extract, *Life Sci* **74**(12), 1503-11 (2004)

66. Sathishsekar D, S Subramanian; Antioxidant properties of *Momordica charantia* (bitter gourd) seeds on streptozotocin induced diabetic rats, *S Asia Pac J Clin Nutr* **14**(2), 153-58 (2005).
67. Sekar DS, K Sivagnanam, S Subramanian; Anti-diabetic activity of *Momordica charantia* seeds on streptozotocin induced diabetic rats, *Pharmazie* **60**(5), 383-87 (2005).
68. Yadav UC, K Moorthy, NZ Baquer; Combined treatment of sodium orthovanadate and *Momordica charantia* fruit extract prevents alterations in lipid profile and lipogenic enzymes in alloxan diabetic rats, *Mol Cell Biochem* **268**(1-2), 111-20 (2005).
69. Reyes BA, ND Bantista, NC Tanquilut, RV Anunciado, AB Leung, GC Sanchez, RL Magtoto, P Castronuevo, H Tsukamura, KL Maeda; Anti-diabetic potentials of *Momordica charantia* and *Andrographis paniculata* and their effects on estrous cyclicity of alloxan-induced diabetic rats, *J Ethnopharmacol* **105**(1-2), 196-200 (2006)
70. Harinantenaina L, M Tanaka, S Takaoka, M Oda, O Mogami, M Uchida, Y Asakawa; *Momordica charantia* constituents and anti-diabetic screening of the isolated major compounds, *Chem Pharm Bull* (Tokyo) **54**(7),:1017-21 (2006)
71. Krawinkel MB, GB Keding; Bitter gourd (*Momordica charantia*): A dietary approach to hyperglycaemia, *Nutr Rev* **64**(7 Pt 1), :331-37 (2006).
72. Xiang L, X Huang, L Chen, P Rao, L Ke; The reparative effects of *Momordica charantia* Linn. extracton HIT-T15 pancreatic *beta* cells, *Asia Pac J Clin Nutr* **16**(Suppl.1), 249-52 (2007)

Momordica cymbalaria Hook. f. (Cucurbitaceae)

Momordica cymbalaria is a species found in some southern States of India. Its tuber is traditionally used as an abortifacient but the extracts of dry fruits and leaves are generally known to have anti-diabetic and hypolipidaemic properties. The effect of *M. cymbalaria* fruit powder on blood glucose and other biochemical parameters was studied in alloxan-induced diabetic rats. After the treatment for 15 days, a significant reduction was observed in fasting blood glucose levels in the treated diabetic rats, but not in the treated normal rats. A significant improvement in hepatic glycogen level was also observed in treated diabetic rats. A considerable lowering of serum cholesterol and triglycerides was also observed in the treated diabetic group. The fruit powder of *M. cymbalaria* was thus proved to possess anti-diabetic and hypolipidemic effects in alloxan-induced diabetic rats (1). The aqueous extract of *M. cymbalaria* fruits, given at a dosage of 0.5 g/kg b.w. after an overnight fast, showed maximum blood glucose lowering effect in diabetic rats. The same dosage did not produce any hypoglycaemic activity in normal rats. The anti-hyperglycaemic activity of *M. cymbalaria* fruits was compared with glibenclamide, an oral hypoglycaemic agent (2). A significant anti-hyperglycaemic as well as anti-hyperlipidaemic effect was observed in the alloxan-induced diabetic rats, treated by oral administration of the extract (0.5 g/kg) for 6 weeks (3).

1. Rao BK, MM Kesavulu, R Giri, C Appa-Rao; Anti-diabetic and hypolipidemic effects of *Momordica cymbalaria* Hook. fruit powder in alloxan-diabetic rats, *J Ethnopharmacol* **67**(1), 103-09 (1999).
2. Rao BK, MM Kesavulu, C Appa-Rao; Anti-hyperglycaemic activity of *Momordica cymbalaria* in alloxan diabetic rats, *J Ethnopharmacol* **78**(1), 67-71 (2001).
3. Kameswarrao B, MM Kesavulu, C Appa-Rao; Evaluation of anti-diabetic effect of *Momordica cymbalaria* fruit in alloxan-diabetic rats, *Fitoterapia* **74**(1-2), 7-13 (2003)

Momordica foetida Schumach. (Cucurbitaceae)

Momordica foetida is found in Southern Nigeia where it is used natively for the treatment of a variety of ailments. It is a perennial climber emitting an unpleasant smell when crushed. From the whole plant and the unripe fruits of *M. foetida*, a homogenous mixture of β-sitosterol β-D-glucoside and 5, 25-stigmastadien-3β-ol glucoside was isolated and shown to be identical with charantin of *Momordica charantia* (1). The effect of foetidin, isolated from *M. foetida*, on blood glucose level of albino rats was studied (2).

1. Olaniyi AA; A neutral constituent of *Momordica foetida*, *Lloydia* **38**(4), 361-62 (1975).
2. Marquis VO, TA Adanlawo, AA Olaniyi; The effect of foetidin from *Momordica foetida* on blood glucose level of albino rats, *Planta Med* **31**(4), 367-74 (1977).

Momordica grosvenori Swingle (Cucurbitaceae). "Lo ha kuo"

Momordica grosvenori, a traditional medicinal herb in China, is used as a substitute for sugar for obese and diabetic patients and known to exhibit an enhancement of immunity. Heme oxygenase-1 is one of the acute phase proteins that show anti-inflammatory activities with their antioxidant properties. The hypothesis that *M grosvenori* could modulate an imbalance of the cellular immune system and prevent the progression of diabetes mellitus, *via* induction of Heme oxygenase-1 protein expression was investigated using alloxan-induced diabetic male Balb/c mice. Administration of *M grosvenori* effectively regulated the immune imbalance in diabetic mice and showed anti-diabetic effects.

Song F, W Chen, W Jia, P Yao, AK Nussler, X Sun, L Liu; A natural sweetener, *Momordica grosvenori*, attenuates the imbalance of cellular immune functions in alloxan-induced diabetic mice, *Phytother Res* **20**(7), 552-60 (2006)

Morinda lucida Benth. (Rubiaceae)

Morinda lucida is a medium-sized tree and is widely used as a medicinal plant in West Africa, especially in Nigeria. In normal rats, a methanol extract of *M. lucida* demonstrated a significant and dose-dependent hypoglycaemic activity within 4 h after oral administration. In streptozotocin-induced hyperglycaemic rats, the extract produced a significant anti-diabetic effect from day 3 after oral administration of the extract (400 mg/kg). The results suggest that the leaves of *Morinda lucida* have a strong glucose lowering property when administered to streptozotocin-treated rats.

Olajide OA, SO Awe, JM Makinde, O Morebise; Evaluation of the anti-diabetic property of *Morinda lucida* leaves in streptozotocin-diabetic rats, *J Pharm Pharmacol* **51**(11), 1321-24 (1999).

Morinda officinalis F. C. How (Rubiaceae)

For centuries, traditional Chinese healers have used the dried roots of *M. officinalis*, as an energy-boosting tonic. The hypoglycaemic and antioxidant activities of this plant drug were investigated in streptozotocin-induced diabetic rats. In the three-hour dose response study, the ethanol extract of the dried roots of the plant reduced the fasting serum glucose levels of the diabetic rats significantly at 150 mg/kg but increased those of the normal rats significantly at 600 mg/kg only. The water-soluble fraction of the extract demonstrated a dose dependent hypoglycaemic effect in the diabetic rats whereas the n-butanol-soluble fraction increased the fasting serum glucose levels of the diabetic rats significantly at 50 mg/kg only within three hours after administration. The 10-day oral administration of the extract reduced the fasting serum glucose, hepatic and renal thiobarbituric acid reactive substances level and significantly increased the hepatic superoxide dismutase and catalase activities as well as reduced glutathione levels. The dried roots of *M. officinalis* were thus proved to possess hypoglycaemic, hyperglycaemic and anti-oxidant properties.

Soon YY, BK Tan; Evaluation of the hypoglycaemic and anti-oxidant activities of *Morinda officinalis* in streptozotocin-induced diabetic rats, *Singapore Med J* **43**(2), 77-85 (2002)

Moringa oleifera Lam (Moringaceae)
(Drumsticks, H. Sahjan, S . Shigru)

It is a highly valued vegetable tree with a variety of potential uses. The immature green pods, called "drumsticks" are commonly consumed in India, The plant, distributed in many countries of the tropics and subtropics, is well known for its medicinal properties but rather less known for its anti-diabetic activities (2). Administration of methanol extract of the root bark of *M. oleifera* (1 and 1.5g/kg b.w.) showed significant fall in fasting blood sugar levels. At a dose of 1.5g/kg, a 43% fall in blood sugar level was observed at the 5th hour of medication, compared to a 45% fall exhibited by tolbutamide (200mg/kg). Glucose tolerance test to albino rats also showed significant activity (1). Anwar and co-authors, in their review article, focused on detailed phytochemical composition, medicinal uses, along with pharmacological properties of different parts of this multipurpose tree (3).

1. Pillai NR; Hypoglycaemic potential of *Moringa oleifera* Linn. *Seminar on Research in Ayurveda and Siddha*, CCRAS, New Delhi, p. 64, March 20-22, 1995
2. Kar A, BK Choudhury, NG Bandyopadhyay; Evaluation of a few Indian folk medicinal plants less known for their hypoglycaemic activity, *Ethnobotany* **11**(1-2), 18-21 (1999)
3. Anwar F, S Latif, M Ashraf, AH Gilani; *Moringa oleifera*: a food plant with multiple medicinal uses, *Phytother Res* **21**(1), 17-25 (2007)

Moringa stenopetala (Baker f.) (Moringaceae)

It is an important food plant in south-western Ethiopia, where it is cultivated as a crop plant. It is an indigenous tree of semiarid and sub-humid Ethiopia, Somalia and Kenya. The tree finds various uses including medicinal uses. Its use for the treatment of diabetes, high blood pressure and heart problems is particularly important.

Mayer FA, E Stelz; Distribution, ecological requirements and uses of the multipurpose tree *Moringa stenopetala* in southern Ethiopia, *Plant Research and Development* **38**, 20-25 (1993)

Morus alba Linn. (Moraceae) Syn. *Morus indica* (White mulberry)

White mulberry trees are extensively grown in southern Europe and India for their leaves as food for silkworms.

A glycoprotein was isolated from the root barks of *M. alba* and designated as Moran A. Its hypoglycaemic activity was studied (1). Moran 20K, a new glycoprotein with a molecular weight of approximately 20 kDa was isolated from the methanol extract of the root bark of the plant. It was found to lower blood glucose level in streptozotocin-induced hyperglycaemic mice model and increase the glucose transport in cultured epididymis fat cells (6).

Administration of a single dose (200 mg /kg, ip) of aqueous extract of mulberry leaves (Folium mori) or mulberry bark (Cortex mori) to fasted and non-fasted sptreptozotocin-induced diabetic mice resulted in a significant lowering of blood sugar levels. Aqueous extract of mulberry leaves exhibited maximum hypoglycaemic effect. Ethanol soluble fractions of the extracts were most potent (3). Ethanol extract of mulberry leaves and its water soluble fraction showed significant glucose lowering effect in alloxan-induced hyperglycaemic mice. The extract prevented the hyperglycaemic responses from an oral load of starch and glucose *in vivo*. The glucose lowering effect of mulberry leaf extract is considered to be related to the inhibition of *alpha*-glucosidase-catalysed enzymatic reaction (2). The effect of prolonged treatment (10 weeks) with a fraction obtained by column chromatography of Mori Folium extract on intestinal *alpha*-glucosidase activity was studied in mice, made hyperglycaemic and hyperinsulinaemic by feeding a high carbohydrate diet. While the fraction had no effect on body weight, it prevented the rise in glycaemia and insulinaemia (4). The ethanol-soluble fraction of Mori Folium at a dose of 500 and 1000 mg/kg, and 5 mg/kg dose of acarbose were administered to db/db mice for 6 weeks. Body weight gain and levels of fasting and non-fasting serum glucose, glycated haemoglobin, and triglycerides were reduced dose dependently, when compared between db/db control group and the drug treated group. In animals receiving 500 mg/kg dose of Mori Folium extract, total activities of sucrase and maltase decreased but in animals receiving 1000mg/kg dose of the extract or acarbose, these enzyme activities were increased (5). Mulberry leaves were found to possess anti-hyperglycaemic and antioxidant properties. Increased lipid peroxidation in erythrocytes, observed in diabetic control, was significantly reduced by mulberry leaves. This effect was better than glibenclamide. Decreased activities of antioxidant enzymes and increased activity of catalase, observed in uncontrolled diabetes, were brought back to normal level by mulberry treatment. This effect was also better than glibenclamide (11). The hypoglycaemic effect of the mulberry leaves was evaluated in a clinical trial with type-2 diabetic patients and compared with that of the standard drug, glibenclamide. Patients with mulberry therapy significantly improved their glycaemic control and showed significant improvement in lipid profiles, while glibenclamide treatment showed only marginal improvement in glycaemic control and the changes in the lipid profile were not statistically significant. Both treatments displayed no apparent effect on the concentrations of the glycosylated hemoglobin (Hb A(1)c) in diabetic patients. In summary, mulberry therapy was found to exhibit potential hypoglycaemic and hypolipidaemic effects in diabetic patients (8). Dried leaf powder of mulberry, given with the diet at 25% level to streptozotocin-induced diabetic male Wistar albino rats for 8 weeks, controlled hyperglycaemia, glycosuria, albuminuria and retarded onset of retinopathy (14). *M. alba* leaves (Folium mori), traditionally used for the treatment of diabetic hyperglycaemia, have been shown to induce enhanced nitric oxide synthase (NOS) expression in the hypothalamus of streptozotocin-induced diabetic rats This effect was investigated *via* nicotinamide adenine dinucleotide phosphate-diaphorase (NADPH-d) histochemistry. Administration of the aqueous extract of *M. alba* leaves to rats with streptozotocin-induced diabetes resulted in decreased NADPH-d positivity. These results suggest that Folium mori treatment is effective in curbing the desire for food under diabetic conditions *via* modulation of NOS expression in the hypothalamus (10). The hypoglycaemic activity of the flavonoid-rich fraction of an alcohol (70%) extract of the Egyptian *Morus alba* root bark was evaluated. Administration of this fraction to streptozotocin-induced diabetic rats for 10 days at a dose of 600 mg/kg/day significantly reduced the amount of the blood glucose from control level to a lower level and significantly increased the insulin level from control to a higher level. A lower dose was not significantly effective. An anti-peroxidative activity of this fraction was indicated from the measurement of thiobarbituric acid reactive substances. Oral administration of this fraction to streptozotocin-diabetic rats significantly decreased the lipid peroxides. The phytochemical investigation of the fraction resulted in the isolation of four hydrophobic flavonoids and two triterpenes, betulinic acid and methyl ursolate. The data obtained from this study revealed that the flavonoid-rich fraction of the alcoholic extract of the root bark of *M. alba* may protect pancreatic *beta* cells from degeneration and diminish lipid peroxidation (15). A galactolipid [2(R) -1-O-octadecanoyl -2-O-(9Z, 12Z, 15Z-octatrienoyl)-3-O-β-D-galactpyranosyl glycerol], isolated from the methanol (80%) extract of *M. alba* leaves showed approximately 16 percent hypoglycaemic activity in streptozotocin-induced diabetic rats (7). Treatment of alloxan diabetic rats on high-calorie chow with Ramulus mori (the extract of mulberry twigs) was found to improve hypoglycaemic symptoms, the blood lipid levels and the ratio of kidney over body weight. It also reduced blood N-acetyl-β-D-glucosaminidase activity and the degree of renal pathological changes (12). The effects of an aqueous extract of Ramulus mori were studied in normal and alloxan diabetic rats and mice, and the results were compared with those for acarbose, an *alpha*-glucosidase inhibitor. After 2 weeks of administration of an aqueous extract of R. mori with high-calorie chow or a normal diet, the fasting and non-fasting blood glucose concentrations in alloxan diabetic mice and rats were decreased. In alloxan rats, the blood fructosamine concentration was lowered. Results for acarbose and R. mori extract were similar. The observations indicate that R. mori has *alpha*-glucosidase inhibitory effects (13). The hot water extract of mulberry leaves was shown to have inhibitory effect against *alpha*-glucosidases, sucrase and maltase enzymes. It has the potential to be consumed as anti-diabetic herbal tea (16). Anti-diabetic effect of protoplast preparation from fresh leaves of *M. alba* was investigated in experimental models. The protoplast preparation, at doses of 200 and 500 mg/kg, inhibited the increase of blood glucose in streptozotocin-induced diabetic rats. The preparation suppressed adrenaline or nor-adrenaline-induced lipolysis in fat cells from rat epididymal adipose tissues. The efficacy of protoplast preparation from fresh leaves was superior to 50 percent ethanol extract of dry leaves (9).

1. Hikino H, T Mizuno, Y Oshima, C Konno; Isolation and hypoglycaemic activity of moran A, a glycoprotein of *Morus alba* root barks, *Planta Med* **2,** 159-60 (1985).

2. Lee JS, MH Choi, SH Chung; Blood glucose lowering effect of Mori folium, *Yakhak Hoeji* **39**(4), 367-72 (1995)

3. Chen F, N Nakashima, I Kimura, M Kimura; Hypoglycaemic activity and mechanism of action of extract from Mulberry leaves (Folium mori) and cortex mori radicis in streptozotocin induced diabetic mice , *Yakugaku Zasshi* **115**(6), 476-82 (1995)

4. Chung SH, MS Kim, RW Choue; Effect of Mori Folium column fraction on intestinal *alpha*-glucosidase activity in mice administered with a high carbohydrate-containing diet, *Yakhak Hoeji* **41**(4), 484-91 (1997)

5. Ryu JW, SH Seo, SH Chung; Anti-diabetic activity of Mori Folium ethanol-soluble fraction in db/db mice, *Yakhak Hoeji* **42**(6), 613-20 (1998)

6. Kim ES, SJ Park, EJ Lee, BK Kim, H Huh, BJ Lee; Purification and characterization of Moran 20K from *Morus alba, Arch Pharm Res* **22**(1), 9-12 (1999).

7. Kim CY, SH Kang, GW Jeong, CS Cheong, BK Kim, H Huh; Galactolipids from Mori Folium and their hypoglycaemic effect, *Korean J Pharmacogn* **31**(1), 95-100 (2000)

8. Andallu B, V Suryakantham, B Lakshmi Srikanthi, GK Reddy; Effect of mulberry (*Morus indica* L.) therapy on plasma and erythrocyte membrane lipids in patients with type-2 diabetes, *Clin Chim Acta* **314**(1-2), 47-53 (2001)

9. Kubo M, Y Ido, H Matsuda, H Mikami; Anti-diabetic effect of protoplast preparation from fresh leaves of mulberry (*Morus alba*), *Natural medicine* **55**(4), 181-86, (2001)

10. Jang MH, H Kim, MC Shin, BV Lim, TH Lee, SB Jung, CJ Kim, EH Kim; Administration of Folium mori extract decreases nitric oxide synthase expression in the hypothalamus of streptozotocin-induced diabetic rats, *Jpn J Pharmacol* **90**(2), 189-92 (2002)

11. Andallu B, NC Varadachaaryulu; Anti-hyperglycaemic and antioxidant role of mulberry (*M. indica* L.) leaves, *Indian J Pharmacol* **34**(2), 145 (2002)

12. Ye F, ZF Shen, FX Qiao, DY Zhao, MZ Xie; Experimental treatment of complications in alloxan diabetic rats with *alpha*-glucosidase inhibitor from the Chinese medicinal herb ramulus mori, *Acta Pharmaceutica Sinica* **37**(2), 108-12 (2002)

13. Ye F, ZF Shen, MZ Xie; *Alpha*-glucosidase inhibition from a Chinese medical herb (Ramulus mori) in normal and diabetic rats and mice, *Phytomedicine* **9**(2), 161-66 (2002)

14. Andallu B, NC Varadachaaryulu; Control of hyperglycemia and retardation of cataract by mulberry (*Morus indica* L.) leaves in streptozotocin diabetic rats, *Indian J Exp Biol* **40**(7), 791-95 (2002)

15. Singab AN, HA El-beshbishy, M Yonekawa, T Nomura, T Fukai; Hypoglycaemic effect of Egyptian *Morus alba* root bark extract: effect on diabetes and

lipid peroxidation of streptozotocin-induced diabetic rats, *J Ethnopharmacol* **100**(3), 333-38 (2005)

16. Hansawasdi C, J Kawabata; *Alpha*-glucosidase inhibitory effect of mulberry (*Morus alba*) leaves on Caco-2, *Fitoterapia* **77**(7-8), 568-73 (2006)

Morus bombysis Koidz. (Moraceae)

Morus bombysis is a variety of mulberry indigenous to East Asia, particularly Japan. The hypoglycaemic activity of *M. bombysis* was significantly affected with anaerobic incubation for 6 hours. The body weight of mice, treated with anaerobic conditioned *M. bombysis* leaves was higher than that of the control group. The treated leaves significantly decreased blood glucose level of alloxan-induced type-1 diabetic mice. Glucose tolerance was also significantly improved by this treatment. The disappearance of insulin secreting *beta* cells in the islets of Langerhans from alloxan-treated diabetic mice was strongly inhibited by treatment with anaerobic conditioned *M. bombysis* leaves.

Kim SY, KS Ryu, WC Lee, HO Ku, HS Lee, KR Lee; Hypoglycaemic effect of mulberry leaves with anaerobic treatment in alloxan-induced diabetic mice, *Korean J Pharmacogn* **30**(2), 123-29 (1999)

Morus indica Linn. (Moraceae) Syn. *Morus alba* (Mulberry)

See ***Morus alba***

Morus insignis Bureau (Moraceae)

Morus insignis is native to South America. Ethyl acetate and n-butanol-soluble fractions of the leaves of *M. insignis* showed significant hypoglycaemic activity in streptozotocin-induced hyperglycaemic rats. Two new compounds (mulberrofuran U and moracin M-3-O-β-D-glucopyranoside) and six known phytochemicals (β-sitosterol, b -sitosterol-3-O-β -glucopyranoside, ursolic acid, moracin M, kaempferol-3-O- β -glucopyranoside and quercetin-3-O-β -glucopyranoside) were isolated from the active fractions.

Basnet P, S Kadota, S Terashima, M Shimizu, T Namba; Two new 2-arylbenzofuran derivatives from hypoglycaemic activity-bearing fractions of *Morus insignis*, *Chem Pharm Bull* (Tokyo) **41**(7), 1238-43 (1993).

Mucuna pruriens (L) DC (Fabaceae) (Velvet bean, H. Kewanch, S. Kapikachu)

The plant is an annual, climbing shrub, which is almost completely covered with fuzzy hairs, when young. Its seed pods are covered in loose orange hairs that cause a severe itch if they come in contact with skin. The seeds are shiny black or brown and rich in L-Dopa, a direct precursor of the neurotransmitter dopamine. It is found in tropical Africa, India and the Caribbean islands.

In normal rabbits, powdered seeds of *M. pruriens* (0.5, 1 and 2 g/kg) significantly decreased the blood glucose levels but in alloxan-induced diabetic rabbits a significant fall was discernible only at a dose of 1 and 2 g/kg body weight. High levels of trace elements like manganese, zinc, and others were found in these seeds. It was, therefore, conjectured that active constituents might be both organic and mineral, which seem to act indirectly by stimulating the release of insulin and/or by a direct insulin-like action (1). Anti-diabetic oligocyclitols, D-*chiro*-inositol and its two galacto-derivatives were isolated from the seeds of *Mucuna pruriens*, The quantities of these compounds detected in the seeds explain its well-established anti-glycaemic effect (2).

1. Akhtar MS, AQ Qureshi, J Iqbal; Anti-diabetic evaluation of *Mucuna pruriens*, Linn seeds, *J Pak Med Assoc* **40**(7), 147-50 (1990).
2. Donati D, LR Lampariello, R Pagani, R Guerranti, G Cinci, E Marinello; Anti-diabetic oligocyclitols in seeds of *Mucuna pruriens*, *Phytother Res* **19**(12), 1057-60 (2005)

Murraya koenigii Spreng (Rutaceae)
(Curry tree, H, Meethee neem, Curry patta)

Curry patta, a commonly used spice, is traditionally consumed by diabetics in southern part of India. Effect of *M. koenigii* on carbohydrate metabolism was studied using rats as experimental animals. The crushed leaves of *M. kkoenigii* were tested for their potential hypoglycaemic activity on rabbits, rats and also on healthy human volunteers. Fasting normal rabbits exhibited hypoglycaemic activity (33%) during the very first hour at a dose level of 10 g/kg. In alloxan diabetic rats, a 17 percent fall in blood sugar level was observed at the 5th hour at the same dose level but the effect was not significant. The same response was observed in glucose tolerance test. Human volunteers showed a peak fall in blood sugar level (24%) three hours after medication at a dose level of 50 g (1).

Feeding of diets containing various doses of curry leaves (5, 10 and 15%) to normal rats for 7 days caused a negligible reduction in blood glucose. However, a fall of 21.4% blood glucose level was observed in alloxan-induced mild diabetic rats receiving diets containing 15% *M koenigii* leaves for 5 weeks. A similar but less significant fall in blood glucose level was observed in streptozotocin-induced moderately diabetic rats. The mechanism of action has been discussed (3).

The plant drug showed significant hypoglycaemic action; it increased the concentration of hepatic glycogen and glycogenesis and decreased glycogenolysis and gluconeogenesis, as evident from the decreased activity of glycogen phosphorylase and gluconeogenic enzymes (2). These effects were found to be comparable to those of *Brassica juncea* (mustard seeds) but unlike the latter, feeding of a diet containing 15% *M. koenigii* leaf powder to fructose-mediated non-genetic model of insulin resistant rats failed to play a role in the management of pre-diabetic state of insulin resistance (6).

Significant reduction in blood glucose levels was observed in alloxan-induced diabetic rats, treated with aqueous (600 mg/kg b.w.) and methanol extracts (200 mg/kg b.w.) of *M. koenigii* leaves for a period of eight weeks. Plasma insulin levels were found to be significantly high on 43rd and 58th days of treatment with these extracts. It has been surmised that the hypoglycaemic effect of *M. koenigii* is mediated through stimulation of insulin synthesis and/or secretion of insulin from the *beta* cells of pancreatic islets of Langerhans (5). Oral administration of different doses of semi-purified aqueous extract of *M. koenigii* led to lowering of blood glucose level in normal rabbits and improvement in glucose tolerance test in sub-diabetic rabbits (4). The hypoglycaemic activity of an aqueous extract of *M. koenigii* leaves was evaluated in normal and alloxan induced diabetic rabbits and also compared with that of a standard hypoglycaemic drug, tolbutamide. A single oral administration of variable dose levels (200, 300 and 400 mg/kg) of aqueous extract led to lowering of blood glucose level in normal as well as in diabetic rabbits. The maximum fall in normal and mild diabetic rabbits were observed after 4 h of oral administration of 300 mg/kg. The same dose also showed a marked improvement in glucose tolerance of sub-diabetic and mild diabetic rabbits after 2 hour (7). Oral administration of an ethanol extract of *M. koenigii* to streptozotocin-induced diabetic rats at a dose of 200 mg/kg/ b.w./day for a period of 30 days significantly decreased their levels of blood glucose, glycosylated haemoglobin, urea, uric acid and creatinine. The plasma insulin levels of treated animals revealed the insulin stimulatory effect of the extract. The *M. koenigii* extract appeared to be more effective than glibenclamide, a known anti-diabetic drug (8).

1. Santhakumari G, RG Pillai, NR Pillai, RB Nair; Hypoglycaemic potential of *Murraya koenigii* Spreng (Karaypak), *Natl Med Ethno-Bot Res* **6**(2-4), 189-95 (1985)
2. Khan BA, A Abraham, S Leelamma; Hypoglycaemic action of *Murraya koenigii* (curry leaf) and *Brassica juncea* (mustard): mechanism of action, *Indian J Biochem Biophys* **32**(8), 106-08 (1995)
3. Yadav S, V Vats, Y Dhunnoo, JK Grover; Hypoglycaemic and anti-hyperglycaemic activity of *Murraya koenigii* leaves in diabetic rats, *J Ethnopharmacol* **82**(2-3), 111-16 (2002)
4. Watal G, AN Kesari, RK Gupta, SK Singh; Anti-diabetic and hypoglycaemic effect of *Murraya koenigii* leaves on experimental animals, *National Seminar on New Millenium Strategies for Quality, Safety & GMP of Herbal Drugs/Products,* NBRI, Lucknow, India, p.85, November 11-13, 2003
5. Vinuthan MK, Girish Kumar, JP Ravindra, Jayaprakash, K Narayana; Effect of extracts of *Murraya koenigii* leaves on the levels of blood glucose and plasma insulin in alloxan-induced diabetic rats, *Indian J Physiol Pharmacol* **48**(3), 348-52 (2004)

6. Yadav SP, V Vats, AC Ammini, JK Grover; *Brassica juncea* (Rai) significantly prevented the development of insulin resistance in rats fed fructose-enriched diet, *J Ethnopharmacol* **93**(1), 113-16 (2004)
7. Kesari AN, RK Gupta, G Watal; Hypoglycaemic effects of *Murraya koenigii* on normal and alloxan-diabetic rabbits, *J Ethnopharmacol* **97**(2), 247-51 (2005)
8. Arulselvan P, GP Senthilkumar, D Sathish Kumar, S Subramanian; Anti-diabetic effect of *Murraya koenigii* leaves on streptozotocin induced diabetic rats, *Pharmazie* **61**(10), 874-77 (2006)

Musa paradisiaca Blanco (Musaceae)
(Plantains, Cooking bananas, H. Kacha kela)

There is lot of confusion between two *Musa* species; *Musa paradisiaca* and *Musa sapientum* and often one has been treated as the sub-species of the other. But generally *Musa paradisiaca* is known by 'plantains' or cooking bananas. The hypoglycaemic effect of methanol extract of mature, green fruits of *M. paradisiaca* was evaluated in normoglycaemic and streptozotocin-treated hyperglycaemic mice, using chlorpropamide as the reference anti-diabetic agent. Oral administration of the extract (100-800 mg/kg) induced significant, dose-related reductions in the blood glucose concentrations of both normal and diabetic mice. The results of the study indicate that *M. paradisiaca* fruit extract possesses hypoglycaemic activity. Although the exact mechanism of the hypoglycaemic action of the plant drug is not clear, it could be due, at least in part, to stimulation of insulin production and subsequent glucose utilization.

Ojewole JA, CO Adewunmi; Hypoglycaemic effect of methanolic extract of *Musa paradisiaca* (Musaceae) green fruits in normal and diabetic mice, *Methods Find Exp Clin Pharmacol* **25**(6), 453-56 (2003)

Musa sapientum Linn (Musaceae)
(Dessert banana, H. Kela)

The pectin, isolated from the juice of the inflorescence stalk of *Musa sapientum*, at a dose of 20 mg/100 g body weight showed significant hypoglycaemic effect both in normoglycaemic and alloxan-induced diabetic rats (1). Free sugar content of banana depends upon the degree of ripening. In under-ripe banana, starch constitutes 80-90% of its total carbohydrate and as it ripens free sugar content increases. The effect of ripening of banana on the postprandial blood glucose and insulin responses was studied on ten type 2 diabetic subjects and compared with white bread. The mean postprandial blood glucose response area to white bread was significantly higher compared with under-ripe and over-ripe bananas. The mean insulin response areas to the three meals were similar. The low glycaemic response of under-ripe compared with over-ripe bananas may be ascribed to the high starch content, which has been found to be hydrolysed only slowly by a-amylase in humans (2).

Hypoglycaemic activity of dried and powdered unripe fruits of *Musa sapientum* was studied in normal and alloxanised rabbits. Administration of a single dose (1.5 g/kg, per os) of the fruit powder caused a significant decrease of blood glucose level in normal rats after 4 hour. However, no anti-hyperglycaemic effect was observed in alloxan-induced diabetic rabbits (3).

Oral administration of 0.25 g/kg of chloroform extract of *M. sapientum* flowers for 30 days to rats resulted in a highly significant reduction in blood glucose, glycosylated haemoglobin and an increase in total haemoglobin. A significant improvement in glucose tolerance was observed in animals treated with banana flower extract and the effect was compared with glibenclamide (4). The extract prevented a decrease in body weight, and also resulted in a decrease in free radical formation in the tissues. The decrease in thiobarbituric acid reactive substances and the increase in reduced glutathione, glutathione peroxidase, superoxide dismutase and catalase clearly indicated the antioxidant property of the banana flower extract (5). Oral administration of the ethanol extract of *M. sapientum* showed significant blood glucose lowering effect at 200 mg/kg in alloxan induced diabetic rats. The extract was also found to significantly scavenge oxygen free radicals. *M. sapientum*-induced blood sugar reduction may possibly be due to inhibition of free radicals and subsequent inhibition of tissue damage induced by alloxan (6).

1. Gomathy R, NR Vijayalaksmi, PA Kurup; Hypoglycaemic action of the pectin present in the juice of the inflorescence stalk of plantain (*Musa sapientum*) – Mechanism of action, *J Biosci* **15**(4), 297-303 (1990)

2. Hermansen K, O Rasmussen, S Gregersen, S Larsen; Influence of ripeness of banana on the blood glucose and insulin response in type 2 diabetic subjects, *Diabet Med* **9**(8), 739-43 (1992)

3. Rao VV, SK Dwivedi, D Swarup; Hypoglycaemic effect of *Musa sapientum*, *Fitoterapia* **65**(1), 65-67 (1994)

4. Pari L, JU Maheswari; Hypoglycaemic effect of *Musa sapientum* L. in alloxan-induced diabetic rats, *J Ethnopharmacol* **68**(1-3), 321-25 (1999)

5. Pari L, J Umamaheswari; Anti-hyperglycaemic activity of *Musa sapientum* flowers: effect on lipid peroxidation in alloxan diabetic rats, *Phytother Res* **14**(2), 136-38 (2000)

6. Dhanabal SP, M Sureshkumar, M Ramanathan, B Suresh; Hypoglycaemic effect of ethanolic extract of *Musa sapientum* on alloxan induced diabetes mellitus in rats and its relation with antioxidant potential, *J Herb Pharmacother* **5**(2), 7-19 (2005)

Musanga cecropioides R.Br. (Urticaceae/ Cecropiaceae) (The African Corkwood Tree)

Musanga cecropioides, a soft-wooded tree with an umbrella-like crown, is found mostly in the tropical forests of Africa. The bark of the tree has many medicinal properties.

The effects of administration of an aqueous extract of the leaves of *M. cecropioides* were studied in normoglycaemic and streptozotocin-induced diabetic rats. The plant extract (30 mg/ml) produced a significant fall in blood sugar level in normoglycaemic rats by the 8th day of treatment but a relatively insignificant fall was observed at a higher concentration of the extract (60 mg/ml). In streptozotocin-induced diabetic rats, a very significant fall of blood sugar level was observed between the 8th and 12th day of treatment with the extract concentration of 60mg/ ml.

Kamanyi A, P Watcho, S Wansi, T Nguelefack, TF Nguegium; Further studies on *Musanga cecropioides* (Cecropiaceae): A possible source active anti-hyperglycaemic principles, *Phytomedicine* **7**(Suppl.II), 67 (2000)

Myrcia multiflora (Lam) DC. (Myrtaceae)

Myrcia multiflora is a medium-sized shrub that grows in drier regions of the Amazon and other parts of Brazil. The plant is a very popular natural remedy for diabetes in South America. Traditionally, its leaf tea with a pleasant, slightly sweet taste is used.

The methanol extract of the leaves of *M. multiflora* and its ethyl acetate-soluble fraction were found to show inhibitory activities on aldose reductase and *alpha*-glucosidase and on the increase of serum glucose level in sucrose-loaded rats and in alloxan-induced diabetic mice. From the ethyl acetate-soluble portion, a number of new and known flavonoid glucosides and two new acetophenone glucosides, myrciaphenones A and B were isolated and fully characterized. Of the isolated phytochemicals, myrciacitrin I (a flavanone glucoside) and myrciaphenone B (an acetophenone glucoside) were found to show potent inhibitory activities on aldose reductase and *alpha*-glucosidase (1). Subsequent work on the plant led to the isolation three more flavanone glucosides myrciacitrins III, IV, and V and their complete characterization. Myrciacitrins were found to show potent inhibitory activity on aldose reductase (2).

1. Yoshikawa M, H Shimada, N Nishida, Y Li, I Toguchida, J Yamahara, H Matsuda; Anti-diabetic principles of natural medicines. II. Aldose reductase and *alpha*-glucosidase inhibitors from Brazilian natural medicine, the leaves of *Myrcia multiflora* DC. (Myrtaceae): structures of myrciacitrins I and II and myrciaphenones A and B, *Chem Pharm Bull* (Tokyo) **46**(1), 113-19 (1998)

2. Matsuda H, N Nishida, M Yoshikawa; Anti-diabetic principles of natural medicines. V. Aldose reductase inhibitors from *Myrcia multiflora* DC. (2): Structures of myrciacitrins III, IV, and V, *Chem Pharm Bull* (Tokyo) **50**(3), 429-31 (2002)

Myrcia uniflora Barb. Rodr. (Myrtaceae)

Myricia uniflora is a plant that is widely used in northern Brazil for treatment of diabetes. *M. uniflora* was compared with placebo for its hypoglycaemic effect in randomized cross over double-blind studies in 2 groups of normal subjects and 2 groups of type-2 diabetic patients. The protocol with the plant lasted for 56 days. Ingestion of an infusion of 3 g *M. uniflora* leaves/day caused no acute or chronic effects on plasma glucose levels or glycated hemoglobin in either group. However, plasma insulin levels in the diabetic group were found to be lower (1).

Percolation of dried leaves of *M. uniflora* with boiled water and subsequent lyophilisation of the aqueous extract furnished a powder (7.5 mg of lyophilized powder, corresponding to about 60 mg of dried leaves). Treatment of streptozotocin-induced diabetic rats with 7.5 mg of this lyophilized powder for 3 weeks did not affect body weight gain but reduced hyperglycaemia. The effect of the extracts of *M. uniflora* on the intestinal absorption of glucose was also investigated. The intestinal absorption of glucose, measured with a perfusion technique *in situ*, was markedly inhibited by *Myrcia* extract (7.5 mg of lyophilized powder per ml of perfusion solution). The results of the detailed investigation revealed that aqueous extract of *Myrcia* possesses a beneficial effect on the diabetic state, mainly by improving metabolic parameters of glucose homeostasis (2).

1. Russo EM, AA Reichelt, JR De-Sa, RP Furlanetto, RC Moises, TS Kasamatsu, AR Chacra; Clinical trial of *Myrcia uniflora* and *Bauhinia forficata* leaf extracts in normal and diabetic patients, *Braz J Med Biol Res* **23**(1), 11-20 (1990)
2. Pepato MT, JR Oliveira, IC Kettelhut, RH Migliorini;, Assessment of the anti-diabetic activity of *Myrcia uniflora* extracts in streptozotocin diabetic rats, *Diabetes Res* **22**(2), 49-57 (1993)

Myrtus communis Linn. (Myrtaceae)
(Common Myrtle)

Intra-gastric administration of an aqueous ethanol extract of the leaves and branches of *M. communis* (2g/kg) to streptozotocin-induced diabetic rats exhibited significant anti-hyperglycaemic activity. Administration of *Myrtus* extract 48 h after streptozotocin significantly reduced the hyperglycaemia and this effect was maintained by its repeated administration. *Myrtus* extract had no effect on the blood glucose level of normal mice (1).

The volatile oil obtained from the leaves of *Myrtus communis* is used to lower the blood glucose level in type-2 diabetic patients in Turkish folk medicine. The oral hypoglycaemic activity of single and multiple doses of *Myrtus* oil were studied in normal and alloxan-induced diabetic rabbits. The oil did not show any effect in normoglycaemic rabbits either in single or multiple dose administrations, but a good hypoglycaemic activity was observed 4 h after the administration to diabetic animals at 50 mg/kg. Repeated administration of *Myrtus* oil in both normal and diabetic rabbits once a day for one week significantly lowered blood glucose in alloxan-diabetic rabbits on the fourth hour and the following days at a dose of 50 mg/kg. However, the volatile oil did not affect serum insulin concentrations in normal and alloxan-diabetic rabbits but reduced the serum triglyceride concentrations. The reduction in blood glucose level is considered to be due to the reversible inhibition of *alpha*-glucosidases present in the brush-border of the small intestinal mucosa (2). The *alpha*-glucosidase inhibitory activity of *Myrtus communis* was also verified by Onal and coworkers (3).

1. Elfellah MS, MH Akhtar, MT Khan; Anti-hyperglycaemic effect of an extract of *Myrtus communis* in streptozotocin-induced diabetes in mice, *J Ethnopharmacol* **11**(3), 275-81 (1984).
2. Sepici A, I Gurbuz, C Cevik, E Yesilada; Hypoglycaemic effects of myrtle oil in normal and alloxan-diabetic rabbits, *J Ethnopharmacol* **93**(2-3), 311-18 (2004)
3. Onal S, S Timur, B Okutucu, F Zihnioglu; Inhibition of *alpha*-glucosidase by aqueous extracts of some potent anti-diabetic medicinal herbs, *Prep Biochem Biotechnol* **35**(1), 29-36 (2005)

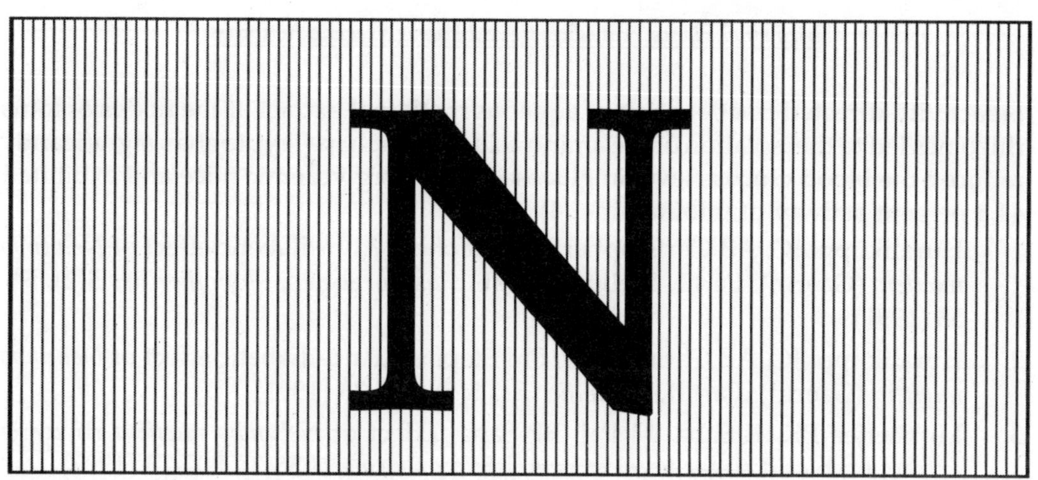

Nelumbo nucifera Gaertn. (Nelumbonaceae)
(Indian lotus, Sacred water lily, H. & S. Kamal)

This plant is an aquatic perennial, widely naturalized in southern Asia and Australia. It is the National flower of India and Vietnam. Sun-dried flowers of *N. nucifera* (test drug) as well as its aqueous and alcoholic extracts were found to produce significant hypoglycaemia in fasting normal albino rabbits. No significant difference in activities was observed between the test drug (1000 mg/kg) and equivalent amounts of extracts; the effect was half of that produced by tolbutamide (250 mg/kg). Oral administration of the extracts equivalent to 1000 mg/kg of the test drug produced significant depression in fasting blood sugar level after glucose load, the effect being comparable to that of tolbutamide. In normal rabbits, the extracts, in doses mentioned above, significantly reduced hyperglycaemia, induced by injection of adrenaline hydrochloride (5 mg/kg, s.c.). Chronic administration of the plant extracts to normal rats did not produce a sustained fall in fasting blood sugar levels though concurrent glucose tolerance tests showed beneficial effects. *In vitro* studies with rat hemi-diaphragms revealed that the test drug treatment of donor animals significantly enhanced the effect of insulin. The improvement of glucose tolerance might, therefore, be due to increased peripheral glucose utilisation caused by increased sensitivity of skeletal muscles to endogenous insulin. The test drugs were, however, proved to be ineffective in severely diabetic rabbits even after four-fold increase of the dose (1, 2).

Oral administration of the ethanol extract of *N. nucifera* rhizomes markedly reduced the blood sugar level of normal, glucose-fed hyperglycaemic and streptozotocin-induced diabetic rats, when compared with control animals. The extract improved glucose tolerance and potentiated the action of exogenously injected insulin in normal rats. The activity of the extract was compared with that of tolbutamide (3).

Bioactivity-directed fractionation of aqueous methanol extract of the nodes of lotus rhizomes led to the isolation of the amino acid, tryptophan. Tryptophan significantly reduced the blood glucose level in glucose-fed hyperglycaemic mice and exhibited 44.3 percent activity of tolbutamide (4)

1. Huralikuppi JC, AB Christopher, PM Stephen; Anti-diabetic effect of *Nelumbo nucifera* (Gaertn). Part I. Preliminary studies in rabbits, *Phytother Res* **5**(2), 54-58 (1991)
2. Huralikuppi JC, AB Christopher, PM Stephen; Anti-diabetic effect of *Nelumbo nucifera* (Gaertn). Part II, *Phytother Res* **5**(5), 217-23 (1991)
3. Mukherjee PK, K Saha, M Pal, BP Saha; Effect of *Nelumbo nucifera* rhizome extract on blood sugar level in rats, *J Ethnopharmacol* **58**(3), 207-13 (1997)
4. Lee MW, JS Kim, SM Cho, JH Kim, JS Lee; Anti-diabetic constituent from the node of lotus rhizome (*Nelumbo nucifera*(Gaertn), *Nat Prod Sci* **7**(2), 107-09 (2001)

Neurolaena lobata (L.) Cass. (Asteraceae / Compositae) (Jackass Bitters)

Neurolaena lobata is a member of the Asteraceae family and a common Central American plant. It has yellow flowers and bitter-tasting leaves. Ethanol extract of the leaves of the plant was found to exhibit hypoglycaemic activity both in normal and alloxan-induced diabetic mice.

Gupta MP, NG Solis, ME Avella, C Sanchez; Hypoglycaemic activity of *Neurolaena lobata* (L.) R. BR, *J Ethnopharmacol* **10**(3), 323-27 (1984)

Nicotiana glutinosa (Tobacco) Linn. (Solanaceae)

Sucrose fatty acid esters are non-ionic surfactants consisting of sucrose as hydrophilic group and fatty acid as lipophilic group. Some sucrose fatty acid esters have been reported to be aldose reductase inhibitors. A sucrose fatty acid ester, isolated from the leaves of *Nicotiana glutinosa*, was found to be a potent aldose reductase inhibitor suitable for use in the treatment of diabetes. The isolated sugar ester may be administered to patients at the dose level of 1-100 mg/kg/day either orally, subcutaneously or intra- peritoneally.

Toshiaki M, K Akira, O Hitoshi; Inhibitors of aldose reductase extracted from plants for treatment of diseases associated with diabetes, JAP. KOKAI TOKKYO KOHO, JP01,26,589 (C1 C07 H13/04)1989, 6PP.

Nigella sativa Linn (Ranunculaceae) (Black cumin, H. Kalonji)

Nigella sativa is an annual flowering plant, native to southwest Asia. The seeds of *N. sativa* are used as spice. It is one of the plants commonly used in Moroccan folk medicine for treatment of various ailments including diabetes mellitus. The intra-peritoneal administration of the volatile oil of *N. sativa* seeds (50 mg/kg) to fasting normal and alloxan-induced diabetic rabbits produced significant and time-dependent hypoglycaemic effects. In normal animals, 15 and 23 percent decreases in fasting plasma glucose levels were observed after 4 and 6 hours, respectively. This effect was relatively less marked in diabetic rabbits. The administration of the volatile oil did not alter the basal insulin levels in all animal groups (1). The effect of *N. sativa* oil on blood glucose concentrations was studied in streptozotocin diabetic rats. In addition, the effect of this oil was also studied on insulin secretion of isolated rat pancreatic islets in the presence of different concentrations of glucose. The oil lowered blood glucose concentrations in diabetic rats after 2, 4 and 6 weeks. The blood sugar lowering effect of *nigella* oil was, however, not proportional to the extent of stimulation of insulin release in the presence of oil or its constituents, thymoquinone and its carbonyl polymer, nigellone. This indicated that the hypoglycaemic effect of *N. sativa* oil might be mediated by extra-pancreatic actions rather than by stimulated insulin release (3). The possible insulinotropic properties of *N. sativa* oil in streptozotocin plus nicotinamide-induced diabetes mellitus were studied in hamsters. Oral treatment with *N. sativa* oil began 4 weeks after induction of diabetes. Significant decrease in blood glucose level together with significant increase in serum insulin level was observed after treatment with *N. sativa* oil for 4 weeks. The hypoglycaemic effect of *N. sativa* oil in streptozotocin plus nicotinamide diabetic hamsters resulted, at least partly, from a stimulatory effect on *beta*-cell function with consequent increase in serum insulin level. The results indicated insulinotropic properties of *N. sativa* oil in type-2 like model (4). The possible protective effects of *N. sativa* against *beta*-cell damage from streptozotocin-induced diabetes in rats were evaluated. It was inferred from the results of the investigation that *N. sativa* exerts a therapeutic protective effect in diabetes by decreasing oxidative stress and preserving pancreatic *beta*-cell integrity. *N. sativa* may, therefore, be clinically useful for protecting *beta*-cells against oxidative stress (5).

The acute and chronic toxicity of *N. sativa* fixed oil were investigated. LD_{50} value, obtained by oral administration of a single dose of oil was 28.8 ml/kg body weight. The same value was 2.06 ml/kg body weight, when administered intra-peritoneally. In chronic toxicity test, rats were treated with an oral dose of the oil (2 ml/kg b.w.) daily for 12 weeks. Changes in key hepatic enzyme levels and histopathological modifications (heart, liver, kidneys and pancreas) were not observed in rats treated with *N. sativa* fixed oils for 12 weeks. The serum total cholesterol, triglyceride and glucose levels and the count of leukocytes and platelets decreased significantly compared to the control values, while haematocrit and haemoglobin levels increased significantly. The low toxicity of *N. sativa* oil, stability of key hepatic enzymes and integrity of organs suggest a wide margin of safety for therapeutic doses of *N. sativa* fixed oil (2).

The mechanisms underlying the hypoglycaemic effect of *N. sativa* oil in streptozotocin-induced diabetic hamsters, in terms of hepatic glucose production were studied. The possible immunopotentiating effect of the oil on peritoneal macrophages was also investigated. The results of detailed investigation indicated that the hypoglycaemic effect of *N. sativa* oil was due to a decrease in hepatic gluconeogenesis, and that the immunopotentiating effect of the oil was mediated through stimulation of macrophage phagocytic activity either directly or *via* activation of lymphocytes (6)

The effects of 4-week intra-gastric gavage with a petroleum ether extract of *Nigella sativa* seeds on blood glucose, insulin and lipids were studied in normal rats. Fasting plasma glucose remained stable throughout treatment. At the end of the treatment, *N. sativa*-treated rats had lower fasting plasma levels of insulin and triglycerides, and higher HDL-cholesterol as compared to pair-fed controls. Response to insulin was evaluated in hepatocytes isolated from animals by Western blot analysis. The results of the investigation demonstrated that *in vivo* treatment with the petroleum ether extract exerts an insulin-sensitizing action (7).

Rchid and coworkers (8) studied the effects of different fractions of *N. sativa* seed extract on insulin secretion. The insulin secretory effects of the extracts were evaluated individually at different concentrations *in vitro* in isolated rat pancreatic islets in the presence of 8.3 mmol/L glucose. Addition of both the defatted whole extract of the seed as well as its basic sub-fraction in the incubation medium significantly increased glucose-induced insulin release from the islets. The stimulatory effect of the acidic and neutral sub-fraction was observed only for the higher concentration. However, only the basic sub-fraction showed a clear concentration-dependent increase in insulin release from isolated pancreatic islets. The anti-diabetic properties of *N. sativa* seeds may be, at least partly, mediated by stimulating insulin release, and that the basic sub-fraction largely contributes to this stimulatory effect.

Oral administration of an ethanol extract of *N. sativa* seeds (300 mg/kg b.w./d) to streptozotocin-induced diabetic rats for 30 days significantly reduced the elevated levels of blood glucose, lipids, plasma insulin and improved altered levels of lipid peroxidation products and antioxidant enzymes like catalase, superoxide dismutase, reduced glutathione and glutathione peroxidase in liver and kidney. The findings confirmed the anti-diabetic activity of *N. sativa* seed extract and suggested its administration to be useful in controlling the diabetic complications because of its antioxidant effects (9).

1. Al-Hader A, M Aqel, Z Hasan; Hypoglycaemic effects of the volatile oil of *Nigella sativa, Int J Pharmacogn* **31**(2), 96-100 (1993)
2. Zaoui A, Y Cherrah, N Mahassini, K Alaoui, H Amarouch, M Hassar; Acute and chronic toxicity of *Nigella sativa* fixed oil, *Phytomedicine* **9**(1), 69-74 (2002)

3. El-Dakhakhny M, N Mady, N Lembert, HP Ammon; The hypoglycaemic effect of *Nigella sativa* oil is mediated by extrapancreatic actions, *Planta Med* **68**(5), 465-66 (2002)
4. Fararh KM, Y Atoji, Y Shimizu, T Takewaki; Isulinotropic properties of *Nigella sativa* oil in Streptozotocin plus Nicotinamide diabetic hamster, *Res Vet Sci* **73**(3), 279-82 (2002)
5. Kanter M, O Coskun, A Korkmaz, S Oter; Effects of *Nigella sativa* on oxidative stress and *beta*-cell damage in streptozotocin-induced diabetic rats, *Anat Rec A Discov Mol Cell Evol Biol* **279**(1), 685-91 (2004)
6. Fararh KM, Y Atoji, Y Shimizu, T Shiina, H Nikami, T Takewaki; Mechanisms of the hypoglycaemic and immunopotentiating effects of *Nigella sativa* L. oil in streptozotocin-induced diabetic hamsters, *Res Vet Sci* **77**(2), 123-29 (2004)
7. Le PM, A Benhaddou-Andaloussi, A Elimadi, A Settaf, Y Cherrah, PS Haddad; The petroleum ether extract of *Nigella sativa* exerts lipid-lowering and insulin-sensitizing actions in the rat, *J Ethnopharmacol* **94**(2-3), 251-59 (2004)
8. Rchid H, H Chevassus, R Nmila, C Guiral, P Petit, M Chokairi, Y Sauvaire; *Nigella sativa* seed extracts enhance glucose-induced insulin release from rat-isolated Langerhans islets, *Fundam Clin Pharmacol* **18**(5), 525-29 (2004)
9. Kaleem M, D Kirmani, M Asif, Q Ahmed, B Bano; Biochemical effects of *Nigella sativa* L seeds in diabetic rats, *Indian J Exp Biol* **44**(9), 745-48 (2006)

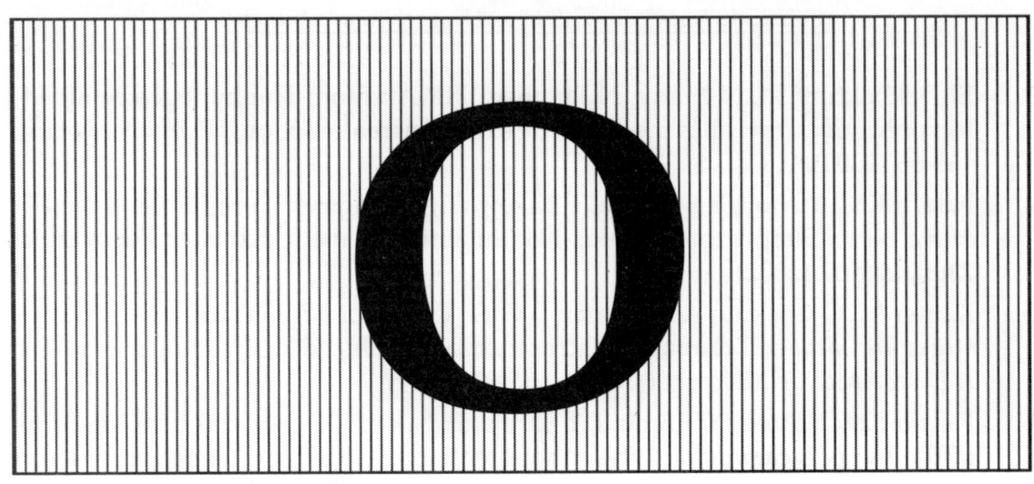

Ocimum canum Sim (Lamiaceae) Syn, *Ocimum americanum* (Hoary basil)

Ocimum canum is one of 35 species of the genus *Ocimum* and is a native of tropical Africa despite being synonymous with *Ocimum americanum*. Hairy seeds of *O. canum* contain a high percentage of dietary fibre and 30 gram of seeds provided some 24 g dietary fibre. Dietary supplementation of this basil seed (30g/day in 3 divided doses for 1 month) to 16 diabetic subjects significantly lowered their fasting plasma glucose levels and consistently improved their glucose tolerance (1, 2).

Aqueous extract of the plant, which is used by some Ghanaians to manage diabetes mellitus, was found to significantly decrease the fasting blood glucose level and body weight of diabetic and non-diabetic C57BL/KsJ mice, In the diabetic mice, fasting blood glucose decreased by 60% compared to 10% in control mice after 13 weeks of extract administration. Body weight, serum total cholesterol and LDL-cholesterol decreased while serum HDL-cholesterol increased in the extract-treated group. The extract significantly enhanced insulin release from isolated rat pancreatic *beta*-islet cells *in vitro*. Insulin release was found to be dependent on glucose concentration and increased with increasing *O. canum* concentration in the incubation medium up to an optimum extract concentration of 0.03 mg/ml. *In vitro* hydroxyl and superoxide radical formation, and lipid peroxidation of isolated human LDL and mouse liver homogenates decreased in extract-treated experimental systems. These results justify the use of *0. canum* in Ghanaian folk medicine to manage diabetes mellitus (3, 4).

1. Tinnarat P, Effect of dietary fibre on blood glucose in diabetics, *J Natl. Res Counc Thail* **15**(2), 67-89 (1983)
2. Viseshakul D, P Premvatana, P Tinnarat; Improved glucose tolerance induced by long term dietary supplementation with hairy basil seed (*Ocimum canum* Sim) in diabetes, *J Med Assoc Thailand* **68**(8), 408 **444** (1983)

3. Nyarko AK, H Asare-Anane, M Ofosuhene, ME Addy; Extract of *Ocimum canum* lowers blood glucose and facilitates insulin release by isolated pancreatic *beta*-islet cells, *Phytomedicine* **9**(4), 346-51 (2002)
4. Nyarko AK, H Asare-Anane, M Ofosuhene, ME Addy, K Teye, P Addo; Aqueous extract of *Ocimum canum* decreases levels of fasting blood glucose and free radicals and increases antiatherogenic lipid levels in mice, *Vascul Pharmacol* **39**(6), 273-79 (2002)

Ocimum gratissimum Linn. (Lamiaceae) (Wild basil)

Intra-peritoneal injection of the methanol extract of *O. gratissimum* (400 mg/kg) significantly reduced plasma levels of glucose both in normal and diabetic rats by 56 and 68%, respectively.

Aguiyi JC, CI Obi, SS Gang, AC Igweh; Hypoglycaemic activity of *Ocimum gratissimum* in rats, *Fitoterapia* **71**(4), 444-46 (2000)

Ocimum sanctum Linn. (Lamiaceae) (Holy basil, H. Tulsi)

O. sanctum is a sacred herb in India but is not much used for culinary purposes like other *Ocimum* species. A tea made from tulsi leaves is used as a remedy for cold in India. Both seeds and leaves of *Ocimum sanctum* are reported to possess hypoglycaemic activity. A comparative study of the hypoglycaemic action of the seeds and fresh leaves of the plant was made (3). Oral administration of an alcoholic extract of leaves of *O. sanctum* led to marked lowering of blood sugar level in normal, glucose fed hyperglycaemic and streptozotocin-induced diabetic rats. The extract was also found to potentiate the action of exogenous insulin in normal rats. The activity of the extract is comparable to that of tolbutamide in normal and diabetic rats (4). Treatment with extracts of holy basil (*Ocimum sanctum*) leaves on fasting and postprandial blood glucose and serum cholesterol levels in humans through randomized, placebo-controlled, crossover single blind trial indicated a significant decrease in fasting and postprandial blood glucose levels during the treatment. Urine glucose levels also showed similar trend. The study suggested that basil leaves might be prescribed as adjunct to dietary therapy and drug treatment in mild to moderate NIDDM (5). Administration of leaf powder of *O. sanctum* as a dietary supplement at 1% level in normal and diabetic rats for a period of one month resulted in a significant reduction of fasting blood sugar, uronic acid, total amino acids, total cholesterol, triglyceride, phospholipids and total lipids. The observations indicated the hypoglycaemic and hypolipidaemic effect of *O. sanctum* leaves in diabetic rats (6). The effect of oral administration of aqueous extract of Tulsi (200 mg/kg b.w.) mixed with diet for eight weeks to diabetic rats was studied.

Significant reductions in fasting blood glucose, serum lipid profile, lipid peroxidation products and improvement in glucose tolerance were observed. The decreased level of thiobarbituric acid reactive substances (TBARS) and increase in antioxidant enzymes clearly showed an antioxidant property of *Ocimum sanctum* (7). Dietary supplementation with fresh leaves of Tulsi (2 g/kg b.w.) for 30 days led to a significant lowering of blood glucose level in test group. Intake of *O. sanctum* leaves also led to a significant increase in the levels of superoxide dismutase, reduced glutathione and total thiols and marked reduction of peroxidised lipid levels in comparison to the untreated control group. The leaves were found to have the ability to scavenge superoxide and hydroxyl free radicals (10)).

The effect of an aqueous extract of *O. sanctum* on ^{14}C-glucose uptake in isolated rat lipocytes was studied. The extract equivalent to 5 mg of dried stems in 2 ml of incubation medium produced 151 percent increase in the uptake of glucose and its conversion to lipids. This insulin-like activity of the extract was found to be dose dependent and it did not require the presence of insulin in the incubation medium (1). Like insulin, an aqueous extract of *O. sanctum* was found to exhibit inhibiting effect on lipolysis and adenylcyclase in rat adipose tissue challenged with nor-adrenaline but no effect was observed under basal condition. This effect was similar to that of insulin (2). .

Ethanol extract of *O. sanctum* leaves was found to exhibit a dose-dependent hypoglycaemic effect and prevent a rise in plasma glucose in normal rats. It also showed significant anti-hyperglycaemic effect in streptozotocin-induced diabetes. The extract also partially corrected the alterations of glucokinase, hexokinase and phosphofructokinase, the three important enzymes of carbohydrate metabolism, in model of diabetes, induced by streptozotocin (8, 9).

1. Crespo S, E Guel, R Menendez, RM Gonzalez; Study of the hypoglycaemic action mechanism of *Ocimum sanctum* L. II. Effect of glucose uptake in isolated rat lipocytes, *Revista Cubana de Farmacia* **22**(1), 86-91 (1988)
2. Gonzalez RM, S Crespo, MD Rodriguez; Study of the hypoglycaemic action mechanism of *Ocimum sanctum* L. III. Effect of lipolysis and adenylcyclase in rat tissue, *Revista Cubana de Farmacia* **22**(1), 92-100 (1988)
3. Sarkar A, MC Pant; A comparative study of the hypoglycaemic action of the seeds and fresh leaves of *Ocimum sanctum* (Tulsi), *Indian J Physiol; Pharmacol* **33**(3), 197-98 (1989)
4. Chattopadhyay RR; Hypoglycaemic effect of *Ocimum sanctum* leaf extract in normal and streptozotocin diabetic rats, *Indian J Exp Biol* **31**(11), 891-93 (1993)
5. Agrawal P, V Rai, RB Singh; Randomized placebo-controlled, single blind trial of holy basil leaves in patients with noninsulin-dependent diabetes mellitus, *Int J Clin Pharmacol Ther* **34**(9), 406-09 (1996)
6. Rai V, U Iyer, UV Mani; Effect of Tulasi (*Ocimum sanctum*) leaf powder sup-

plementation on blood sugar levels, serum lipids and tissue lipids in diabetic rats, *Plant Foods Hum Nutr* **50**(1), 9-16 (1997)

7. Halim EMA, KJ Hussain, M Rao; Hypoglycaemic, hypolipidaemic and anti-oxidant properties of Tulsi (*Ocimum sanctum* Linn.) in streptozotocin-induced diabetes in rats, *Indian J Clin Biochem* **16**(2), 190-94 (2001)
8. Vats V, JK Grover, SS Rathi; Evaluation of anti-hyperglycaemic and hypoglycaemic effect of *Trigonella foenum-graecum* Linn, *Ocimum sanctum* Linn and *Pterocarpus marsupium* Linn in normal and alloxanized diabetic rats, *J Ethnopharmacol* **79**(1), 95-100 (2002)
9. Vats V, SP Yadav, JK Grover; Ethanolic extract of *Ocimum sanctum* leaves partially attenuates streptozotocin-induced alterations in glycogen content and carbohydrate metabolism in rats, *J Ethnopharmacol* **90**(1), 155-60 (2004)
10. Sethi J, S Sood, S Seth, A Talwar; Evaluation of hypoglycaemic and antioxidant effect of *Ocimum sanctum, Indian J Clin Biochem* **19**(2), 152-55 (2004)

Oenanthe javanica (Blume) DC (Apiaceae) (Water parsley)

A single intra-gastric administration of *Oenanthe javanica* flavone (200 mg/kg) reduced the blood glucose in normal mice. Administration of the flavone (200 and 400 mg/kg) daily for 10 days decreased the blood glucose in alloxan-induced hyperglycaemic mice. The flavone promoted the release of insulin both in normal and in diabetic mice. It also decreased serum triglyceride and raised the lowered pancreatic amylases in diabetic mice. The hypoglycaemic and hypo-triglyceride actions of the flavone were mainly concerned with promoting release of insulin from *beta*-cells in islets of Langerhans.

Yang XB, ZM Huang, WB Cao, M Zheng, HY Chen, JZ Zhang; Anti-diabetic effect of *Oenanthe javanica* flavone, *Acta Pharmacol Sin* **21**(3), 239-42 (2000)

Olea europaea Linn. (Oleaceae) (Olive)

Olea europaea is native to the Mediterranean region from Lebanon, Syria and northern Iran at the south end of the Caspian sea. Its fruit, the olive, is of major agricultural importance in the Mediterranean region as the source of olive oil. A study of the hypoglycaemic activity of olive leaf showed that the leaves collected in winter months, particularly in February, showed maximum hypoglycaemic activity. Oleuropeoside, a constituent of the leaves, was recognized to be the active constituent and it showed activity at a dose of 16 mg/kg. This compound also demonstrated anti-diabetic activity in animals with alloxan-induced diabetes. The possible mechanisms, by which the compound shows its hypoglycaemic activity, were discussed (1).

The glycerol-alcoholic macerates of shoots and leaves of *O. europaea* showed hypoglycaemic effects in normal and alloxan-induced diabetic rats. An increase in glucose tolerance was also observed. The iridoid, oleuropin, also showed similar activity (2).

African wild olive leaves were found to be different from those of *Olea europaea* from Greece and a cultivar of *O. europaea* grown in Cape Town, in triterpenoid constituents. The African wild olive leaves were found to contain a 1:1 mixture of oleanolic acid and ursolic acid but no ursolic acid was found in either of the remaining two plants. The anti-hypertensive, diuretic, anti-atherosclerotic, antioxidant and hypoglycaemic effects of authentic oleanolic and ursolic acids and of the isolates from the leaves of three different varieties of olives were studied on Dahl salt-sensitive, insulin-resistant rat genetic model of hypertension. All three isolates, in a dose 60 mg/kg b.w. for 6 weeks, prevented the development of severe hypertension and atherosclerosis and improved the insulin resistance of the experimental animals indicating that the absence of ursolic acid in *Olea europaea* from Greece and Cape Town had nothing to do with the activity (3).

The long-term effects of an olive oil-enriched diet on glucagon-like peptide-1 (GLP-1) content of the intestinal tract, as well as the plasma D-glucose, insulin, and GLP-1 pattern during an oral glucose tolerance test were studied in normal rats. The intake of an olive oil-enriched diet was found to increase GLP-1 release in normal rats. A long-term exposure to the olive oil-enriched diet led to higher body weight gain, increased secretory response of insulin-producing cells to oral glucose administration, and, after 36 days, improved glucose tolerance (4).

1. Gonzalez M, A Zarzuelo, MJ Gamez, MP Utrilla, J Jimenez, I Osuna; Hypoglycaemic activity of olive leaf, *Planta Med* **58**(6), 513-15 (1992)
2. Trovato A, AM Forestieri, L Link, R Barbera, MT Monforte, EM Galati; Hypoglycaemic effect of different extracts of *Olea europaea* L. in the rats, *Plantes Medicinales Phytotherapie* **26**(4), 300-08 (1993)
3. Somova LI, FO Shode, P Ramnanan. A Nadar; Antihypertensive, antiatherosclerotic and antioxidant activity of triterpenoids isolated from *Olea europaea*, subspecies *africana* leaves, *J Ethnopharmacol* **84**(2-3), 299-305 (2003)
4. Prieto PG, J Cancelas, ML Villanueva-Penacarriillo, I Valverde, WJ Malaisse; Effects of an olive oil-enriched diet on plasma GLP-1 concentration and intestinal content, plasma insulin concentration, and glucose tolerance in normal rats, *Endocrine* **26**(2), 107-115 (2005)

Olea europea L. var. ***oleaster*** (Hoff. et Lk) (Oleaceae) (Olive tree)

Sand rats submitted to a high cholesterol diet for four months developed hyperglycaemia, glucose intolerance, hypercholesterolaemia and moderate hyperinsulinaemia. The treatment of the rats with a decoction of the leaves of the plant for a period of two months produced hypoglycaemic, anti-hyperglycaemic and hypoinsulinaemic activities. A hypocholesterolaemic effect accompanied by a lowering of oxidized LDL was also observed by the treatment (1). The beneficial effects of *olea europea* var. *oleaster* leaves to regulate unbalanced metabolism were studied in sand rats, which are known to develop obesity, insulin-resistance, hyperlipidaemia and pre-diabetes even when given a standard laboratory chow diet. Sand rats, fed on hyper-caloric diet during 7 months, were treated by plant decoction (1.5 ml/100g during 3 months) as well as by simvastatin; a hypocholesterolaemic drug. The plant drug exhibited a hypocholesterolaemic effect related to decreases in LDL and VLDL cholesterol in addition to hypoglycaemic and anti-hyperglycaemic effects accompanied by a decrease in insulin. No significant reduction in plasma levels of triglycerides and HDL cholesterol was observed by either of the treatments. (2).

1. Bennani-Kabehi N, H Edhil, Y Cherrah, L Kehel, F El-Bouayadi, A Amarti, M Saïdi, G Marquie; Effects of *Olea europea* var. *oleaster* leaves in hypercholesterolemic insulin-resistant sand rats, *Therapie* **54**(6), 717-23 (1999)
2. Bennani-Kabehi N, H Edhil, Y Cherrah, F El-Bouayadi, L Kehel, G Marquie; *Ann Pharm Fr* **58**(4), 271-77 (2000) [Article in French]

Oplopanax horridum (Smith) Miq. (Araliaceae) (Devil's club)

Devil's club is found from south-central Alaska and along the coast of California. Devil's club is closely related to American ginseng, and the plant was traditionally used by Native Americans to treat adult-onset diabetes and a variety of tumors. The findings of pharmacological investigations of *Oplopanax horridum*, known to exhibit hypoglycaemic activity, have been reviewed.

Smith GW, Arctic Pharmacognosis II. Devil's Club, *Oplopanax horridum*, *J Ethnopharmacol* **7**(3), 313-20 (1983)

Ononis pubescens Linn. (Fabaceae)

Five different extracts of *Ononis pubescens* were screened by a multidimensional pharmacological test in conscious rats. While all the five extracts exhibited depressive action on the central nervous system, some fractions exhibited hypoglycaemic activity.

Montero MJ, A Moran, ML Martin, LS Roman; Pharmacological screening of *Ononis pubescens* L., *Int J Crude Drug Res* **26**(4), 215-19 (1988)

Ophiopogon japonicus Ker-Gawl. (Ruscaceae) (Mondo grass)

Radix Ophiopogonis is the dried root tuber of *Ophiopogon japonicus.* The n-butanol extract of rhizomes of Ophiopogonis tuber (100 mg/kg) reduced the blood glucose of normal mice 4h after intra-peritoneal administration and also significantly lowered the blood glucose of streptozotocin-induced diabetic mice under similar conditions. The extract also tended to suppress epinephrine-induced hyperglycaemia in mice. It was inferred that the hypoglycaemic effect of the extract does not alter the insulin concentration.

Kako M, T Miura, M Usami, A Kato, S Kadowaki; Hypoglycaemic effect of the rhizomes of ophiopogonis tuber in normal and diabetic mice, *Biol Pharm Bull* **18**(5), 785-87 (1995)

Opuntia ficus indica (L.) Mill. (Cactaceae) (Prickle-pear cactus, Indian Fig Opuntia, Nopal)

Opuntia ficus-indica, a species of cactus, is a long-domesticated crop plant important in agricultural economies throughout arid and semiarid parts of the world. Most of the *Opuntia* species have been described as 'prickly pear' or 'nopal'. Reports of reduced blood glucose and insulin level by administration of this cactus extract and the mechanism for its hypoglycaemic action was postulated (1, 2). Dehydrated extract of nopal (*O. ficus indica*) stems did not reduce fasting glycaemia in diabetic subjects but diminished the increase of serum glucose level after a dextrose load. Dehydrated extract of nopal did not show acute hypoglycaemic effect, although it could attenuate postprandial hyperglycaemia (3).

Oral intake of *O. ficus indica* stems (500 g) in different forms (broiled, blended broiled, blended crude, blended crude and heated at 60° C) by diabetic patients decreased their glycaemia, which reached statistically significant levels afer 120 and 180 min, From the findings, it was inferred that *O. ficus indica* exerts hypoglycaemic effects in non-insulin dependent diabetic patients and heating or blending does not affect the activity of this herbal drug (4).

In order to assess whether commercial capsules with dried nopal extracts may have a role in the management of diabetes mellitus, 30 capsules were given in fasting condition to 10 diabetic subjects and serum glucose was measured through 3 hours; a control test was performed with 30 placebo capsules. Oral glucose tolerance test with previous intake of 30 nopal or placebo capsules was performed in ten healthy individuals. A crossover and single blinded study was also made with 14 diabetic patients, who withdrew the oral hypoglycaemic treatment and received 10 nopal or placebo capsules tds. during one week. *Opuntia* capsules did not show acute hypoglycaemic effect and did not influence oral glucose tolerance test. In diabetic patients, serum glucose, cholesterol and tryglyceride levels did not change with *Opuntia*, but they increased with placebo. The intake of *Opuntia* capsules daily in patients with diabetes mellitus had a discrete beneficial effect on glucose and cholesterol. (5).

Hypoglycaemic activity of the polysaccharide isolated from *Opuntia ficus-indica* has been reported (6).

Fruits and leaves of *Opuntia ficus-indica* var. *sabotan* inhibited intestinal *alpha*-glucosidase of rats as well as glucose elevation in the blood of normal mice. It also exhibited inhibitory activities on streptozotocin-induced rather than on alloxan-induced diabetic mice, loaded with maltose and sucrose. Leaves were found to be more effective than fruits (7).

1. Frati-Munari AC, JA Fernandez-Harp, M Banales-Ham, CR Ariza-Andraca; Decreased blood glucose and insulin by nopal (*Opuntia* sp.), *Arch Invest Med* (Mex) **14**(3), 269-74 (1983) [Article in English, Spanish]
2. Frati-Munari AC, A Yever-Garces, S Andrade, CR Ariza-Andraca; A Chavez-Negrete; Studies on the mechanism of "hypoglycaemic" effect of nopal (*Opuntia* sp.), *Arch Invest Med* (Mex) **18**(1), 7-12 (1987) [Article in English, Spanish]
3. Frati-Munari AC, C de Leon, R Ariza-Andraca; MB Banales-Ham, R Lopez-Ledesma, X Lozoya; Effect of a dehydrated extract of nopal (*Opuntia ficus indica* Mill.) on blood glucose, *Arch Invest Med* (Mex) **20**(3), 211-16 (1989) [Article in Spanish]
4. Frati AC, E Jimenez, CR Ariza; Hypoglycaemic effect of *Opuntia ficus indica* in non-insulin dependent diabetes mellitus patients, *Phytother Res* **4**(5), 195-97 (1990)
5. Frati-Munari AC, O Vera-Lastra, CR Ariza-Andraca; Evaluation of nopal capsules in diabetes mellitus, *Gac Med Mex* **128**(4), 431-36 (1992) [Article in Spanish]
6. Alarcon-Aguilar FJ, A Valdes-Arzate, S Xolalpa-Molina, T Banderas-Dorantes, M Jhnenez-Estrada, E Hernandez-Galicia, R Roman-Ramos; Hypoglycaemic activity of two polysaccharides isolated from *Opuntia ficus-indica* and *O. streptacantha*, *Proc West Pharmacol Soc* **46**, 139-42 (2003)
7. Shin J, MJ Han, LK Lee, YI Moon, DH Kim; Hypoglycaemic activity of *Opuntia ficus-indica* var. *sabotan* on alloxan- or streptozotocin-induced diabetic mice, *Korean J Pharmacogn* **34**(1), 75-79 (2003)

Opuntia fuliginosa Griffiths (Cactaceae)

This cactus, also known as prickly pear cactus, is native to Mexico. The hypoglycaemic activity of a purified extract from *Opuntia fuliginosa* was evaluated on strptozotocin-induced diabetic rats. Blood glucose and glycated haemoglobin levels were reduced to normal values by a combined treatment of insulin and

Opuntia extract. Withdrawal of insulin from this combination therapy maintained normoglycaemic state in the diabetic rats. The blood glucose response to administered glucose also showed similar results. Combination treatment of insulin and *Opuntia* extract for 7 weeks followed by *Opuntia* extract alone was capable of rapidly returning blood glucose to the levels of the non-diabetic rats. The magnitude of glucose control by the small amount of *Opuntia* extract (1 mg/kg body weight per day) warrants clinical studies with humans.

Trejo-Gonzalez A, G Gabriel-Ortiz, AM Puebla-Perez, MD Huizar-Contreras, MR Munguia-Mazariegos, S Mejia-Arreguin, E Calva; A purified extract from prickly pear cactus (*Opuntia fuliginosa*) controls experimentally induced diabetes in rats, *J Ethnopharmacol* **55**(1), 27-33 (1996)

Opuntia lindheimeri Engelm. (Cactaceae)

Both oral and parenteral administration of the aqueous extract of *O. lindheimeri* produced hypoglycaemic effect in streptozotocin-induced diabetic rats. The dialysate of a dilute aqueous solution of *O. lindheimeri* also produced hypoglycaemic effect when administered intravenously. The concentration and/or potency of the active hypoglycaemic principle in *Opuntia* cacti has been reported to be species specific (1) The hypoglycaemic activity of *O. lindheimeri* extract was investigated in non-diabetic and streptozotocin-induced diabetic pigs. While the blood glucose concentrations in non-diabetic pigs fluctuated around initial baseline concentrations following oral administration of the extract (0, 250 or 500 mg/kg b.w.), a significant decrease in blood glucose concentration was observed in strptozotocin-induced diabetic pigs and the effect was both dose-and time-dependent. These results confirm the hypoglycaemic effect of *O. lindheimeri* extract in a diabetic pig model (2).

1. Enigbokan MA, TB Felder, Jjo Thompson, JO Kim, KJ Ekpenyong; Hypoglycaemic effects *Opuntia ficus-indica* Mill, *Opuntia lindheimeri* Englem and *Opuntia robusta* Wendl. in streptozotocin-indiced diabetic rats, *Phytother Res* **10**(3), 379-82-(1996)
2. Laurenz JC, CC Collier, JO Kuti; Hypoglycaemic effect of *Opuntia lindheimeri* Englem in a diabetic pig model, *Phytother Res* **17**(1), 26-29 (2003)

Opuntia megacantha Salm-Dyck (Cactaceae)
Syn. *Opuntia ficus-indica* (L) Mill

Streptozotocin-induced diabetic and non-diabetic rats were orally administered extracts of *O. megacantha* leaves (20 mg/100 g b.w.) daily for 5 weeks and respective control rats were administered normal saline (0.1 ml/100 mg b.w.). Plasma glucose concentrations in streptozotocin-induced diabetic and non-diabetic rats were reduced by the administration of leaf extracts of *O. megacantha*. The results of detailed investigation suggest that leaf extracts of *O. megacantha* not only reduce blood glucose levels, but may be toxic to the kidney as shown by the elevation in plasma urea and creatinine concentrations and the reduction of plasma Na^+ concentration.

Bwititi P, CT Musabayane, CF Nhachi; Effects of *Opuntia megacantha* on blood glucose and kidney function in streptozotocin diabetic rats, *J Ethnopharmacol* **69**(3), 247-52 (2000)

Opuntia robusta JC Wendl. (Cactaceae)

Intravenous administration of the aqueous extract of *O. robusta* produced hypoglycaemic effect in streptozotocin-induced diabetic rats but oral administration failed to produce this effect (1). Pectin, a soluble fibre, has been reported to be effective in lowering cholesterol levels in both animals and men with hyperlipidaemia. It is also capable to slow down carbohydrate absorption and thus reduce the postprandial rise in blood glucose and serum insulin in patients with type-2 diabetes. The influence of prickly pear (*O. robusta*)-pectin intake on glucose- and lipid metaolism was examined in 24 non-diabetic, non-obese males suffering from primary isolated hypercholesterolemia or combined hyperlipidaemia. Consumption of prickly pear led to a decrease of total cholesterol, low-density lipoprotein-cholesterol, apolipoprotein B, triglycerides, fibrinogen, blood glucose, insulin and uric acid (2).

1. Enigbokan MA, TB Felder, Jjo Thompson, JO Kim, KJ Ekpenyong; Hypoglycaemic effects *Opuntia ficus-indica* Mill, *Opuntia lindheimeri* Englem and *Opuntia robusta* Wendl. in streptozotocin-indiced diabetic rats, *Phytother Res* **10**(3), 379-82-(1996)

2. Wolfram RM, H Kritz, Y Efthimiou, J Stomatopoulos, H Sinzinger; Effect of prickly pear (*Opuntia robusta*) on glucose- and lipid- metabolism in non-diabetics with hyperlipidemia—a pilot study, *Wien Klin Wochenschr* **114**(19-20), 840-46 (2002)

Opuntia streptacantha Lemaire(Cactaceae)

Opuntia species has traditionally been used by the Mexican population for the treatment of diabetes mellitus. The effect of the extracts from *Opuntia streptacantha* in healthy and pancreatectomized rabbits was studied and from preliminary results it was concluded that this cactus possesses hypoglycaemic properties when orally administered in animals with experimentally induced diabetes as well as in healthy ones with physiological hyperglycaemia. The hypoglycaemic effect of *O. streptacantha* sap was also studied in three different animal species using several experimental conditions and the results validated the popular use of this plant for treatment of diabetes mellitus symptomatology (1-3). The complementary daily administration of *O. streptacantha* sap to a diabetic volunteer, being under treatment with chlorpropamide, remarkably improved the general symptomatology of the patient as well as his insulin and blood glucose levels (4).

Frati-Munari and co-workers did considerable work on the hypoglycaemic effect of this cactus. The hypoglycaemic effect of nopal (*Opuntia streptacantha*) was studied in patients with non-insulin-dependent diabetes mellitus. The study revealed that the stems of *O. streptacantha* caused a hypoglycaemic effect in patients with NIDDM. A significant direct correlation was also noticed between the doses of broiled stems of the plant and the hypoglycaemic effect. Though the exact mechanism for the observed hypoglycaemic effect is not clear, increased insulin sensitivity has been suggested to be a plausible mechanism (5-7, 10). The duration of hypoglycaemic effect with an intake of 500 g of broiled *Opuntia* stems using 400 ml of water as control was assessed in eight type-2 diabetics. The decrease of serum glucose level was more pronounced at the fourth hour of treatment but it remained unchanged the following two hours (8). It was further observed that the intake of broiled *Opuntia* stems rather than raw extract caused a significant decrease of serum glucose level and it was logically assumed that heating of *O. streptacantha* is necessary to obtain the hypoglycaemic effect (9). Hypoglycaemic effect of *O. streptacantha* was observed not only in diabetic subjects but also in healthy subjects with induced hyperglycaemia (11). Serum glucose and insulin levels were measured at 0, 60, 120 and 180 minutes after ingestion of *O. streptacantha* stems by 14 healthy volunteers and to 14 patients with NIDDM. The intake of the plant drug by the NIDDM group was followed by a significant reduction of serum glucose and insulin concentration. No significant changes were noticed in the healthy group as compared with the control group. The mechanisms of this effect appear to differ from conventional hypoglycaemic agents. (12). Tests were performed to find out whether a second dose of *O. streptacantha* (500 g of broiled stems) enhances its hypoglycaemic effect in type-2 diabetic subjects and healthy individuals. It was observed that a second dose of the plant drug two hours after the first one, did not improve its hypoglycaemic activity (13). Hypoglycaemic activity of the polysaccharide isolated from *O. streptacantha* was studied (14).

1. Ibanez-Camacho R, R Roman-Ramos; Hypoglycaemic effect of *Opuntia* cactus, *Arch Invest Med* (Mex) **10**(4), 223-30 (1979) [Article in English, Spanish]

2. Ibanez-Camacho R, M Meckes-Lozoya, V Mellado-Campos; The hypoglycaemic effect of *Opuntia streptacantha* studied in different animal experimental models, *J Ethnopharmacol* **7**(2), 175-81 (1983)

3. Ibanez-Camacho R, M Meckes-Lozoya; Effect of a semipurified product obtained from *Opuntia streptacantha* L. (a cactus) on glycaemia and triglyceridemia of rabbit, *Arch Invest Med* (Mex) **14**(4), 437-43 (1983) [Article in English, Spanish]

4. Meckes-Lozyoa M, R Roman-Ramos; *Opuntia streptacantha*: a coadjutor in the treatment of diabetes mellitus, *Am J Chin Med* **14**(3-4), 116-18 (1986)

5. Frati-Munari AC, A Yever-Garces, S Islas-Andrade, CR Ariza-Andraca, A Chavez-Negrete; Studies on the mechanism of "hypoglycaemic" effect of nopal (*Opuntia* sp.), *Arch Invest Med* (Mex) **18**(1), 7-12 (1987) [Article in English, Spanish

6. Frati-Munari AC, BE Gordillo, P Altamirano, CR Ariza; Hypoglycaemic effect of *Opuntia streptacantha* Lemaire in NIDDM, *Diabetes Care* **11**(1), 63-66 (1988)

7. Frati-Munari AC, LM Del Valle-Martinez, CR Ariza-Andraca, S Islas-Andrade, A Chavez-Negrete; Hypoglycaemic action of different doses of nopal (*Opuntia streptacantha* Lemaire) in patients with type II diabetes mellitus, *Arch Invest Med* (Mex) **20**(2), 197-201 (1989) [Article in Spanish]

8. Frati-Munari AC, U Rios-Gil, CR Ariza-Andraca, S Islas-Andrade, R Lopez-Ledesma; Duration of the hypoglycaemic action of *Opuntia streptacantha* Lem., *Arch Invest Med* (Mex) **20**(4), 297-300 (1989) [Article in Spanish]

9. Frati-Munari AC, E Altamirano-Bustamante, N Rodriguez, CR Ariza-Andraca, R Lopez-Ledesma; Hypoglycaemic action of *Opuntia streptacantha* Lemaire: study using raw extracts, *Arch Invest Med* (Mex) **20**(4), 321-25 (1989) [Article in Spanish]

10. Frati AC, BE Gordillo, P Altamirano, CR Ariza, R Cortes-Franco, A Chavez-Negrete; Acute hypoglycaemic effect of *Opuntia streptacantha* Lemaire in NIDDM, *Diabetes Care* **13**(4), 455-56 (1990)

11. Frati-Munari AC, R Licona-Quesada, CR Araiza-Andraca, R Lopez-Ledesma, A Chavez-Negrete; Activity of *Opuntia streptacantha* in healthy individuals with induced hyperglycemia, *Arch Invest Med* (Mex) **21**(2), 99-102 (1990) [Article in Spanish]

12. Frati AC, BE Gordillo, P Altamirano, CR Ariza, R Cortes-Franco, A Chavez-Negrete, S Islas-Andrade; Influence of nopal intake upon fasting glycemia in type II diabetics and healthy subjects, *Arch Invest Med* (Mex) **22**(1) 51-56 (1991)

13. Frati AC, N Xilotl-Diaz, P Altamirano, R Ariza, R Lopez-Ledesma; The effect of two sequential doses of *Opuntia streptacantha* upon glycaemia, *Arch Invest Med* (Mex) **22**(3-4) 333-36 (1991)

14. Alarcon-Aguilar FJ, A Valdes-Arzate, S Xolalpa-Molina, T Banderas-Dorantes, M Jimenez-Estrada, E Hernandez-Galicia, R Roman-Ramos; Hypoglycaemic activity of two polysaccharides isolated from *Opuntia ficus-indica* and *O. streptacantha*, *Proc West Pharmacol Soc* **46**, 139-42 (2003)

Origanum vulgare Linn. (Lamiaceae)

The effect of an aqueous extract of *O. vulgare* leaves on blood glucose levels was investigated in normal and streptozotocin-induced diabetic rats. Oral administration of a single dose of an aqueous extract of *O. vulgare* (20 mg/kg) produced a significant decrease on blood glucose levels in streptozotocin diabetic rats. In these rats, the blood glucose levels were normalised from the fourth day after daily repeated oral administration of this aqueous extract. However, this effect was less pronounced 2 weeks after daily repeated oral administration of the extract. No changes were observed in basal plasma insulin concentrations after treatment in either normal or streptozotocin-induced diabetic rats indicating that the aqueous extract of the plant drug acted without changing insulin secretion.

Lemhadri A, NA Zeggwagh, M Maghrani, H Jouad, M Eddouks; Anti-hyperglycaemic activity of the aqueous extract of *Origanum vulgare* growing wild in Tafilalet region, *J Ethnopharmacol* **92**(2-3), 251-56 (2004)

Orthosiphon stamineus Benth (Lamiaceae) (Java Tea.)

Java tea is a medicinal plant native to South East Asia and some parts of tropical Australia. Orthosiphon is a popular garden plant because of its unique flowers, which are white and bluish with filaments resembling a cat's whiskers. The plant is traditionally used to treat diabetes, kidney and urinary disorders.

Oral administration of an aqueous extract *O. stamineus* (1.0 g/kg) caused significant hypoglycaemic effect in normal rats. Hyperglycaemic effect induced by streptozotocin was also inhibited by the same dose (1). The aqueous extract was also found to be effective in alleviating hyperglycaemia and improving lipid profile in diabetic rats. The extract (0.2–1.0 g/kg) significantly decreased plasma glucose concentration in a dose-dependent manner in both normal and diabetic rats. Repeated daily oral administrations of the extract (0.5 g/kg) for 14 days not only significantly reduced plasma glucose concentration in diabetic rats but also reduced plasma triglyceride concentration and increased plasma HDL-cholesterol concentration in diabetic rats. In perfused rat pancreas, the extract did not increase insulin secretion in the presence of 5.5 mM glucose, but the extract (100 μg/ml) potentiated glucose-induced insulin secretion (2).

1. Marian A, MZ Asmawi, A Sadikun; Hypoglycaemic activity of the aqueous extract of *Orthosiphon stamineus, Fitoterpia* **67**(5), 465-68 (1996)
2. Sriplang K, S. Adisakwattana, A. Rungsipipat, S. Yibchok-anun; Effects of *Orthosiphon stamineus* aqueous extract on plasma glucose concentration and lipid profile in normal and streptozotocin-induced diabetic rats, *J Ethnopharmacol* **109**(3), 510-14 (2007)

Oryza sativa Linn.(Poaceae) (Rice)

Rice is an extensively grown food crop in the World. Rice is a staple diet for a large part of the world's human population, making it the most consumed cereal grain. Rice is mainly produced and consumed in the Asian region. India has the largest area under paddy cultivation in the world and ranks second in the production after China. The major part of rice consists of carbohydrate in the form of starch. Rice provides more than one fifth of the calories consumed worldwide by humans. Being a source of starch, which breaks down to glucose after digestion, it cannot be expected to be hypoglycaemic but its glycaemic index depends upon various factors and these have been pointed out here.

See glycans in Appendix (1, 2)

The effects of thermal processing of rice on plasma glucose and insulin responses were examined in healthy subjects. Rice boiled in salted water and that baked for 10 min at 160°C prior to boiling showed clear difference in viscosity and in *in vitro* hydrolytic rates but their plasma glucose and insulin responses in the volunteers differed to a smaller extent. In particular the 60-min incremental area for glucose was significantly lower in the case of baked rice, compared to boiled rice. The findings suggest that thermal processing of complex carbohydrates may differently affect glycaemic responses in man (3).

Three high-amylose rice varieties, IR42, IR36, and IR62, with similar chemical composition and amylose content, were cooked under the same conditions and tested for *in vitro* digestibility as well as blood glucose and insulin responses in healthy human volunteers. The starch-digestion rate and the glycaemic and insulin responses were the highest in IR42, followed by IR36 and then IR62. The differences were not due to unabsorbed carbohydrate but were related to their physicochemical properties. When the three varieties were cooked for their minimum cooking time, they had the same degree of gelatinization and their starch-digestion rates and glycaemic responses were similar. It was inferred that amylose content alone is not a good predictor of starch-digestion rate or glycaemic response and rice varieties with similar high-amylose contents can differ in physicochemical (gelatinization) properties and this, in turn, can influence starch digestibility and blood glucose response (4).

To test whether the glycaemic index is altered by the amount of carbohydrate meals containing 25 and 50 g carbohydrate as white rice and white bread were taken by seven non-insulin-dependent diabetic subjects. The incremental areas of blood glucose (above basal) to parboiled white rice (25 g carbohydrate) were significantly lower than that for white bread (25 g carbohydrate). Similar insulin response areas to 25 g carbohydrate, given as parboiled white rice and white bread, were observed. However, 50 g carbohydrate as white bread caused a significantly higher insulin response area than parboiled white rice (5).

The glycaemic and insulin-index values for 12 rice products were examined, using eight healthy subjects. These results indicated that rice varieties, whether white, brown, or parboiled, should be classified as high glycaemic index foods. Only high-amylose varieties are potentially useful as low- glycaemic index diets (6).

The dose-response relationships between postprandial blood glucose, insulin, and glucagon responses and the amount of starch ingested in non-insulin-dependent diabetic (NIDDM) subjects were examined. Mixed meals of 23, 46, and 69 g parboiled white rice containing approximately 20, 40, and 60 g available carbohydrate, cooked with 167 g meat sauce, were served to patients after a 12-hour fast on 3 separate days. Glucose response areas to meals of 20, 40, and 60 g carbohydrate as white rice differed significantly. Insulin response areas to meals of 23 g rice were significantly lower compared with response areas to 46 g and 69 g rice. Glucagon response areas showed an inverse pattern to glucose response areas (7).

The influence of parboiling, amylose content and gelatinisation-temperature of rice on the postprandial blood glucose and insulin responses was studied in non-insulin-dependent diabetic subjects. From the results of the investigation it was concluded that mild parboiling process used did not influence glycaemic index. The study also showed that the amylose content, rather than the gelatinisation temperature, might be a useful criterion in selection of rice with low glycaemic index (8).

The influence of parboiling and the severity of the process on glycaemic and insulinaemic responses to rice were studied in type-2 diabetes. It was observed that rice processed by traditional parboiling method had no effect on glycaemic index but rice processed by pressure parboiling reduced the glycaemic index by almost 30% compared to non-parboiled rice (9).

The effect of resistant starch from corn and rice on blood glucose and insulin levels was examined in streptozotocin-induced diabetic rats. No significant effect of resistant starch feeding on blood glucose and insulin was found (10).

The influence of the physical form of processed rice products (garaeduk, bagsulgi, and cooked rice) on the enzymatic hydrolysis of rice starch *in vitro* and on the postprandial glucose and insulin responses in patients with type-2 diabetes mellitus was studied. It was inferred that the specific surface area of different forms of a food are different with the same degree of maceration and this in turn affects the rate of rice starch hydrolysis both *in vitro* and *in vivo* (11).

The starch in parboiled rice was found to be less susceptible to digestion *in vitro*, exogenous glucose availability was not significantly different after ingestion of large amounts of polished or parboiled rice. Glucose absorption remains incomplete 8 h after ingestion of both types of rice (12).

Glucagon-like peptide-1 (GLP-1) is the most potent physiological insulinotropic hormone in humans. A GLP-1 analogue, derived from trypsin-digested genetically modified rice seeds, stimulated insulin secretion from a mouse pancreatic *beta*-cell line, MIN6 (13).

1. Hikino H, M Murakami, Y Oshima, C Konno; Isolation and hypoglycaemic activity of oryzarans A, B, C, and D: glycans of *Oryza sativa* roots, *Planta Med* (6), 490-92 (1986)

2. Hikino H, M Takahashi, Y Oshima, C Konno; Isolation and hypoglycaemic activity of oryzabrans A, B, C and D, glycans of *Oryza sativa* bran, *Planta Med* **54**(1), 1-3 (1988)

3. Gatti E, G Testolin, D Noe, F Brighenti, GP Buzzetti, M Porrino, CR Sirtori; Plasma glucose and insulin responses to carbohydrate food (rice) with different thermal processing, *Ann Nutr Metab* **31**(5), 296-303 (1987)

4. Panlasigui N, LU Thompson, BO Juliano, CM Perez, SH Yiu, GR Greenberg; Rice varieties with similar amylose content differ in starch digestibility and glycaemic response in humans, *Am J Clin Nutr* **54**(5), 871-77 (1991)

5. Rasmussen O, S Gregersen, K Hemansen; Influence of the amount of starch on the glycaemic index to rice in non-insulin-dependent diabetic subjects, *Br J Nutr* **67**(3), 371-77 (1992)

6. Miller JB, E Pang, L Bramall; Rice: a high or low glycaemic index food, *Am J Clin Nutr* **56**(6), 1034-36 (1992)

7. Rasmussen O, Dose-dependency of the glycaemic response to starch-rich meals in non-insulin-dependent diabetic subjects: studies with varying amounts of white rice, *Metabolism* **42**(2), 214-17 (1993)

8. Larsen HN, C Christensen, OW Rasmussen, IH Tetens, NH Choudhury, SH Thilsted, K Hermansen; Influence of parboiling and physico-chemical characteristics of rice on the glycaemic index in non-insulin-dependent diabetic subjects, *Eur J Clin Nutr* **50**(1), 22-27 (1996)

9. Larsen HN, OW Rasmussen, PH Rasmussen, KK Alstrup, SK Biswas, I Tetens, SH Thilsted, K Hermansen; Glycaemic index of parboiled rice depends on the severity of processing: study in type-2 diabetic subjects, *Eur J Clin Nutr* **54**(5), 380-85 (2000)

10. Kim WK, MK Chang, NF Kang, MH Kim, OJ Park; Effect of resistant starch from corn or rice on glucose control, colonic events, and blood lipid concentrations in streptozotocin-induced diabetic rats, *J Nutr Biochem* **14**(3), 166-72 (2003)

11. Kim JC, JI Kim, BW Kong, MJ Kang, MJ Kim, IJ Cha; Influence of the physical form of processed rice products on the enzymatic hydrolysis of rice starch *in vitro* and on the postprandial glucose and insulin responses in patients with type-2 diabetes mellitus, *Biosci Biotechnol Biochem* **68**(9), 1831-36 (2004)

12. Korach-Andre M, H Roth, D Barnoud, M Pean, F Peronnet, X Leverve; Glucose appearance in the peripheral circulation and liver glucose output in men after a large ^{13}C starch meal, *Am J Clin Nutr* **80**(4), 881-86 (2004)

13. Sugita K, S Endo-Kasahara, Y Tada, H Yasuda, Y Hayashi, T Jomori, H Ebinuma, F Takaiwa; Genetically modified rice seeds accumulating GLP-1 analogue stimulate insulin secretion from a mouse pancreatic *beta*-cell line, *FEBS Lett* **579**(5), 1085-88 (2005)

Otholobium pubescens (Poir.) J.W. Grimes (Fabaceae)

Otholobium pubescens is a Peruvian medicinal plant used for the treatment of diabetes. Oral administration of bakuchiol, isolated from an extract of *O. pubescens* by bioassay-guided fractionation, using db/db mouse model for type-2 diabetes, reduced blood glucose levels in a dose-dependent fashion but did not display a hypoglycaemic effect when tested in lean mice at 250 mg/kg q.d. In fat-fed, streptozotocin-treated rat, an oral dose of bakuchiol at 150 mg/kg q.d. significantly lowered plasma glucose and triglyceride levels.

Krenisky JM, J Luo, MJ Reed, JR Camey; Isolation and anti-hyperglycaemic activity of bakuchiol from *Otholobium pubescens* (Fabaceae), a Peruvian medicinal plant used for the treatment of diabetes, *Biol Pharm Bull* **22**(10), 1137-40 (1999)

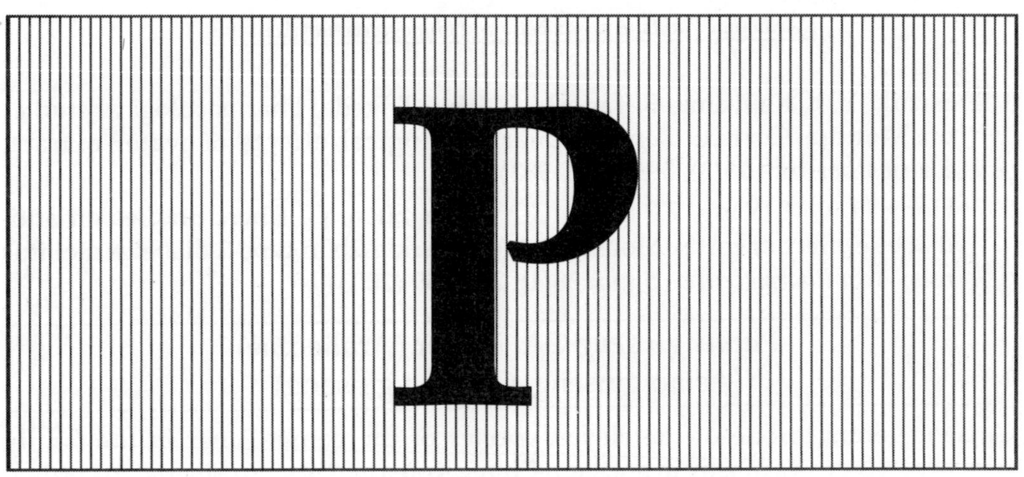

Paeonia lactiflora Pall. (Paeoniaceae / Ranunculaceae) (Chinese Peony)

Paeonia lactiflora is a herbaceous perennial flowering plant, native to central and eastern Asia from eastern Tibet across northern China to eastern Siberia. It is used as a medicinal herb in traditional Chinese medicine. Paeoniflorin and 8-debenzoylpaeoniflorin, isolated from the dried root of the plant produced a significant blood sugar lowering effect in streptozotocin-treated rats and showed a maximum effect at 25 min after treatment. This hypoglycaemic action was also observed in normoglycaemic rats only at 1 mg/kg. Paeoniflorin appeared to be more active than 8-debenzoylpaeoniflorin. Plasma insulin was not changed in paeoniflorin-treated normoglycaemic rats indicating an insulin-independent action. Increase in glucose utilization by paeoniflorin was thus considered to be the mechanism of action.

Hsu FL, CW Lai, JT Cheng; Anti-hyperglycaemic effects of paeoniflorin and 8-debenzoylpaeoniflorin, glucosides from the root of *Paeonia lactiflora*, *Planta Med* **63**(4), 323-25 (1997)

Paeonia suffruticosa Andrews (Paeoniaceae) (Tree Paeony)

Moutan Cortex is the root bark of *Paeonia suffruticosa* .The water extract of the dried root bark of *P. suffruticosa* was found to exhibit hypoglycaemic activity (1). The effect of oral administration of Moutan polysaccharide-2b, isolated from the cortex of *P. suffruticosa*, to type-2 diabetic rats was examined. Oral administration of the polysaccharide-2b daily for 4-5 weeks significantly decreased water and food intake, fasting blood glucose, total cholesterol and triglyceride in type-2 diabetic rats. The treatment also remarkably improved the impaired glucose tolerance and raised the number of low affinity insulin receptors and insulin sensitivity index in type-2 diabetic rats (2).

1. Suzuki Y, K Kajiyama, K Taguchi, Y Ishii, T Ikeda; Pharmacological studies on Moutan Cortex: General pharmacological effects of water. extract, *Pharmacometrics* **25**(3), 393-404 (1983).
2. Hong H, QM Wang, ZP Zhao, GQ Liu, Y Shen, GI Chen; Studies on anti-diabetic effect of cortex Moutan Polysaccharide-2b in type-2 diabetes mellitus rats, *Acta Pharmaceutica Sinica* **38**(4), 255-259 (2003)

Panax ginseng CA. Meyer (Araliaceae) (Asian ginseng, Chinese ginseng)

Ginseng refers to one of the eleven species of the genus *Panax* in the family Araliaceae. It grows mostly in northern China, Korea and eastern Siberia. According to Traditional Chinese Medicine, *Panax ginseng* promotes energy, improves circulation, increases blood supply, revitalizes and aids recovery from weakness after illness and stimulates the body. Asiatic ginseng (*Panax ginseng*) is different from American ginseng (*P. quinquefolius*) and Siberian ginseng (*Eleutherococcus senticosus*).

Several glycans, isolated from *Panax ginseng*, have been reported to exhibit hypoglycaemic activity. These are mentioned under "Hypoglycaemic glycans" in Appendix.

Effects of ginseng saponins on the actions of adrenaline, ACTH and insulin on lipolysis and lipogenesis in adipose tissue were studied (1). Ginseng fruit saponins were found to improve experimental insulin resistance in rats (23).

Bioactivity directed fractionation of *Panax ginseng* led to the isolation of an active hypoglycaemic component from the non-saponin fraction of the plant drug. The fraction was about 100-fold more effective than the original water-soluble extract of the ginseng radix. The ED_{50} value was 0.4 mg/kg in lowering the blood glucose level of alloxan diabetic mice. It was demonstrated that some ginseng fractions, other than saponins, inhibited epinephrine-induced transient hyperglycaemia in mice, increased glycogen content in rat liver, decreased the blood level of acetone bodies in alloxan diabetic mice, and inhibited the release of free fatty acid from rat epididymal fat pad (2). These fractions also stimulated insulin release, especially glucose-induced insulin release from pancreatic islets and thereby lowered the blood glucose level (3).

DPG-3-2, a component derived from the water extract of ginseng, which lowers the blood glucose level and stimulates insulin release in diabetic animals, was studied for its effects on insulin biosynthesis in different preparations of pancreas from animals with normoglycaemia and with hyperglycaemia (alloxan diabetic rats and genetically diabetic mice, KK-CAy). From the results of detailed investigation, DPG-3-2 was proved to stimulate insulin biosynthesis in different preparations of pancreas from animals with hyperglycaemia (4).

Ginsenoside–Rb_2, a constituent of *P, ginseng*, decreased the blood sugar levels in streptozotocin-induced diabetic rats significantly and also elicited moderate but insignificant increase in hepatic glycogen contents. The treated diabetic rats exhibited a significant increase in hepatic glucokinase along with a significant decrease of glucose-6-phosphatase activity. These changes in the activity of enzymes glucokinase and glucose-6-phosphatase might probably be one of the mechanisms responsible for the hypoglycaemic activity of ginsenoside Rb_2 (5). The effects of ginsenoside Rb_2 on albumin mRNA in streptozotocin-induced diabetic rats were studied. The level of albumin mRNA, which in diabetic control rats is significantly lower than that of normal rats, was elevated following treatment with ginsenoside Rb_2, (12).

Administration of a tincture of *P. ginseng* to alloxan-induced diabetic animals significantly reduced the blood sugar levels. This tincture also effectively lowered blood sugar in immobilization stressed rats (6).

An acidic substance from Korean red ginseng powder that inhibited epinephrine-induced lipolysis and stimulated insulin-mediated lipogenesis from glucose was recognised as pyro-glutamic acid (7).

Ginseng polypeptide, isolated from the roots of *P. ginseng,* was demonstrated to decrease the levels of blood sugar and liver glycogen upon intravenous injection to rats at doses of 50-200 mg/kg. The polypeptide also produced similar effect in mice, injected subcutaneously daily at doses of 50 and 100 mg/kg for 7 successive days. It was found to decrease experimental hyperglycaemia induced by injection of adrenaline, glucose and alloxan. The polypeptide, however, exhibited inhibiting effect on the glycogen enhancement induced by glucose, but strengthened the effect on the glycogen decrease induced by adrenaline (8).

Intra-peritoneal or subcutaneous administrations of ginseng polysaccharides (50-200 mg/kg) reduced blood glucose and liver glycogen of mice. The polysaccharides accelerated oxidative-phosphorylation of carbohydrate and also stimulated the release of insulin. It has been suggested that the reduction of blood glucose and liver glycogen induced by ginseng polysaccharides are primarily due to the increase of carbohydrate utilization and the decrease of glycogenesis (10).

The adaptogenic agents, derived from the roots and leaves of *P. ginseng* and tissue culture of ginseng root, displayed a significant anti-diabetic and hepatoprotective activity in experimental mice and rats. The adaptogens prevented alloxan-induced lipid peroxidation in the pancreas and demonstrated definite insulinogenic properties. The increase of basal content of insulin in blood and the glucose-dependent secretion of this hormone were also achieved by these adaptogens (9).

The hypoglycaemic activity of ginseng glycopeptide was studied using normal mice or rabbits and alloxan or streptozotocin-induced hyperglycaemic rats or mice. Ginseng glycopeptide injection (sc or ip) resulted in pronounced decreases in blood glucose and liver glycogen levels in both normal and hyperglycaemic animals in a dose-dependent manner. The hypoglycaemic activity of ginseng glycopeptide may be attributed to the enhancement of aerobic glycolysis through stimulation of *beta*-adrenoceptor and increase of various rate-limiting enzyme activities related to tricarboxylic acid cycle (17, 18).

The oral administration of an aqueous extract of ginseng radix to normal and epinephrine-induced hyperglycaemic mice caused a significant decrease in the blood glucose level 4 h after its administration with concomitant increase in GLUT-2 protein content in mouse liver. It has been suggested that the hypoglycaemic activity of ginseng radix is due, at least in part, to the increment of GLUT-2 protein content (11).

White ginseng is grown for four to six years, and then peeled and dried to reduce the water content to 12% or less. The mechanisms responsible for the anti-diabetic activity of white ginseng radix (Ginseng Radix Alba) as well as of the rootlet (Ginseng Radix Palva) were investigated. Oral administration of the drugs to KKAy mice for a period of 4 weeks lowered the fasting blood glucose levels in comparison to control group. In order to elucidate the mechanism(s) for hypoglycaemic activity of the ginseng radices, glucose absorption from the small intestine, hepatic hexokinase and glucose-6-phosphatase activities, in addition to PPAR-gamma expression in adipose tissue were examined. It was inferred from the results that while white ginseng radix improves hyperglycaemia in KKAy mice by blocking intestinal glucose absorption and inhibition of hepatic glucose-6-phosphatase, the rootlet does so through the up-regulation of adipocytic PPAR-gamma protein expression as well as by inhibition of intestinal glucose absorption (13).

Intra-peritoneal administration of *Panax ginseng* berry extract (150 mg/kg) to adult obese C57BL/Ks db/db mice for 12 consecutive days significantly decreased fasting blood sugar levels as compared to vehicle treated mice on 5th day. The extract-treated db/db mice became virtually normoglycaemic on 12th day. The extract, however, failed to decrease the fasting blood sugar levels of lean mice. After treatment of db/db mice for 12 days with the extract, glucose tolerance of the mice increased significantly. Furthermore, the extract-treated db/db mice and their lean littermates exhibited a loss of body weight. The observation suggested that *Panax ginseng* berry extract could be useful in obese diabetic patients. A comparison between intra-peritoneal and oral administrations of ginseng berry extract was also made (14, 15). The improvement in blood glucose levels in the extract-treated ob/ ob mice was associated with a significant reduction in serum insulin levels in fed and fasting mice. Additional studies demonstrated that ginsenoside Re, a major constituent of *P. ginseng,* plays a significant role in anti-hyperglycaemic action. This anti-diabetic effect of ginsenoside Re was, however, not associated with body weight changes, suggesting that other constituents in the extract must be responsible for it (16).

Both ginseng root and ginseng berry possess anti-diabetic activity and a direct comparison between the root and the berry under the same experimental conditions was conducted. The results of the investigation suggest that, compared to ginseng root, ginseng berry exhibits more potent anti-hyperglycaemic activity, and only ginseng berry shows marked anti-obesity effects in ob/ob mice (19).

Wild ginseng is anecdotally thought to be superior to cultivated ginseng as far as its pharmacological properties are concerned but no scientific report on anti-diabetic effect of wild ginseng is on record. It is for this reason that Yun and coworkers investigated the preventative anti-diabetic and anti-obese effects of wild ginseng. Ethanol extract of wild ginseng administered with a high fat diet significantly inhibited body weight gain, fasting blood glucose, triglyceride, and free fatty acid levels in a dose dependent manner. The extract at doses of 250 and 500 mg/kg improved the insulin resistance index of mice by 55% and 61% respectively, compared to the high fat diet control. Ethanol extract of wild ginseng has potential as a preventive agent for type-2 diabetes mellitus and also obesity (21).

Oral administration of *P. ginseng* root (125 mg/kg) to rats three times daily for three days after receiving fructose-rich chow for four weeks reversed the increased glucose-insulin index, which is the product of the areas under the curve of glucose and insulin during the intra-peritoneal glucose tolerance test. The observation indicated the ability of ginseng root to improve insulin sensitivity. Further the plasma glucose concentrations in rats, repeatedly treated with ginseng root, were not elevated as markedly as those of the vehicle-treated group during the fructose-rich chow-feeding period. The time in which the plasma glucose-lowering response to tolbutamide (10 mg/kg ip) receded in fructose-rich chow fed rats was markedly delayed by repeated ginseng root treatment compared to the vehicle-treated group. The plasma glucose-lowering activity of tolbutamide is believed to depend on the secretion of endogenous insulin, which is widely used as an indicator of insulin resistance development. Thus, it provided supportive data that oral administration of *Panax ginseng* root could delay the development of insulin resistance in rats (22).

Results of clinical studies demonstrate that *Panax ginseng* may improve immune function, and conditions associated with diabetes. *Panax ginseng* appears to be well tolerated, although caution is advised about concomitant use with some pharmaceuticals, such as warfarin, oral hypoglycaemic agents, insulin, and phenelzine (20).

The anti-lipolytic effect of ginseng extract in rat adipocytes was studied and it showed that both insulin and ginseng extract inhibited lipolysis. The results of the detailed study suggest that ginseng exerts its anti-lipolytic effect through a signaling pathway different from that of insulin and that anti-lipolytic action of ginseng extract is mediated in part by activating phosphodiesterase 4 in rat adipocytes (24).

1. Ohminami H, Y Kimura, H Okuda, T Tani, S Arichi, T Hayashi; Effects of ginseng saponins on the actions of adrenaline, ACTH and insulin on lipolysis

and lipogenesis in adipose tissue, *Planta Med* **41**(4), 351-58 (1981)

2. Kimura M, I Waki, O Tanaka, Y Nagai, S Shibata; Pharmacological sequential trials for the fractionation of components with hypoglycaemic activity in alloxan diabetic mice from ginseng radix, *J Pharmacobiodyn* **4**(6), 402-09 (1981)
3. Kimura M, I Waki, T Chujo, T Kikuchi, C Hiyama, K Yamazaki, O Tanaka; Effects of hypoglycaemic components in ginseng radix on blood insulin level in alloxan diabetic mice and on insulin release from perfused rat pancreas, *J Pharmacobiodyn* **4**(6), 410-17 (1981)
4. Waki I, H Kyo, M Yasuda, M Kimura; Effects of a hypoglycaemic component of ginseng radix on insulin biosynthesis in normal and diabetic animals, *J Pharmacobiodyn* **5**(8), 547-54 (1982)
5. Yokozawa T, T Kobayashi, H Oura, Kawashima Y; Studies on the mechanism of the hypoglycaemic activity of ginsenoside-Rb2 in streptozotocin-diabetic rats, *Chem Pharm Bull* (Tokyo) **33**(2), 869-72 (1985)
6. Molokovsky DS, OD Barnaulov; Protective properties of tincture of *Panax ginseng* C A Mey leaves in cases of immobilizational stress and alloxan induced diabetes, *Rastit Resurg* **22**(3), 387-95 (1986)
7. Takaku T, K Kameda, Y Matsuura, K Sekiya, H Okuda; Studies on insulin-like substances in Korean red ginseng, *Planta Med* **56**(1), 27-30 (1990)
8. Wang BX, M Yang, YL Jin, ZY Cui, Y Wang; Studies on the hypoglycaemic effect of ginseng polypeptide, *Yao Xue Xue Bao* **25**(6), 401-05 (1990) .[Article in Chinese]
9. Davydov VV, DS Molokovskii, Alu Limarenko; Efficacy of ginseng drugs in experimental insulin-dependent diabetes and toxic hepatitis, *Patol Fiziol Eksp Ter* (5), 49-52 (1990) [Article in Russian]
10. Yang M, BX Wang, YL Jin, Y Wang, ZY Ciu; Effects of ginseng polysaccharides on reducing blood glucose and liver glycogen, *Zhongguo Yao Li Xuo Bao* **11**(6), 520-24 (1990) [Article in Chinese]
11. Ohnishi Y, S Takagi, T Miura, M Usami, M Kako, E Ishihara, H Yano, K Tanigawa, Y Seino; Effect of ginseng radix on GLUT2 protein content in mouse liver in normal and epinephrine-induced hyperglycaemic mice, *Biol Pharm Bull* **19**(9), 1238-40 (1996)
12. Yokozawa T, T Yasui, H Oura; Molecular biological analysis of the effects of ginsenoside-Rb2 on albumin mRNA in streptozotocin-induced diabetic rats, *J Pharm Pharmacol* **48**(7), 763-67 (1996)
13. Chung SH, CG Choi, SH Park; Comparisons between white ginseng radix and rootlet for anti-diabetic activity and mechanism in KKAy mice, *Arch Pharm Res* **24**(3), 214-18 (2001)
14. Xie JT, YP Zhou, L Dey, AS Attele, JA Wu, M Gu, KS Polonsky, CS Yuan; Ginseng berry reduces blood glucose and body weight in db/db mice,

Phytomedicine **9**(3), 254-58 (2002)

15. Dey L, L Zhung, CS Yuan; Anti-diabetic and anti-obese effects of ginseng berry extract: comparison between intra-peritoneal and oral administrations, *Am J Chin Med* **30**(2-3), 187-94 (2002)
16. Attele AS, YP Zhou, JT Xie, JA Wu, L Zhang, L Dey, W Pugh, PA Rue, KS Polonsky, CS Yuan; Anti-diabetic effects of *Panax ginseng* berry extract and the identification of an effective component, *Diabetes* **51**(6), 1851-58 (2002)
17. Wang BX, QL Zhou, M Yang, Y Wang, ZY Cui, YQ Liu, T Ikejima; Hypoglycaemic activity of ginseng glycopeptide, *Acta Pharmacol Sin* **24**(1), 50-54 (2003)
18. Wang BX, QL Zhou, M Yang, Y Wang, ZY Cui, YQ Liu, T Ikejima; Hypoglycaemic mechanism of ginseng glycopeptide, *Acta Pharmacol Sin* **24**(1), 61-66 (2003)
19. Dey L, JT Xie, A Wang, J Wu, SA Maleckar, CS Yuan; Anti-hyperglycaemic effects of ginseng: comparison between root and berry, *Phytomedicine* **10** (6-7), 600-05 (2003)
20. Kiefer D, T Pantuso; *Panax ginseng, Am Fam Physician* **68**(8),*1539-42 (2003)*
21. Yun SN, SJ Moon, SK Ko, BO Im, SH Chung; Wild ginseng prevents the onset of high-fat diet induced hyperglycaemia and obesity in ICR mice, *Acta Pharm Res* **27**(7), 790-96 (2004)
22. Liu TP, JM Liu, JT Cheng; Improvement of insulin resistance by *Panax ginseng* in fructose-rich chow-fed rats, *Horm Metab Res* **37**(3), 146-51 (2005)
23. Luo L, HJ Yin, Y Zhang, YR Jiang, Y Liu, DZ Shi; Effect of ginseng fruit saponins on insulin sensitivity index in high fat-fed rats, *Zhong Xi Yi Jie He Xue Bao* **3**(6), 463-65 (2005) [Article in Chinese]
24. Wang H, LA Reaves, NK Edens; Ginseng extract inhibits lipolysis in rat adipocytes *in vitro* by activating phosphodiesterase 4, *J Nutr* **136**(2), 337-42 (2006)

Panax notoginseng(Burkill) FH Chen (Araliaceae) (Notoginseng, Pseudoginseng, Sanchi)

Notoginseng grows naturally in China and Japan. It is not an adaptogen like ginseng but it is said to invigorate and build blood. In Chinese Medicine, it has acquired reputation for treatment of blood disorders, blood deficiency and particularly for its haemostatic property.

In alloxan-induced diabetic mice, the hypoglycaemic effect of sanchinoside C-1 (ginsenoside Rg-1), one of the major components of *Panax notoginseng*, was evaluated and compared with that of insulin. This compound effectively lowered blood sugar levels of diabetic animals in a dose dependent manner. The action was strengthened with repeated administration and tended to be dose-dependent; its effect lasted for more than four hours and no synergism or antagonism between sanchinoside C-1 and insulin was observed (1, 2).

The role and mechanism of saponins of *Panax notoginseng* in treating patients of type-2 diabetic macroangiopathy were investigated. Serum level of MMP-9 (matrix metallopeptidase 9) and lipid in patients and healthy subjects were measured before and after treatment with *P. notoginseng* saponins. The serum levels of MMP-9, triglyceride, total cholesterol, LDL-cholesterol, VLDL-cholesterol in patients with type 2 diabetic macroangiopathy were improved, while the levels of HDL-cholesterol were decreased. (3).

1. Jiang JX, ZJ Zhang, LH Zhang, MX Huang; Effects of general saponin of *Panax notoginseng* and Sanchinoside C1 on blood sugar in experimental animals, *Yao Xue Xue Bao* **17**(3), 222-25 (1982) [Article in Chinese]
2. Gong YH, JX Jiang, Z Li, LH Zhu, ZZ Zhang; Hypoglycaemic effect of sanchinoside C-1 in alloxan diabetic mice, *Acta Pharmaceutica Sinica* **26**(2), 81-85 (1991) [Article in Chinese]
3. Liu KZ, JB Li, HL Lu, M Han; Effects of Astragalus and saponins of *Panax notoginseng* on MMP-9 in patients with type 2 diabetic macroangiopathy, *Zhongguo Zhong Yao Za Zhi* **29**(3), 264-66 (2004) [Article in Chinese]

Panax quinquefolius Linn. (Araliaceae)
(American ginseng)

Panax quinquefolius is an herbaceous perennial that is native to eastern North America, though it is also cultivated in China. American Ginseng, once widespread in forested regions of Pennsylvania and New York State has become rather rare in most parts of the United States due to over-harvesting. The plant's forked root and leaves were traditionally used for medicinal purposes by Native Americans. Like *Panax ginseng*, American ginseng contains dammarane type ginsenosides as the major biologically active constituents. The ginsenoside Rg1 was found to be present in American ginseng. Plasma glucose levels in resting rats were decreased by saponin extracts of this plant (1).

Like *P. ginseng, P. quinquefolius* also yields some glycans with hypoglycaemic activity (2). These may be seen under "Hypoglycaemic glycans" in the Appendix.

A preliminary short-term clinical study was undertaken to assess whether American ginseng affects postprandial glycaemia in humans. In non-diabetic subjects, no difference was found in postprandial glycaemia between placebo and ginseng when administered together with the glucose challenge. When *P. quinquefolius* (3g) was taken 40 minutes before 25-g oral glucose challenge, significant reductions were observed. In subjects with type-2 diabetes mellitus, the same was true whether ginseng capsules were taken before or together with the glucose challenge (3). The effect of escalating the dose and time of administration of American ginseng in non-diabetic individuals was studied to achieve further improvements in glucose tolerance in a 25 g glucose challenge. In non-diabetic individuals, 3, 6 or 9 g of the drug taken 40, 80 or 120 minutes before a glucose challenge improved glucose tolerance (4).

American ginseng, with a specific ginsenoside profile, was found to decrease postprandial glycaemia significantly. However, a batch of American ginseng was unable to reproduce the postprandial hypoglycaemic effects that were earlier observed. Possible explanations for this discrepancy include marked decrements in total ginsenosides and the key ratios of protopanaxadiol: protopanaxatriol, Rb_1:Rg_1, and Rb_2:Rc. These data suggest that the ginsenoside profile of American ginseng might play a role in its hypoglycaemic effects. The involvement of other components cannot, however, be precluded (6). In contrast to the findings with American ginseng, Asian ginseng (*Panax ginseng*) showed both null and opposing effects on indices of acute postprandial plasma glucose and insulin. Marked differences in ginsenoside content of the two ginsengs might be the explanation (7).

The anti-hyperglycaemic effects of American ginseng berry extract were evaluated in diabetic ob/ob mice. Animals receiving intra-peritoneal injections of the extract (150 mg/kg) for 12 consecutive days showed significantly lower fasting blood glucose levels. Glucose tolerance of the treated animals also improved significantly. In addition, a significant reduction in body weight and a significant increase in body temperature were noticeable. The *in vivo* anti-hyperglycaemic and anti-obese activity of American ginseng berry extract may prove to be of clinical importance in the prevention and treatment of type-2 diabetes (5). The anti-hyperglycaemic effect of a polysaccharide fraction from American ginseng berry extract was evaluated in diabetic ob/ob mice. Animals receiving intra-peritoneal injections of the polysaccharides (150 mg/kg and 50 mg/kg b.w.) for 10 consecutive days showed significantly lower fasting blood glucose levels compared to the vehicle-treated animals on day 5. On day 10, the 150 mg/kg dose group became virtually normoglycaemic. Interestingly, the fasting blood glucose levels stayed lower even after cessation of polysaccharide treatment and returned to control concentration on day 30. Data from the intra-peritoneal glucose tolerance test revealed a significant improvement in glucose tolerance in animals, receiving both 50 and 150 mg/kg polysaccharide doses. The findings of the investigation revealed a potential clinical utility of the polysaccharide fraction from American ginseng berry extract in treating diabetic patients (9).

High performance liquid chromatography of American ginseng leaf extract detected the presence of six major ginsenosides (Rb_1, Rb_2, Rc, Rd, Re, and Rg_1). Like American ginseng root and berry extracts, the leaf extract of the plant also showed a significant anti-hyperglycaemic and thermogenic activity in diabetic ob/ob adult mice and was considered to be beneficial in the management of type-2 diabetes (8).

The effects of eight popular ginseng types (American, American-wild, Asian, Asian-red, Vietnamese-wild, Siberian, Japanese-rhizome, and Sanchi ginsengs) on postprandial plasma glucose and insulin indices were assessed linking effects to ginsenoside profiles. Ginseng was found to have variable glycaemic effects, in which the protopanaxadiol : protopanaxatriol ginsenoside ratio might be involved. But the low variance suggests the involvement of other unmeasured ginsenoside or non-ginsenoside components (10).

1. Martinez B, EJ Staba; The physiological effects of Aralia, Panax and Eleutherococcus on exercised rats, *Jpn J Pharmacol* .**35**(2), 79-85 (1984)
2. Oshima Y, K Sato, H Hikino; Isolation and hypoglycaemic activity of quinquefolans A, B, and C, glycans of *Panax quinquefolium* roots, *J Nat Prod* **50**(2), 188-90 (1987)
3. Vuksan V, JL Sievenpiper, VY Koo, T Francis, U Beljan-Zdravkovic, Z Xu, E Vidgen; American ginseng (*Panax quinquefolius* L) reduces postprandial glycaemia in nondiabetic subjects and subjects with type-2 diabetes mellitus, *Arch Intern Med* **160**(7), 1109-13 (2000)
4. Vuksan V, MP Stavro, JL Sievenpiper, VY Koo, F Wong, U Beljan-Zdravkovic, T Francis, AL Jenkins, LA Leiter, RG Josse, Z Xu; American ginseng improves glycaemia in individuals with normal glucose tolerance: effect of dose and time escalation, *J Am Coll Nutr* **19**(6), 738-44 (2000)
5. Xie JT, HH Aung, JA Wu, AS Attel, CS Yuan; Effects of American ginseng berry extract on blood glucose levels in ob/ob mice, *Am J Chin Med* **30**(2-3), 187-94 (2002)
6. Sievenpiper JL, JT Arnason, LA Leiter, V Vuksan; Variable effects of American ginseng: a batch of American ginseng (*Panax quinquefolius* L.) with a depressed ginsenoside profile does not affect postprandial glycaemia, *Eur J Clin Nutr* **57**(2), 243-48 (2003)
7. Sievenpiper JL, JT Arnason, LA Leiter, V Vuksan; Null and opposing effects of Asian ginseng (*Panax ginseng* C.A. Meyer) on acute glycaemia: results of two acute dose escalation studies, *J Am Coll Nutr* **22**(6), 524-32 (2003)
8. Xie JT, SR Mehendale, A Wang, AH Han, JA Wu, J Osinski, CS Yuan; American ginseng leaf: ginsenoside analysis and hypoglycaemic activity, *Pharmacol Res* **45**(2), 113-17 (2004)
9. Xie JT, JA Wu, S Mehendale, HH Aung, CS Yuan' Anti-hyperglycaemic effect of the polysaccharides fraction from American ginseng berry extract in ob/ob mice, *Phytomedicine* **11**(2-3), 182-87 (2004)
10. Sievenpiper JL, JT Arnason, LA Leiter, V Vuksan; Decreasing, null and increasing effects of eight popular types of ginseng on acute postprandial glycaemic indices in healthy humans: the role of ginsenosides, *J Am Coll Nutr* **23**(3), 248-58 (2004)

Pandanus odorus **Ridl. (Pandanaceae)**
(Fragrant Screwpine, Thai name: Bai Toey)

Pandanus odorus is the only *Pandanus* species with fragrant leaves. Like *Murraya koenigii* commonly known as curry leaves in India, the fragrant pandan leaves are very much needed for their culinary usages in Malaysia, Indonesia, Thailand, Singapore and Sri Lanka.

Hypoglycaemic effect of aqueous extract of the root of *P. odorus* was examined in normal and streptozotocin-induced-diabetic rats. Oral administration of the extract (0.5g/kg) significantly lowered the plasma glucose level in diabetic rats but not significantly in normal rats. In oral glucose tolerance test, an administration of the extract at a dose of 0.5g/kg p.o. significantly lowered the plasma glucose level in normal as well as in diabetic rats. Repeated administration of the extract at doses of 0.25 and 0.5 g/kg p.o. for 7days produced a significant hypoglycaemic effect in diabetic rats. The LD_{50} after oral administration was over 8 g/kg in both sexes of rat and mice (1). Oral administration of 4-hydroxybenzoic acid, a constituent of *P. odorus*, caused a decrease in plasma glucose levels dose-dependently in diabetic rats. The constituent did not affect serum insulin level and liver glycogen content in the diabetic model, but increased glucose consumption in normal and diabetic rat diaphragms. The results suggest that 4-hydroxybenzoic acid produces a hypoglycaemic effect mediated by an increase in the peripheral glucose consumption (2). Oral administration of 4-hydroxybenzoic acid (5 mg/kg) also showed a hypoglycaemic effect in normal rats. Additionally, the compound increased serum insulin levels and hepatic glycogen content in normal rats (3).

1. Peungvicha P, SS Thirawarapan, H Watanabe; Hypoglycaemic effect of water extract of the root of *Pandanus odorus* RIDL, *Biol Pharm Bull* **19**(3), 364-66 (1996)
2. Peungvicha P, SS Thirawarapan, H Watanabe; Possible mechanism of hypoglycaemic effect of 4-hydroxybenzoic acid, a constituent of *Pandanus odorus* root, *Jpn J Pharmacol* **78**(3), 395-98 (1998)
3. Peungvicha P, R Temsiririrkkul, JK Prasain, Y Tezuka, S Kadota, SS Thirawarapan, H Watanabe; 4-Hydroxybenzoic acid: a hypoglycaemic constituent of aqueous extract of *Pandanus odorus* root, *J Ethnopharmacol* **62**(1), 79-84 (1998)

Parkia speciosa **Hassk. (Fabaceae)**
(Stink bean)

Parkia speciosa is a plant that bears long, flat edible beans with bright green seeds with a rather peculiar smell. They are popular in southern Thailand, Burma, Malaysia, Indonesia and North-eastern India. Oral administration of the chloroform extract of the empty pods significantly reduced the blood sugar levels of alloxan-induced diabetic rats. Activity-guided fractionation of the extract gave stigmast-4-

en-3-one, which produced 84% lowering of blood sugar levels at a dose of 100 mg/kg body weight. The minimum effective dose, capable of producing significant decrease of blood sugar levels, was found to be 50 mg/kg. However, it did not affect blood sugar levels of normal rats.

Jamaluddin F, S Mohamed, Md. N Lajis, Hypoglycaemic effect of Stigmast-4-en-3-one, from *Parkia speciosa* empty pods, *Food Chem* **54**(1), 9-13 (1995)

Parmentiera edulis DC (Bignoniaceae) (Candle tree)

This is an ornamental tree of Mexico and Guatemala but it grows in a wide range of climatic conditions, particularly in high-rainfall forests. The interesting shape of its leaves and the greenish cream flowers that grow directly from the stems makes the plant interesting. Its fruits are juicy with a sweet flavour of sugar cane and resemble a greenish yellow cucumber.

The administration of chloroform extract of the dried fruits of *P. edulis* (300 mg/kg) to diabetic mice decreased the blood glucose levels by 43.75% compared to a fall by 29.61% in normal mice (1). Hypoglycaemic activity-guided fractionation of the extract led to the isolation of one guaianolide (lactucin-8-O-methylacrylate), which was found to lower blood sugar levels after administration to alloxan-induced diabetic mice (2).

1. Perez-Gutierrez RM, C Perez-Gonzalez, MA Zavala-Sanchez, S Perez-Gutierrez; Hypoglycaemic activity of *Bouvardia terniflora, Brickellia veronicaefolia,* and *Parmentiera edulis, Salud Publica Mex* **40**(4), 354-58 (1998) [Article in Spanish]
2. Perez RM, C Perez, MA Zavala, S Perez, H Hernandez, F Lagunes; Hypoglycaemic effects of lactucin-8-O-methylacrylate of *Parmentiera edulis* fruit, *J Ethnopharmacol* **71**(3), 391-94 (2000)

Paronychia argentea Lam. (Caryophyllaceae)

Paronychia argentea is one of the plants widely used for their hypoglycaemic activity in Jordan. The plant was tested for its *alpha*-amylase inhibitory activity *in vitro* and for its hypoglycaemic activity in normoglycaemic and streptozotocin-induced hyperglycaemic rats. Although the plant has been advocated for its hypoglycaemic effects in Jordanian traditional herbal medicine; it failed to show significant hypoglycaemic activity compared to the untreated animals but showed significant *alpha* amylase inhibitory activity (1). No hypoglycaemic activity was also observed in normoglycaemic and alloxan-induced hyperglycaemic rabbits by intranasal administration of the crude plant extract (10%) in a vehicle containing 5% (w/w) Pluronic F127 (2).

1. Hamdan II, FU Afifi; Studies on the *in vitro* and *in vivo* hypoglycaemic activities of some medicinal plants used in treatment of diabetes in Jordanian traditional medicine, *J Ethnopharmacol* **93**(1), 117-21 (2004)

2. Afifi FU, B Al-Khalidi, E Khalil; Studies on the *in vivo* hypoglycaemic activities of two medicinal plants used in the treatment of diabetes in Jordanian traditional medicine following intranasal administration, *J Ethnopharmacol* **100**(3), 314-18 (2005)

Petiveria alleaceae Linn. (Phytolaccaceae) (Anamu))

Petiveria alliacea is a perennial bush plant that grows widely in Brazil. The roots and leaves of the plant have been used in folk medicine for the management of a variety of ailments. Oral administration of extracts from leaves and stem powder of the plant in male Balb/C mice (20 g), fasted for 48 hours, was found to produce a decrease of blood sugar concentration one hour after oral administration. The existence of possible hypoglycaemic active principle in the leaves and stems of the plant was thus verified.

Lores RI, M Cires Pujol; *Petiveria alleaceae* L. (anamu): Study of the hypoglycaemic effect, *Med Interne* **28**(4), 347-52 (1990)

Petroselinum crispum (Mill.) Nyman ex A.W.Hill (Apiaceae / Umbelliferae) (Parsley)

Parsley is used for its leaf in the same way as coriander, which is also known as Chinese parsley, although it has a milder flavour. The herbs have similar-shaped leaves and can be used similarly. Parsley is one of the medicinal herbs used by diabetics in Turkey. The effect of feeding parsley on diabetes-induced impairments in rat skins was investigated. Administration of parsley extract failed to inhibit non-enzymatic glycosylation of skin proteins and lipid peroxidation but inhibited the increase in blood glucose (1). The effect of administration of parsley extract on diabetes-induced impairments in rat lenses was investigated. Administration of parsley extract did neither prevent a decrease in glutathione nor an increase in protein glycation, although it did significantly prevent an increase in blood glucose (2). Further study on this plant drug suggested that Parsley extract can provide blood glucose homeostasis but cannot regenerate *beta*-cells of the endocrine pancreas (3).

The morphological and biochemical effects of parsley on liver tissue were studied. Degenerative changes, observed in the hepatocytes of diabetic rats, were significantly reduced or absent in the hepatocytes of diabetic rats, treated with parsley. Diabetic rats treated with parsley also showed significantly lower levels of blood glucose, alanine transaminase and alkaline phosphatase indicating the hepatoprotective effect of parsley (4).

1. Tunali T, A Yarat, R Yanardag, F Ozcelik, O Ozsoy, G Ergenekon, N Emekli; Effect of parsley (*Petroselinum crispum*) on the skin of STZ induced diabetic rats, *Phytother Res* **13**(2), 138-41 (1999)
2. Ozcelik F, A Yarat, R Yanardag, T Tunali, O Ozsoy, N Emekli, A Ustuner; Limited effects of parsley (*Petroselinum crispum*) on protein glycation and glutathione in lenses of streptozotocin-induced diabetic rats, *Pharmaceut Biol* **39**(3), 230-33 (2001)
3. Yanardag R, S Bolkent, A Tabakoglu-Oguz, O Ozsoy-Sacan; Effects of *Petroselinum crispum* extract on pancreatic B cells and blood glucose of streptozotocin-induced diabetic rats, *Biol Pharm Bull* **26**(8), 1206- 10 (2003)
4. Bolkent S, R Yanardag, O Ozsoy-Sacan, O Karabulut-Bulan; Effects of parsley (*Petroselinum crispum*) on the liver of diabetic rats: a morphological and biochemical study, *Phytother Res* **18**(12), 996-99 (2004)

Peucedanum japonicum Thunb. (Apiaceae / Umbelliferae)

The plant grows in China, Japan, Korea and the Phillipines. While some members of the genus are known to cause photo-sensitivity and/or dermatitis, no toxicity has yet been reported for this species. Anti-diabetic activity-guided fractionation of the ethanol extract of the plant led to the isolation of peucedanol-7-O-β-D-glucopyranoside and myo-inositol as active compounds. Both the compounds significantly inhibited postprandial hyperglycaemia.

Lee SO, SZ Choi, JH Lee, SH Chung, SH Park, HC Kang, EY Yang, HJ Cho, KR Lee; Anti-diabetic coumarin and cyclitol compounds from *Peucedanum japonicum, Arch Pharm Res* **27**(12), 1207-10 (2004)

Phaseolus vulgaris Linn. (Fabaceae) (Kidney bean, H. Rajmah)

Phaseolus vulgaris, is an annual plant that is now grown worldwide for its edible bean. Twenty five patients with diabetes mellitus showed a highly significant reduction in blood glucose response when carbohydrates were taken in the form of 'Rajmah' (*Phaseolus vulgaris*), compared with equivalent amount of carbohydrates in the form of wheat or rice (1). An *alpha*-amylase inhibitor prepared from cranberry bean was examined for its *in vivo* action on pancreatic *alpha*-amylase in rat small intestine. The purified preparation from cranberry bean served as a potent inhibitor of rat pancreatic *alpha*-amylase (2). The acute oral administration of the purified inhibitor (50 mg/kg b.w.) to adult Wistar rats together with a starch load (2 g/kg b.w. suspended in saline) reduced the increase in glycaemia over the basal value without modifying the insulin response. The prolonged administration of this *alpha*-

amylase inhibitor was found to reduce blood glucose levels and body-weight gain in Wistar rats (9).

Alterations in the level of insulin receptor and GLUT-4 mRNA in skeletal muscle from rats, fed a kidney bean (*P. vulgaris*) diet, were studied. A decline in the level of circulating insulin was observed in rats fed a diet containing kidney bean. The diet caused an increase in the level of mRNAs for the insulin receptor and GLUT-4 in the gastrocnemius muscle. From the results of the investigation it has been proposed that a component of kidney beans, most likely the lectin phytohaemagglutinin, has systemic effects which lead to changes in expression of the insulin receptor and GLUT-4 genes and to the sensitivity of muscle to insulin (3).

Oral administration of an aqueous extract of *P. vulgaris* pods (200 mg/kg b.w.) for 45 days significantly reduced the elevated blood glucose, serum triglycerides, free fatty acids, phospholipids, total cholesterol, VLDL-cholesterol, and LDL-cholesterol in rats with streptozotocin-induced diabetes. The extract also caused a significant reduction in thiobarbituric acid reactive substances and hydroperoxides, vitamin E, and ceruloplasmin. A significant increase in reduced glutathione, superoxide dismutase, catalase, glutathione peroxidase and glutathione-S-transferase in the liver and kidneys of rats was also observed in streptozotocin-induced diabetic rats, treated with the extract. The extract thus showed antioxidant and anti-hyperlipidaemic properties in addition to anti-diabetic action (4, 5).

Changes in the structural and functional properties of collagen caused by advanced glycation might be of importance for the etiology of late complications in diabetes. In diabetic rats, collagen content as well as its degree of cross-linking was increased. Investigation showed that administration of *P. vulgaris* pod extract (200 mg/kg b.w.) for 45 days to streptozotocin-diabetic rats significantly reduced the accumulation and cross-linking of collagen. *P. vulgaris* pod extract was thus found to show a positive influence on the content of collagen and its properties in streptozotocin-diabetic rats (6). Oral administration of aqueous extract of *P, vulgaris* pods (200 mg/kg) to diabetic animals for 45 days resulted in a significant decrease in blood glucose, glycosylated haemoglobin and significant increase in total haemoglobin and plasma insulin. The decreased activities of the lipogenic enzyme and hexokinase and the increased activities of gluconeogenic enzymes in the diabetic liver were reversed to near normal levels by administration of the extract to diabetic animals (7). Oral administration of the aqueous extract of *P. vulgaris* pods (200 mg/kg b.w.) for 45 days to diabetic rats also prevented the fatty acid changes produced during diabetes (8).

1. Dilwari JB, VK Ajit Kumar, S Khurana, R Bhatnagar, RJ Dash; Effect of legumes on blood sugar in diabetes mellitus, *Indian J Med Res* **85**(Feb), 184-87 (1987)

2. Kotaru M, K Iwami, HY Yeh, F Ibuki; *In vivo* action of *alpha*-amylase inhibitor

from cranberry bean (*Phaseolus vulgaris*) in rat small intestine, *J Nutr Sci Vitaminol* (Tokyo) **35**(6), 579-88 (1989)

3. Knott RM, G Grant, S Bardocz, A Pusztai, AF de-Carvalho, JE Hesketh; Alterations in the level of insulin receptor and GLUT-4 mRNA in skeletal muscle from rats fed a kidney bean (*Phaseolus vulgaris*) diet, *Int J Biochem* **24**(6), 897-902 (1992)
4. Venkateswaran S, L Pari, G Saravanan; Effect of *Phaseolus vulgaris* on circulatory antioxidants and lipids in rats with streptozotocin-induced diabetes, *J Med Food* **5**(2), 97-103 (2002)
5. Venkateswaran S, L Pari; Antioxidant effect of *Phaseolus vulgaris* in streptozotocin-induced diabetic rats, *Asia Pac J Clin Nutr* **11**(3), 206-09 (2002)
6. Pari L, S Venkateswaran; Effect of an aqueous extract of *Phaseolus vulgaris* on the properties of tail tendon collagen of rats with streptozotocin-induced diabetes, *Braz J Med Biol Res* **36**(7), 861-70 (2003)
7. Pari L, S Venkateswaran; Effect of an aqueous extract of *Phaseolus vulgaris* on plasma insulin and hepatic key enzymes of glucose metabolism in experimental diabetes, *Pharmazie* **58**(12), 916-19 (2003)
8. Pari L, S Venkateswaran; Protective role of *Phaseolus vulgaris* on changes in the fatty acid composition in experimental diabetes, *J Med Food* **7**(2), 204-09 (2004)
9. Tormo MA, I Gil-Exojo, A Romero de Tejada, JE Campillo; Hypoglycaemic and anorexigenic activities of an *alpha*-amylase inhibitor from white kidney beans (*Phaseolus vulgaris*) in Wistar rats, *Br J Nutr* **92**(5), 785-90 (2004)

***Phoenix dactylifera* Linn. (Arecaceae)
(Date palm, H. Khajur)**

Phoenix dactylifera, the second most well-known palm after the cocoanut (*Cocos nucifera*), produces dates. It is rather common in the Middle-east, and northern African desert regions. Of the different varieties, Khalas dates are the favourites for their delicious taste and succulence. The glycaemic index of Khalas variety of date, alone and in mixed meals with plain full-milk yoghurt was examined. Results of investigation showed that Khalas dates, when eaten alone or in mixed meals with plain yoghurt have low glycaemic indices. The consumption of dates may be of benefit in glycaemic and lipid control of diabetic patients. The consumption of dates in mixed meals with yoghurt appears to have a minimal effect on the glycaemic index.

Miller CJ, EV Dunn, IB Hashim; The glycaemic index of dates and date/yoghurt mixed meals: Are dates 'the candy that grows on trees', *Eur J Clin Nutr* **57**(3), 427-30 (2003)

Phyllanthus amarus Schumach. & Thonn. (Phyllanthaceae / Euphorbiaceae) (Shatterstone, S. Bahupatra)

Phyllanthus amarus is now officially known as a variety of *Phyllanthus niruri*. It has also been reported to be synonymous with *P. niruri*. Phyllanthus grows in India, China, and tropical regions ranging from the Philippines to Cuba. The plant is a traditional ayurvedic herb used in southern India for the treatment of jaundice.

Hypoglycaemic, diuretic and hypotensive effects of a preparation of whole plant of *Phyllanthus amarus* were evaluated in nine mild hypertensive patients four of which were also suffering from diabetes mellitus. These patients exhibited significant lowering of blood sugar levels and systolic blood pressure along with an increase in 24 hours urine volume following 10 days of treatment. No adverse effects were noted in these patients (1).

Aqueous extract of aerial parts of *P. amarus* (0.1 and 1 g/kg b.w.) significantly enhanced the clearance of glucose from the blood during oral glucose tolerance test in normal fasted rabbits. However, the extract did not affect the blood sugar levels in unfed rabbits. Methanol extract of the aerial parts (1 g/kg b.w.) of the plant was ineffective during oral glucose tolerance test. It was suggested that aqueous extract of the plant contained hypoglycaemic principles as claimed by traditional healers (2).

The effect of *P. amarus* aqueous extract on blood glucose level was studied in non-insulin dependent diabetic patients. From the results of the investigation it was concluded that one week treatment with the aqueous extract of the plant was incapable of lowering both fasting and postprandial blood glucose levels of non-insulin dependent diabetic patients (3).

Methanol extract of *P. amarus* was found to have potential anti-oxidant activity as it could inhibit lipid peroxidation, and scavenge hydroxyl and superoxide radicals *in vitro*. The amount required for 50% inhibition of lipid peroxide formation was 104 μg/ml and the concentrations needed to scavenge hydroxyl and superoxide radicals were 117 and 19 μg/ml, respectively. The extract was found to reduce the blood sugar in alloxan diabetic rats. Continued administration of the extract (1000 mg/kg b.w.) for 15 days produced significant reduction in blood sugar. On 18th day after alloxan administration, blood sugar level was almost similar to normal (4).

1. Srividya N, S Periwal; Diuretic, hypotensive and hypoglycaemic effect of *Phyllanthus amarus*, *Indian J Exp Biol* **33**(11), 861-64 (1995)
2. Moshi MJ, FC Uiso, RLA Mahunnah, SR Malele, ABM Swai; A study of the effect of *Phyllanthus amarus* extracts on blood glucose in rabbits, *Int J Pharmacogn* **35**(2), 167-73 (1997)

3. Moshi MJ, JJ Lutale, GH Rimoy, ZG Abbas, RM Josiah, AB Swai; The effect of *Phyllanthus amarus* aqueous extract on blood glucose in non-insulin dependent diabetic patients, *Phytother Res* **15**(7), 577-80 (2001)

4. Raphael KR, MC Sabu, R Kuttan; Hypoglycaemic effect of methanol extract of *Phyllanthus amarus* Schum & Thonn on alloxan induced diabetes mellitus in rats and its relation with antioxidant potential, *Indian J Exp Biol* **40**(8), 905-09 (2002)

Phyllanthus fraternus G L Webster (Phyllanthaceae/Euphorbiaceae)

It is probably native to Western India and Pakistan. The flowers and fruits of the plant are borne on the lower side of the leaf-stalk. Oral administration of flavonoids FG-1 and FG-2, isolated from the water-soluble fraction of the ethanol extract of *Phyllanthus fraternus*, exhibited significant hypoglycaemic activity in alloxan-induced diabetic rats. The flavonoid FG-2 was found to be comparatively more effective than FG-1.

Hukari VI, GA Kalyani, HK Kakarani; Hypoglycaemic activity of the flavonoids of *Phyllanthus fraternus* in rats, *Fitoterapia* **59**(1), 68-70 (1988)

Phyllanthus niruri Linn. (Phyllanthaceae) Syn. *P. amaras* (H. Bhuiamla)

Alcoholic extract of leaves of *Phyllanthus niruri* (250 mg/kg p.o.) significantly lowered the blood sugar levels of alloxan-induced diabetic rabbits (1). The alcoholic extract reduced the blood sugar level of normal rats dose dependently. The extract also reduced the blood sugar level of alloxan-induced diabetic rats. Continuous administration of the extract, at a dose of 1000 mg/kg b.w., brought down the blood sugar levels of alloxan-induced diabetic rats to near normal levels on the 15th day. The potential anti-diabetic effect of the plant extract was thus confirmed (2).

1. Kumar NG, MC Nair, VR Raghunandan, MK Rajgopalan; effect of *Phyllanthus niruri* leaves in rabbits, *Kerala J Vet Sci* **20**(1), 77-80 (1989)

2. Raphael KR, MC Sabu, R Kuttan; Anti-diabetic activity of *Phyllanthus niruri*, *Amla Res Bull* **20**, ,19-25 (2000)

Phyllanthus sellowianus Muller Arg. (Phyllanthaceae)

Phyllanthus sellowianus is used widely as a hypoglycaemic and diuretic agent in South American folk medicine. Hnatyszyn and co-workers worked on the hypoglycaemic activity of this plant and reported their findings in four different publications. Fresh extracts of the plant was initially reported to exhibit moderate hypoglycaemic activity. Daily oral administration of the aqueous extract (5% w/v) of the stem bark and leaves of *P. sellowianus*, to streptozotocin-induced diabetic rats for 3 weeks significantly lowered their blood glucose levels (1, 2). An aqueous extract (5% w/v) of the stem bark of *P. sellowianus* (400 mg/kg b.w.) produced a significant increase in the urinary excretion after 8 h (3). The aqueous extract of the stem barks of *P. sellowianus* was sequentially extracted with dichloromethane and butanol. The butanol-soluble fraction and the remaining aqueous extract (200 mg/kg p.o.) caused a significant reduction in blood glucose concentration at 6 and 9 h. The reduction in blood glucose levels obtained with these fractions was similar to that observed with glibenclamide (10 mg/kg), a reference hypoglycaemic drug. Phytochemical analysis of the fractions revealed the presence of rutin and isoquercitrin (quercetin-3-O-β-glucopyranoside). The possible involvement of these flavonoids in the hypoglycaemic effect of the active fractions has been discussed (4).

1. Hnatyszyn O, V Martino, G Ferraro, J Coussio; *Phyllanthus sellowianus*: Bioassay in the search for biological activities, *Phytomedicine* **3**(Suppl. 1), p. 232 (1996-97)
2. Hnatyszyn O, J Mino, S Gorzalczany, J Coussio, C A Acevedo, G Ferraro; Anti-diabetic activity of *Phyllanthus sellowianus, International Joint Symposium: Chemistry, Biological and Pharmacological Properties of Medicinal Plants from the Americas, Panama, Republic of Panama,* B-26, February 23-26, 1997
3. Hnatyszyn O, J Mino, S Gorzalczany, J Opezzo, G Ferraro, J Coussio, C Acevedo; Diuretic activity of an aqueous extract of *Phyllanthus sellowianus, Phytomedicine* **6**(3), 177-79 (1999)
4. Hnatyszyn O, J Mino, G Ferraro, C Acevedo; The hypoglycaemic effect of *Phyllanthus sellowianus* fractions in streptozotocin-induced diabetic mice, *Phytomedicine* **9**(6), 556-59 (2002)

Phyllanthus urinaria Linn. (Phyllanthaceae) (Chamber bitter)

Phyllanthus urinaria is a common weed in Suriname and closely related in appearance to *Phyllanthus amarus* and *Phyllanthus niruri*. *P. urinaria* has larger leaves than the latter and its fruit is wart-like. Oral administration of a 50% methanol extract (30 mg/kg) of Siamese *P. urinaria* decreased the blood glucose level by 24% at 3 h after administration. The n-butanol-soluble fraction of the extract was found to decrease blood glucose level by 23% and 39% at the doses of 10 and 30 mg/kg, respectively. In the oral glucose tolerance test, this extract (30 mg/kg, p.o.) inhibited initial increase in blood glucose level but failed to do so in the intra-peritoneal glucose tolerance test. The extract may act *via* facilitation of glucose metabolism and/or the inhibition of glucose absorption in the gut, like biguanides.

Higashino H, A Suzuki, Y Tanaka, K Pootakham; Hypoglycaemic effects of Siamese *Momordica charantia* and *Phyllanthus urinaria* extracts in streptozotocin-induced diabetic rats (the 1st report), *Nippon Yakurigaku Zasshi* **100**(5), 415-21 (1992) [Article in Japanese]

Phytolacca americana Linn. (Phytolaccaceae) (American nightshade)

Activity-guided fractionation of chloroform extract of the roots of *Phytolacca americana* yielded *alpha*-spinasterol, which was proved to be a potent inhibitor of glomerular mesangial cell proliferation caused by high-ambient glucose. *Alpha*-spinasterol also significantly reduced the increases of serum triglycerides, renal weight and urinary protein excretion in streptozotocin-induced diabetic mice. The findings suggest that *alpha*-spinasterol has a significant therapeutic potential to modulate the development and/or progression of diabetic nephropathy.

Jeong SI, KJ Kim, MK Choi, KS Keum, S Lee, SH Ahn, SH Back, JH Song, YS Ju, BK Choi, KY Jung; *Alpha*-spinasterol isolated from the root of *Phytolacca americana* and its pharmacological property on diabetic nephropathy, *Planta Med* **70**(8), 736-39 (2004)

Picralima nitida, (Staph) (Apocynaceae) (Akuamma)

Administration of an aqueous extract *Picralima nitida* seeds, at a dose of 648 mg/kg body weight, produced maximum lowering of blood sugar levels both in normal and alloxanised diabetic rabbits. While the mean fasting blood sugar level of normoglycaemic rabbits was reduced by 19.46 percent within 3 h, that of alloxan-induced diabetic rabbits was reduced by 75.5 percent within 6 hours.

Aguwa CN, CV Ukwe, SL Inya-Agha, JM Okonta; Anti-diabetic effect of *Picralima nitida* aqueous seed extract in experimental rabbit model, *J Nat Remedies* **1**(2), 135-39 (2001)

Picrorrhiza kurroa Royle ex Benth (Scrophulariaceae) (S. Katuka, H. Kutki)

Picrorhiza kurroa has a long, creeping rootstock that is bitter in taste, and grows in rock crevices and moist, sandy soil. The plant is naturally distributed in alpine and temperate regions of the Himalayas from 2500 to 3500 m. It grows in China, Nepal, Sikkim, Bhutan and India. An alcoholic extract of *P. kurroa* was found to lower blood glucose in basal conditions and after a heavy glucose load in normal rats, the maximum reduction in serum glucose being observed after 2 h at a dose level of 75 mg /kg of body weight. The extract was also found to reduce the increase of blood sugar in alloxan-induced diabetic rats (60% reduction at 150 mg/kg b.w.). Chronic administration of the extract significantly reduced the blood sugar in alloxan-induced diabetic rats for 10 days. The extract was also found to reduce the increased serum lipid peroxides in alloxan-induced diabetic animals. *P. kurroa* extract was thus found to ameliorate biochemical damages induced by alloxan in diabetic rats.

Joy KL, R Kuttan; Anti-diabetic activity of *Picrorrhiza kurroa* extract, *J Ethnopharmacol* **67**(2), 143-48 (1999)

Pinus pinaster ssp. ***atlantica*** Villar (Pinaceae) (French maritime pine)

Pinus pinaster ssp. *atlantica* is a pine native to the western Mediterranean region. Pycnogenol is the registered trade name for a special standardized extract from the bark of the French maritime pine and the extract contains a specific mixture of procyanidins. A double-blind, placebo-controlled, randomized, multi-centre study was performed with 77 type-2 diabetic patients to investigate anti-diabetic effects of pycnogenol. Supplementation with pycnogenol (100 mg) for 12 weeks, during which a standard anti-diabetic treatment was continued, significantly lowered plasma glucose levels as compared to placebo. HbA1(c) was also lowered. Pycnogenol significantly decreased endothelin-1 but elevated the level of 6-ketoprostaglandin F1a in plasma compared to placebo. It was observed that supplementation of pycnogenol to conventional diabetes treatment lowers glucose levels and improves endothelial function.

Liu X, J Wei, F Tan, S Zhou, G Wurthwein, P Rhodewald; Anti-diabetic effect of Pycnogenol, French maritime pine bark extract in patients with diabetes type II, *Life Sci* **75**(21), 2505-13 (2004)

Piper sarmentosum Roxb. (Piperaceae) (Thai betel, Thai name: Cha-phloo)

Thai betel leaves are used to make 'miang kham' a delicious Thai recipe. The water extract of the whole plant of *P. sarmentosum* was examined for hypoglycaemic effect in normal and streptozotocin-induced diabetic rats. A single oral administration of the water extract (0.125 and 0.25 g/kg) significantly lowered the plasma glucose level in the normal rats, very much like glibenclamide, at a dose of 5 mg/kg (p.o.) but both the extract as well as glibenclamide failed to show this effect in the diabetic rats. However, repeated oral administration of the water extract (0.125 g/kg) for 7 days produced a significant hypoglycaemic effect in diabetic rats.

Peungvicha P, SS Thirawarapan, R Temsiririrkkul, H Watanabe, J Kumar Trasain, S Kadota; Hypoglycaemic effect of the water extract of *Piper sarmentosum* in rats, *J Ethnopharmacol* **60**(1), 27-32 (1998)

Pisonia morindifolia R. Br. (Nyctaginaceae)

The glycoside, 4'-O-methyl-5'-O-acetylmyricetin-3-O-gluco(2→1) rhamnoside, isolated from the methanol (80%) extract of fresh leaves of *Pisonia morindifolia* , exhibited significant hypoglycaemic activity.

Manogaran S, N Sulochana; Phytochemical and pharmacological activity of *Pisonia morindifolia* Linn., *National Symposium on Emerging Trends in Indian Medicinal Plants*, Lucknow, p.27 (4-O/2), October 10-12, 2003

Pithecellobium jiringa (Jack) Prain (Fabaceae/ Leguminosae)

Aqueous extract of *Pithecellobium jiringa* was found to induce hypoglycaemia in fasted cats.

Thevathasan OI; Hypoglycaemia induced in fasted cats by aqueous extracts of *Pithecellobium jiringa*, *Med J Malaya* **26**(3), 217-19 (1972)

Plantago asiatica Linn. (Plantaginaceae) (Chinese Plantain)

Water-soluble micilages, obtained from plants of different plant families, and their modified products were tested for hypoglycaemic activity in normal mice. The de-acetylated product of Plantago mucilage A, the main mucilage present in the seed of *Plantago asiatica*, showed remarkable hypoglycaemic activity

Tomoda M, N Shimizu, Y Oshima, M Takahashi, M Murakami, H Hikino; Hypoglycaemic activity of twenty plant mucilages and three modified products, *Planta Med* **53**(1), 8-12 (1987)

Plantago ovata Forssk. (Plantaginaceae) (Psyllium, H. Isabgol, Isapgol)

Plantago ovata, a bushy herb growing in sandy, salty soil, is believed to be native to Asia, the Mediterrian Region and North Africa. The plant is now cultivated on large scale in western India because of its wide use in pharmaceutical, cosmetics and food grade industries worldwide. Psyllium seeds have characteristics of mucilage formation and are largely used as dietary fibre to control irregular bowel syndrome and constipation.

Effect of addition of 'Isapgol' (25 g) to control diets (rice, dhal, curds) of 8 normal and 6 non-insulin dependent diabetic volunteers was studied. A negative correlation between the level of dietary fibre and blood glucose levels, in terms of mean percent peak rise, AUC, and percent glycaemic response was observed (1). *Plantago ovata* has been reported to reduce postprandial glucose concentrations in diabetic patients. The efficacy and possible modes of action of hot-water extracts of husk of *P. ovata* were evaluated. The administration of *P. ovata* (0.5 g/kg b.w.) significantly improved glucose tolerance in normal, type-1 and type-2 diabetic rat models. Oral administration of the extract together with sucrose solution suppressed postprandial blood glucose and retarded small intestinal absorption without inducing the influx of sucrose into the large intestine. The extract significantly reduced glucose absorption in the gut during *in situ* perfusion of small intestine in non-diabetic rats. The extract did not stimulate insulin secretion in perfused rat pancreas, isolated rat islets or clonal *beta* cells. Neither did the extract affect glucose transport in 3T3 adipocytes. Aqueous extract of *P. ovata* was thus found to reduce hyperglycaemia in diabetes *via* inhibition of intestinal glucose absorption and enhancement of motility (2).

1. Sreedevi, A Chaturvedi; Effect of vegetable fibre on post prandial glycaemia, *Plant Food Hum Nutr* **44**(1), 71-78 (1993)

2. Hannan JM, L Ali, J Khaleque, M Akhter, PR Flatt, YH Abdel-Wahab; Aqueous extracts of husks of *Plantago ovata* reduce hyperglycaemia in type-1 and type-2 diabetes by inhibition of intestinal glucose absorption, *Br J Nutr* **96**(1), 131-37 (2006)

Plantago psyllium Linn. (Plantaginaceae) (Sand plantain)

Plantago seed, known commercially as black, French or Spanish psyllium, is obtained from *P. psyllium*. It is mainly used as a dietary fibre, which is not absorbed by the small intestine. *P. psyllium* seed husks become mucilaginous and is used when wet and is used as bulk laxative and fibre supplement products. Beneficial effect of vegetable protein diet supplemented with psyllium fibre was studied in 8 diabetic patients with chronic portal-systemic encephalopathy. The use of vegetable diet plus fibre was found to facilitate the treatment of patients with both diabetes and hepatic encephalopathy (1).

The effect of acarbose (an *alpha*-glucosidase inhibitor) and *Plantago psyllium* mucilage on glycaemic index of bread was studied. The study revealed that addition of acarbose or *P. psyllium* to meals may reduce glycaemic index of carbohydrate foods and may help diabetic control (2).

1. Uribe M, M Dibildox, S Malpica, E Guillermo, A Villallobos, L Nieto, F Vargas, G Garcia Ramos; Beneficial effect of vegetable protein diet supplemented with *psyllium plantago* in patients with hepatic encephalopathy and diabetes mellitus, *Gastroenterology* **88**(4), 901-07 (1985)

2. Frati-Munari AC, W Benitez-Pinto, C Raul Ariza Andraca, M Casarrubias; Lowering glycaemic index of food by acarbose and *Plantago psyllium* mucilage, *Arch Med Res* **29**(2), 137-41 (1998)

Pollichia campestris Aiton (Caryophyllaceae)

The plant is distributed in Africa from Ethiopia to South Africa and also in Arabia. Methanol (80%) extract of *P. campestris* (300 mg/kg) reduced the blood-glucose level of normal mice from 2 to 7 h after oral administration and decreased hyperglycaemia 4 h after oral administration in streptozotocin-induced diabetic mice. The extract strongly increased glucose uptake in adipose tissues. Further, the petroleum ether-soluble fraction of the extract inhibited aldose reductase activity.

The findings suggest the anti-diabetic activity of *P. campestris* and support its use in traditional medicine.

Miura T, A Kato; Hypoglycaemic and aldose reductase activity of *Polichia campestris*, *Biol Pharm Bull* **19**(6), 852-54 (1996)

Polygala senega Linn. (Polygalaceae) (Senega snakeroot)

Polygala senega is a perennial herb that grows throughout central and western North America. Senegin-II, the main component of *Polygala senega,* at a dose of 2.5 mg/kg, reduced the level of blood glucose in normal mice 4 hours after intra-peritoneal administration. It also significantly lowered the blood glucose of KK-Ay mice, one of the model animals of non-insulin-dependent diabetes mellitus.

Kako M, T Miura, M Usami, Y Nishiyama, M Ichimaru, M Moriyasu, A Kao; Effect of senegin-II on blood glucose in normal and NIDDM mice, *Biol Pharm Bull* **18**(8), 1159-61 (1995)

Polygala senega* L.** var. ***latifolia Torrey et Gray (Polygalaceae)

E- and *Z*-isomers of Senegasaponins a and b were isolated from the roots of the plant and their structures were fully elucidated. The saponins were found to exhibit potent hypoglycaemic activity in the oral D-glucose tolerance tests in rats. Some structure-activity relationship was also advanced for these saponins (1). The chemical structures of *E* and *Z*-senegasaponins c and *Z*-senegins II, III, and IV, isolated from this plant, were also elucidated. These compounds were found to exhibit hypoglycaemic activity in the oral D-glucose tolerance test. (*E*) and (*Z*)-Senegins II also showed an inhibitory effect on alcohol absorption in rats (2). The n-butanol extract (5 mg/kg) of Senega rhizomes as well as Senegins II and III, isolated from the rhizomes, reduced the blood glucose level of normal mice 4 hours after intra-peritoneal administration. A significant decrease in the glucose level of KK-Ay mice was also observed under similar conditions. The hypoglycaemiceffect of the butanol extract was found to occur without altering the insulin concentration. However, streptozotocin-induced diabetic mice did not experience a change in the blood glucose level after administration of this extract. Senegin IV and desmethoxysenegin II as well as senegose A, an oligosaccharide ester, were inactive when tested against normal mice (3, 4)

1. Yoshikawa M, T Murakami, T Ueno, M Kadoya, H Matsuda, J Yamahara, N Murakami; Bioactive saponins and glycosides. I. Senegae radix. (1): *E*-senegasaponins a and b and *Z*-senegasaponins a and b, their inhibitory effect on alcohol absorption and hypoglycaemic activity, *Chem Pharm Bull* (Tokyo) **43**(12), 2115-22 (1995)
2. Yoshikawa M, T Murakami, H Matsuda, T Ueno, M Kadoya, J Yamahara, N Murakami; Bioactive saponins and glycosides. II. Senegae Radix. (2): Chemi-

cal structures, hypoglycaemic activity, and ethanol absorption-inhibitory effect of *E*-senegasaponin c, *Z*-senegasaponin c, and *Z*-senegins II, III, and IV, *Chem Pharm Bull* (Tokyo) 44(7), 1305-13 (1996)

3. Kako M, T Miura, Y Nishiyama, M Ichimaru, M Moriyasu, A Kato; Hypoglycaemic effect of the rhizomes of *Polygala senega* in normal and diabetic mice and its main component, the triterpenoid glycoside senegin-II, *Planta Med* **62**(5), 440-43 (1996)
4. Kako M, T Miura, Y Nishiyama, M Ichimaru, M Moriyasu, A Kato; Hypoglycaemic activity of some triterpenoid glycosides, *J Nat Prod* **60**(6), 604-05 (1997)

Polygonatum odoratum (Mill.) Druce. (Ruscaceae / Liliaceae) (Fragrant Solomon's-seal)

Polygonatum odoratum (Syn. *Polygonatum officinale* All.) is a colonizing herbaceous plant. Its tubular, scented, green-tipped, white flowers appear in late spring. It is one of three native species of the genus, found in Britain, the others being common Solomon's-seal and whorled Solomon's-seal.

Oral administration of ether extract of *P. officinale* exhibited significant hypoglycaemic activity after one hour. However, its ethanol extract did not elicit hypoglycaemic effect (1). The methanol extract of rhizomes of *P. officinale* (800 mg/kg) reduced the blood glucose of normal mice 4 hours after intra-peritoneal administration, and also significantly lowered the blood glucose of streptozotocin-induced diabetic mice under similar conditions. The extract also suppressed epinephrine-induced hyperglycaemia in mice. The n-butanol-soluble fraction of the methanol extract elicited a significant decrease in the blood glucose level of streptozotocin-induced diabetic mice after 4 hours (2).

Water-soluble extract of Rhizoma Polygonati Odorati significantly lowered hyperglycaemia caused by starch loading in both normal and diabetic mice. Administration of the extract for four weeks reduced fasting blood glucose, decreased glycosylated haemoglobin, and improved the glucose tolerance in diabetic mice. It also reduced both hyperglycaemia and hypertriglyceridaemia of diabetic rats complicated with hyperlipaemia. The aqueous extract of the plant drug was assumed to influence glucose or carbohydrate metabolism of diabetic animals in many ways including inhibiting the activity of *alpha*-glucosidase in digestive canal, and improving the metabolism of glucose and triglyceride (3).

The effects of three steroidal glycosides (SG-100, SG-280, and SG-460), obtained from *P. odoratum,* were studied on insulin secretion, insulin action, and relative glucose uptake in various tissues of 90% pancreatectomized male Sprague-Dawley rats. The study revealed that the glycoside, SG-100 exerts its anti-hyperglycaemic activity by promoting peripheral insulin sensitivity without changing insulin secretion (4).

1. Lee WH, UK Jee, TH Ahu; *Polygonatum officinale* extracts and their interaction with oral hypoglycaemic agents, *J Korean Pharm Sci* **12**(1), 12–22 (1982)
2. Kato A, T Miura; Hypoglycaemic action of the rhizomes of *Polygonatum officinale* in normal and diabetic mice, *Planta Med* **60**(3), 201-03 (1994)
3. Chen H, R Feng, Y Guo, L Sun, J Jiang; Hypoglycaemic effects of aqueous extract of Rhizoma Polygonati Odorati in mice and rats, *J Ethnopharmacol* **74**(3), 225-29 (2001)
4. Choi SB, S Park; A steroidal glycoside from *Polygonatum odoratum* (Mill.) Druce. improves insulin resistance but does not alter insulin secretion in 90% pan-createctomized rats, *Biosci Biotechnol Biochem* **66**(10), 2036-43 (2002)

Polygonatum officinale All. Syn. *Polygonatum odoratum* (Mill.) Druce. (Ruscaceae / Liliaceae)

See *Polygonatum odoratum* (Mill.) Druce.

Polygonatum sibricum Red (Ruscaceae / Liliaceae) (Polygonati rhizoma)

The methanol extract of Polygonati Rhizoma (800 mg/kg) reduced the blood glucose of normal and streptozotocin-induced diabetic mice 4 h after intra-peritoneal administration. However, the hypoglycaemic effects were not accompanied by any alteration in the serum insulin in these mice. The extract also suppressed epinephrine-induced hyperglycemia in mice. One of the active components of the extract of Polygonati Rhizoma was identified as a spirostanol glycoside (1). Using the perfused rat liver *in vitro*, a significant decrease of the hepatic glucose output was observed by the infusion of this plant extract. In addition, the hepatic content of facilitative glucose transporter isoform 2 (GLUT2) mRNA and its protein content in the total membrane fraction from rat liver significantly decreased in the rats, treated intra-peritoneally with the extract when compared to that in the controls. The extract exhibited no apparent stimulatory effect on the insulin secretion from the isolated rat pancreatic islets. From the results it was inferred that the hypoglycaemic effect of methanol extract of Polygonati Rhizoma is derived, at least in part, from the decrease in hepatic glucose output, due presumably to the reduction of GLUT2 mRNA expression and its protein content in total membrane of the liver (2). The methanol extracts of the rhizomes of both *P. sibricum* and *P. officinale* (800 mg/kg) reduced the blood glucose levels in KK-Ay mice (one of the animal models of non-insulin dependent diabetes mellitus) 4 h after intra-peritoneal administration but the hypoglycaemic effect of the latter was more than that of the former. The blood glucose level of mice treated with *P. officinale* significantly decreased in an insulin tolerance test, but those treated with *P. sibricum* did not change. The hypoglycaemic effect of *P. officinale* raised insulin sensitivity (3).

1. Kato A, T Miura; Hypoglycaemic activity of Polygonati rhizoma in normal and diabetic mice, *Biol Pharm Bull* **16**(11), 1118-20 (1993)
2. Kato A, T Miura, H Yano, K Masuda, H Ishida, Y Seino; Suppressive effects of Polygonati rhizoma on hepatic glucose output, GLUT2 mRNA expression and its protein content in rat liver, *Endocr J* **41**(2), 139-44 (1994)
3. Miura T, A Kato; The difference in hypoglycaemic action between Polygonati rhizoma and *Polygonati officinalis* rhizoma, *Biol Pharm Bull* **18**(11), 1605-06 (1995)

Polymnia sonchifolia Poeppig & Endl. (Asteraceae //Compositae) (Yacon, Peruvian ground apple)

Yacon (*P. sonchifolia*) grows in temperate, subtropical and tropical regions and yields sweet, juicy tubers that can be eaten raw or cooked. Yacón tubers store carbohydrates in the form of inulin, a polymer of sucrose that the human body cannot metabolize. It has been suggested that efforts be made to preserve this species as it is claimed to be a promising food for diabetics though it is of little food value.

Zardini E , Ethnobotanical notes on Yacon, *Polymnia sonchifolia* (Asteraceae), *Econ Bot* **45**(1),72 -85 (1991)

Pongamia pinnata (L.) Pierre (Fabaceae./ Leguminosae) (Indian Beech, S. Karanj, H. Sukchain)

It is a tree thought to have originated in India and is found throughout Asia. Small clusters of white, purple, and pink flowers blossom on its branches throughout the year, maturing into brown seed pods. The hypoglycaemic effect of *P. pinnata* flowers was assessed in normal persons (volunteers) as well as in patients suffering from non-insulin dependent diabetes mellitus. The intake of dry flower powder of *P. pinnata* (5 g) with water (200 ml) by normal persons significantly decreased their blood glucose level at 1, 2 and 3 hours. In NIDDM patients, 4 and 5 g of flower powder produced a dose dependent decrease in blood glucose levels. The hypoglycaemic effect in NIDDM patients has been attributed to increased insulin secretion as well as direct insulin-like action.

Akhtar MS; Hypoglycaemic effect of dried (Sukhchain) *Pongamia pinnata* flowers in normal volunteers and non-insulin dependent diabetes mellitus patients, *Hamdard Medicus* **42**(1), 33-36 (1999)

Portulaca oleracae Linn. (Portulacaceae) (Purslane, Pigweed, Urdu: Kulfa)

The weed is a native of India and the Middle East but also found elsewhere. Effects of *P. oleracae* in normoglycaemic and alloxan-treated hyperglycaemic rabbits have been studied.

Akhtar MS, QM Khan, T Khaliq; Effects of *Portulaca oleracae* (Kulfa) and *Taraxacum officinale* (Dhudhal) in normoglycaemic and alloxan-treated hyperglycaemic rabbits, *J Pak Med Assoc* **35**(7), 207-10 (1985)

Potentilla fulgens Wall. ex Lehm (Rosaceae)

Tap roots of *P. fulgens* are traditionally chewed along with betel nut (*Areca catechu*) and betel leaves (*Piper betel*), for various types of ailments. Hypoglycaemic activity of the crude methanol extract of the roots of *P. fulgens* was tested in normoglycaemic and alloxan-induced diabetic mice and it was observed to be dose- and time-dependent. Blood glucose level of both normal and alloxan-induced diabetic mice was significantly reduced following administration of an effective dose of the extract; the effect being more pronounced in alloxan-induced diabetic mice. A prolonged anti-hyperglycaemic action was also observed in the diabetic mice. Glucose tolerance was also improved in both normal and diabetic mice. The results were compared against those of insulin, glibenclamide, metformin, and the probable mechanism of action has been discussed.

Syiem D, G Syngai, PZ Khup, BS Khongwir, B Kharbuli, H Kayang; Hypoglycaemic effects of *Potentilla fulgens* L in normal and alloxan-induced diabetic mice, *J Ethnopharmacol* **83**(1-2), 55-61 (2002)

Poterium ancistroides Desf. (Rosaceae)

Tormentic acid, a triterpene acid, was isolated from *P. ancistroides* and it showed potent hypoglycaemic activity. The activity was compared with glibenclamide (1). A decrease in blood sugar levels along with an increase in circulating insulin levels was observed in normoglycaemic and hyperglycaemic rats following administration of tormentic acid. This triterpene acid also improved the glucose tolerance possibly by enhancing the insulin secretion in response to glucose load. Tormentic acid, however, failed to affect the glucose and insulin levels in streptozotocin-induced diabetic rats. It was inferred from these observations that tormentic acid, like glibenclamide, might be acting by stimulating insulin secretion from islets of Langerhans (2).

1. Villar A, M Paya, MD Hortiguela, D Cortes; Tormentic acid, a new hypoglycaemic agent from *Poterium ancistroides, Planta Med* (1), 43-45 (1986)
2. Ivorra MD, M Paya, A Villar; Hypoglycaemic and insulin release effects of tormentic acid : a new hypoglycaemic natural product, *Planta Med* **54**(4), 282-86 (1988)

Poterium spinosum Linn. (Rosaceae)

Poterium is a genus of thorny herbs or shrubs of the family Rosaceae. *Poterium spinosum* is characteristic of the more humid highlands of the Western mountain range of Lebanon. The plant is used in Bedouin folklore medicine as an anti-diabetic

(4). A triterpene, isolated from the extract of the plant, has been found to affect blood glucose levels (1). Oral administration of the purified chemical as well as of the plant extract (25% water solution) was found to reduce all symptoms of type-2 diabetes (2, 3).

1. Mishkinsky J, E Menezel, FG Sulman; Hypoglycaemic effect of *Poterium spinosum* L. (Rosaceae), *Arch Int Pharmacodyn Ther* **161**(2), 306-13 (1966)
2. Quisenberry TM, G Gyersted; *Poterium spinosum*: A potential cure for diabetes, *Q J Crude Drug Res* **7**, 957-67 (1967)
3. Shani J, B Joseph, FG Sulman; Fluctuations in the hypoglycaemic effect of *Poterium spinosum* L. (Rosaceae), *Arch Int Pharmacodyn Ther* **185**(2), 344-49 (1970)
4. Soumyanath Amla, Traditional Medicine for Modern Times Anti-diabetic plants, CRC Press, 2006

Poupartia birrea (Hochst.) Aubr. (Anacardiaceae) (Marula)

Marula occurs throughout most of sub-Saharan Africa outside the humid forest zone. It is also present in Madagascar and has been introduced to Mauritius. It has also been introduced to Australia and India The main product of the plant is its fruit ('marula plum'), which is a dietary item. Considerable medicinal significance has been attached to the tree, especially to its leaves and bark. The anti-diabetic activity of *P. birrea* leaf extract in normoglycaemic and hyperglycaemic rats was confirmed.

Laurens A, O Giono-Barber, J Mosser, O Sylla; Anti-diabetic activity of leaf extracts of *Poupartia birrea* (Hochst.) Aubr., *Ann Pharm Fr* **42**(6), 547-51 (1984) [Article in French]

Premna integrifolia (Linn.) Roxb. (Lamiaceae / Verbenaceae)

The effect of *P. integrifolia* on blood glucose level in streptozotocin-induced type-1 and type-2 diabetic rats was studied (1). Comparative evaluation of the hypoglycaemic activity of some 30 Indian medicinal plants was made by Kar and co-workers and *P. integrifolia* showed considerable hypoglycaemic activity (2).

1. Alamgir M, B Rokeya, JM Hannan, MS Choudhuri; The effect of *Premna integrifolia* Linn. (Verbenaceae) on blood glucose in streptozotocin induced type 1 and type 2 diabetic rats, *Pharmazie* **56**(11), 903-04 (2001)
2. Kar A, BK Choudhary, NG Bandyopadhyay; Comparative evaluation of hypoglycaemic activity of some Indian medicinal plants in alloxan diabetic rats, *J Ethnopharmacol* **84**(1), 105-08 (2003)

Prosopis farcta (Banks & Sol.) J.F. Macbr. (Fabaceae/Leguminosae) (Syrian mesquite)

Prosopis farcta is used as a hypoglycaemic and hypotensive agent in Jordonian folklore medicine. The hypoglycaemic activity of a lyophilized root extract of the plant was evaluated in normoglycaemic and streptozotocin-induced diabetic rats. Oral administration of the root extract caused significant lowering of blood sugar levels in these animals.

Afifi FU, Hypoglycaemic effects of *Prosopis fracta, Int J Pharmacogn*, **31**(2), 161-64 (1993)

Prunus amygdalus Batsch (Rosaceae) (Almond, H. Badam)

Administration of almond seed (2.5 g) to albino rabbits showed a definite hypoglycaemic action during a two months study. Similar effects were also observed by administration of defatted almond seed (1.22 g) and almond oil (1.28 g), derivable from 2.5 g almond seed. The active factor appeared to be a non-oil fraction, which is only partly soluble in ethyl ether (1).

The effects of almond-enriched diets on insulin sensitivity and lipids in patients with normoglycaemia or type-2 diabetes were studied. The effect of almonds on insulin sensitivity was studied in 20 free-living healthy volunteers who received 100 g almonds/d for 4 weeks. The result showed that almond consumption did not significantly change insulin sensitivity but the body weight increased and total and LDL-cholesterol decreased. It also failed to alter glycaemia in patients with diabetes. It, however, had beneficial effects on serum lipids in healthy adults and produced changes similar to high monounsaturated fat/oils in diabetic patients (2).

1. Teotia S, M Singh; Hypoglycaemic effect of *Prunus amygdalus* seeds in albino rabbits, *Indian J Exp Biol* **35**(3), 295-96 (1997)
2. Lovejoy Jc, MM Most, M Lefevre, FL Greenway, JC Rood; Effect of diets enriched in almonds on insulin action and serum lipids in adults with normal glucose tolerance or type 2 diabetes, *Am J Clin Nutr* **76**(5), 1000-06 (2002)

Prunus davidiana Franch (Rosaceae)

Intra-peritoneal administrations of a methanol extract of *P. davidiana* stems for 6 days not only produced a significant decrease of blood triglycerides and total cholesterol but also reduced an elevated level of glucose in rats with high fat-fed hyperlipaemia. However, rats fed with stock diet were not affected by administration of this extract. It has been suggested that this methanol extract probably increases the metabolic utilization only when fed with excess fat (1). Intra-peritoneal administration of the methanol extract of *P. davidiana* stems as well as prunin (naringenin 7-O-β-D-glucoside), the main flavanone glycoside of the extract, produced a significant hypoglycaemic effect in streptozotocin-induced diabetic rats. It has been suggested that this methanol extract contains one or more hypoglycaemic principles including prunin, which can significantly reduce the levels of blood glucose and total lipids in streptozotocin-diabetic rats (2).

1. Choi JS, SS Suh, HS Young, HJ Park; Hypolipaemic and hypoglycaemic activities of *Prunus davidiana* in high fat-fed rats, *Arch Pharm Res* **14**(1), 44-47 (1991)

2. Choi JS, T Yokozawa, H Oura; Improvement of hyperglycaemia and hyperlipaemia in streptozotocin-diabetic rats by a methanolic extract of *Prunus davidiana* stems and its main component, prunin, *Planta Med* **57**(3), 208-11(1991)

Psacalium decompositum (Gray) H.E. Robbins.& Brett (Asteraceae)

Psacalium decompositum is a Mexican medicinal shrub with anti-diabetic properties. The decoction of the roots of the plant reduced the blood sugar levels of normal mice along with a significant lowering of glycaemic peak in diabetic rabbits (1). The freeze-dried water decoction significantly reduced the blood glucose in normal and mild diabetic mice 240 min after intra-peritoneal administration. It also diminished fasting glycaemia in severe diabetic mice, but the effects were minor. While the main sesquiterpenoid constituents from *P. decompositum* roots failed to show a hypoglycaemic effect on healthy mice, the polysaccharide fractions (F1 and F3) obtained from the freeze-dried water extract significantly reduced the fasting glycaemia in healthy mice. The best results were obtained with the F1 fraction (3). Maceration of the aqueous extract of the roots of *P. decompositum* with methanol yielded a precipitate, which showed significant hypoglycaemic activity in healthy and mild diabetic mice but no significant fall in the levels of blood glucose was observed in animals with severe diabetes. Two polysaccharide components isolated from this fraction showed hypoglycaemic effect when tested in healthy mice (4).

In vivo bioassay-guided fractionation of an aqueous extract of the roots of *P. decompositum* led to the isolation of two new sesquiterpene lactones (3-hydroxycacalolide and *epi*-3-hydroxycacalolide). A 1:1 mixture of the two compounds (1.09 mmol/kg) exhibited anti-hyperglycaemic activity, when tested in ob/ob mice. The known compounds cacalone and epicacalone, isolated from this plant, were found to be inactive but cacalol was active (2).

1. Alarcon-Aguilar FJ, Roman-Ramos R, Jimenez-Estrada M, Ryes-Chilpa R, Gonzalez-Paredes B, Flores-Saenz JL: Effects of three Mexican medicinal plants (Asteraceae) on blood sugar levels in healthy mice and rabbits, *J Ethnopharmacol* **55**(3), 171-77 (1997)

2. Inman WD, J Luo, SD Jolad, SR King, R Cooper; Anti-hyperglycaemic sesquiterpenes from *Psacalium decompositum*, *J Nat Prod* **62**(8), 1088-92 (1999)

3. Alarcon-Aguilar FJ, M Jimenez-Estrada, R Reyes-Chilpa, R Roman-Ramos; B Gonzalez-Paredes, CC Contreras, R Roman-Ramos; Hypoglycaemic activity of root water decoction, sesquiterpenoids, and one polysaccharide fraction from *Psacalium decompositum* in mice, *J Ethnopharmacol* **69**(3), 207-15 (2000)

4. Alarcon-Aguilar FJ, M Jimenez-Estrada, R Reyes-Chilpa, R Roman-Ramos; Hypoglycaemic effect of extracts and fractions from *Psacalium decompositum* in healthy and alloxan-diabetic mice, *J Ethnopharmacol* **72**(1-2), 21-27 (2000)

Psacalium peltatum (Kunth) Cass (Asteraceae)

Psacalium peltatum is a Mexican folk medicinal plant, traditionally used for the treatment of diabetes mellitus. Like *Psacalium decompositum*, aqueous decoction of the roots of *P. peltatum* also reduced the blood sugar levels of normal mice and lowered glycaemic peak in diabetic rabbits but the effect was less prounced than the former (1). Intra-peritoneal administration of aqueous decoction of the plant to normoglycaemic and diabetic mice exhibited hypoglycaemic activity in the studied mice. The methanol and aqueous extracts of the plant also showed similar activity. Chromatographic resolution of methanol extract of the plant led to the separation of two fractions (SFII and SFIII), which significantly reduced blood glucose levels in healthy mice (2).

The aqueous ethanol extract of *P. peltatum* significantly diminished glycaemia in healthy mice at 240 min. In mildly diabetic mice, this extract lowered the basal blood glucose level 120 (16%) and 240 min (54%) after intra-peritoneal administration. The administration of the extract to animals with severe hyperglycaemia did not cause a significant decrease (3). A new carbohydrate, isolated from aqueous extract of roots and rhizomes of the plant, has been determined to have hypoglycaemic activity at doses of 100 mg/kg, comparable to that of tolbutamide and insulin in alloxan diabetic mice. The skeletal structure of the new compound has been established (4).

1. Alarcon-Aguilar FJ, Roman-Ramos R, Jimenez-Estrada M, Ryes-Chilpa R, Gonzalez-Paredes B, Flores-Saenz JL: Effects of three Mexican medicinal plants (Asteraceae) on blood sugar levels in healthy mice and rabbits, *J Ethnopharmacol* **55**(3), 171-77 (1997)

2. Contreras-Weber C, S Perez-Gutierrez, F Alarcon-Aguilar, R Roman-Ramos; Anti-hyperglycaemic effect of *Psacalium peltatum*, *Proc West Pharmacol Soc* **45**, 134-36 (2002)

3. Alarcon-Aguilar FJ, R Roman-Ramos, JL Flores-Saenz, F Aguirre-Garcia; Investigation on the hypoglycaemic effects of extracts of four Mexican medicinal plants in normal and alloxan-diabetic mice, *Phytother Res* **16**(4), 383-86 (2002)

4. Contreras C, R Roman, C Perez, F Alarcon, M Zavala, S Perez; Hypoglycaemic activity of a new carbohydrate isolated from the roots of *Psacalium peltatum*, *Chem Pharm Bull* (Tokyo) **53**(11), 1408-10 (2005)

Psidium guajava **Linn. (Myrtaceae)**
(Guava, H. Amrud)

The apple guava or common guava (*P. guajava*) is a small tree, native to Brazil but it has now spread widely throughout the tropics. The leaf of *Psidium guajava* is used traditionally in African folk medicine to treat a plethora of human ailments, including diabetes mellitus. Anti-diabetic effect of aqueous ethanol (1:1) extract of *P. guajava* leaves was studied in alloxan-induced diabetic rats by Maruyama and co-workers. The extract (200 mg/kg p.o.) significantly inhibited the increase in the plasma sugar levels in alloxanised animals without affecting the insulin levels. It also prevented the increase of sugar levels in diabetic animals during glucose tolerance test. The n-butanol-soluble fraction of aqueous ethanol extract prevented the increase of blood sugar levels and improved the glucose tolerance in diabetic animals at a lower dose (1). A similar observation was made by using a water extract of *P. guajava* leaves. In both acute and sub-acute tests, the water extract, at an oral dose of 250 mg/kg, showed statistically significant hypoglycaemic activity in alloxan-induced diabetic rats (2).

An extract from *P. guajava* leaves exhibited significant inhibitory effect on protein tyrosine phosphatase 1B (PTP 1B). Significant blood glucose lowering effects of the extract were observed after intra-peritoneal injection of the extract at a dose of 10mg/kg in both 1- and 3-month-old Lepr(db)/Lepr(db) mice. Histological analysis of the livers of these mice, treated with the butanol-soluble fraction of the extract, revealed a significant decrease in the number of lipid droplets compared to the control mice. Taken together, it was suggested that the extract from *P. guajava* leaves possesses anti-diabetic effect in type-2 diabetic mice model and these effects are, at least in part, mediated *via* the inhibition of PTP 1B (3).

The hypoglycaemic effect of the plant extract was examined in normal and diabetic rats, using streptozotocin-induced diabetes mellitus model and chlorpropamide (250 mg/kg, p.o.) as the reference hypoglycaemic agent for comparison. Acute oral administrations of the plant extract (50-800 mg/kg, p.o.) caused dose-related, significant hypoglycaemia in normal and streptozotocin-treated diabetic rats. The numerous tannins, polyphenolic compounds, flavonoids, pentacyclic triterpenoids, and other chemical compounds present in the plant are speculated to account for the observed hypoglycaemic effects of leaf extract of the plant (4).

Ethanol extract of the stem bark of the plant exhibited statistically significant hypoglycaemic activity in alloxan-induced hyperglycaemic rats but was devoid of significant hypoglycaemic effect in normal and normal glucose loaded rats (5).

1. Maruyama Y, H Matsuda, R Matsuda, M Kubo, T Hatano, T Okuda; Study on *Psidium guajava* L. (1): Anti-diabetic effect and effective components of the leaf of *Psidium guajava* L. (Part 1), *Shoyakugaku Zasshi* **39**(4), 261-69 (1985)
2. Mukhtar HM, SH Ansari, M Ali, T Naved, ZA Bhat; Effect of water extract of

Psidium guajava leaves on alloxan-induced diabetic rats, *Pharmazie* **59**(9), 734-35 (2004)

3. Oh WK, CH Lee, MS Lee, EY Bae, CB Sohn, H Oh, BY Kim, JS Ahn; Anti-diabetic effects of extracts from *Psidium guajava, J Ethnopharmacol* **96**(3), 411-15 (2005)
4. Ojewole JA; Hypoglycaemic and hypotensive effects of *Psidium guajava* Linn. (Myrtaceae) leaf aqueous extract, *Methods Find Exp Clin Pharmacol* **27**(10), 689-95 (2005)
5. Mukhtar HM, SH Ansari, ZA Bhat, T Naved, P Singh; Anti-diabetic activity of an ethanol extract obtained from the stem bark of *Psidium guajava* (Myrtaceae), *Pharmazie* **61**(8), 725-27 (2006).

Psoralea corylifolia Linn. (Fabaceae Papilionaceae) (Babachi, H. Bawchi, S. Sugandha kantak)

The inhibition of protein tyrosine phosphatase 1B (PTP-1B) is regarded as a viable approach for the treatment and prevention of obesity-associated insulin resistance and type-2 diabetes. The ethyl acetate-soluble extract of the seeds of *P. corylifolia* afforded two protein tyrosine phosphatase 1B inhibitory compounds, psoralidin and bakuchiol, which inhibited PTP-1B activity in a dose-dependent manner.

Kim YC, H Oh, BS Kim, TH Kang, EK Ko, YM Han, BY Kim, JS Ahn; *In vitro* protein tyrosine phosphatase 1B inhibitory phenols from the seeds of *Psoralea corylifolia, Planta Med* **71**(1), 87-89 (2005)

Pterocarpus marsupium Roxb. (Fabaceae) (Indian Kino Tree, H. Vijayasar)

Pterocarpus marsupium is native to India, Nepal, and Sri Lanka. Different parts of the tree have been used for their medicinal properties in Ayurveda. The dark red heartwood of the plant is astringent and well known for its anti-diabetic activity. Clinical and experimental observations on the hypoglycaemic properties of the plant were recorded (1, 2, 8). Anti-hyperglycaemic activity of the extract of *P. marsupium* was studied in experimental albino rats. The extract exhibited significant blood sugar lowering activity and normaoglycemia was maintained till the end of experiment (6). The aqueous extract of the heartwood exhibited anti-diabetic activity in diabetic rats and human beings at a dose of 2 mg/kg (10). Administration of ethyl acetate-soluble fraction of ethanol extract of *P. marsupium* wood to alloxan-induced diabetic rats for 5 days significantly reduced the blood sugar levels along with an increase in insulin levels (9). Vats *et al* reported that the aqueous extract of the plant (1 g/kg p.o.) significantly reduced the blood sugar levels of rats 2 h after oral administration of the extract and also significantly lowered the blood glucose in alloxan-induced diabetic rats from 21 days after daily oral administration of the extract (12). This group also reported increase in activity of hepatic glucokinase, phosphofructokinase and muscle hexokinase and tissue glycogen content in test animals, treated with *P. marsupium*. This can be due to enhanced insulin release or due to insulinomimetic activity of the components, present in the plant (14). An aqueous extract of *P. marsupium* wood was screened for hypoglycaemic activity on alloxan-induced diabetic rats. During both acute and sub-acute tests, the water extract, at an oral dose of 250 mg/kg, showed statistically significant hypoglycaemic activity (17).

Chakravarthy and coworkers reported hypoglycaemic activity of *P marsupium* and located the activity in the flavonoid fraction of its heartwood extract. The active constituent was recognised by these workers as (-)-epicatechin, which showed hypoglycaemic activity in alloxan-induced hyperglycaemic rats (3). However, it was later observed that (-)-epicatechin reversed hyperglycaemia in alloxan-induced diabetic rats, only when given before or within 24 h after the dose of alloxan. No significant difference in blood glucose levels was observed between control and (-)-epicatechin (30 mg/kg, ip, bd)-treated rats when the treatment began 92 h after alloxan. From the findings, the usefulness of (-)-epicatechin in the treatment of diabetes was considered minimal (4). The anti-diabetic effect of (-)-epicatechin, isolated from *P, marsupium* bark, was assessed in streotozotocin-induced diabetic and spontaneously diabetic BB/E rats. This compound failed to reverse established diabetes in either of these experimental models (5). (-) Epicatechin, has been found to be insulinogenic. *In vitro* study also shows its insulin like activities. Like insulin, (-) epicatechin stimulates oxygen uptake in fat cells and tissue slices of various organs, increases glycogen content of rat diaphragm in a dose-dependent manner with corresponding increase in U ^{14}C glucose uptake, and inhibits theophylline-induced lipolysis in isolated fat pads in a dose-dependent manner. Experiments on competitive binding of ^{125}I-insulin and (-) epicatechin to liver cell plasma membrane indicate that insulin does not share binding site with (-) epicatechin. (-) Epicatechin at a concentration of up to 1 mM does not release glucagon from the islets *in vitro*. Thus, (-) epicatechin has insulinogenic as well as insulin-like properties (7). The activity of erythrocyte Ca^{++}-ATPase was found to be significantly lower in type-2 diabetes. Treatment with epicatechin (1mM) resulted in increase of activity of Ca^{++}-ATPase in both normal individuals and type-2 diabetic patients (13).

The effect of the anti-diabetic plant, *P. marsupium*, on the development of cataract was assessed in rats. An aqueous extract of *P. marsupium* (1 g/kg/day) was given to alloxan (120 mg/kg)-induced diabetic rats until the development of cataract. Administration of the plant extract exerted a favourable effect on body weight, blood glucose and anti-cataract effect as evident from decreased opacity index (16).

Water extract of the latex of *P. marsupium* was found to have a potential *alpha*-glucosidase inhibitory activity (15).

Glucose levels in streptozotocin-induced hyperglycaemic rats were measured after intra-peritoneal administration of marsupsin, pterosupin, and pterostilbene, three important phenolic constituents of the heartwood of *P. marsupium*. Marsupsin and pterostilbene significantly lowered the blood glucose level of hyperglycaemic rats, and the effect was comparable to that of metformin (11).

1. Bose SN, GC Sepaha; Clinical observations on the anti-diabetic properties of *Pterocarpus marsupium* and *Eugenia jambolana*, *J Indian Med Assoc* **27**(11), 388-91 (1956)
2. Shah DS; A preliminary study of the hypoglycaemic action of heartwood of *Pterocarpus marsupium* Roxb, *Indian J Med Res* **55**(2), 166-68 (1967)
3. Chakravarthy BK, S Gupta, SS Gambhir, KD Gode; *l*-Epicatechin – A novel anti-diabetic drug, *Indian Drug* **18**(5), 184-85 (1981)
4. Sheehan EW, MA Zemaitis, DJ Slatkin, PL Schiff Jr; A constituent of *Pterocarpus marsupium*, (-)-epicatechin, as a potential anti-diabetic agent, *J Nat Prod* **46**(2), 232-34 (1983)
5. Bone JT, CS T Hii, D Brown, W Smith, SL Howell, Assessment of the anti-diabetic activity of (-)-epicatechin in streptozotocin diabetic and spontaneously diabetic BB/E rats, *Biosci Rep* **5**(3), 215 21 (1985)
6. Apte IC, IP Vaishwanar, B Khannade, SN Jadhav; Studies on anti-hyperglycaemic effect of some indigenous plants, *Indian Drugs* **25**(11), 461–63 (1988)
7. Ahmad F, P Khalid, MM Khan, AK Rastogi, JR Kidwai; Insulin like activity in (-) epicatechin, *Acta Diabetol Lat* **26**(4), 291-300 (1989)
8. Singh DC, BP Sharma; Management of Madhumeha (Diabetes mellitus)by indigenous drugs; Bijayasar and Kushtha, *Aryavaidyan* **4**(1), 21-23 (1990)
9. Ahmad F, P Khalid, MM Khan, M Chaubey, AK Rastogi, JR Kidwai; Hypoglycaemic activity of *Pterocarpus marsupium* wood, *J Ethnopharmacol* **35**(1), 71-75 (1991)
10. Chakrabarti D, A Ghosh, N Banerji, PC Majumder, M Gupta; The hypoglycaemic and anti-ulcerogenic effect of the aqueous extract of the heartwood of *Pterocarpus marsupium* Roxb. (Invited lecture), *Int Conf Curr Prog Med Aromatic Plant Res* , Calcutta, India , p. 21-23 Dec.30, 1994 – Jan. 1, 1995
11. Manickam M, M Ramanathan, MA Jahromi, JP Chansouria, AB Ray; Anti-hyperglycaemic activity of phenolics from *Pterocarpus marsupium, J Nat Prod* **60**(6), 609-10 (1997)
12. Vats V, JK Grover, SS Rathi; Evaluation of anti-hyperglycaemic and hypoglycaemic effect of *Trigonella foenum-graecum* Linn, *Ocimum sanctum* Linn and *Pterocarpus marsupium* Linn in normal and alloxanized diabetic rats, *J Ethnopharmacol* **79**(1), 95-100 (2002)

13. Zaid M, KK Sharma, SJ Rizvi; Effect of epicatechin in modulating Calcium ATPase activity in normal and diabetic human erythocytes, *Indian J Clin Biochem* **17**(2), 27-32 (2002)

14. Vats V, JK Grover, S Yadav; Anti-hyperglycaemic/hypoglycaemic effect of *Pterocarpus marsupium* Linn. in normal and diabetic rats, *National Convention on Current Trends in Herbal Drugs & Annual Conference of Indian Society of Pharmacognosy. Herb: The Natural Alternative,* Gandhinagar, Gujrat, India, p. A-08, Jan. 17-18, 2003

15. Abesundara KJ, T Matsui, K Matsumoto; *alpha*-Glucosidase inhibitory activity of some Sri Lanka plant extracts, one of which, *Cassia auriculata*, exerts a strong anti-hyperglycaemic effect in rats comparable to the therapeutic drug acarbose, *J Agric Food Chem* **52**(9), 2541-45 (2004)

16. Vats V, SP Yadav, NR Biswas, JK Grover; Anti-cataract activity of *Pterocarpus marsupium* bark and *Trigonella foenum-graecum* seeds extract in alloxan diabetic rats, *J Ethnopharmacol* **93**(2-3), 289-94 (2004)

17. Mukhtar HM, SH Ansari, M Ali, ZA Bhat, T Naved; Effect of aqueous extract of *Pterocarpus marsupium* wood on alloxan-induced diabetic rats, *Pharmazie* **60**(6), 478-79 (2005)

Pterocarpus santalinus Linn. (Fabaceae) (Red Sandalwood, S. Rakta chandana)

Pterocarpus santalinus is native to India. It is most commonly found in south and south western India, notably in the state of Karnataka. Ethanol extract of *P. saintalinus* bark (0.25 g/kg b.w.) showed anti-hyperglycaemic activity in diabetic rats but failed to show any hypoglycaemic activity in normal rats. The extract at this dose level was found to be more effective than that of glibenclamide.

Kameswara Rao B, R Giri, MM Kesavulu, C Apparao; Effect of oral administration of bark extracts of *Pterocarpus santalinus* L. on blood glucose level in experimental animals, *J Ethnopharmacol* **74**(1), 69-74 (2001)

Pterospermum acerifolium (L.) Willd. (Malvaceae /Sterculaceae) (Dinner Plate Tree)

Pterospermum acerifolium is a native of North East India; Bangla Desh, Burma and Malayasia and is cultivated in Pakistan and N. America. The tree bears fragrant nocturnal white flowers and yields a reddish wood. A subfraction (E4b) of the ethanol extract of the bark of the plant was tested both for its acute and chronic effects on glycaemic status as well as on lipid levels in type-2 diabetic model rats. The fraction was found to decrease both hyperglycaemia and atherogenic lipids in the plasma of type-2 diabetic model rats.

Murshedd S, B Rokeya, L Ali, N Nahar, A.K. Azad Khan, M. Mosihuzzaman; Chronic effect of *Pterospermum acerifolium* bark on glycaemic and lipidemic status of Type-2 diabetic model rats, *Diab Res Clin Pract* **50**(Suppl.1), 224 (2000)

Pterospermum semisagittatum Buch. Ham (Malvaceae/ Sterculaceae)

The plant grows in India, Bangladesh, Sri Lanka, Myanmar, Thailand and other adjoining countries. Mosihuzzaman and coworkers of Bangladesh published three papers reporting the anti-hyperglycaemic, insulin-like and insulin releasing activity of *Pterospermum semisagittatum* leaves (1-3). The leaves of the plant yielded three megastigmane glycosides of which (*E*)-4-hydroxy-4-[3'-(α-D-glucopyranosyloxy)-butylidene]-3,5,5-trimethyl-2-cyclohexen-1-one showed a significant insulin releasing effect on rat pancreatic islets (3).

1. Rokeya B, SH Khan, NS Chowdhury, L Ali, N Nahar, AK Azad Khan, M Mosihuzzaman; Insulin releasing effects of some pure compounds from *Pterospermum semisagittatum* leaves on isolated rat islets, *Diabetologia* **874,** A 227 (2001)
2. Mamun MIR, B Rokeya, NS Chowdhury, M Muniruzz aman, N Nahar, MU Ahmed, M Mosihuzzaman, L Ali, AK Azad Khan, SH Khan; Anti-hyperglycaemic effect of *Pterospermum acerifolium* Willd. and *Pterospermum semisagittatum* Ham., *Diab Res* **35,** 163-70 (2001)
3. Khan SH; M Mosihuzzaman; N Nahar; MA Rashid, B Rokeya, L Ali; AK Azad Khan; Three megastigmane glycosides from the leaves of *Pterospermum semisagittatum*, *Pharmaceut Biol* **41**(7), 512-15 (2003)

Pueraria lobata (Willd.) Ohwi (Fabaceae / Leguminosae) (Kudzu)

Kudzu is a climbing, woody or semi-woody, perennial vine capable of reaching heights up to 98 ft on trees. It produces purple and highly fragrant flowers. It is native to southern Japan and southeast China in eastern Asia. The name comes from the Japanese word for this plant, *kuzu*.

Effects of puerarin, an active principle contained in the roots of *P. lobata*, on the regulation of glucose metabolism in an insulin deficient state were investigated in cultured myoblast C 2 C 12 cells using glucose uptake as indicator. Puerarin enhanced the uptake of radioactive glucose into C 2 C 12 cells in a concentration-dependent manner but this stimulatory action of puerarin on glucose uptake was reduced in C 2 C 12 cells pre-incubated with the antagonists that block *alpha* 1A - adrenoceptor. The results of the detailed investigation suggest that an activation of *alpha* 1A -AR by puerarin in C 2 C 12 cells may increase the glucose uptake *via* the phospholipase C - protein kinase C pathway (1). The anti-hyperglycaemic action of puerarin, an active principle of the roots of *P. lobata*, was studied in streptozotocin-induced diabetic rats. Bolus intravenous injection of puerarin decreased the plasma glucose concentrations in a dose-dependent manner in streptozotocin-induced diabetic rats, although the effect was much less pronounced in normal rats. Puerarin at a dose of 15.0 mg/kg significantly attenuated the increase of plasma glucose induced by an intravenous glucose challenge test in normal rats. The results of the detailed investigation suggest that puerarin can increase the glucose utilization to lower plasma glucose in diabetic rats lacking insulin (2). Puerarin, at a dose which effectively reduced plasma glucose levels, increased plasma β-endorphin-like immunoreactivity in streptozotocin-induced diabetic rats. Both these effects of puerarin were, however, abolished by pretreatment with prazosin and also by bilateral adrenalectomy in streptozotocin-diabetic rats. Puerarin is considered to activate α_1-adrenoceptors on the adrenal gland to enhance the secretion of β-endorphin to result in a decrease of plasma glucose in streptozotocin-induced diabetic rats (3).

1. Hsu HH, CK Chang, HC Su, IM Liu, JT Cheng; Stimulatory effect of puerarin on *alpha* 1A-adrenoceptor to increase glucose uptake into cultured C2C12 cells of mice, *Planta Med* **68**(11), 999-1003 (2002)
2. Hsu FL, LM Liu, DH Kuo, WC Chen, HC Su, JT Cheng; Anti-hyperglycaemic effect of puerarin in streptozotocin-induced diabetic rats, *J Nat Prod* **66**(6), 788-92 (2003)
3. Chen WC, S Hayakawa, T Yamamoto, HuiChen Su, IM Liu; Mediation of â-endorphin by the isoflavone puerarin to lower plasma glucose in streptozotocin-induced diabetic rats, *Planta Med* **70**(2), 113-16 (2004)

Pueraria thomsonii Benth (Fabaceae / Leguminosae) (Mealy kudzu)

The influence of *Pueraria thomsonii* on insulin resistance of rats, induced by dexamethasone, was investigated. 3T3-L1 adipocytes model of insulin resistance was made by dexamethasone and the change of glucose concentration in cell culture was determined after action of drugs. *P. thomsonii* decreased the concentration of glucose in 3T3-L1 adipocytes culture significantly and improved the sensitivity of 3T3-L1 adipocytes to insulin. The plant drug improved the sensitivity of rats to insulin and diminished the fasting serum insulin and insulin resistance index (1). Compounds that target the peroxisome proliferator-activated receptors PPARα and PPAR gamma are used to correct dyslipidaemia and to restore glycaemic balance, respectively. Because the majority of diabetic patients suffer from atherogenic lipid abnormalities, in addition to insulin resistance, ligands are required that can activate both PPARα and PPAR *gamma*. Extract of *P. thomsonii* was found to significantly activate both PPARα and PPAR *gamma*. Bioassay-guided fractionation resulted in the isolation of daidzein from *P. thomsonii* as the PPAR-activating compound. At low doses, however, daidzein was not sufficiently active (2).

1. Bai HY, WJ Zou, XP Gao; Influence of *Pueraria thomsonii* on insulin resistance induced by dexamethasone, *Zhongguo Zhong Yao Za Zhi* **29**(4), 356-58 (2004) [Article in Chinese]
2. Shen P, MH Liu, TY Ng, YH Chan, EL Yong; Differential effects of isoflavones, from *Astragalus membranaceus* and *Pueraria thomsonii* on the activation of PPAR α, PPAR*gamma*, and adipocyte differentiation *in vitro*, *J Nutr* **136**, 899-905 (2006)

Pueraria thunbergiana (Siebold & Zucc.) Benth. (Fabaceae / Leguminosae)

Pueraria thunbergiana flowers (Puerariae Flos) are used as a therapeutic agent for diabetes mellitus in traditional Korean medicine. 6"-O-Xylosyltectoridin and tectoridin, the flower constituents of *P. thunbergiana*, are metabolized to tectorigenin by human intestinal bacteria. Tectorigenin was found to possess potent hypoglycaemic activity. The flower constituents of *P. thunbergiana* are, therefore, regarded as pro-drugs, which can be transformed to the active agents by human intestinal bacteria (1).

Tectorigenin and kaikasaponin III were isolated from the flowers of *P. thunbergiana*. Intra-peritoneal administration of tectorigenin (5 mg/kg) and kaikasaponin III (10 mg/kg) to streptozotocin-induced diabetic rats for 7 days significantly reduced the blood glucose, total cholesterol, LDL- and VLDL-cholesterol and triglycerides in comparison to the control rats. Tectorigenin also showed *in vitro* antioxidant activity. Tectorigenin and kaikasaponin III also protected vero cell line from injury by hydrogen peroxide. Antioxidant action of these two compounds may contribute to the hypoglycaemic and hypolipidaemic effects. Tectoridin, the glycoside of tectorigenin did not improve hyperglycaemia and hyperlipidaemia (2). Kaikasaponin III, the flower constituent of *P. thunbergiana,* inhibited the formation of malondialdehyde and hydroxy radicals in serum and liver, but promoted superoxide dismutase activity. Low malondialdehyde concentrations and low xanthine oxidase and aldehyde oxidase activities were observed in the kaikasaponin III-treated rats, suggesting that such Phase I enzyme activities are the major source of lipid peroxidation. However, this saponin increased Phase II enzyme activities such as superoxide dismutase, glutathione peroxidase, and catalase, suggesting the activation of free radical-scavenging enzymes. These results suggest that kaikasaponin III may exhibit its hypoglycaemic and hypolipidaemic effects by up-regulating or down-regulating antioxidant mechanisms *via* the changes in Phase I and II enzyme activities (3).

1. Bae EA, MJ Han, KT Lee, JW Choi, HJ Park, DH Kim; Metabolism of 6"-O-xylosyltectoridin and tectoridin by human intestinal bacteria and their hypoglycaemic and *in vitro* cytotoxic activities, *Biol Pharm Bull* **22**(12), 1314-18 (1999)
2. Lee KT, IC Sohn, DH Kim, JW Choi, SH Kwon, HJ Park; Hypoglycaemic and

hypolipidaemic effects of tectorigenin and kaikasaponin III in the streptozotocin-induced diabetic rat and their antioxidant activity *in vitro, Arch Pharmacal Res* **23**(5), 461-66 (2000)

3. Choi J, MH Shin, KY Park, KT Lee, HJ Jung, MS Lee, HJ Park; Effect of kaikasaponin III obtained from *Pueraria thunbergiana* flowers on serum and hepatic lipid peroxides and tissue factor activity in the streptozotocin-induced diabetic rat, *J Med Food* 7(1), 31-37 (2004)

Pulsatilla chinensis (Bunge.) Reg. (Ranunculaceae) (Pulsatillae Radix)

Pulsatilla chinensis is a perennial that grows in dry grassy places and rocky hillsides of North China to Eastern Siberia. Ethyl acetate extract of dried roots of *P. chinensis* showed significant hypoglycaemic effect on alloxan diabetic mice. Bioassay guided chromatographic fractionation of the extract resulted in the isolation of 2β, 3β, 14α, 20, 22R, 25-hexahydroxy-cholest-7-en-6-one as the hypoglycaemic constituent.

Kim HJ, HT Kim, CH Bae, GJ Oh, SK Park, SG Chung, EH Cho; Studies on the hypoglycaemic constituent of Pulsatillae Radix (I), *Yakhak Hoeji* **41**(6), 709-13 (1997)

Punica granatum Linn. (Lythraceae / Punicaceae) (Pomegranate, H. Anar, S. Dadim)

The pomegranate is native to the region from Afghanistan, Iran, and Pakistan and has been cultivated and naturalised over the whole Mediterranean region and also in other countries for its fruits. The extract of *Punica granatum* rind (250 mg/kg b.w.) exhibited significant hypoglycaemic activity in mild diabetic albino rats (1).

Oral administration of the methanol extract of *P. granatum* seed (150, 300 and 600 mg/kg) caused a significant reduction of blood glucose levels in streptozotocin-induced diabetic rats at the end of 12 hours (3).

The effect of concentrated pomegranate juice consumption on lipid profiles of type II diabetic patients with hyperlipidaemia was studied. From the results of the study it was concluded that pomegranate juice consumption may modify heart disease risk factors in hyperlipidaemic patients, and its inclusion in their diets may be beneficial (4).

Male abortive flowers of *P.granatum* (Gulnar farsi) are used for the treatment of diabetes mellitus in Unani system of medicine. Oral administration of its aqueous-ethanol (1:1) extract (400 mg/kg, b.w.) led to significant blood glucose lowering effect in normal, glucose-fed hyperglycaemic and alloxan-induced diabetic rats. The extract showed maximum effect at 400 mg/kg, b.w. (2). Oral administration of methanol extract of pomegranate flowers markedly lowered plasma glucose levels in non-fasted Zucker diabetic fatty rats (a genetic model of obesity and type 2 diabetes), whereas it had little effect in the fasted animals, suggesting that it affected postprandial hyperglycaemia in type-2 diabetes. Pomegranate flower extract demonstrated a potent inhibitory effect on *alpha*-glucosidase activity *in vitro*. The findings strongly suggest that pomegranate flower extract improves postprandial hyperglycaemia in type-2 diabetes and obesity, at least in part, by inhibiting intestinal *alpha*-glucosidase activity (5). Peroxisome proliferator-activated receptor (PPAR)-*gamma* activators are widely used in the treatment of type-2 diabetes, because they improve the sensitivity of insulin receptors. The anti-diabetic activity of pomegranate flower extract may result from improved sensitivity of the insulin receptor as it has been found, by *in vitro* studies, to increase PPAR-*gamma*-dependent mRNA expression in human THP-1-differentiated macrophage cells. The findings indicate that PPAR-*gamma* is a molecular target for *P.granatum* flower extract and gallic acid, the prominent component of the extract (6).

1. Zafar R, J Singh, Anti-diabetic activity of *Punica granatum* Linn., *Sci &Cult* **56**(7), 303-*04* (1990)
2. Jafri MA, M Aslam, K Javed, S Singh; Effect of *Punica granatum* Linn. (flowers) on blood glucose level in normal and alloxan-induced diabetic rats, *J Ethnopharmacol* **70**(3), 309-14 (2000)
3. Das AK, SC Mandal, SK Banerjee, S Sinha, BP Saha, M Pal; Studies on the hypoglycaemic activity of *Punica granatum* seed in streptozotocin induced diabetic rats, *Phytother Res* **15**(7), 628-29 (2001)
4. Esmaillzadeh A, F Tahbaz, I Gaieni, H Alavi-Majd, L Azadbakht; Concentrated pomegranate juice improves lipid profiles in diabetic patients with hyperlipidemia, *J Med Food* **7**(3), 305-08 (2004)
5. Li Y, S Wen, BP Kota, G Peng, GQ Li, J Yamahara, BD Raufogalis; *Punica granatum* flower extract, a potent *alpha*-glucosidase inhibitor, improves postprandial hyperglycemia in Zucker diabetic fatty rats, *J Ethnopharmacol* **99**(2), 239-44 (2005)
6. Huang TH, G Peng, BP Kota, GQ Li, J Yamahara, BD Roufogalis, Y Li; Anti-diabetic action of *Punica granatum* flower extract: activation of PPAR-*gamma* and identification of an active component, *Toxicol Appl Pharmacol* **207**(2), 160-69 (2005)

Pycnanthus angolensis (Welw.) Warb (Myristicaceae)

Pycnanthuquinone A and pycnanthuquinone B (SP-18904 and SP-18905) were isolated from leaves and stems of *P. angolensis* by bioasay-guided fractionation of their ethanol extract, using a diabetic mouse model. The compounds significantly lowered plasma glucose concentration, when given orally to ob/ob or db/db mice both of which are hyperglycaemic and hyperinsulinaemic. The anti-hyperglycaemic actions of the compounds were associated with significant decreases in plasma insulin concentrations, suggesting that both compounds lowered glucose by enhancing insulin-mediated glucose uptake. Pycnanthuquinones A and B are the first representatives of novel terpenoid-type quinones (1. 2).

1. Luo J, J Cheung, EM Yevich, JP Clark, J Tsai, P Lapresca, RP Ubillas, DM Fort, TJ Carlson, RF Hector, SR King, CD Mendez, SD Jolad, GM Reaven; Novel terpenoid-type quinones isolated from *Pycnanthus angolensis* of potential utility in the treatment of type 2 diabetes, *J Pharmacol Exp Ther* **288**(2), 529-34 (1999)
2. Fort DM, RP Ubillas, CD Mendez, SD Jolad, WD Inman, JR Carney, JL Chen, TT Ianiro, C Hasbun, RC Bruening, J Luo, MJ Reed, M Iwu, TJ Carlson, SR King, DF Bierer, R Cooper;, Novel anti-hyperglycaemic terpenoid-quinones from *Pycnanthus angolensis*, *J Org Chem* **65**(20), 6534-39 (2000)

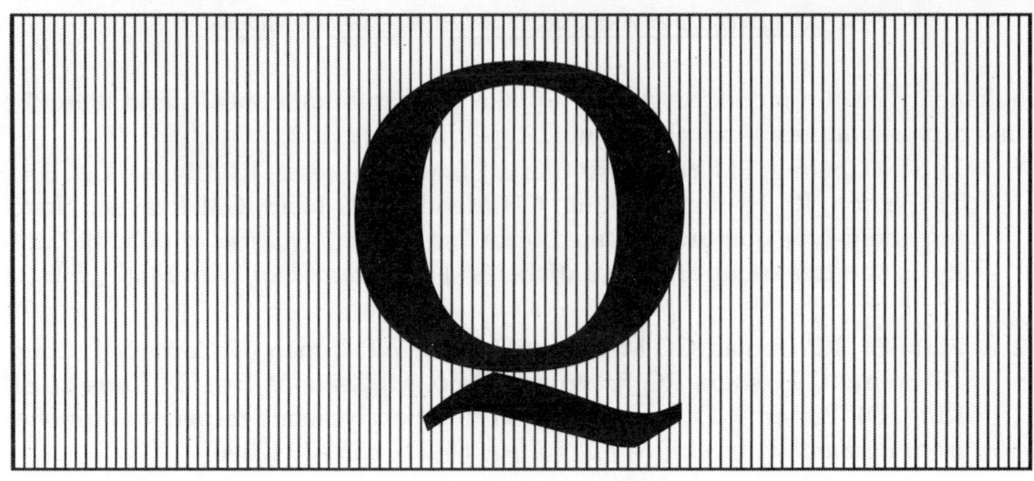

Quercus infectoria Oliv. (Fagaceae) (Cyprus oak, H. Manjuphal)

Quercus infectoria is a commonly available plant in Iran. The galls of the plant were tested pharmacologically and a fraction obtained from the methanol extract of the galls of *Q. infectoria* was found to significantly reduce the blood sugar levels in rabbits (1). Hexagalloylglucose (3-O-digalloyl-1,2,4,6-tetra-O-galloyl-b-D- glucose), isolated from the methanol extract of the galls of *Q. infectoria,* significantly inhibited *alpha*-glycosidases such as sucrase, maltase and isomaltase. Its inhibitory activity was found to be comparable to that of acarbose, which is used as a hypoglycaemic agent (2).

1. Dar MS, M Ikram, T Fakouhi; Pharmacology of *Quercus infectoria, J Pharm Sci* **65**(12), 1791-94 (1976)
2. Hwang JK, TW Kong, NI Baek, YR Pyun; *alpha*-Glycosidase inhibitory activity of hexagalloylglucose from the galls of *Quercus infectoria, Planta Med* **66**(3), 273-74 (2000)

Quillaja saponaria Molina (Quillajaceae) (Soap bark tree)

It is an evergreen tree, native to warm temperate central Chile north to Peru. The inner bark of *Q. saponaria* can be reduced to powder and employed as a substitute for soap, since it forms a lather with water, owing to the presence of a glucoside saponin. DS-1, a modified Quillaja saponin, was found to enhance ocular and nasal absorption of insulin. Anesthetized rats receiving eye drops or nose drops formulated with regular pork insulin in saline showed no hypoglycaemic response, indicating no systemic absorption of insulin. However, rats receiving eye drops or nose drops formulated with insulin plus DS-1 (0.025-0.10%) showed rapid absorption of insulin and a concomitant decrease in serum D-glucose levels. No response was observed following sublingual or buccal delivery of insulin.

1. Pillion DJ, J Recchia, P Wang, DJ Marciani, CR Kensil; DS-1, a modified *Quillaja* saponin, enhances ocular and nasal absorption of insulin, *J Pharm Sci* **84**(11), 1276-79 (1995)
2. Pillion DJ, JA Amsden, CR Kensil, J Recchia; Structure-function relationship among *Quillaja* saponins serving as excipients for nasal and ocular delivery of insulin, *J Pharm Sci* **85**(5), 518-24 (1996)

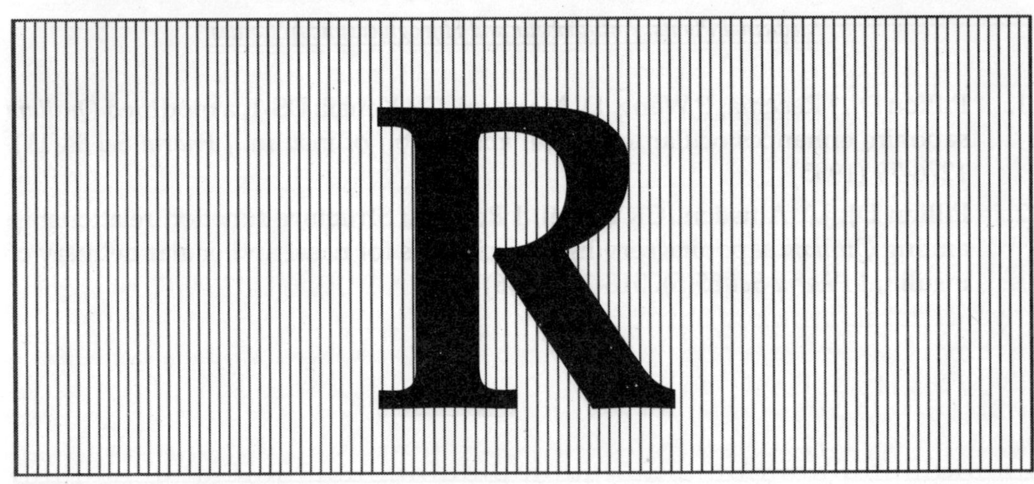

Rehmannia glutinosa (Gaertn.) (Phyrmaceae/Scrophulariaceae) (Korean foxglove)

R. glutinosa is a perennial herb with reddish-violet flowers native to China, Japan and Korea. The hypoglycaemic and anti-diabetic effects of *R. glutinosa* oligosaccharide in glucose-induced hyperglycaemic and alloxan-induced diabetic rats were investigated. It was observed that pre-treatment of normal rats with the oligosaccharide (100 mg/kg ip, for 3 days) induced a partial prevention of hyperglycaemia caused by glucose (2g/kg, ip), but when hyperglycaemia was induced in adrenalectomized rats, the preventive effect of the oligosaccharide on hyperglycaemia was lost. In alloxan-induced diabetic rats, the oligosaccharide (100 mg/kg, i.p., for 15 days) showed a significant decrease in blood glucose level and hepatic glucose-6-phosphatase activity with an increase in hepatic glycogen content. It also raised plasma insulin level and lowered plasma corticosterone level in alloxan-induced diabetic rats. The regulatory mechanism of the oligosaccharide on glucose metabolism was adrenal dependent and had a close relation with the neuroendocrine system (1). Water extract of the plant and a fraction (Part III), which contains mainly stachyose, a tetrasaccharide, showed a significant hypoglycaemic effect in glucose- and adrenaline-induced hyperglycaemic and alloxan-induced diabetic rats (2).

1. Zhang R, J Zhou, Z Jia, Y Zhang, G Gu; Hypoglycaemic effect of *Rehmannia glutinosa* oligosaccharide in hyperglycaemic and alloxan-induced diabetic rats and its mechanism, *J Ethnopharmacol* **90**(1), 39-43 (2004)
2. Zhang RX, ZP Jia, LY Kong, HP Ma, J Ren, MX Li, X Ge; Stachyose extract from *Rehmannia glutinosa* Libosch. to lower plasma glucose in normal and diabetic rats by oral administration, *Pharmazie* **59**(7), 552-56 (2004)

Rehmannia glutinosa var. *hueichingensis* (Phrymaceae/Scrophulariaceae) (Chinese foxglove)

In addition to known iridoid glycosides, several new glycosides (Rehmanniosides A, B, C, and D) were isolated from *R. glutinosa* var. *hueichingensis* and *R. glutinosa* var *purpurea*. Of these compounds, Rehmannioside D exhibited mild hypoglycaemic activity in spontaneously diabetic mice (1). The precipitate, obtained by addition of ethanol to hot water extract of *R. glutinosa* var. *hueichingensis*, produced hypoglycaemia in normal and streptozotocin-induced diabetic mice. It also significantly increased the activities of hepatic glucokinase and glucose-6-phosphate dehydrogenase along with a reduction of hepatic glucose-6-phosphatase and phosphofructokinase in normal mice. It stimulated the insulin secretion and lowered the hepatic glucose contents of normal mice. Chemical modification and proteinase treatment of the precipitate revealed that the hypoglycaemic activity resided in polysaccharide moiety (2).

1. Oshio H, H Inouye; Iridoid glycosides of *Rehmannia glutinosa*, *Phytochemistry* **21**(1), 133-38 (1982)

2. Kiho T, T Watanabe, K Nagai, S Ukai; Hypoglycaemic activity of polysaccharide fraction from rhizome of *Rehmannia glutinosa* Libosch. f *hueichingensis* Hsiao and the effect on carbohydrate metabolism in normal mouse liver, *Yokugaku Zasshi* **112**(6), 393-400 (1992)]

Retama raetam (Forssk.) Webb & Berthel (Fabaceae)

Retama raetam is a desert shrub of Syria and Arabia having small white flowers. The aqueous extract of *R. raetam* at a dose of 20mg/kg significantly reduced the blood glucose level in normal rats 6 h after a single oral administration and two weeks after repeated oral administration. This hypoglycaemic effect was more pronounced in streptozotocin-induced diabetic rats. The extract showed no effect on basal plasma insulin levels indicating the activity to be extra-pancreatic (1). The hypoglycemic effect of intravenous administration of an aqueous extract of *R. raetam* (10 mg /kg/h) to normal and streptozotocin induced diabetic rats, produced a significant lowering of blood glucose levels, the decrease being relatively more marked in diabetic rats. However, the basal insulin levels remained unchanged which suggested that hypoglycaemic activity of this plant might be due to its extrapancreatic action. The treated normal and diabetic rats also exhibited an increase in glycosuria which could be due to its potent inhibitory action on renal glucose reabsorption (2).

1. Maghrani M, A Lemhadri, H Jouad, JB Michel, M Eddouks; Effect of the desert plant *Retama raetam* on glycaemia in normal and streptozotocin-induced diabetic rats, *J Ethnopharmacol* **87**(1), 21-25 (2003)

2. Maghrani M, JB Michel, M Eddouks; Hypoglycaemic activity of *Retama raetam* in rats, *Phytother Res* **19**(2), 125-28 (2005)

Rhazya stricta Decne. (Apocynaceae)

Rhazya stricta is a small glabrous shrub, widely distributed throughout Western Asia. It is abundantly found in various regions of Pakistan. *R. stricta*, a medicinal plant in the United Arab Emirates, exhibits a variety of biological activities. Acute treatment of rats with the lyophilized extract at doses of 4 g/kg produced a significant rise in insulin concentration. In streptozotocin-induced diabetic rats, loaded orally with glucose (1 g/kg), *R. stricta* at doses of 8 g/kg produced significant decreases in plasma glucose concentration at 0.5 and 1 h after treatment. However, chronic treatment of rats and mice for 28 days with the lyophilized extract of *R. stricta* did not affect the plasma glucose or insulin concentration or any of the haematological or biochemical indices measured (1). Treatment of control rats with the extract at oral doses of 2.0 and 4.0 g/kg did not significantly affect the concentration of glucose, insulin or glucagon for up to 4 h after administration of the extract. However, the same doses in diabetic rats reduced the glucose level 1 h and 2 h after administration of the extract. This was accompanied by significant increases in insulin concentration 1, 2 and 4 h after administration of the extract. Treatment of normal and diabetic rats simultaneously with the plant extract (0.5, 2.0 and 5.0 g/kg) and glibenclamide (5.0 mg/kg) significantly exacerbated the effects on glucose, insulin and glucagon induced by the extract or by glibenclamide when given separately. The results imply that co-administration of the extract with glibenclamide might adversely interfere with glycaemic control in diabetic patients (2).

1. Tanira MO, BH Ali, AK Bashir, I Chandranath; Some pharmacologic and toxicologic studies on *Rhazya stricta* Decne in rats, mice and rabbits, *Gen Pharmacol* **27**(7), 1261-67 (1996)
2. Ali BH; The effect on plasma glucose, insulin and glucagon levels of treatment of diabetic rats with the medicinal plant *Rhazya stricta* and with glibenclamide, alone and in combination, *J Pharm Pharmacol* **49**(10), 1003-07 (1997)

Rheum emodi Wall. (Polygonaceae)
(Rhubarb, H. Amla-vetasa, S. Aml parni)

Rheum emodi is a leafy perennial herb, found mostly in rocky and sandy places where moisture remains for long time. The hypoglycaemic action of stilbene glycoside E, isolated from ethyl alcohol (95%) extract of *R. emodi*, was studied and its utility was assessed.

Li J, Z Wang, J Li; Studies on hypoglycaemic action of *Rheum emodi*, *Zhong Yao Cai* **20**(5), 249-50 (1997) [Article in Chinese]

Rheum undulatum Linn. (Polygonaceae)

The anti-diabetic-activity-guided fractionation of ethanol (80%) extract of Korean Rhubarb rhizomes (*R. undulatum*) led to the isolation of desoxyrhapontigenin (a stilbene), emodin and chrysophanol. The compounds inhibited postprandial hyperglycaemia by 35.8, 29.5 and 42.3%, respectively.

Choi SZ, SO Lee, KU Jang, SH Chung, SH Park, HC Kang, EY Yang, HJ Cho, KR Lee; Anti-diabetic stilbene and anthraquinone derivatives from *Rheum undulatum*, *Arch Pharm Res* **28**(9), 1027-30 (2005)

Rhodiola sachalinensis Boriss. (Crassulaceae)

Of the two polysaccharides (RSP-A and RSP-B), isolated from *R. sachalinensis*, RSP-B was proved to be the effective hypoglycaemic ingredient of the plant by intra-peritoneal administration to mice at dosages of 50 mg/kg and 100 mg/kg. RSP B failed to exhibit significant hypoglycaemic effect through absorption in the intestine but was found to possess significant hypoglycaemic effect when administrated subcutaneously, intramuscularly, intra-peritoneally and intravenously.

Chem X, L Di, Y Wu, X Liu, Q Ren; Hypoglycaemic effect of *Rhodiola sachalinensis* A. Bor. polysaccharides: comparison of administration in different ways, *Zhongguo Zhong Yao Za Zhi* **21**(11), 685-87 (1996) [Article in Chinese]

Rhus aromatica Aiton (Anacardiaceae)
(Fragrant Sumac)

Rhus aromatica has been reported as one of effective plant drugs for the treatment of diabetes mellitus.

Kapoor KK, Diabetes mellitus, *Indian J Homoeopath Med* **19**(3), 114-20 (1984)

Rhus coriaria Linn. (Anacardiaceae)
(Sumac)

The hypoglycaemic efficacy of sumac extract was investigated through inhibition of a glycoside hydrolase: *alpha*-amylase. The ethyl acetate extract of sumac is of interest in the treatment and prevention of hyperglycaemia, diabetes and obesity,

Giancarlo S, LM Rosa, F Nadjafi, M Francesco; Hypoglycaemic activity of two spices extracts: *Rhus coriaria* L. and *Bunium persicum* Boiss, *Nat Prod Res* **20**(9), 882-86 (2006)

Rhynchelytrum repens (Willd.) C.E. Hubb. (Poaceae)
(Natal Grass)

Rhynchelytrum repens is a pan tropical grass species popularly used for diabetes treatment. The effects of irradiance on non-structural carbohydrate contents and composition, as well as on the hypoglycaemic activity of the grass were assessed. Intra-peritoneal administration of the precipitate obtained from the aqueous extracts of the plants, growing under natural or low irradiance of light, showed a reduction in the blood sugar level but the supernatant fraction showed no hypoglycaemic effect (1). The presence of *beta*-glucan in the leaf blades, sheaths, stems, and young leaves of *R. repens* was confirmed and *beta*-glucan is considered to be responsible for the hypoglycaemic activity of the plant (2).

1. Souza A, AC Paula, RC Figueiredo-Ribeiro; Effects of irradiance on non-structural carbohydrates, growth, and hypoglycaemic activity of *Rhynchelytrum repens* (Willd.) C.E. Hubb. (Poaceae), *Braz J Biol* **64**(3B), 697-706 (2004)
2. De-Paula AC, RV Sousa, RC Figueiredo-Ribeiro, MS Buckeridge; Hypoglycaemic activity of polysaccharide fractions containing *beta*-glucans from extracts of *Rhynchelytrum repens* (Willd.) C.E. Hubb., Poaceae, *Braz J Med Biol Res* **38**(6), 885-93 (2005)

Rosmarinus officinalis Linn. (Lamaceae / Labiatae) (Rosemary)

Rosemary is a member of the mint family. It is a perennial herb with fragrant evergreen needle-like leaves and is native to the Mediterranean region. The effects of leaf extract of *R. officinalis* on plasma glucose levels in normoglycaemic and diabetic mice were studied,

Erenmemisoglu A, R Saraymen, S Ustun; Effect of a *Rosmarinus officinalis* leaf extract on plasma glucose levels in normoglycaemic and diabetic mice, *Pharmazie* **52**(8), 645-46 (1997)

Rubus fruticosus Linn. (Rosaceae) (Common Blackberry)

Alonso *et al* made a preliminary investigation of the hypoglycaemic activity of the plant (1). Jouad and coworkers (2) observed that acute or chronic oral administration of aqueous extract of *R. fructicosus* significantly decreased the blood sugar levels in normal and streptozotocin-induced diabetic rats. However, this plant extract did not affect the insulin secretion in normal or diabetic rats indicating that the mechanism of action of the drug was extra-pancreatic in nature. Acute toxicity study showed that the extract was safe.

1. Alonso R, I Cadavid, JM Calleja; A preliminary study of hypoglycaemic activity of *Rubus fruticosus*, *Planta Med* (Suppl) 102-06 (1980)
2. Jouad H, M Maghrani, M Eddouks; Hypoglycaemic effect of *Rubus fructicosis* L. and *Globularia alypum* L. in normal and streptozotocin-induced diabetic rats, *J Ethnopharmacol* **81**(3), 351-56 (2002)

Rubus imperialis Cham & Schltdl. (Rosaceae)

The plant is in popular use as an anti-diabetic in Brazil. *In vivo* assays confirmed the hypoglycaemic activity of a methanol extract of roots of the plant and validated its popular use as an anti-diabetic agent.

Kanegusuku M, JC Benassi, RC Pedrosa, RA Yunes, VC Filho, AA Maia, MM de Souza, F Delle Monache, R Niero; Cytotoxic, hypoglycaemic activity and phytochemical analysis of *Rubus imperialis* (Rosaceae), *Z Naturforsch* {C] **57**(3-4), 272-76 (2002)

Rumex patientia Linn. (Polygonaceae)

It is a North American plant and has been found in some parts of Canada. The effects of acarbose and *Rumex patientia* on liver ultra-structure and on the morphological changes in *beta* cells in streptozotocin induced diabetic (type-2) rats were investigated. Administration of acarbose (40 mg/100 g feed) and *Rumex patientia* grain (2% decoction) to diabetic rats lowered the blood glucose and HbA1c levels. Electron microscopic examination of the *beta* cells of streptozotocin induced diabetic rats showed mitochondrial vacuolization and swelling with dilatation of endoplasmic reticulum. Reduction of the secretory granules of the *beta* cells was also observed in diabetic rats. However, streptozotocin + acarbose treated group did not show any pathological changes in the *beta* cells. In streptozotocin + *Rumex patientia* treated group comparatively lesser swelling was noted in some of the mitochondria (1, 2).

1. Deginmenci I, S Kalender, MC Ustuner, Y Kalender, HV Gunes, N Unal, A Basaran; The effects of acarbose and *Rumex patientia* on liver ultrastructure in streptozotocin-induced diabetic (type II) rats, *Drugs Exp Clin Res* **28**(6), 229-34 (2002)
2. Deginmenci I, MC Ustuner, Y Kalender, S Kalender, HV Gunes; The effects of acarbose and *Rumex patientia* L. on ultrastructural and biochemical changes of pancreatic B cells in streptozotocin-induced diabetic rats, *J Ethnopharmacol* **97**(3), 555-59 (2005)

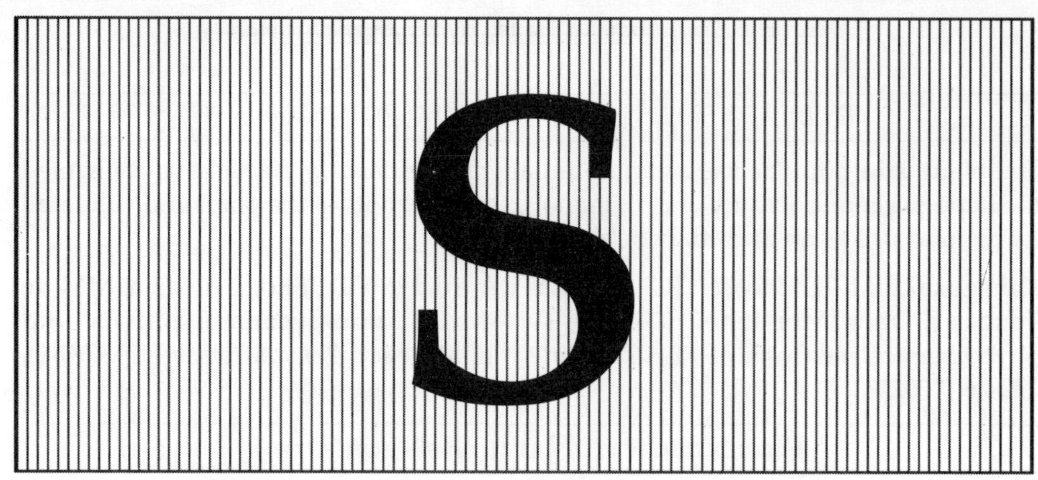

Saccharum officinarum Linn. (Poaceae)
(Sugar cane, H..Ganna S. Ikshu)

Sugar-cane juice was not found to have a protective factor with regard to glucose tolerance curves. See hypoglycaemic glycans in Appendix for glycans, isolated from stalks of *S. officinarum*.

Kloppers PJ, L Meiring, GD Campbell; A protective factor in sugar-cane juice, *S Afr Med J* **57**(19), 781-82 (1980) [Article in Afrikaans]

Salacia chinensis Linn. (Celastraceae / Hippocerateaceae)

Methanol extract of *S. chinensis* stems showed potent anti-hyperglycaemic effects in oral sucrose or maltose-loaded rats, inhibitory effects on intestinal *alpha*-glucosidase, rat lens aldose reductase, formation of Amadori compounds and advanced glycation end-products. The principal *alpha*-glucosidase inhibitor, salacinol, was isolated from the stems of *S. chinensis*.

Yoshikawa M, Y Pongpiriyadacha, A Kishi, T Kageura, T Wang, T Morikawa, H Matsuda; Biological activities of *Salacia chinensis* originating in Thailand: the quality evaluation guided by *alpha*-glucosidase inhibitory activity, *Yakugaku Zasshi* **123**(10), 871-80 (2003) [Article in Japanese]

Salacia diandra Thwaites (Celastraceae)

Methanol extract of *S. diandra* significantly reduced fasting serum glucose levels, area under curve of sucrose tolerance test and oral glucose tolerance test. The methanol extract yielded on fractionation L-diandrol, epicatechin and salacinol, a known *alpha*-glucosidase inhibitor. While the reduction in glycaemic response after sucrose load is considered to be due to salacinol, the reduction of fasting serum glucose is due to L-diandrol, which either inhibited gluconeogenesis or increased peripheral utilisation of blood glucose or sensitized glucose-induced insulin release from the cells of pancreas.

Kumara NKVM, MIFP Jayawardane, C Pathirana; Anti-diabetic activity of *Salacia diandra* on glucose homeostasis of diabetic rats, *IUPAC International Conference on Biodiversity and Natural Products Chemistry and Medical Applications,* New Delhi, OP-13, Jan.26-31, 2004

Salacia oblonga Wall. (Celastraceae) (Saptrangi)

Salacia oblonga is a woody plant found in the forests of Sri Lanka and India. The roots and stems of the plant have been used extensively in Ayurveda and traditional Indian Medicine for the treatment for diabetes. The petroleum ether extract of the root bark of *S. oblonga* significantly prevented the streptozotocin-induced hyperglycaemia and hypoinsulinaemia in rats. It also produced a significant decrease in peroxidation products *viz.* thiobarbituric acid reactive substances, conjugated dienes and hydroperoxides. Chromatographic resolution of the extract yielded fractions having more than half of the hypoglycaemic potency of an equal dose of tolbutamide (250 mg/kg) in albino rats (1, 2). The root bark of *S. oblonga* has been suggested to possess anti-diabetic and anti-peroxidative principles, useful in the treatment of diabetes and associated renal complications (4)

An aqueous methanol extract of *S. oblonga* roots was found to show inhibitory activity on the increase in serum glucose level in sucrose- and maltose-loaded rats. The water-soluble fraction of the extract showed inhibitory activities on *alpha*-glucosidase and potent *alpha*-glucosidase inhibitors, salacinol and kotalanol, were isolated from this fraction. The ethyl acetate-soluble fraction of aqueous methanol extract was found to be an aldose reductase inhibitor. The fraction yielded a new friedelane-type triterpene, kotalagenin 16-acetate along with known diterpenes and triterpenes, which were found to be components responsible for the inhibitory activity on aldose reductase (3).

The addition of *S oblonga* extract in test meals tended to lower postprandial glycaemia and reduced the postprandial insulin response in healthy subjects. The increase in breath hydrogen excretion suggested a mechanism similar to prescription *alpha*-glucosidase inhibitors (5).

1. Augusti KT, P Joseph, TD Babu; Biologically active principles isolated from *Salacia oblonga* Wall, *Indian J Physiol Pharmacol* **39**(4), 415-17 (1995)
2. Krishnakumar K, KT Augusti, PL Vijayammal; Hypoglycaemic and anti-oxidant activity of *Salacia oblonga* Wall. extract in streptozotocin-induced diabetic rats, *Indian J Physiol Pharmacol* **43**(4), 510-14 (1999)
3. Matsuda H, T Murakami, K Yashiro, J Yamahara, M Yoshikawa; Anti-diabetic principles of natural medicines. IV. Aldose reductase and *alpha*-glucosi-

dase inhibitors from the roots of *Salacia oblonga* Wall. (Celastraceae): structure of a new friedelane-type triterpene, kotalagenin 16-acetate, *Chem Pharm Bull* (Tokyo) **47**(12), 1725-29 (1999)

4. Krishnakumar K, KT Augusti, PL Vijayammal; Anti-peroxidative and hypoglycaemic activity of *Salacia oblonga* extract in diabetic rats, *Pharmaceut Biol* **38**(2), 101-05 (2000)
5. Heacock PM, SR Hertzler, JA Williams, BW Wolf; Effects of a medical food containing an herbal *alpha*-glucosidase inhibitor on postprandial glycaemia and insulinemia in healthy adults, *J Am Diet Assoc* **105**(1), 65-71 (2005)

Salacia macrosperma Wight, (Celastraceae)

The ethanol extract of *S. macrosperma* showed significant hypoglycaemic activity in fasted rabbits and also in alloxan-induced hyperglycaemic albino rats. The effect of oral administration (for 8 days) of various fractions of the alcoholic extract of the roots of *S. macrosperma* was studied by estimating various biochemical parameters in blood. The biologically active fractions of the extract exhibited significant anti-diabetic activity and were able to correct the metabolic aberrations in diabetic rats (1, 2).

1. Venkateswarlu V, CK Kokate, G Peddanna, C Veeresham, D Rambhau; Pharmaceutical investigations on *Salacia macrosperma* I, *Ancient Sci Life* **9**(4), 215-19 (1990)
2. Venkateswarlu V, CK Kokate, D Rambhau, C Veeresham; Anti-diabetic activity of roots of *Salacia macrosperma Planta Med* **59**(5), 391-93 (1993)

Salacia prenoides (Willd.) DC. (Celastraceae)

The commercially available Saptarangi was correctly identified as *Salacia prenoides* (yellow variety). Pillai and co-workers studied the hypoglycaemic activity of the root bark of *S. prenoides* and it evinced hypoglycaemic acivity comparable to tolbutamide (1). Relative efficacy of *S. prenoides* as an anti-diabetic agent with that of *S. fruticosa* and *S. macrosperma* was studied. Of these plants, *S. prenoides* was most active (2)

1. Pillai NR, C Seshadri, G Santhakumari; Hypoglycaemic activity of the root bark of *Salacia prenoides, Indian J Exp Biol* **17**(11), 1279-80 (1979)
2. Nair RB, AV Bhat, G Santhakumari; Comparative study of the hypoglycaemic activity of the *Salacia* species, *J Res Ayur Siddha* **3**(1-2), 53-68 (1982)

Salacia reticulata Wight (Celastraceae)

Kotalanol, an inner salt and a potent natural *alpha*-glucosidase inhibitor, was isolated from the roots and stems of *Salacia reticulata*. Kotalanol was found to show more potent inhibitory activity against sucrase than salacinol and acarbose (1). Salacinol, a most potent *alpha*-glucosidase inhibitor, was also isolated from this plant by bioassay-guided search. Salacinol showed potent inhibitory activities on several *alpha*-glucosidases, such as maltase, sucrase, and isomaltase. The inhibitory effects on serum glucose levels in maltose- and sucrose-loaded rats were found to be more potent than that of acarbose, a commercial *alpha*-glucosidase inhibitor (2).

Chronic oral administration (twice a day for 120 days) of the precipitate, obtained from the methanol extract of roots and stems of *S. reticulate* var. *beta-diandra*, to alloxan-induced diabetic rats improved glucose tolerance and significantly reduced fasting blood glucose, fructosamine and and glycosylated haemoglobin levels. The polydypsia, hyperphagia and weight loss of the alloxan diabetic rats were also reduced by the treatment (3).

1. Yoshikawa M, T Murakami, K Yashiro, H Matsuda; Kotalanol, a potent alpha-glucosidase inhibitor with thiosugar sulfonium sulfate structure, from anti-diabetic Ayurvedic medicine *Salacia reticulata, Chem Pharm Bull* (Tokyo) **46**(8), 1339-40 (1998)
2. Yoshikawa M, T Morikawa, H Matsuda, G Tanabe, O Muraoka; Absolute stereostructure of potent *alpha*-glucosidase inhibitor, Salacinol, with unique thiosugar sulfonium sulfate inner salt structure from *Salacia reticulata, Bioorg Med Chem* **10**(5), 1547-54 (2002)
3. Ruvin Kumara NKVM, RN Pathirana, C Pathirana, Hypoglycaemic activity of the root and stem of *Salacia reticulata* var. *beta-diandra* in alloxan diabetic rats, *Pharmaceut Biol* **43**(3), 219-25 (2005)

Salvia fruticosa Mill. (Lamiaceae / Labiatae) (Greek Sage)

Salvia fruticosa is a dwarf shrub that exhibits typical hairy or tomentose coverings on its leaves and stems. It is used as a folk medicine in the eastern Mediterranean region for the treatment of diabetes. In order to confirm this claim, a 10% infusion of its leaves was tested, at an oral dose of 0.250 g/kg body weight, on normoglycaemic and alloxan-induced hyperglycaemic rabbits. This oral dose caused a statistically significant reduction in blood glucose levels in alloxan-induced hyperglycaemic rabbits. However, in normoglycaemic animals this effect was observed only after repeated administrations of the infusion (once a day for 7 consecutive days). The hypoglycaemic effect was, however, evoked by a single oral dose of the infusion in both normoglycaemic and alloxan-induced hyperglycaemic rabbits, orally loaded with glucose. However, in these animals *S. fruticosa* infusion did not modify plasma insulin levels. Moreover, the hypoglycaemic effect of the drug was not evoked in rabbits receiving the glucose load intravenously. These data strongly suggest that *S. fruticosa* treatment produces hypoglycaemia mainly by reducing intestinal absorption of glucose.

Perfumi M, N Arnold, R Tacconi; Hypoglycaemic activity of *Salvia fruticosa* Mill from Cyprus, *J Ethnopharmacol* **34**(2-3), 135-40 (1991)

Salvia lavandulifolia Vahl (Lamiaceae / Labiatae) (Spanish sage)

Hypoglycaemic activity of *Salvia lavandulifolia* and of *S. lavandulifolia* ssp. *oxydon* was studied by Jimenez and co-workers (1-3). After establishing the hypoglycaemic action of the plant, its mechanism of action was studied. The results indicated that several mechanisms [(i) potentiation of insulin release induced by glucose, (ii) increased peripheral uptake of glucose, (iii) decreased intestinal absorption of glucose and (iv) hyperplasia of the pancreatic islet *beta* cells] operate simultaneously for exhibiting hypoglycaemic activity. The dry residue of the plant extract, at a dose of 10 mg/kg, produced an increase in the number and size of islets of Langerhans and also an increase in pancreatic insulin content. When both the plant extract (10 mg/kg) and glibenclamide (1 mg/kg) were administered concurrently to streptozotocin diabetic rats, a significant decrease in glycaemic level and mortality index was achieved.

1. Jimenez J, S Risco, T Ruiz, A Zarzuelo; Hypoglycaemic activity of *Salvia lavandulifolia*, *Planta Med* (4), 260-62 (1986)
2. Zarzuelo A, S Risco, MJ Gamez, J Jimenez, M Camara, MA Martinez; Hypoglycaemic action of *Salvia lavandulifolia* Vahl. ssp. *oxyodon*: a contribution to studies on the mechanism of action, *Life Sci* **47**(11), :909-15 (1990)
3. Jimenez I, J Jimenez, MJ Gamez, M Gonzalez, FS de Medina, A Zarzuelo, I Osuna; Effects of *Salvia lavandulifolia* Vahl. ssp. *oxyodon* extract on pancreatic endocrine tissue in streptozotocin-diabetic rats, *Phytother Res* **9(7)**, 536-37 (1995)

Salvia officinalis Linn. (Lamiaceae) (Common sage)

Common sage is a small perennial shrub, native to the Mediterranean region. It is cultivated mainly as a kitchen and medicinal herb. An aqueous ethanol extract of *S. officinalis* of Mexican origin significantly reduced the blood glucose of fasting normal mice 120 and 240 min after intra-peritoneal administration. The extract also significantly diminished the hyperglycaemia in mildly diabetic mice at 240 mins.

Alarcon-Aguilar FJ, R Roman Ramos, JL Flores-Saenz, F Aguirre-Garcia; Investigation on the hypoglycaemic effects of extracts of four Mexican medicinal plants in normal and alloxan-diabetic mice, *Phytother Res* **16**(4), 383-86 (2002)

Sambucus nigra Linn. (Adoxaceae) (Elderberry)

Sambucus nigra is native to most of Europe, northwest Africa and southwest Asia. It yields dark purple to black berry in drooping clusters. The fruits are an important food for many fruit-eating birds, notably Blackcaps. *Sambucus nigra* has been documented as a traditional treatment of diabetes. In an acute 20-min test, an aqueous extract of *S. nigra* (1 g/l) in absence of added insulin, significantly increased transport of 2-deoxy-glucose, oxidation of glucose and glycogenesis of mouse abdominal muscle. The extract (0.25-1 g/l) evoked a stepwise stimulation of insulin secretion from clonal pancreatic *beta*-cells. The insulin releasing effect of the extract (0.5 g/l) was significantly potentiated by glucose and significantly reduced by diazoxide. It did not further enhance insulin secretion in cells stimulated by L-alanine, 3-isobutyl-1-methylxanthine or a depolarizing concentration of KCl (25 mmol/l). Sequential extraction with solvents revealed activity in both methanol and water fractions, indicating a cumulative effect of more than one plant constituent. The known constituents of plant (lectin, rutin, lupeol and β-sitosterol) did not stimulate insulin secretion. The results demonstrate the presence of insulin-releasing and insulin-like activity in this traditional anti-diabetic plant.

Gray AM, YH Abdel-Wahab, PR Flatt; The traditional plant treatment, *Sambucus nigra* (elder), exhibits insulin-like and insulin-releasing actions *in vitro*, *J Nutr* **130**(1), 15-20 (2000)

Sarcopoterium spinosum (L) Spach (Rosaceae) (Thorny Burnet)

The triterpene and tannin constituents of *Sarcopoterium spinosum* were isolated and characterised. A combination of tannins and triterpenes in the ratio of 95:5 significantly lowered the blood sugar level at a concentration of 300 mg/kg.

Reher G, M Slijepeevic, L Kraus; Hypoglycaemic activity of triterpenes and tannins from *Sarcopoterium spinosum* and two *Sanguisorba* species, *Planta Med* **57**(Suppl.2), A57-A58 (1991)

Saussurea lappa (Decne.)C.B.Clarke. (Asteraceae / Compositae) (Costus, H. Kuth, S. Kushtha)

Saussurea is a genus of about 300 species of flowering plants, native to cool temperate regions of Asia, Europe, and North America. *Saussurea lappa* is found in the Himalayas. Administration of *Saussurea lappa* (500 mg) and its decoction (100 ml) each for 30 days was found to be effective in the management of Madhumeha (Diabetes mellitus). No side effect was observed (1). Treatment of albino rats with alcoholic extract of *S. lappa* for 7 days showed significant hypoglycaemic response without an increase in plasma insulin. The acute response showed the accumulation of glycogen in the liver, followed by its depletion. The histology of the thyroid showed stimulation. Liver sections showed no toxic effects up to a dose of 400 mg/kg body weight. No morphological change was observed in adrenal gland and pancreas (2).

1. Singh DC, BP Sharma; Management of Madhumeha (Diabetes mellitus) by indigenous drugs; Bijayasar and Kushtha, *Aryavaidyan* **4**(1), 21-23 (1990)

2. Chaturvedi P, P Tripathi, S Pandey, U Singh, YB Tripathi; Effect of *Saussurea lappa* alcoholic extract in endocrine glands in relation to glucose metabolism in the rat, *Phytother Res* 7(2), 205-07 (1993)

Satureja khuzestanica Jamzad (Lamiaceae)

Satureja khuzestanica is an endemic plant of Iran and is famous for its various medicinal uses. Treatment of rats with the essential oil of *S. khuzestanica* decreased the normal blood lipid peroxidation level and increased total antioxidant power. The essential oil significantly decreased the fasting blood glucose and triglyceride levels in diabetic and hyperlipidaemic rats, respectively. The antioxidant properties of the essential oil of the plant may explain its anti-diabetic and triglyceride-lowering effects (1). The effect of the essential oil of the plant on rat hepatic key enzymes of glycogenolysis and gluconeogenesis was studied. The essential oil did not affect blood glucose concentrations but decreased hepatic phosphoenolpyruvate carboxy kinase activity and increased hepatic glycogen phosphorylase. Disturbance of hepatic glucose metabolism is proposed to be the mechanism of anti-diabetic action of the essential oil of the plant (2).

1. Abdollahi M, A Salehnia, SH Mortazavi, M Ebrahimi, A Shafiee, F Fouladian, K Keshavarz, S Sorouri, R Khorasani, A Kazemi; Antioxidant, anti-diabetic, anti-hyperlipidaemic, reproduction stimulatory properties and safety of essential oil of *Satureja khuzestanica* in rat *in vivo*: a toxicopharmacological study, *Med Sci Monit* **9**(9), BR331-35 (2003)

2. Saadat M, S. Pournourmohammadi, M. Donyavi, R Khorasani, G Amin, Ali N Salehnia, M Abdollahi; Alteration of rat hepatic glycogen phosphorylase and phosphoenolpyruvate carboxykinase activities by *Satureja khuzestanica* Jamzad essitial oil, *J Pharm Pharmaceut Sci* **7**(3), 327-31 (2004)

Schefflera leucantha Viguier (Araliaceae).

Water extract of *Schefflera leucantha* exhibited hypoglycaemic activity in normal and diabetic rats.

Satayavivad J, N Bunyapraphatsara, A Thiantanawat, U Kositchaiwat; Hypoglycaemic activity of the aqueous extract of *Schefflera leucantha* Viguier in rats, *Thai J Phytopharm* **3**(1), 1-5 (1996)

Schizonepeta tenuifolia Briq.(Lamiaceae) (Japanese catnip)

This annual aromatic herb with long spikes of delicate, lavender coloured blooms is native to China and Japan. The aerial parts of the plant are used in Chinese medicine. Phytosterols and hesperidin were isolated respectively, from ether and n- butanol extracts of the spikes of the plant. These compounds significantly reduced the blood glucose level of mice and lessened their loss of body weight dose dependently when administered at i.p. doses of 10 and 20 mg/kg for 4 days after the i.v. injection of streptozotocin. The compounds also showed protective activity on the pancreatic islets, especially *beta*-cells from the degenerative effects of streptozotocin.

Kim CJ, JS Lim, SK Cho; Anti-diabetic agents from medicinal plants: inhibitory activity of *Schizonepeta tenuifolia* spikes on the diabetogenesis by streptozotocin in mice, *Arch Pharmacol Res* **19**(6), 441-46 (1996)

Sclerocarya birrea (A. Rich.) Hochst. ssp. *caffra* (Sond.) Kokwaro (Anacardiaceae)

The plant finds folkloric use in the management and/or control of adult-onset, type-2 diabetes mellitus in some African communities. The decoction of *S. birrea* bark exhibited hypoglycaemic activity, an increase in plasma immunoactive insulin in normal rats and an incremented oral glucose tolerance. The decoction was also active against diet-induced hypercholesterolaemia (1). Following acute treatment, relatively moderate to high doses of aqueous extract of *S. birrea* stem-bark (100-800 mg/kg p.o.) produced dose-dependent, significant reductions in the blood glucose concentrations of both fasted normal and fasted diabetic rats. The action was found to be comparable to that of chlorpropamide. Administrations of a single dose of the plant extract (800 mg/kg p.o.) also significantly reduced the blood glucose levels of both fasted normal (normoglycemic) and fasted streptozotocin-treated, diabetic rats. The hypoglycaemic properties of the plant drug were thus confirmed (2, 3).

1. Trovato A, S Kirjavainen, EM Gulati, AM Forestieri; Effect of *Sclerocarya birrea* Hochst. extract on some metabolic activities in the rat, *Phytother Res* **9**(8), 591-93 (1995)
2. Ojewole JA; Hypoglycaemic effect of *Sclerocarya birrea* [(A. Rich.) Hochst. [Anacardiaceae] stem-bark aqueous extract in rats, *Phytomedicine* **10**(8), 675-81 (2003)
3. Ojewole JA; Evaluation of the analgesic, anti-inflammatory and anti-diabetic properties of *Sclerocarya birrea* (A. Rich.) Hochst. stem-bark aqueous extract in mice and rats, *Phytother Res* **18**(8), 601-08 (2004)

Scoparia dulcis Linn. (Scrophulariaceae) (Sweet broomweed')

Scoparia dulcis is widely used in Indian folk medicine for the treatment of diabetes mellitus. Latha, Pari and co-workers made extensive investigation on the anti-diabetic activity of the plant. Oral administration of the aqueous extract of *S. dulcis* leaves (0.15, 0.30 and 0.45 g/kg b.w.) to alloxan-induced diabetic rats for 45 days resulted in a significant reduction in blood glucose, glycosylated haemoglobin and an increase in total haemoglobin; the effect being highly significant at a dose of 0.45 g/kg body weight. A significant improvement in glucose tolerance was also observed in animals treated with this plant extract and the effect was comparable to that of glibenclamide (1). Aqueous, ethanol, and chloroform extracts of *S. dulcis* showed significant increases in the activities of insulin, superoxide dismutase, catalase, glutathione peroxidase, glutathione-S-transferase, reduced glutathione, vitamin C, and vitamin E in liver, kidney, and brain of streptozotocin-induced diabetic rats. The treated rats also showed significant decreases in blood glucose, thiobarbituric acid-reactive substances, and hydroperoxide formation in tissues, suggesting the role of the extracts of *S. dulcis* in protection against lipid peroxidation-induced membrane damage. Of the different extracts, the aqueous extract was particularly effective (2).

The insulin-receptor-binding effect of *S. dulcis* plant extract in streptozotocin-induced male Wistar rats was studied using circulating erythrocytes as a model system. The mean specific binding of insulin to erythrocytes was significantly lower in diabetic control rats than in diabetic rats, treated with the plant extract-(200 mg/kg, p.o.) and glibenclamide. The decrease in insulin binding in diabetic control rats was accounted for by a lower number of insulin receptor sites per cell when compared with drug-treated rats. The results of the study revealed that *S. dulcis* plant extract and glibenclamide increase total erythrocyte membrane insulin binding sites with a concomitant increase in plasma insulin (3). Administration of *S. dulcis* plant extract (200 mg/kg/day) and glibenclamide (600 mg/kg/day) by gavage to diabetic rats for 6 weeks significantly reduced blood glucose, sorbitol dehydrogenase, glycosylated hemoglobin, thiobarbituric acid reactive substances, and hydroperoxides, and significantly increased plasma insulin, glutathione peroxidase, glutathione-S-transferase and reduced glutathione activities in liver. The effect of the plant extract, which compared well with that of glibenclamide, might be due to the decreased influx of glucose into the polyol pathway leading to increased activities of antioxidant enzymes and plasma insulin and decreased activity of sorbitol dehydrogenase. These results indicated that the plant extract was effective in attenuating hyperglycaemia in rats and their susceptibility to oxygen free radicals (4).

Oxidative stress is implicated in the pathogenesis of diabetic complications and an aqueous extract of *S. dulcis* was found to protect against streptozotocin induced oxidative stress and apoptosis both *in vitro* and *in vivo*. Oral administration of an aqueous extract of *S. dulcis* (200 mg/kg b.w.) for 6 weeks to streptozotocin-induced diabetic rats significantly increased the plasma insulin and plasma antioxidants and significantly decreased lipid peroxidation. The effect of this plant extract at 200 mg/kg body weight was better than that of glibenclamide, a reference drug. The protective effect of this plant extract against streptozotocin induced oxidative stress and apoptosis was also studied both *in vitro* and *in vivo* (5, 6). The plant extract, at this dose, also significantly decreased the blood glucose with significant increase in plasma insulin level in streptozotocin diabetic rats at the end of 15 days treatment. The insulin secretagogue action of the extract was also confirmed by using isolated pancreatic islets from mice. The extract, at a dose of 10µg/ml, evoked six fold stimulation of insulin secretion from isolated islets. The glucose lowering effect of the extract of *S. dulcis* was thus found to be associated with potentiation of insulin release from pancreatic islets (7). The effect of aqueous extract of *S. dulcis* on the occurrence of oxidative stress in the brain of rats during diabetes was investigated by measuring the extent of oxidative damage as well as the status of the antioxidant defense system. The findings suggested a possible anti-peroxidative role for *Scoparia dulcis* plant extract. The antioxidant properties of *S. dulcis* extract, in addition to its anti-diabetic effect, make the plant extract a very useful drug for the treatment of diabetes and its complications (8, 9).

1. Pari L, S Venkateswaran; Hypoglycaemic activity of *Scoparia dulcis* L. extract in alloxan induced hyperglycaemic rats, *Phytother Res* **16**(7), 662-64 (2002)
2. Latha M, L Pari; Modulatory effect of *Scoparia dulcis* in oxidative stress-induced lipid peroxidation in streptozotocin diabetic rats, *J Med Food* **6**(4), 379-86 (2003)
3. Pari L, M Latha, CA Rao; Effect of *Scoparia dulcis* extract on insulin receptors in streptozotocin induced diabetic rats: studies on insulin binding to erythrocytes, *J Basic Clin Physiol Pharmacol* **15**(3-4), 223-40 (2004)
4. Latha M, L Pari; Effect of an aqueous extract of *Scoparia dulcis* on blood glucose, plasma insulin and some polyol pathway enzymes in experimental rat diabetes, *Braz J Med Biol Res* **37**(4), 577-86 (2004)
5. Pari L, M Latha; Effect of *Scoparia dulcis* (Sweet Broomweed) plant extract on plasma antioxidants in streptozotocin-induced experimental diabetes in male albino Wistar rats, *Pharmazie* **59**(7), 557-60 (2004)
6. Latha M, L Pari, S Sitasawad, R Bhonde; *Scoparia dulcis*, a traditional anti-diabetic plant, protects against streptozotocin induced oxidative stress and apoptosis *in vitro* and *in vivo*, *J Biochem Mol Toxicol* **18**(5), 261-72 (2004)
7. Latha M, L Pari, S Sitasawad, R Bhonde; Insulin-secretagogue activity and cytoprotective role of the traditional anti-diabetic plant *Scoparia dulcis* (Sweet Broomweed), *Life Sci* **75**(16), 2003-14 (2004)
8. Pari L, M Latha; Protective role of *Scoparia dulcis* plant extract on brain anti-

oxidant status and lipid peroxidation in STZ diabetic male Wistar rats, *BMC Compliment Altern Med* **4**, 16 (2004)

9. Pari L, M Latha; Anti-diabetic effect of *Scoparia dulcis*: effect on lipid peroxidation in streptozotocin diabetes, *Gen Physiol Biophys* **24**(1), 13-26 (2005)

Scrophularia deserti Delile (Scrophulariaceae)

Several iridoid glycosides were isolated from the aerial parts of *S. deserti*. Of these compounds scropolioside-D2 and harpagoside-B were found to possess significant anti-diabetic activity. The biological activity and the structure-activity relationship of the compounds were studied.

Ahmed B, AJ Al-Rehaily, TA Al-Howiriny, KA El-Sayed, MS Ahmad; Scropolioside-D2 and harpagoside-B: two new iridoid glycosides from *Scrophularia deserti* and their anti-diabetic and antiinflammatory activity, *Biol Pharm Bull* **26**(4), 462-67 (2003)

Secale cereale M. Bieb.(Poaceae)
(Rye)

Rye is grown extensively as a grain and forage crop. It is closely related to barley and wheat. Rye grain is used for flour, rye bread, rye beer, and some other alcoholic drinks, Alloxan diabetic rats, fed a basic diet made from a mixture of rye bread and milk containing raw bran for 14 days, were found to have a lower urinary glucose excretion than those fed a basic diet containing processed bran. The effects of the two brans on weight, serum insulin levels, and non-fasting blood glucose levels were similar in control and diabetic animals with the exception of the lower non-fasting blood glucose level in control animals receiving raw bran than in control animals receiving processed bran (1).

Rye flakes, rye bread and white wheat bread were given as suspensions to rats and in standardised breakfast meals to non-insulin-dependent diabetics. In both cases the postprandial glucose response was lower after rye bread than after wheat bread. Delayed gastric emptying might be one of the factors for the lower response after rye bread as a larger amount of starch remained in the stomach of the rats 15 min after ingestion of rye bread compared to wheat bread. The absorption pattern and metabolic response after rye bread seems preferable to that after wheat bread. The flaked rye on the other hand was not effective in reducing postprandial glycaemia despite a lower availability of starch *in vitro* (2). Whole-kernel rye bread was found to produce lower postprandial insulin response than wheat bread, but no difference in glucose response was observed. Postprandial glucose and insulin may also be affected by type of rye bread. Characteristics of different types of rye breads must be further investigated to develop health properties of rye breads (3).

1. Nygren C, G Hallmans; Effects of processed rye bran and raw rye bran on glucose metabolism in alloxan diabetic rats, *J Nutr* **112**(1), 17-20 (1982)

2. Hagander B, I Bjorck, NG Asp, S Efendic, J Holm, P Nilsson-Ehle, I Lundquist, B Schersten; Rye products in the diabetic diet. Postprandial glucose and hormonal responses in non-insulin-dependent diabetic patients as compared to starch availability *in vitro* and experiments in rats, *Diabetes Res Clin Pract* **3**(2), 85-96 (1987)

3. Leinonen K, K Liukkonen, K Poutanen, M Uusitupa, H Mykkanen; Rye bread decreases postprandial insulin response but does not alter glucose response in healthy Finnish subjects, *Eur J Clin Nutr* **53**(4), 262-67 (1999)

Securigera securidaca (L.) Deg. et Dorf. (Fabaceae)

Securigera securidaca is an anti-diabetic Egyptian folk medicine. The total aqueous extract of the seeds of *S. securidacea* showed a marked diuretic and severe hypokalemic effects on the K^+-level in serum. The hypoglycaemic effect of the seeds was also confirmed. Isolation of several phytochemicals from the seeds of the plant has also been reported. The total aqueous extract of the seeds and the new cardenolide (14-methoxyhyrcanoside), isolated from the extract showed marked chronotropic activity (1).

The intra-peritoneal and oral administration of the aqueous and ethanol extracts of the seeds of the plant significantly reduced blood glucose level in alloxan-induced diabetic mice but not significantly in normoglycaemic and glucose-induced hyperglycaemic mice. The mechanism by which the extract reduces blood glucose level in alloxan-induced diabetic mice appears to be different from that of sulfonylurea agents (2).

1. Ali AA, MH Mohamed, MS Kamel, MA Fouad, O Spring; Studies on *Securigera securidacea* (L.) Deg. et Dorfl. (Fabaceae) seeds, an anti-diabetic Egyptian folk medicine, *Pharmazie* **53**(10), 710-15 (1998)

2. Hosseinzadeh H, M Ramezani, AR Danaei' Anti-hyperglycaemic effect and acute toxicity of *Securigera securidacea* L. seed extracts in mice, *Phytother Res* **16**(8), 745-47 (2002)

Securinega virosa (Roxb. ex Willd.) Baill. (Phyllanthaceae / Euphorbiaceae)

An aqueous extract of roots of *S. virosa* is used by traditional healers in Tanzania for the treatment of impotence, which is one of the manifestations of diabetes mellitus. The extract at doses of 0.1, 0.2, 0.4, and 1.0 g/kg body weight lowered the area under the oral glucose tolerance curve in normal albino rabbits. The extract, at a dose of 0.4 g/kg body weight, had no effect on fasting blood glucose (FBG) when compared to controls, except at 4 h, when the FBG for treated animals was higher.

Moshi MJ, MC Kapingu, FC Uiso, ZH Mbwambo, RLA Mahunnah; Some pharmacological properties of an aqueous extract of *Securinega virosa* roots, *Pharmaceut Biol* **38**(3), 214-21 (2000)

Semecarpus anacardium Linn. (Anacardiaceae) (Marking nut, S. Bhallataka, H. Bhilawa)

Semecarpus anacardium is a native of India and is closely related to the cashew, which is native to northeastern Brazil. The ethanol extract of dried nuts of *S. anacardium* (100 mg/kg) reduced the blood glucose levels of normal, streptozotocin-induced as well as of alloxan induced diabetic rats 3 h after oral administration of the extract. The anti-hyperglycaemic activity of *S. anacardium* was compared with that of tolbutamide, an oral hypoglycaemic agent (1, 2).

1. Arul B, R Kothai, AJ Christina; Hypoglycaemic and anti-hyperglycaemic effect of *Semecarpus anacardium* Linn in normal and streptozotocin-induced diabetic rats, *Methods Find Exp Clin Pharmacol* **26**(10), 759-62 (2004)
2. Kothai R, Arul B, KS Kumar, AJ Christina; Hypoglycaemic and anti-hyperglycaemic effects of *Semecarpus anacardium* Linn in normal and alloxan-induced diabetic rats, *J Herb Pharmacother* **5**(2), 49-56 (2005)

Senecio species (Asteraceae)

The antioxidant and anti-diabetic properties of different extracts of two *Senecio* species (*Senecio inaequidens* DC, and *Senecio vulgaris* Linn.) were studied. Methanol and dichloromethane extracts of both the species showed appreciable *alpha*-amylase inhibition and this property of the plant extracts might be responsible for their anti-diabetic properties. The extracts were also found to possess antioxidant activity but the activity of *S. inaequidens* was greater than that of *S. vulgaris*.

Conforti F, MR Loizzo, GA Statti, PJ Houghton, F Menichini; Biological properties of different extracts of two Senecio species, *Int J Food Sci Nutr* **57**(1-2), 1-8 (2006)

Sesamum indicum Linn. (Pedaliaceae) (Sesame, H. Til, S. Tila)

Numerous wild relatives of sesame occur in Africa and a smaller number in India. It is widely naturalised in tropical regions around the world and is cultivated for its edible seeds. Hypoglycaemic effect of a hot-water extract from defatted sesame seed and its fractions were tested in genetically diabetic KK-Ay mice. The fractions were obtained by chromatographic resolution of hot water extract on HP-20 resin and eluting with water and methanol. Genetically diabetic (type-2) KK-Ay mice were divided into four groups. Group one received basal diet, the remaining three groups received, in addition to the basal diet, either a 4.0% of the hot-water extract or 1.4% of the water eluent fraction or 0.7% of the methanol eluent fraction. After a feeding period of 4 weeks, the plasma glucose concentration and amount of urinary excreted glucose were lower in groups receiving hot water extract or methanol eluted fraction compared to the other groups. This effect was suggested to have been caused by the delayed glucose absorption.

Takeuchi H, LY Mooi, Y Inagaki, P He; Hypoglycaemic effect of a hot-water extract from defatted sesame (*Sesamum indicum* L.) seed on the blood glucose level in genetically diabetic KK-Ay mice, *Biosci Biotechnol Biochem* **65**(10), 2318-21 (2001)

Sesbania sesban (L) Merr.(Fabaceae / Leguminosae) (Egyptian riverhemp)

Sesbania sesban is thought to be native to Egypt. The plant is known to have the ability to improve soil through the fixation of atmospheric nitrogen. Oral administration of the unsaponifiable matter of the seed fat of *S. sesban*, at a dose level of 300 mg/kg, produced a fall (20%) in blood sugar in rats. No toxicity was observed in rats even after 73 hours at a dose 1 g/kg.

Jayalaxmi S, R Shrivastava, D Kohli,; Antibacterial and pharmacological studies of unsaponifiable matter of seeds of *Sesbania sesban* Merr. *Indian J Hosp Pharm* **19**(2), 67-69 (1981)

Sida cordifolia Linn. (Malvaceae) (H. Bala)

The methanol extract of the roots of *S. cordifolia* was found to possess significant hypoglycaemic activity.

Kanth VR, PV Diwan; Analgesic, antiinflammatory and hypoglycaemic activities of *Sida cordifolia, Phytother Res* **13**(1), 75-77 (1999)

Silybum marianum (L.) Gaertn. (Asteraceae) (Milk Thistle)

The hypoglycaemic effect of the aqueous extract of aerial part of *Silybum marianum* was investigated in normal and streptozotocin-induced diabetic rats. After a single dose or 15 daily doses, oral administration of this aqueous extract (20 mg/kg) produced a significant decrease of blood glucose levels in both normal and streptozotocin-induced diabetic rats. No changes were observed in basal plasma insulin concentrations after treatment with this extract in either normal or streptozotocin induced diabetic rats indicating that the plant extract exerts its pharmacological activity without affecting insulin secretion.

Maghrani M, NA Zeggwagh, A Lemhadri, M Amraoui, JB Michel, M Eddouks; Study of the hypoglycaemic activity of *Fraxinus excelsior* and *Silybum marianum* in an animal model of type-1 diabetes mellitus, *J Ethnopharmacol* **91**(2-3), 309-16 (2004)

Smallanthus sonchifolius(Poeppig & Endlicher) H. Robinson (Asteraceae) (Yacon)

Smallanthus sonchifolius (yacon), originating from South America, has become popular in Japan and in New Zealand for its tubers which contain β-1,2-oligofructans as the main saccharides. The plant is also successfully cultivated in Central Europe in the Czech Republic in particular.

A 10% decoction of *S. sonchifolius* (yacon) leaves produced a significant decrease in plasma glucose levels in normal rats when administered by intra-peritoneal injection or gastric tube. In a glucose tolerance test, a single administration of the decoction lowered the plasma glucose levels in normal rats. In contrast, a single oral or intra-peritoneal administration of the decoction produced no effect on the plasma glucose levels of streptozotocin-induced diabetic rats. However, the administration of 2% yacon tea *ad libitum* instead of water for 30 days produced a significant hypoglycaemic effect on streptozotocin-induced diabetic rats. After 30 days of tea administration, diabetic rats showed improved plasma glucose, plasma insulin levels and renal parameters in comparison with the diabetic controls (1).

Hot water extract of aerial parts of yacon suppressed the elevation of glucose levels after loading starch in normal rats. Bioactivity directed fraction of the extract led to the isolation of three known dicaffeoylquinic acids, which showed *alpha*- amylase inhibitory activities. 3,4- and 3,5- dicaffeoylquinic acids dose dependently exhibited hypoglycaemic activity after loading starch. The dicaffeoylquinic acids were thus recognised to be active hypoglycaemic constituents of yacon (2).

Aqueous extracts of yacon leaves, rich in phenolic compounds with antioxidant activity, have been studied for their hypoglycaemic activity in normal and diabetic rats. The effects of two organic fractions and two aqueous extracts from the leaves of *S. sonchifolius* on rat hepatocyte viability, on oxidative damage induced by tert-butyl hydroperoxide and allyl alcohol, and on glucose metabolism and their insulin-like effect on the expression of cytochrome P450 mRNA were studied. All the extracts tested exhibited strong protective effect against oxidative damage to rat hepatocyte primary cultures in concentrations ranging from 1 to 1000 μg/ml, and reduced hepatic glucose production *via* gluconeogenesis and glycogenolysis at 1000 μg/ml. The effects of the organic fractions (200 and 250 μg/ml) and to a lesser extent, the tea infusion (500 μg/ml) on rat CYP2B and CYP2E mRNA expression, were comparable to those observed with insulin. The combination of radical scavenging, cytoprotective and anti-hyperglycaemic activity of *S. sonchifolius* leaves makes it suitable for use in prevention and treatment of chronic diseases involving oxidative stress, particularly diabetes (3).

The dried leaves of *S. sonchifolius* were found to contain a total of 0.97% of the anti-diabetic sesquiterpene lactone, enhydrin. For quantitative determination of this compound, a simple, reliable and rapid reversed-phase HPLC procedure was developed (4)

1. Aybar MJ, AN Sanchez-Riera, A Grau, SS Sanchez; Hypoglycaemic effect of the water extract of *Smallantus sonchifolius* (yacon) leaves in normal and diabetic rats, *J Ethnopharmacol* **74**(2), 125-32 (2001)

2. Terada S, K Ito, M Taka, N Ogose, N Naguchi, Y Koide; *Alpha*-glucosidae inhibitory active components and glucose level lowering effect of Yacon aerial part extract, *Nat Medicine* **57**(3), 89-94 (2003)
3. Valentova K, A Moncion, J de Waziers, J Ulrichova; The effect of *Smallanthus sonchifolius* leaf extracts on rat hepatic metabolism, *Cell Biol Toxicol* **20**(2), 109-20 (2004)
4. Schon K, FB da-Costa; Quantitative determination of enhydrin in leaf rinse extracts and in glandular trichomes of *Smallanthus sonchifolius* (Asteraceae) by reversed-phase high-performance liquid chromatography, *Phytochem Anal* **16**(3), 161-65 (2005)

Smilax glabra Roxburgh (Smilacaceae / Liliaceae)

The plant grows in Ease Asia, from China to the Himalayas. The methanol extract of rhizomes of *S. glabra* (100 mg/kg b.w.) reduced the blood glucose of normal mice 4 h after intra-peritoneal administration, and also significantly lowered the blood glucose of KK-Ay mice under similar conditions. However, the extract did not affect the blood glucose in streptozotocin-induced diabetic mice, one of the animal models of insulin-dependent diabetes mellitus (IDDM) with hypoinsulinaemia. The extract also suppressed epinephrine-induced hyperglycaemia in KK-Ay mice. The extract significantly decreased the blood glucose in an insulin tolerance test. The hypoglycaemic effect of the extract of the rhizomes of *S. glabra* was considered to be due to a rise in insulin sensitivity.

Fukunaga T, T Miura, K Furuta, A Kato; Hypoglycaemic effect of the rhizomes of *Smilax glabra* in normal and diabetic mice, *Biol Pharm Bull* **20**(1), 44-46 (1997)

Solanum lycocarpum (St. Hill.) (Solanaceae) (Wolf Apple)

The *Solanum lycocarpum* is common in the Brazilian savanna. It bears yellow fruits resembling a medium sized tomato (wolf apple), The potential hypoglycaemic activity of the starch of *S. lycocarpum* was evaluated (1). The powder of *Solanum lycocarpum* fruit is used as a hypoglycaemic agent by diabetic patients in Brazil. The hypoglycaemic effect induced by the starch obtained from the unripe fruits of *S. lycocarpum* was investigated. Per os administration of the starch (1000 or 2000 mg/kg, twice daily for 7 days) did not change glycaemia levels of non-diabetic female Swiss mice. In streptozotocin-induced diabetic mice, similar treatment with the starch did not change the elevated glycaemia 3 h after the last dose. Administration of glucose (600 mg/kg) in animals fasted for 15 h, significantly increased glycaemia 1 h later. Previous (30 min) treatment of the animals with the starch (1000 or 2000 mg/kg) did not change the increase of glycaemia. The chemical analysis of the starch indicated the presence of glycoalkaloids, many of which are known to be toxic. The results of the present study failed to provide evidence for a hypoglycaemic effect associated with the polysaccharide fraction of *S. lycocarpum* in either normal or hyperglycaemic mice (2).

The extract of *S. lycocarpum* reduced glycaemia in alloxan induced diabetic rats and reduced nitrate generation in diabetic animals indicating its antioxidant activity. It also restored haemoglobin and haematocrit to normal values in diabetic animals (3).

1. Souza Araujo RJP, MM Coelho, MGL Brandao; Evaluation of the potential hypoglycaemic activity of the starch of *Solanum lycocarpum* St. Hill. in mice, *Phytomedicine* 7(Suppl. II), 68 (2000)
2. Oliveira AC, DC Endringer, RJ Araujo, MG Brandao, MM Coelho; The starch from *Solanum lycocarpum* St. Hill. fruit is not a hypoglycaemic agent, *Braz J Med Biol Res* **36**(4), 525-30 (2003)
3. Perez AC, V Franca, VM Daldegan, LDG Duarte; Effect of *Solanum lycocarpum* St. Hill on various haematological parameters in diabetic rats, *J Etnopharmacol* **106** (3), 442-44 (2006)

Solanum tuberosum Linn. (Solanaceae)
(Potato)

It has been observed that in normal subjects, ingestion of butter with potato results in a considerably lower blood glucose level than that observed in the same subjects after potato ingestion alone, insulin levels were, however, similar or slightly higher in the butter-potato group. The observation prompted the investigators to determine whether butter ingested with potato would result in a greater stimulation in insulin secretion than ingestion of potato alone in subjects with NIDDM. The mean plasma glucose area response after ingestion of potato with or without various amounts of butter were all similar and were 82% of that observed after ingestion of 50 g glucose. The mean insulin areas for potato plus 50 g of fat meals were greater than for ingestion of potato alone, and a maximal response was observed with addition of 15 g fat. The C-peptide data did not confirm an increase in insulin secretion. Overall the area responses after ingestion of meals containing fat were not different from the response to potato ingestion alone. In contrast to the results in normal subjects after ingestion of butter with potato, the glucose response was not smaller in subjects with NIDDM.

Gannon MC, N Ercan, SA Westphal, FQ Nuttall; Effect of added fat on plasma glucose and insulin response to ingested potato in individuals with NIDDM, *Diabetes Care* **16**(6), 874-80 (1993)

Spathodea campanulata P.Beauv.(Bignoniaceae)
(African tulip tree)

A decoction of *S. campanulata* stem bark exerted hypoglycaemic activity in streptozotocin-induced diabetic mice (1). Different fractions, obtained by chromatographic resolution of the decoction, were evaluated for their hypoglycaemic, anti-complement and anti-HIV activities. The most polar fraction exerted by far the most prominent effect in different biological models (2).

1. Niyonzima G, S Scharpe, L von Becck, AJ Vhetlnck, GM Lackeman, T Mets; Hypoglycaemic activity of *Spathodea campanulata* stem bark decoction in mice, *Phytother Res* 7(1), 64-67 (1993)
2. Niyonzima G, G Laekeman, M Witvrouw, B van Poel, L Pieters, D Paper, E de Clercq, G Franz, AJ Vlietinck; Hypoglycaemic, anticomplement and anti-HIV activities of *Spathodea campanulata* stem bark, *Phytomedicine* **6**(1), 45-49 (1999)

Spergularia purpurea (Pers.) G. Don f. (Caryophyllaceae) (Purple sandspurry)

Aqueous extract of *S. purpurea* decreased significantly the plasma glucose levels of normal rats 4 h after single oral administration, and one week after repeated oral administration. In case of severe hyperglycaemic rats, such decrease of plasma glucose levels was observed 6 h after a single oral administration of the extract. Repeated oral administration of the water extract of *S. purpurea* in diabetic rats normalised their plasma glucose levels after two weeks (1). The underlying mechanism of the hypoglycaemic activity of this aqueous extract of the plant was studied in diabetic mice and streptozotocin-induced diabetic rats. The aqueous extract (10 mg/kg i.v.) produced a significant decrease in blood glucose levels in normal rats and even more in diabetic rats. This hypoglycaemic effect might be due to an extra-pancreatic action of the aqueous extract of *S. purpurea,* since the basal plasma insulin concentrations remained unchanged after this plant drug treatment. In diabetic mice, a similar effect was observed and the results showed that aqueous extract of *S. purpurea* caused a potent inhibitory effect on basal endogenous glucose production. It was inferred that perfusion of aqueous extract of *S. purpurea* inhibits endogenous glucose production in mice. This inhibition is at least one of the mechanisms for the observed hypoglycaemic activity of this plant in diabetic animals (2).

1. Jouad H, M Eddouks, MA Lacaille-Dubois, B Lyoussi; Hypoglycaemic effect of *Spergularia purpurea* in normal and streptozotocin-induced diabetic rats, *J Ethnopharmacol* **71**(1-2), 169-77 (2000)
2. Eddouks M, H Jouad, M Maghrani, A Lemhadri, R Burcelin; Inhibition of endogenous glucose production accounts for hypoglycaemic effect of *Spergularia purpurea* in streptozotocin mice, *Phytomedicine* **10**(6-7), 594-99 (2003)

Stephania tetrandra S. Moore (Menispermaceae)

S, tetrandra Radix was found to increase the blood insulin level and decrease the blood glucose level in streptozotocin-diabetic ddY mice. The actions of bis-benzylisoquinoline alkaloids, isolated from *S. tetrandra,* were also studied in the hyperglycaemia of streptozotocin-induced diabetic mice. The main bis-benzylisoquinoline alkaloid, fangchinoline (0.3-3 mg/kg) significantly reduced the blood glucose level of the diabetic mice in a dose-dependent manner. The effect of fangchinoline was 3.9-fold greater than that of water extract of *S. tetrandra*. However, another main alkaloid of the plant, tetrandrine (1-100 mg/kg) did not have any effect. Some structure-activity relationship of these alkaloids has been studied.

Tsutsumi T, S Kobayashi, YY Liu, H Kontani; Anti-hyperglycaemic effect of fangchinoline isolated from *Stephania tetrandra* Radix in streptozotocin-diabetic mice, *Biol Pharm Bull* **26**(3), 313-17 (2003)

Stevia rebaudiana Bertoni (Asteraceae / Compositae) (Sweet leaf)

The genus *Stevia* is native to subtropical and tropical South America and Central America. *Stevia rebaudiana* or sweet leaf is used as a sugar substitute but its taste has a slower onset and longer duration than that of sugar. *S. rebaudiana* extracts, having up to 300 times the sweetness of sugar, are in demand for low-carbohydrate, low-sugar food alternatives. It is an attractive natural sweetener to diabetics and others on carbohydrate-controlled diets.

The leaves of *Stevia rebaudiana,* used as sweetening agent by Paraguayan Indians and other tribes, are also used for the treatment of diabetes mellitus (1). Jeppesen and coworkers studied anti-hyperglycaemic, insulinotropic and glucagonostatic properties of the plant and of the diterpene glycosides present in the plant (2-5, 7).

The natural sweetener stevioside, present in *S. rebaudiana,* has been used for many years in the treatment of diabetes among Indians in Paraguay and Brazil. Both stevioside and its aglucon, steviol (1 nmol/l to 1 mmol/l) dose-dependently enhanced insulin secretion from incubated mouse islets in the presence of 16.7 mmol/l glucose. The insulinotropic effects of stevioside and steviol were found to be critically dependent on the prevailing glucose concentration. Both stevioside and steviol potentiated insulin secretion from INS-1 cells. Neither stevioside nor steviol influenced the plasma membrane K^+-adenosine triphosphate (K^+ ATP)-sensitive channel activity, nor did they alter cyclic adenosine monophosphate levels in islets. Stevioside and steviol were thus found to stimulate insulin secretion *via* a direct action on *beta* cells. The results indicate that the compounds may have a potential role as anti-hyperglycaemic agents in the treatment of type-2 diabetes mellitus (2). Stevioside significantly suppressed the glucose response to the i.v. glucose tolerance test in type-2 diabetic Goto-Kakizaki (GK) rats and concomitantly increased the insulin response. Interestingly, the glucagon level was suppressed by stevioside during the glucose tolerance test. In the normal Wistar rats, stevioside enhanced insulin above basal level during the i.v. glucose tolerance test; without altering the blood glucose response or the glucagon levels. Stevioside was thus proved to exert anti-hyperglycaemic, insulinotropic, and glucagonostatic actions in the type-2 diabetic GK rats (3). The anti-hyperglycaemic and blood pressure-lowering effects of stevioside were examined in a long-term study in the type-2 diabetic GK rats. Results revealed that stevioside enjoys a dual positive effect by acting as an anti-hyperglycaemic and a blood pressure-lowering substance (4). Stevioside was found to reduce postprandial blood glucose levels in type-2 diabetic patients, indicating beneficial effects on the glucose metabolism (5). In addition to stevioside, the leaves of *S. rebaudiana* contain another diterpene glycoside, rebaudioside A. The influence of rebaudioside A on the insulin release from mouse islets was studied using static incubations, as well as perfusion experiments. Rebaudioside A was found to stimulate insulin secretion in a glucose-dependent manner and only potentiated insulin secretion at a glucose concentration above 6.6 mmol/l. The effect of rebaudioside A was, however, found to be critically dependent on the presence of extra-cellular Ca^{2+}, i.e., rebaudioside A-induced insulin stimulation at high glucose level disappeared in the absence of extra-cellular Ca^{2+}. The findings suggest that rebaudioside A may serve a potential role in the treatment of type-2 diabetes mellitus (7).

The effect of stevioside on glucose and insulin metabolism was investigated in streptozotocin-induced diabetic and NIDDM diabetic rats, induced by fructose feeding. Stevioside (0.5 mg/kg) reduced the blood sugar levels in streptozotocin-induced diabetic rats. Administration of stevioside twice daily to rats of both diabetic models caused lowering of blood glucose in a dose dependent manner. In normal rats, this glycoside prevented the rise of blood sugar during glucose tolerance test. Following 15 days of treatment, stevioside decreased protein levels of phosphoenol pyruvate carboxykinase (PEPCK) and PEPCK mRNA. Stevioside also decreased insulin resistance in diabetic rats. It was suggested that stevioside regulated blood glucose levels by enhancing secretion of insulin and its utilization in insulin deficient rats (8).

Experiments provided supportive data that repeated oral administration of stevioside delayed the development of insulin resistance in rats on a high-fructose diet. The observation that oral administration of stevioside (0.2 mg/kg three times daily) to streptozotocin-induced diabetic rats for ten days increased the plasma glucose-lowering action of exogenous insulin suggested that stevioside also increased insulin sensitivity (9).

The effect of oral treatment (gavage) with *Stevia rebaudiana* was compared with that of stevioside on glycaemia and gluconeogenesis of 15-h fasted rats. Liver perfusion and isolated hepatocytes were used to measure hepatic gluconeogenesis. Glycaemia and gluconeogenesis from L-alanine (5 mM), L-glutamine (5 mM) and L-lactate (2 mM) were decreased after pre-treatment with the leaf extract of the plant but stevioside did not influence glycaemia and gluconeogenesis. In order to secure information about the mechanism by which leaf extract inhibit gluconeogenesis, its potential role as a PPAR *gamma* agonist was investigated but the data showed absence of activation of PPAR *gamma* receptors. The results showed that the reduction of glycaemia promoted by the treatment with *S. rebaudiana* leaves was mediated, at least in part, by an inhibition of hepatic gluconeogenesis but this effect did not involve stevioside and the activation of PPAR *gamma* receptors (10).

The effects of pre-treatment of mice with two commercial products of *Stevia rebaudiana* [Stevita (Stevita Co, INC, Arlington Texas) and Clear Steviosides liquid (Stevita Co, INC, Herbal supplement, Brazil)] on the blood glucose concentration were studied. One group of mice was pre-treated four days with 200 mg/kg of Stevita and the other with 20 mg/kg of Clear Steviosides liquid whereas the animals of the control group received at the same time physiological solution. Pre-treatment with Stevioside liquid caused no significant increase in blood glucose concentration after administering adrenaline, which was not the case with the animals pre-treated with Stevita and control. Pre-treatment with Stevita, and to a greater extent with Stevioside liquid, protected test animals from the toxic action of alloxan compared with controls (6).

1. Lewis WH, Early uses of *Stevia rebaudiana* (Asteraceae) leaves as a sweetner in Paraguay, *Econ Bot* **46**(3), 336-37 (1992)

2. Jeppesen PB, S Gregersen, CR Poulsen, K Hermansen; Stevioside acts directly on pancreatic *beta* cells to secrete insulin: actions independent of cyclic adenosine monophosphate and adenosine triphosphate-sensitive K^+-channel activity, *Metabolism* **49**(2), 208-14 (2000)

3. Jeppesen PB, S Gregersen, KK Alstrup, K Hermansen; Stevioside induces anti-hyperglycaemic, insulinotropic and glucagonostatic effects *in vivo*: studies in the diabetic Goto-Kakizaki (GK) rats, *Phytomedicine* **9**(1), 9-14 (2002)

4. Jeppesen PB, S Gregersen, SE Rolfsen, M Jepsen, M Colombo, A Agger, J Xiao, M Kruhoffer, T Orntoft, K Hermansen; Anti-hyperglycaemic and blood pressure-reducing effects of stevioside in the diabetic Goto-Kakizaki rat, *Metabolism* **52**(3), 372-8 (2003)

5. Gregersen S, PB Jeppesen, JJ Holst, K Hermansen; Anti-hyperglycaemic effects of stevioside in type-2 diabetic subjects, *Metabolism* **53**(1), 73-76 (2004)

6. Rascovic A, M Gavrilovic, V Jakovljevic, J Sabo; Glucose concentration in the blood of intact and alloxan-treated mice after pretreatment with commercial preparations of *Stevia rebaudiana* (Bertoni), *Eur J Drug Metab Pharmacokinet* **29**(2), 87-90 (2004)

7. Abudula R, PB Jeppesen, SE Rolfsen, J Xiao, K Hermansen; Rebaudioside A potently stimulates insulin secretion from isolated mouse islets: studies on the dose-, glucose-, and calcium-dependency, *Metabolism* **53**(10), 1378-81 (2004)

8. Chen TH, SC Chen, P Chan, YL Chu, HY Yang, JT Cheng; Mechanism of the hypoglycaemic effect of stevioside, a glycoside of *Stevia rebaudiana*, *Planta Med* **71**(2), 108-13 (2005)

9. Chang JC, MC Wu, IM Liu, JT Cheng; Increase of insulin sensitivity by stevioside in fructose-rich chow-fed rats, *Horm Metab Res* **37**(10), 610-16 (2005)

10. Ferreira EB, F de Assis Rocha Neves, MA da Costa, WA do Prado, L Araujo Funari Ferri, RB Bazotte; Comparative effects of *Stevia rebaudiana* leaves and stevioside on glycaemia and hepatic gluconeogenesis, *Planta Med* **72**(8), 691-96 (2006)

Strychnos potatorum Linn. (Loganiaceae / Strychnaceae) (Clearing Nut Tree, H. Nirmali)

Fruits of *Strychnos potatorum* are used in folklore medicine for the treatment of diabetes mellitus, though not amply reported in Ayurveda. Planned pharmacological studies revealed its significant hypoglycaemic effect in streptozocin-induced diabetic animal models. A time course study revealed its immediate as well as long duration of action. A profound influence of the plant on carbohydrate metabolism was established from insulin estimation and specific histopathological tests (1). The effect of *S. potatorum* in the treatment of non-insulin dependent diabetics was clinically evaluated and the result analysed (2). The seeds of *S. potatorum* showed no hypoglycaemic activity in glucose loaded animal models and it was suggested to have potential activity in IDDM model (3)

1. Das J, DP Basu, R Banerjee, P Tripathi; Observation on hypoglycaemic effects of *Strychnos potatorum* in experimental animal model, *International Seminar: Traditional medicine*, Calcutta, p. 136, November 7-9, 1992

2. Islam SS, RJ Prasad, PC Tripathi; Clinical evaluation of *Strychnos potatorum* in the treatment of non-insulin dependent diabetes mellitus, *Proceedings of International Congress on "Ayurveda 2000"* Chennai, TN, India, p. 101, January 28-30, 2000

3. Mandal TK, TK Biswas, PC Tripathi; An experimental study on anti-diabetic effect of *Strychnos potatorum* Linn. *Aryavaidyan* **15**(3 & 4), 178-186 (2002)

Suaeda fruticosa Forssk. (Chenopodiaceae)

The effect of *S. fruticosa* on lipid and carbohydrate metabolism was studied in the hypercholesterolaemic and insulin resistant sand rats. 25 rats were subjected to a high cholesterol diet for 90 days. On the 45th day, the animals were divided into two groups: control and treated. The treated group received a 10 per cent aqueous extract of *S. fruticosa* (1.5 ml/100 g body weight, p.o. per day). On the 90th day, the control group developed a severe hyperlipidaemia, impaired glucose tolerance test and insulin resistance, while the treated group showed hypoglycaemic and anti-hyperglycaemic effects. Furthermore, the plant extract led to a decrease in plasma levels of insulin, total cholesterol, LDL cholesterol, VLDL cholesterol, oxidized LDL, lecithin cholesterol acyl transferase, triglycerides and free fatty acids (1).

The hypoglycaemic activity of the aqueous extract of the aerial part of *S. fruticosa* was examined in normal and streptozotocin-induced diabetic rats. The blood glucose changes as well as the levels of plasma insulin, cholesterol and triglycerides in the animals were determined within 4 h after intravenous administration of aqueous extract. The aqueous extract at a dose of 192 mg/kg produced a significant decrease in blood glucose levels in normal rats, and even more in diabetic rats. This hypoglycaemic effect might be due to an extra-pancreatic action of the plant extract, since the levels of plasma insulin remained unchanged before and after treatment. The effect of the aqueous extract on the plasma cholesterol was also significant in both normal and diabetic rats but not so on plasma triglycerides in both groups (2).

1. Bennani-Kabchi N, F el-Bouayadi, L Kehel, H Fdhil, G Marquie; Effect of *Suaeda fruticosa* aqueous extract in the hypercholesterolaemic and insulin-resistant sand rat, *Therapie* **54**(6), 725-30 (1999)

2. Benwahhoud M, H Jouad, M Eddouks, B Lyoussi; Hypoglycaemic effect of *Suaeda fruticosa* in streptozotocin-induced diabetic rats, *J Ethnopharmacol* **76**(1), 35-38 (2001)

Sutherlandia frutescens (L.) R. Br. (Fabaceae / Leguminosae) (Balloon pea)

Sutherlandia frutescens is widely used in South African traditional medicine for the management and/or control of a plethora of human ailments including diabetes. The hypoglycaemic effect of aqueous extract of the shoots of *S. frutescens* (var. *incana*) was investigated in streptozotocin-induced diabetic rats. The plant extract (50-800 mg/kg p.o. or i.p.) caused significant hypoglycaemia in rats. The study justifies the folkloric uses of the herb in the management and/or control of adult-onset, type-2 diabetes mellitus in some communities of South Africa (1). The usefulness of *S. frutescens* for the treatment of diabetes has also been highlighted (2). *S. frutescens* leaf extract shows promise as a type-2 anti-diabetes medication because of its ability to normalise insulin levels and glucose uptake in peripheral tissues and suppress intestinal glucose uptake, with no weight gain noted. The exact mechanism of action and the extract's efficacy in humans need further confirmation (3).

1. Ojewole JA; Analgesic, antiinflammatory and hypoglycaemic effects of *Sutherlandia frutescens* R. BR. (variety Incana E. MEY.) [Fabaceae] shoot aqueous extract, *Methods Find Exp Clin Pharmacol* **26**(6), 409-16 (2004)

2. Sia C; Spotlight on ethnomedicine: usability of *Sutherlandia frutescens* in the treatment of diabetes, *Rev Diabet Stud* **1**(3), 145-49 (2004)

3. Chadwick WA, S Roux, M van de Venter, J Louw, W Oelofsen; Anti-diabetic effects of *Sutherlandia frutescens* in Wistar rats fed a diabetogenic diet, *J Ethnopharmacol* **109**(1), 121-27(2007)

Swertia chirayita (Roxb ex Flem) Karst. (Gentianaceae) (Chiretta, S. Kirata, H. Chirayita)

Swertia chirayita is a medicinal plant indigenous to temperate Himalayas and used in different traditional systems of medicines such as the Ayurveda, Unani and Siddha. An ethanol (95%) extract of *S. chirayita* (250 mg/kg b.w.) was found to be effective in lowering blood sugar in fasted, fed, and glucose-loaded experimental albino rats. Oral administration of the extract caused enhancement of blood sugar lowering effect of tolbutamide in healthy albino rats (1). The ethanol extract of *S. chirayita* and four of its fractions were tested for their blood sugar lowering activity in rats by oral administration. The hexane-soluble fraction caused maximum lowering of blood sugar at the optimum dose level of 250 mg/kg, although the ethanol extract was clearly active. The optimum dose produced significant lowering of blood sugar in fed, glucose-loaded and tolbutamide-pre-treated animal models, but not in fasted rats (2). Oral administration of hexane fraction of *S. chirayita* (250 mg /kg) to albino rats lowered blood sugar levels and increased plasma insulin levels without affecting hepatic glycogen contents. Chronic treatment for 28 days significantly decreased blood sugar along with an increase of plasma insulin and hepatic glycogen contents. Intestinal glucose absorption remained unaffected by hexane fraction of *S. chirayita,* which was suggested to act by increasing insulin secretion (3). Fractionation of this hexane extract yielded a xanthone, identified as 1,8-dihydroxy-3,5-dimethoxyxanthone (swerchirin). Swerchirin showed a very significant blood sugar lowering effect in fasted, fed, glucose loaded, and tolbutamide-pre-treated albino rat models (4). Single oral administration of crude swerchirin (50 mg/kg, b.w.) to fed CF rats induced about 60% fall in blood glucose level 7 h after-treatment. This was associated with marked depletion of aldehyde-fuchsin-stained *beta*-granules and immuno-stained insulin in the pancreatic islets. From the results of detailed investigation, it was concluded that crude swerchirin lowers blood glucose level by stimulating insulin release from islets of Langerhans (5). The anti-hyperglycaemic effect of three structurally unrelated compounds, tolbutamide, centipiperalone (2-piperazino-3 (H)-4-quinazolone) and crude swerchirin, was examined in normal and streptozotocin-induced mild and severe diabetic rats. Analysis of the data revealed that centpiperalone was more active than tolbutamide and crude swerchirin (6).

Commercially available ethnomedicines; Semburi from Japan, Chirayita from Nepal and Zanyinchen from China, were identified to be *Swertia chirayita* mixed up with small amounts of *S. alata* and *S. mussoti*. The hypoglycaemic activity of 70% ethanol extract of these plant drugs was evaluated in streptozotocin-induced diabetic rats. Semburi and Chirayita significantly decreased blood sugar levels of diabetic animals; Semburi being relatively more effective (7).

1. Mukherjee B, SK Mukherjee; Blood sugar lowering activity of *Swertia chirata* (Buch-Ham) extract, *Int J Crude Drug Res* **25**(2), 97-102 (1987)

2. Chandrasekar B, B Mukherjee, RB Chakravarti, SK Mukherjee; Effect of different fractions of *Swertia chirayita* on the blood sugar level of albino rats, *J Ethnopharmacol* **21**(2), 175-81 (1987)
3. Chandrasekar B, MB Bajpai, SK Mukherjee; Hypoglycaemic activity of *Swertia chirayita* (Roxb ex Flem) Karst., *Indian J Exp Biol* **28**(7), 616-18 (1990)
4. Bajpai MB, RK Asthana, NK Sharma, SK Chatterjee, SK Mukherjee; Hypoglycaemic effect of swerchirin from the hexane fraction of *Swertia chirayita*, *Planta Med* **57**(2), 102-04 (1991)
5. Saxena AM, MB Bajpai, PS Murthy, SK Mukherjee; Mechanism of blood sugar lowering by a swerchirin-containing hexane fraction (SWI) of *Swertia chirayita*, *Indian J Exp Biol* **31**(2), 178-81 ((1993)
6. Saxena AM, PS Murthy, SK Mukherjee; Mode of action of three structurally different hypoglycaemic agents: a comparative study, *Indian J Exp Biol* **34**(4), 351-55 ((1996)
7. Komatsu K, B Purusotam, S Yamaji, S Kadota, T Namba; A comparative study on *Swertia herba* from Japan ,Nepal and China and their hypoglycaemic activities in streptozotocin-induced diabetic rats, *Nat Medicines* **51**(3), 265-68 (1997).

Swertia japonica (Roem.&Schult.) Makino (Gentianaceae)

S. japonica grows in lowland and hills all over Japan. The anti-hyperglycaemic activity of aqueous ethanol extract of *S. japonica* and of its various solvent-soluble fractions was studied in streptozotocin-induced diabetic rats. The aqueous ethanol extract of this plant was found to be more effective in lowering the blood sugar levels than the mixture of tolbutamide and buformine and an ethanol extract of *Swertia chirayita*. The ethyl acetate soluble fraction of *S. japonica* and its ether insoluble fraction elicited potent hypoglycaemic activity (1).

Hypoglycaemic activity-guided fractionation of the ethyl acetate-soluble fraction of *S. japonica* led to the isolation of five known xanthones and two triterpenoids. Both oral and intra-peritoneal administration of one of these xanthones, bellidifolin, elicited potent hypoglycaemic activity in streptozotocin-induced diabetic rats in a dose dependent manner. Bellidifolin significantly lowered the loaded glucose level in normal as well as in diabetic rats. It also significantly reduced the blood triglycerides levels. Glucose uptake by rat fibroblasts was enhanced by bellidifolin (2, 3)

1. Basnet P, S Kadota, T Namba, M Shimizu; The hypoglycaemic activity of *Swertia japonica* extracts in streptozotocin induced hyperglycaemic rats, *Phytother Res* **8**(1), 55-57 (1994)
2. Basnet P, S Kadota, M Shimizu, T Namba; Bellidifolin: a potent hypoglycaemic agent in streptozotocin (STZ)-induced diabetic rats from *Swertia japonica*, *Planta Med* **60**(6), 507-11 (1994)

3. Basnet P, S Kadota, M Shimizu, Y Takata, M Kobayashi, T Namba; Bellidifolin stimulates glucose uptake in rat 1 fibroblasts and ameliorates hyperglycaemia in streptozotocin (STZ)-induced diabetic rats, *Planta Med* **61**(5), 402-05 (1995)

Synsepalum dulcificum (Schumach & Thonn.) Daniell (Sapotaceae) (Miracle fruit)

Miracle fruit, native to West Africa, has the ability to turn bitter and sour foods taste sweet, when chewed prior to tasting sour and bitter food. Single oral administration of the powder of this miracle fruit decreased the plasma glucose in a dose-dependent manner for 150 min in rats fed fructose-rich chow for 4 weeks. Oral administration of this fruit (0.2 mg/kg) to fructose-rich chow fed rats, three times daily for 3 days, reversed the raised value of the glucose-insulin index, indicating the ability of miracle fruit to improve insulin sensitivity. The results of the investigation suggested the use of miracle fruit as an adjuvant for treating diabetic patients with insulin resistance because this fruit has the ability to improve insulin sensitivity.

Chen CC, IM Lin, JT Cheng; Improvement of insulin resistance by miracle fruit (*Synsepalum dulcificum*) in fructose-rich chow-fed rats, *Phytother Res* **20**(11), 987-92 (2006)

Syzygium alternifolium (Wight.) Walp. (Myrtaceae) (Mogi)

S. alternifolium is endemic to Andhra Pradesh, Tamil Nadu and Karnataka in India. The water, ethanol and hexane extracts (0.75 g / kg) of *S. alternifolium* seeds exhibited blood sugar lowering effect in normal and alloxan-induced diabetic rats. Maximum hypoglycaemic and anti-hyperglycaemic activity was noted in the aqueous extract. The anti-hyperglycaemic effect of *S. alternifolium* was compared with that of glibenclamide.

Rao BK, CH Rao; Hypoglycaemic and anti-hyperglycaemic activity of *Syzygium alternifolium* (Wt.) Walp. seed extracts in normal and diabetic rats, *Phytomedicine* **8**(2), 88-93 (2001)

Syzygium aromaticum (L.) Merrill and Perry (Myrtaceae) (Clove, H. Laung, S. Lavanga)

Insulin action is impaired in diabetic patients, which leads to increased hepatic glucose production. The extract of clove acts like insulin in hepatocytes and hepatoma cells by reducing phosphoenolpyruvate carboxykinase and glucose 6-phosphatase gene expression. Very much like insulin, clove extract-mediated repression is reversed by PI3K inhibitors and N-acetylcysteine. The findings indicate a potential role for compounds derived from clove as insulin-mimetic agents.

Prasad RC, B Herzog, B Boone, L Sims, M Waltner-Law; An extract of *Syzygium aromaticum* represses genes encoding hepatic gluconeogenic enzymes, *J Ethnopharmacol* **96**(1-2), 295-301 (2005)

Syzygium cordatum (L.) Hochst. (Myrataceae) (Water berry)

S. cordatum is a water-loving tree, found near streams or in swampy spots. The fruits are oval berries, red to dark-purple when ripe and with a crisp, crunchy texture and tart taste. The hypoglycaemic activity of *S. cordatum* leaf extract was evaluated in normal and streptozotocin-induced diabetic rats. Administration of the extract significantly reduced the blood sugar levels in normal and diabetic rats.

Musabayane CT, N Mahalalela, FO Shode, JAO Ojewole; Effects of *Syzygium cordatum* (Hochst) Myrtaceae leaf extract on plasma glucose and hepatic glycogen in streptozotocin induced diabetic rats, *J Ethnopharmacol* **97**(3), 485-90 (2005)

Syzygium cumini (L.) Skeels (Myrtaceae)

See *Eugenia jambolana* Lam. (Myrtaceae)

Syzygium samarangense (Blume) Merr. and Perry (Myrtaceae) (Water apple)

Two chalcones and a flavanone were isolated from the leaves of *S. samarangense*. Administration of 2',4'-dihydroxy-3',5'-dimethyl-6'-methoxychalcone and its isomeric flavanone 5-O-methyl-4'-desmethoxymatteucinol, at a dose of 1.0 mg/20 g body weight, significantly lowered the blood glucose levels in glucose-fed hyperglycaemic mice when administered 15 min after a glucose load. Of the two compounds, only the chalcone, co-administered with glucose, showed a significant lowering of blood glucose level 45 min after its oral administration. Only this compound also significantly lowered the blood sugar levels in alloxan-induced diabetic mice.

Resurreccion-Magno MH, IM Villasenor, N Harada, K Monde; Antihyperglycaemic flavonoids from *Syzygium samarangense* (Blume) Merr and Perry, *Phytother Res* **19**(3), 246-51 (2005)

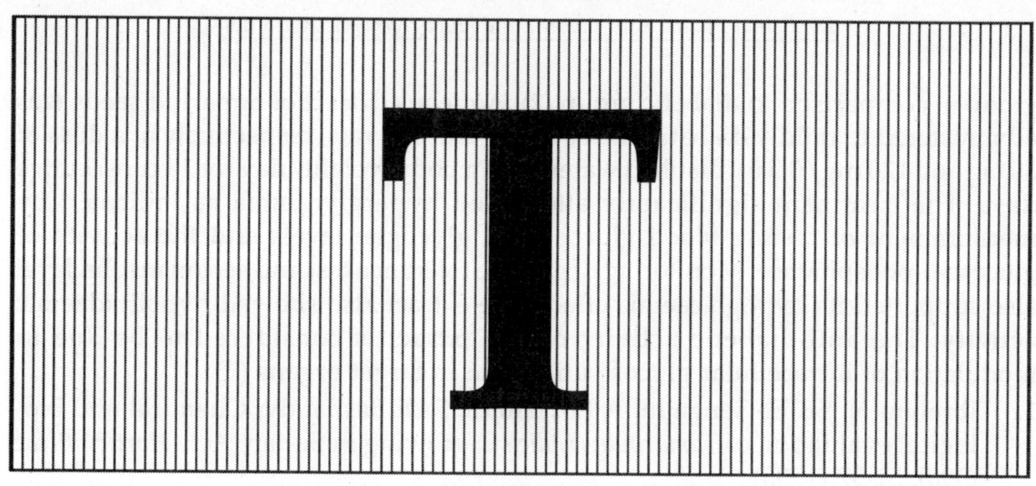

Talauma ovata St. Hil. (Magnoliaceae)

Chemical analysis demonstrated the presence of phytosteroids, saponins, alkaloids and tannins in the crude extract of the plant. Pharmacological studies failed to demonstrate hypoglycaemic effect of this plant in normoglycaemic, hyperglycaemic or alloxan-induced diabetic rats.

Morato GS, JB Calixto, L Cordeiro, TC de Lima, EF Morato, M Nicolau, GA Rae, RN Takahashi, RM Valle, RA Yunes; Chemical and pharmacological studies on *Talauma ovata* St. Hil. (Magnoliaceae), *J Ethnopharmacol* **26**(3), 277-86 (1989)

Tamarindus indica Linn. (Fabaceae /Ceasalpiniaceae) (Tamarind, H. Imalee, S. Amlika)

The tamarind, a large tropical tree, originally native to eastern Africa, has been naturalized in the tropics throughout the world. The pulp in its fruit pods is both sweet and extremely sour. The hypoglycaemic and hypocholesterolaemic properties of the seed pectin and the mucilages of seeds and fruits of *T. indica* were tested in alloxan-induced diabetic rats. Administration of tamarind seed and mesocarp mucilages significantly decreased blood glucose concentration. Tamarind seed pectin also showed hypoglycaemic but no hypocholesterolaemic properties (1). Aqueous extract of *T. indica* seeds was found to have potent anti-diabetogenic activity that reduces blood sugar level in streptozotocin-induced diabetic male rats. Supplementation of this aqueous extract (80 mg/0.5 ml distilled water/100 g b.w./ day) by gavage in streptozotocin-induced diabetic rats resulted in a significant reduction of fasting blood sugar level after 7 days. Continuous supplementation of this extract for 14 days brought down the fasting blood sugar level to that of the control animals. Further, this supplementation produced a significant elevation of glycogen content in liver and skeletal muscle and of liver glucose-6-phosphate dehydrogenase. Activities of liver glucose-6-phosphatase, liver and kidney GOT and GPT activities were decreased significantly in the aqueous extract supplemented group in comparison to diabetic group (2). Aqueous extract of tamarind seeds was administered to mildly diabetic and severely diabetic rats, respectively at a dose of 80 mg and 120 mg/0.5 ml distilled water/ 100 g body weight/ day for 14 consecutive days. The treatment significantly attenuated hyperglycaemia as indicated by measurement of fasting blood glucose and glycogen levels and the activity of glucose-6-phosphatase. Monitoring of glucose tolerance test and serum insulin level also supported its hypoglycaemic effect. The extract also showed hypolipidaemic activity. The anti-diabetic activity of the extract is considered to be due to modulation of intracellular glucose utilisation in target organs (3).

1. Ibrahim N, SE El-Gengaihi, A El-Hamidi, SAE Bashandy; Chemical and biological evaluation of *Tamarindus indica* L. growing in Sudan, *Acta Horticulturae* (390), 51-57 (1995)
2. Maiti R, D Jana, UK Das, D Ghosh; Anti-diabetic effect of aqueous extract of seed of *Tamarindus indica* in streptozotocin-induced diabetic rats, *J Ethnopharmacol* **92**(1), 85-91 (2004)
3. Maiti R, UM Das, D Ghosh; Attenuation of hyperglycaemia and hyperlipidaemia in streptozotocin-induced diabetic rats by aquepous extract of seed of *Tamarindus indica, Biol Pharm Bull* **28**(7), 1172-76 (2005)

Taraxacum officinale F.H. Wigg (Asteraceae / Compositae) (Dandelion, Dhudhal)

Dandelion is a nearly cosmopolitan weed that grows along roadsides and other areas with moist soils. It is best known for its yellow flower heads that turn into round balls of silver tufted fruits that blow away on the wind. The hypoglycaemic effects of *Taraxacum officinale* were studied in normoglycaemic and alloxan-treated hyperglycaemic rabbits (1). Agents with *alpha*-glucosidase inhibitory activity are known to be useful as oral hypoglycaemic drugs for the control of hyperglycaemia in patients with type-2; non-insulin-dependent diabetes mellitus (NIDDM). *Alpha* glucosidase inhibitory activity of Dandelion was studied *in vitro* and compared with different source of this enzyme (baker's yeast, rabbit liver and small intestine) to establish its *alpha* ghicosidase inhibitory activity (2).

1. Akhtar MS, QM Khan, T Khaliq; Effects of *Portulaca oleracae* (Kulfa) and *Taraxacum officinale* (Dhudhal) in normoglycaemic and alloxan-treated hyperglycaemic rabbits, *J Pak Med Assoc* **35**(7), 207-10 (1985)
2. Onal S, S Timur, B Ocutucu, F Zihnioglu; Inhibition of *alpha*-glucosidase by aqueous extracts of some potent anti-diabetic medicinal herbs, *Prep. Biochem. Biotchnol* **35**(1), 29-36 (2005)

Taxus cuspidata Siebold &Zucc (Taxaceae) (Japanese Yew)

Taxus cuspidata is native to Japan, Korea, northeast China and the extreme southeast of Russia. The plant has a rather long life and some are known to be 1000 years old.

Air-dried leaves and stems of the plant, which are used in folk medicine for the treatment of diabetes, yielded an ecdysteroid, taxisterone.

Nakano K, T Nohara, T Tomimatsu, M Nishikawa; A phytoecdysteroid, taxisterone, from *Taxus cuspidata, Phytochemistry* **21**(11), 2749-51 (1982)

Taxus yunnanensis W. C. Cheng & L. K. Fu (Taxaceae) (Chinese Yew)

Aqueous, aqueous methanol and methanol extracts of *T. yunnanensis* wood were found to possess potent radical scavenging effects and significant nitric oxide production inhibitory activity. From the active water extract of the wood, three lignans, isotaxiresinol, secoisolariciresinol and taxiresinol, were isolated as major components. The DPPH radical scavenging activity of the extract was due to these lignans, which also partly contributed to NO inhibitory activity in LPS activated 1774.1 cells. Hypoglycaemic effects of the water and methanol extracts of the wood of *T. yunnanensis* were examined in streptozotocin induced diabetic rats. The water extract significantly lowered the fasting blood glucose level at a dose of 100mg/kg (ip). The isolated lignans were also tested for their hypoglycaemic effects on the same experimental model. At a dose of 100mg/kg (ip), isotaxiresinol reduced the fasting blood glucose level of diabetic rats by 34.5%, while secoisolariciresinol and taxiresinol reduced by 33.4% and 20.9%, respectively. The blood glucose lowering effects of the first two liganas were stronger than the mixture of tolbutamide (200mg/kg) and buformine (1mg/kg) used as a positive control (1, 2).

1. Kadota S, AH Banskota, Y Tezuka, NT Nguyen, T Nobukawa; Chemical constituents and biological activities of the wood of *Taxus yunnanensis, IUPAC International Conference on Biodiversity and Natural Products Chemistry and Medical Applications,* New Delhi, p. ML 31, Jan. 26-31, 2004.
2. Banskota A, N Nguyen, Y Tezuka, T Nobukawa S Kadota; Hypoglycaemic effects of the wood of *Taxus yunnanensis* on streptozotocin-induced diabetic rats and its active components, *Phytomedicine* **13**(1-2), 109-14 (2006)

Tecoma stans (L.) Juss. ex Kunth. (Bignoniaceae) (Yellow trumpetbush)

Tecoma stans is a Mexican medicinal plant traditionally used for the treatment of diabetes. Oral administration of a decoction of the plant to streptozotocin-induced diabetic rats showed statistically significant reduction of glycaemia and improvement of body weight after 2 weeks of therapy (4). In an attempt to elucidate the popularly attributed anti-diabetic properties of this Mexican medicinal plant, Lozoya-Meckes and co-worker studied the effects of an infusion/extract of stems and leaves of *T. stans* on dogs. An intravenous administration of *T. stans* infusion in normal anaesthetised dogs produced a transient hyperglycaemic response and arterial hypotension followed by a slow decrease of the blood glucose values with a concomitant hypertriglyceridaemia. No important changes in immunoreactive insulin were detected. The effects observed on blood parameters appear to be related to hepatic glycogen metabolism, involving an activation of glycogenolysis. The early transient hypotensive and hyperglycaemic response is attributed to the presence of histamine-releasing substances in the plant. The late hypoglycaemic effect of *T. stans* extract was found to persist and it supported the existence of a specific hypoglycaemic principle in the plant (2, 3). The stability of tecomine, the alkaloid considered to be the major anti-diabetic factor of the plant, was assessed (1). The anti-hyperglycaemic activity of tecostanine, an alkaloid isolated from *T. stans* leaves, was also elucidated (5). In view of the reported hypoglycaemic activity of the plant, the major alkaloids, present in the plants growing in Egypt and Brazil, were isolated and tested *in vivo* on db/db mice. However, contrary to the popular belief, the major alkaloid, tecomine was unable to modify glycaemia; the only effect being a decrease in plasma cholesterol levels. The alkaloids, 5b-hydroxyskitanthine and boschniakine were also found to be inactive both *in vivo* and *in vitro* assays (6).

1. Hammouda Y, N Khalafallah; Stability of tecomine, the major anti-diabetic factor of *Tecoma stans* (Juss.) f. Bignoniaceae, *J Pharm Sci* **60**(8), 1142-45 (1971)
2. Lozoya-Meckes M, Mellado-Campos V; Is the *Tecoma stans* infusion an anti-diabetic remedy? *J Ethnopharmacol* **14**(1), 1-9 (1985)
3. Meckes-Lozoya M, X Lozoya; Histaminic response induced by the intravenous administration of *Tecoma stans* crude extract in the dog, *Herba Hungarica* **28**(1-2), 117-22 (1989)
4. Aguilar LC, S Macias, A Chagoya, A Cardenas, P Diaz, JM Cantu; Anti-diabetic activity of *Tecoma stans* in rats, *Fitoterapia* **64**(4), 304-05 (1993)
5. Costantino L, AP Lins, D Barlocco F Celotti, SA el-Abady, T Brunetti, R Maggi, L Antolini; Characterization and pharmacological actions of tecostanine, an alkaloid of *Tecoma stans, Pharmazie* **58**(2), 140-42 (2003)
6. Costantino L, L Raimondi, R Pirisino, T Brunetti, P Pessotto, F Giannessi, AP Lins, D Barlocco, L Antolini, SA El-Abady; Isolation and pharmacological activities of the *Tecoma stans* alkaloids, *Farmaco* **58**(9), 781-85 (2003)

Telfairia occidentalis Hook.f. (Cucurbitaceae)
(Fluted pumpkin)

Telfairia occidentalis is a tropical vine grown in West Africa and it is used as a leaf vegetable and for its edible seeds. Oral administration of an aqueous extract of the leaves of the plant (1 g/kg) did not alter the blood glucose level in normoglycaemic mice but in glucose-induced hyperglycaemia, anti-diabetic activity was seen when the extract and glucose were administered simultaneously and when the extract was given to the mice 60 minutes before glucose. In streptozotocin-induced diabetic mice, a reduction in the blood glucose level was seen from day two of the administration of the extract. The hypoglycaemic effect of the aqueous extract compared well with that of an oral dose of chlorpropamide (200 mg/kg) under the same conditions (1). The beneficial effect of aqueous extract of the leaves of *T. occidentalis* in diabetes mellitus was validated from the observation of a gradual but significant reduction in blood glucose in streptozotocin treated hyperglycaemic rats over a period of eight days compared to the normoglycaemic or chlorpropamide treated controls (2).

1. Aderibigbe AO, BA Lawal, JO Oluwagbemi; The anti-hyperglycaemic effect of *Telfaria occidentalis* in mice, *Afr J Med Sci* **28**(3-4), 171-75 (1999)
2. Emudianughe TS; The hypoglycaemic effect of *Telfaria occidentalis* aqueous leaf extract in rats, *West Afr J Pharmacol and Drug Res* **18**, 14-16 (2002)

Tephrosea purpurea (Linn.) Pers. (Fabaceae / Leguminosae) (Auhuhu, H. Sarphoka)

Tephrosea purpurea is a tropical plant which grows in arid regions of Hawaii. It also grows in other tropical countries. The leaves and seeds of the plant contain tephrosin, which paralyzes fish. Oral administration of an aqueous extract of seeds of *T. purpurea* led to marked lowering of blood glucose levels in normal and alloxan-induced diabetic rabbits. The hypoglycaemic effect of the extract was found to be comparable to that of tolbutamide in normal rabbits.

Rahman H, Kashfudduja, M Tyeb, M Saleemuddin; Hypoglyaemic activity of *Tephrosea purpurea* Linn. Seeds, *Indian J Med Res* **81**, 418-21 (1985)

Teramnus labialis (L.) Spreng. (Fabaceae) (Blue wiss)

Bioassay-guided fractionation of the aqueous alcohol extract of the aerial parts of the plant using C57BL/Ks-db/db mice as a model for type-2 diabetes yielded an active fraction containing a mixture of coumarins. The major coumarin present in the active fraction was identified as fraxidin.

Fort DM, K Rao, SD Jolad, J Luo, TJ Carlson, SR King; Anti-hyperglyaemic activity of *Teramnus labialis* (Fabaceae), *Phytomedicine* **6**(6), 465-67 (2000)

Terminalia catappa Linn (Combretaceae) (Indian almond)

The native range of *Terminalia catappa* is uncertain. It has long been naturalised in a broad belt extending from Northern Australia and New Guinea through South-East Asia into the Indian subcontinent. Petroleum ether, methanol, and aqueous extracts of *T. catappa* fruits produced significant anti-diabetic activity in alloxan-induced diabetic rats at 1/5 of their lethal doses. Histological studies revealed partial regeneration of the pancreas of these animals, which were necrosed by alloxan. Aqueous and methanol extracts were particularly effective.

Nagappa AN, PA Thakurdesai, N Venkat Rao, J Singh; Anti-diabetic activity of *Terminalia catappa* Linn fruits, *J Ethnopharmacol* **88**(1), 45-50 (2003)

Terminalia chebula Retz. (Combretaceae) (Black Myrobalan, H. Harda, S. Haritaki)

Terminalia chebula is native to southern Asia from India and Nepal to southwestern China and to Sri Lanka, Malaysia and Vietnam. The plant has been widely used in Ayurveda for the treatment of diabetes. Water extract of dry fruits of *T. chebula* was found to improve glucose tolerance and bring down the level fasting blood glucose in streptozotocin-induced diabetic rats (1). The anti-diabetic activity of the chloroform extract of *T. chebula* seed powder was studied in streptozotocin-induced diabetic rats using short term and long term study protocols. The chloroform extract of *T. chebula* seeds produced dose-dependent reduction in blood glucose of diabetic rats and the effect was comparable with that of glibenclamide, in short term study. It also produced significant reduction in blood glucose level in a long term study. Significant renoprotective activity was also observed in *T. chebula* treated rats. The results indicate that the hypoglycaemic activity is probably mediated through enhanced secretion of insulin from the *beta*-cells of Langerhans or through extra pancreatic mechanism. The mechanism of potent renoprotective actions of *T. chebula* needs evaluation (2).

1. Murali YK, Ramesh Chandra, PS Murthy; Anti-hyperglycaemic effect of water extract of dry fruits of *Terminalia chebula* in experimental diabetes mellitus, *Indian J Clin Biochem* **19**(2), 202-04 (2004)
2. Rao NK, S Nammi; Anti-diabetic and renoprotective effects of the chloroform extract of *Terminalia chebula* Retz. seeds in streptozotocin-induced diabetic rats, *BMC Complement Altern Med* **6**,17 (2006)

Terminalia pallida Brand (Combretaceae)

Oral administration of an ethanol extract of *T. pallida* fruits (0.5 g/kg b.w.) exhibited a significant anti-hyperglycaemic activity in alloxan-induced diabetic rats. The extract, however, failed to show any hypoglycaemic activity in normal rats.

Kameswara Rao B, P Renuka Sudarshan, MD Rajasekhar, N Nagaraju, Ch Appa Rao; Anti-diabetic activity of *Terminalia pallida* fruit in alloxan induced diabetic rats, *J Ethnopharmacol* **85**(1), 169-72 (2003)

Terminalia superba Engl. & Diels (Combretaceae) (Superb Terminalia)

The plant, native to tropical western Africa, is well known for its wood, which is used for making furniture and musical instruments and prized for its workability and excellent colour and finish. The administration of methanol/methylene chloride extract of the stem bark of *T. suberba* (300 mg/kg) to stretozotocin-induced diabetic rats, by gavage, daily for 14 days, significantly reduced their blood glucose levels. The results of detailed investigation showed that the plant extract was able to reverse hyperglycaemia, polyphagia and polydipsia provoked by streptozotocin.

Kamtchuing P, SM Kahpur; Anti-diabetic activity to methanol/methylene chloride stem bark extracts of *Terminalia superba* and *Canarium schweinfurthii* on streptozotocin-induced diabetic rats, *J Ethnopharmacol* **104**(3), 366-69 (2006)

Tetrapleura tetraptera Taub (Fabaceae / Mimosaceae)

The plant is used in West Africa as a spice, a medicine and as a dietary supplement rich in vitamin. The plant, known as Aridan in Southwest Nigeria, is a medicinal plant with many folkloric uses. The fruits of *T. tetraptera* are frequently used in Tropical African traditional medicine for the management and control of an array of human ailments, including arthritis, asthma, diabetes mellitus etc. The hypoglycaemic effects of an aqueous extract of *T. tetraptera* fruit were studied in rats using chlorpropamide (250 mg/kg p.o.) as the reference hypoglycaemic agent. The plant extract (50-800 mg/kg p.o.) produced dose-dependent, significant reductions in the blood glucose concentrations of both fasted normal and fasted diabetic rats. The findings lent pharmacological credence to the suggested folkloric uses of the plant's fruit in the management and/or control of adult-onset, type-2 diabetes mellitus.

Ojewole JA, CO Adewunmi; Anti-inflammatory and hypoglycaemic effects of *Tetrapleura tetraptera* (Taub) [Fabaceae] fruit aqueous extract in rats, *J Ethnopharmacol* **95**(2-3), 177-82 (2004)

Teucrium polium Linn. (Lamiaceae / Labiatae) (Felty Germander)

Native to the Mediterranean region and the Middle East, this lovely sub-shrub forms a woolly-looking foliage. In traditional Persian medicine, *T. polium* (locally called 'kalpooreh') is used for the treatment of a variety of ailments including diabetes mellitus. The hypoglycaemic activity of an aqueous decoction of aerial parts of the plant was tested in normoglycaemic and streptozotocin-induced hyperglycaemic rats. The extract caused significant reductions in blood glucose concentration 4 h after intravenous administration and 24 h after intra-peritoneal administration. This effect was considered to be due to enhancement of peripheral metabolism of glucose rather than an increase in insulin release (1).

Oral administration of the crude aqueous extract (0.5 g plant powder/kg b.w.) to a group of streptozotocin-induced diabetic rats for six consecutive weeks showed a significant decrease in blood glucose concentration in the treated animals compared to the untreated diabetic rats, without any measurable effect on the major biochemical factors. The extract also significantly enhanced the blood insulin level. The insulinotropic property of *T. polium* extract was further verified by an *in vitro* investigation using isolated pancreatic rat islets. The results of the investigation clearly revealed that the plant extract, probably without metabolic transformation, is able to reduce high blood glucose levels through enhancing insulin secretion by the pancreas (2).

Intranasal administration of the crude plant extract (10%) in a vehicle containing 5% (w/w) Pluronic F127, however, failed to show any significant difference between the extract treated and control animals receiving only water (3).

1. Gharaibeh MN, HH Elayan, AS Salhab; Hypoglycaemic effects of *Teucrium polium*, *J Ethnopharmacol* **24**(1), 93-99 (1988)
2. Esmaeili MA, R Yazdanparast; Hypoglycaemic effect of *Teucrium polium*: studies with rat pancreatic islets, *J Ethnopharmacol* **95**(1), 27-30 (2004)
3. Afifi FU, B Al-Khalidi, E Khalil; Studies on the *in vivo* hypoglyaemic activities of two medicinal plants used in the treatment of diabetes in Jordanian traditional medicine following intranasal administration, *J Ethnopharmacol* **100**(3), 314-18 (2005)

Theobroma cacao Linn. (Malvaceae /Sterculiaceae)

Theobroma cacao or the cocoa plant is a small evergreen tree, native to the deep tropical region of the Americas. It was hypothesized by Brand-Miller and his colleagues that chocolate products (products having cocoa powder) elicit higher insulin responses than matched products with alternate flavouring. An investigation was made to verify this hypothesis and the study showed that the presence of cocoa powder in foods (chocolate bars, cakes, breakfast cereals, ice creams, flavoured milks and puddings) leads to greater postprandial insulin secretion than alternate flavourings. The greatest difference occurred within the flavoured milk category in which the chocolate version elicited 45% greater insulinaemia than the strawberry flavoured milk

Brand-Miller J, SH Holt, V de Jong, P Petocz; Cocoa powder increases postprandial insulinemia in lean young adults, *J Nutr* **133**(10), 3149-52 (2003)

Thunbergia laurifolia Linn. (Acanthaceae) (Laurel clock vine)

Laurel clock vine, used as an ornamental plant, is native to Brazil. The hypoglycaemic properties of the aqueous extract of *T. laurifolia* leaves (60 mg/ml/day) were evaluated in normoglyaemic and alloxan-induced diabetic rats. The 15-day-treatment with *T. laurifolia* extract decreased levels of blood glucose in diabetic rats. The insulin-secreting *beta*-cells in the islet of Langerhans, severely damaged in diabetic rats, were also partially recovered in diabetic rats treated with the extract. Whether *T. laurifolia* leaf contains insulin-like substance(s), which directly act as hypoglycaemic agents, or contains substances that induce the regenerative process of *beta*-cells remains to be investigated.

Aritajat S, S Wutteerapol, K Saenphet; Anti-diabetic effect of *Thunbergia laurifolia* Linn. aqueous extract, *Southeast Asian J Trop Med Public Health* **35**(Suppl 2), 53-58 (2004)

Tillandsia usneoides Linn. (Bromeliaceae) (Spanish moss)

Spanish moss resembles *Usnea* or beard lichen but it is neither a moss nor a lichen but is a flowering plant. It ranges from the south-eastern United States to Argentina. Of the different compounds, isolated by bioactivity directed fractionation of an ethanol extract of *Tillandsia usneoides*, 3- hydroxy-3-methylglutaric acid (HMG) elicited significant hypoglycaemic responses in fasting normal mice. Further evaluation of HMG and other potential inhibitors of HMG CoA lyase, in the treatment of symptoms of diabetes mellitus, is suggested.

Witherup KM, JL McLaughlin, RL Judd, MH Ziegler, PJ Medon, WJ Keller; Identification of 3-hydroxy-3-methylglutaric acid (HMG) as a hypoglyaemic principle of Spanish moss (*Tillandsia usneoides*), *J Nat Prod* **58**(8), 1285-90 (1995)

Tinospora cordifolia (Thunb.) Miers (Menispermaceae) (Gulanshe Tinospara, H. Giloya, S. Amrita, Guduchi)

Tinospora cordifolia is indigenous to the tropical areas of India, Myanmar and Sri Lanka. It is widely used in Indian Ayurvedic medicine for treating diabetes mellitus. Gupta and co-workers studied the effects of the plant on fasting blood sugar level, glucose tolerance and adrenaline-induced hyperglycaemia (1). Administration of aqueous, alcoholic, and chloroform extracts of the leaves of *T. cordifolia* in doses of 50, 100, 150 and 200 mg/kg body weight to normal and alloxan-diabetic rabbits and estimation of blood glucose and total lipid levels before and 2, 4, 6, and 8 h after administration of the extract revealed hypoglycaemic effect of the extract in normal as well as in alloxan-treated rabbits. The extracts, however, had no significant effect on total lipid levels in normal as well as in alloxan-treated diabetic rabbits. From this study, *Tinospora cordifolia* was considered to have an insulin-like action (2). Oral administration of an extract of *T. cordifolia* at a dose of 20 mg/100g body weight showed moderate hypoglycaemic effect in normal and diabetic rats. Propranolol, insulin and tolbutamide in combination with *T. cordifolia* extract showed synergistic effect. A significant fall in glycaemic levels was also observed in glucose-induced hyperglycaemic rats. While the extract was effective in alloxan-induced moderately diabetic rats, it was virtually ineffective in severely diabetic rats (3). The effect of aqueous leaf digest (10 g/200 ml water) of *T. cordifolia* on postprandial blood glucose levels was studied in non-insulin dependent diabetic subjects using the method of glucose tolerance test. The leaf digest was found to significantly reduce blood sugar levels in human subjects (7).

The root extract (5 g/kg b.w.) also showed significant hypolipidaemic effect in alloxan-diabetic rats (4). Oral administration of an aqueous extract of *T. cordifolia* root to alloxan-induced diabetic rats caused a significant reduction in blood glucose and brain lipids. The extract caused an increase in body weight, total haemoglobin and hepatic hexokinase. The root extract also lowered hepatic glucose-6-phosphatase and serum acid phosphatase, alkaline phosphatase, and lactate dehydrogenase in diabetic rats (5). Oral administration of the root extract of *T. cordifolia* for 6 weeks resulted in a significant reduction of blood and urine glucose and of lipids in serum and tissues in alloxan-induced diabetic rats (8). Oral administration of an alcoholic extract of *T. cordifolia* roots (100 mg/kg) to diabetic rats for six weeks normalized the antioxidant status of heart and brain. The effect was more pronounced than that of glibenclamide (9). The anti-hyperglycaemic effect of aqueous and alcoholic extracts as well as lyophilized powder of the plant was evaluated in diabetic animals using different doses of diabetogenic agents for varying duration (21-120 days) so as to assess their effect in mild, moderate and severe diabetes mellitus. In the pilot study (mild diabetes), maximum reduction of glucose levels was seen in animals receiving 400 mg/kg per day of aqueous extract of the plant after 15 weeks of treatment. The percent reduction in glucose decreased significantly in animals having moderate and severe diabetes. The mechanism of action was also discussed (6).

1. Gupta SS, SC Verma, VP Garg, M Rai; Anti-diabetic effects of *Tinospora cardifolia*. I. Effect on fasting blood sugar level, glucose tolerance and adrenaline induced hyperglycaemia, *Indian J Med Res* **55**(7), 733-45 (1967)
2. Wadood N, A Wadood, SA Shah; Effect of *Tinospora cordifolia* on blood glucose and total lipid levels of normal and alloxan-diabetic rabbits, *Planta Med* **58**(2), 131-36 (1992)
3. Prasad HC, R Majumder, R Chakraborty; Hypoglycaemic and anti-hyperglycaemic effect of medicinal plant from Assam, *International Seminar: Traditional Medicine*, Calcutta, p.158, November 7-9, 1992
4. Prince PSM, VP Menon, G Gunasekaran; Hypoglycaemic activity of *Tinospra cordifolia* roots in alloxan diabetic rats, *J Ethnopharmacol* **64**(1), 53-57 (1999)
5. Prince PSM, VP Menon; Hypoglycaemic and other related actions of *Tinospora cordifolia* roots in alloxan-induced diabetic rats, *J Ethnopharmacol* **70**(1), 9-15 (2000)
6. Grover JK, V Vats, SS Rathi; Anti-hyperglycaemic effect of *Eugenia jambolana* and *Tinospora cordifolia* in experimental diabetes and their effects on key metabolic enzymes involved in carbohydrate metabolism, *J Ethnopharmacol* **73**(3), 461-70 (2000)
7. Sai KS, N Srividya; Blood glucose lowering effect of the leaves of *Tinospora cordifolia* and *Sauropus androgynus* in diabetic subjects, *J Nat Remedies* **2**(1), 28-32 (2002)

8. Prince PSM,, VP Menon; Hypoglycaemic and hypolipidaemic action of alcohol extract of *Tinospora cordifolia* roots in chemical induced diabetes in rats, *Phytother Res* **17**(4), 410-13 (2003)
9. Prince PSM, N Kamalakkannan, VP Menon; Restoration of antioxidants by ethanolic *Tinospora cordifolia* in alloxan-induced diabetic Wistar rats, *Acta Pol Pharm* **61**(4), 283-87 (2004)

Tinospora crispa L. Hook f. & Thompson (Menispermaceae) (H. Faridbel)

In Malaysia, *Tinospora crispa* extract is taken orally by patients of non-insulin-dependent diabetes for treating hyperglycaemia. Noor and co-workers (1-4) studied various aspects of the claimed hypoglycaemic property of the plant. Addition of the aqueous extract of the plant to the drinking water of normal and alloxan-induced diabetic rats significantly lowered fasting blood glucose levels and increased serum insulin levels in treated diabetic animals compared to untreated diabetic controls. The insulinotropic action of *T. crispa* was further investigated *in vitro* using isolated human or rat islets of Langerhans and HIT-T15 cells. The extract induced a dose dependent stimulation and potentiation of basal and glucose-stimulated insulin secretion, respectively. This insulinotropic effect was also evident in perifused human and rat islets and HIT-T5 B-cells. The findings substantiated the traditional claims for an oral hypoglycaemic effect of *Tinospora crispa*, and showed the association of hypoglycaemic effect with increased insulin secretion (1). After a 2-week treatment with the extract (4 g/l in the drinking water), these rats also showed improvement in glucose tolerance. Moreover, acute intravenous treatment with the extract (50 mg/kg) caused an increase in plasma insulin levels (2). In order to substantiate the anti-diabetic effect of the plant, its effect on intestinal glucose absorption and glucose uptake into adipocytes was studied. The results of detailed investigation clearly revealed that the anti-hyperglycaemic effect of the plant is not due to interference with intestinal glucose uptake or uptake of the sugar into the peripheral cells but is probably due to stimulation of insulin release *via* modulation of *beta*-cell Ca^{2+} concentration. The extract was found to sensitise the *beta*-cell to extra-cellular Ca^{2+} and promote intra-cellular Ca^{2+} accumulation, which, in turn, caused increased insulin release. That the mechanism of insulinotropic action of *Tinospora crispa* is physiological, suggests that the insulin secretagogue(s) present in the extract could indeed be a potential source of specific oral hypoglycaemic agent for the treatment of non-insulin dependent diabetes mellitus (3, 4).

A randomized double blind placebo controlled trial was conducted to determine the efficacy of *T. crispa* as an additional treatment in patients with type-2 diabetes mellitus who did not respond to oral hypoglycaemic drugs and refused insulin injection. No evidence in support of the use of *Tinospora crispa* powder (1 g, thrice daily for 6 months) as additional therapy in patients with type-2 diabetes mellitus, who did not respond to oral hypoglycaemic drugs, could be secured. It was further suggested that the patients receiving *T. crispa* might have an increased risk of hepatic dysfunction (5).

1. Noor H, SJ Ashcroft; Anti-diabetic effects of *Tinospora crispa* in rats, *J Ethnopharmacol* **27**(1-2), 149-61 (1989)
2. Noor H, P Hammonds, R Sutton, SJ Ashcroft; The hypoglycaemic and insulinotropic activity of *Tinospora crispa*: studies with human and rat islets and HIT-T15 B cells, *Diabetologia* **32**(6), 354-59 (1989)
3. Noor H, SJ Ashcroft; Pharmacological characterisation of the anti-hyperglycaemic properties of *Tinospora crispa* extract, *J Ethnopharmacol* **62**(1), 7-13 (1998)
4. Noor H, SJH Ashcroft; Insulinotropic activity of *Tinospora crispa* extract: Effect on *beta* cell Ca^{2+} handling, *Phytother Res* **12**(2), 98-102 (1998)
5. Sangsuwan C, S Udompanthurak, S Vannasaeng, V Thamlikitkul; Randomized controlled trial of *Tinospora crispa* for additional therapy in patients with type 2 diabetes mellitus, *J Med Assoc Thai* **87**(5), 543-46 (2004)

Tithonia diversifolia (Hemsl) A. Gray (Asteraceae) (Mexican Sunflower, Jpn. Nitobegiku)

Nitobegiku, the herb of *Tithonia diversifolia*, has been used as a medicinal plant for diabetes in Japan. Anti-diabetic effect of the water extract of the plant was investigated in KK-Ay-mice, an animal model of type-2 diabetes. The extract (1,500 mg/kg b.w.) reduced the blood glucose of KK-Ay mice and also lowered the plasma insulin 7 hours after single oral administration. No change in blood glucose level was, however, observed in the extract-treated normal mice (ddY). The results support that *Tithonia diversifolia* improves glucose metabolism by reducing insulin resistance (1). An 80% ethanol extract of the plant (500 mg/kg b.w.) reduced blood glucose in KK-Ay mice after a single oral dose and also significantly lowered plasma insulin. In an insulin tolerance test, the blood glucose level of the extract-treated KK-Ay mice was significantly decreased. These results supported the hypothesis that *T. diversifolia* improves glucose metabolism by reducing insulin resistance (2).

1. Miura T, K Furuta, A Yasuda, N Iwamoto, M Kato, E Ishihara, T Ishida, K Tanigawa; Anti-diabetic effect of nitobegiku in KK-Ay diabetic mice, *Am J Chin Med* **30**(1), 81-86 (2002)
2. Miura T, K Nosaka, H Ishii, T Ishida; Anti-diabetic effect of Nitobegiku, the herb *Tithonia diversifolia*, in KK-Ay diabetic mice, *Biol Pharm Bull* **28**(11), 2152-54 (2005)

Toona sinensis (A Juss.) M Roem. (Meliaceae) (Chinese Mahogany, H. Daaraluu)

Toona sinensis is native to eastern and southeastern Asia and found in North Korea, China, Nepal, northeastern India, Myanmar, Thailand, Malaysia and Indonesia. The effects of an aqueous alcohol extract of *T. sinensis* leaves on cellular [^{3}H]-2-deoxyglucose uptake in differentiated cultured 3T3-L1 adipocytes were investigated. Treatment of the cells with plant extract for 60 minutes increased [^{3}H]-2-deoxyglucose uptake. Similar observation was also made in insulin-stimulated cells. Cellular glucose uptake was also enhanced by *T. sinensis* leaf extract after incubation of cells with 20 mM glucose for 48 hours. Cellular glucose uptake with a combination of *T. sinensis* leaf extract and insulin was significantly inhibited by pre-treatment of cells with the protein synthesis inhibitor cycloheximide and the protein kinase C inhibitor calphostin C in normal-, medium- and high-glucose media. However, the glucose uptake-enhancing effect of *T. sinensis* leaf extract was not diminished by cycloheximide and calphostin C in the absence of insulin.

Yang YC, HK Hsu, JH Hwang, SJ Hong; Enhancement of glucose uptake in 3T3-L1 adipocytes by *Toona sinensis* leaf extract, *Kaohsiung J Med Sci* **19**(7), 327-33 (2003)

Tournefortia hartwegiana Steud (Boraginaceae)

The plant is used in traditional medicine for the treatment of diabetes, diarrhoea and kidney pain in Morelos, Mexico. Administration of a methanol extract from aerial parts of the plant (310 mg/kg b.w./day) for 10 days, to normoglycaemic and alloxan-induced diabetic rats, significantly lowered their blood glucose levels. The anti-diabetic and hypoglycaemic activities due to the methanol extract were similar to those produced by metformin (120 mg/kg). A study was undertaken to establish the possible modes of action of the extract to induce anti-diabetic activity. The plant extract inhibited *alpha*-glucosidase activity *in vitro*, in a concentration-dependent manner. It was inferred that the extract might exert its anti-diabetic effect by suppressing carbohydrate absorption from intestine, and thereby reducing the post-prandial increase of blood glucose (1, 2).

1. Ortiz-Andrade RR, V Rodriguez-Lopez, ML Garduno-Ramirez, P Castillo-Espana, S Estrada-Soto; Anti-diabetic effect on alloxanized and normoglycaemic rats and some pharmacological evaluations of *Tournefortia hartwegiana*, *J Ethnopharmacol* **101**(1-3), 37-42 (2005)
2. Ortiz-Andrade RR, S Garcia-Jimenez, P Castillo-Espana, G Ramirez-Avila, R Villalobos-Molina, S Estrada-Soto; *Alpha*-glucosidase inhibitory activity of the methanolic extract from *Tournefortia hartwegiana*: an anti-hyperglycaemic agent, *J Ethnopharmacol* **109**(1), 48-53 (2007)

Tournefortia hirsutissima Linn. (Boraginaceae) (Chiggery grapes)

The hypoglycaemic effect of aqueous and butanol extracts from *T. hirsutissima* was determined on neonatal induced streptozotocin diabetic rats. Oral administration of these extracts significantly lowered the plasma glucose levels in streptozotocin-induced diabetic rats within 3 h. Glibenclamide, used as reference, showed similar hypoglycaemic effect.

Andrade-Cetto A, Revilla-Monsalve C, Wiedenfeld H; Hypoglycaemic effect of *Tournefortia hirsutissima* L., on *n*-streptozotocin diabetic rats, *J Ethnopharmacol* **112**(1), 96-100 (2007)

Trema micrantha (L.) Blume (Cannabaceae / Ulmaceae) (Jamaican nettletree)

The acute treatment with *T. micrantha* leaf extract (250-1,000 mg/kg) caused a significant decrease in the blood glucose levels in alloxan-induced diabetic rats, but no effect was observed among the treated normal and hyperglycaemic normal rats. *T. micrantha* leaves are regarded as a good candidate for alternative and/or complementary medicine in the management of diabetes mellitus due to the beneficial effects of ethanol extract of leaves on blood glucose levels.

Schoenfelder T, TM Cirimbelli, V Citadini-Zanette; Acute effect of *Trema micrantha* (Ulmaceae) on serum glucose levels in normal and diabetic rats, *J Ethnopharmacol* **107**(3), 456-59 (2006)

Trema orientalis (Linn) Blume (Cannabaceae / Ulmaceae)

The glucose-lowering efficacy of the aqueous extract of *T. orientalis* stem bark was evaluated both in normal and streptozotocin-induced diabetic rats. Oral administration of a single dose (38-300 mg/kg) of the aqueous extract failed to reduce blood glucose levels in normoglycaemic rats, but exhibited a significant hypoglycaemic activity in streptozotocin-induced diabetic rats. The hypoglycaemic property of *T. orientalis* was also assessed by an oral glucose tolerance test in streptozotocin-diabetic rats. One week after repeated administration of the extract, blood glucose levels were significantly decreased and remained low even after 2 weeks. The results of the investigation indicated that *T. orientalis* stem bark extract exhibits hypoglycaemic activity by a mechanism different from that of sulfonylurea agents.

Dimo T, FT Ngueguim, P Kamtchouing, E Dongo, PV Tan; Glucose lowering efficacy of the aqueous stem bark extract of *Trema orientalis* (Linn) Blume in normal and streptozotocin diabetic rats, *Pharmazie* **61**(3), 233-36 (2006)

***Tribulus terrestris* Linn. (Zygophyllaceae) (S. Gokshura)**

It is a flowering plant native to warm temperate and tropical regions; in southern Europe, southern Asia, throughout Africa, and in northern Australia. The decoction of *T. terresteis* was found to significantly inhibit the gluconeogenesis and influence glycometabolism in normal mice. It also reduced the level of triglyceride and cholesterol in the plasma. The saponin, isolated from the plant, significantly reduced the level of serum glucose in normal and diabetic mice. It also reduced the level of serum triglyceride and cholesterol and increased the activity superoxide dismutase in mice (1, 2).

1. Li M, W Qu, S Chu, H Wang, C Tian M Tu; Effect of the decoction of *Tribulus terrestris* on mice gluconeogenesis, *Zhong Yao Cai* **24**(8), 586-88 (2001) [Article in Chinese]
2. Li M, W Qu, Y Wang, H Wan, C Tian; Hypoglycaemic effect of saponin from *Tribulus terrestris, Zhong Yao Cai* **25**(6), 420-22 (2002) [Article in Chinese]

***Trichosanthes kirilowii* Maxim. (Cucurbitaceae) (Snake gourd, Chinese cucumber)**

See "HYPOGLYCAEMIC GLYCANS' in Appendix

***Tridax procumbens* Linn. (Asteraceae) (Coat buttons, H, Ghamra, S. Jayanti veda)**

It is a widespread weed, native to the tropical Americas but has been introduced to tropical, subtropical, and mild temperate regions worldwide. Oleanolic acid, isolated from the plant and its derivatives showed positive response against the enzyme, *alpha*-glucosidase.

Shaiq Ai M, M Jahangir, S Shazad-ul-Hussan, MI Choudhary; Inhibition of *alpha*-glucosidase by oleanolic acid and its derivatives, *Phytochemistry* **60**(3), 295-99 (2002)

***Trifolium alexandrium* Linn. (Fabaceae) (Berseem)**

T. alexandrium whole seed diet significantly lowered blood sugar levels of normal as well as of alloxan-induced diabetic rats. The petroleum ether, alcohol and water extracts of the seeds were effective.

Singhal PC, RK Gupta, LD Joshi; Effect of feeding *Trifolium alexandrium* (Berseem) on blood sugar levels, *Indian J Pharm* **44**(2), 26-28 (1982).

Trigonella foenum graecum L. (Fabaceae / Leguminosae) (Fenugreek, H. Methi)

The seeds of *Trigonella foenum-graecum*, used as a spice in Indian kitchen, are also employed as herbal medicine. The seeds are known for their carminative, tonic, anti-ulcer and anti-diabetic effects, in particular. Considerable work on the hypoglycaemic activity of different parts of the plant, especially of its seeds, has been carried out using different solvent extracts, their fractions and different animal models. Efforts have also been made to postulate the mechanisms of action of this herbal drug. Mishkinsky and co-workers (1) studied the hypoglycaemic effect of *Trigonella foenum graecum* seeds and of its major alkaloids in normal and alloxan-induced diabetic rats. Of the different extracts of fenugreek seeds, tested for their hypoglycaemic effect in rabbits, the alkaloid-rich fraction showed maximum effect within two hours of its administration (6)

The stems, leaves and seeds of the plant were extracted at room temperature for three days with water or acetone or carbon tetrachloride. The extracts were evaporated below 30° C under reduced pressure, and the residues obtained were dissolved in distilled water containing Tween 80 for oral administration to rats. Hypoglycaemic activity of these extracts was tested on 20-hour fasted normal as well as on alloxan- and cadmium-treated rats. (Cadmium has been shown to cause hyperglycaemia by releasing epinephrine in intact rats and inhibiting insulin release in the isolated perfused rat pancreas). Carbon tetrachloride extract of the seed as well as water and acetone extracts of stems and leaves were inactive in normal animals. However, acetone extract of seeds exhibited dose related hypoglycaemic effects. The hyperglycaemia induced by cadmium or alloxan was antagonized by acetone extracts of seed or stem and leaves. From the results it was inferred that *Trigonella* acetone extract acts, at least in part, at the cellular level to produce its hypoglycaemic effects on normal rats or those treated with cadmium or alloxan (2). Aqueous extract of *Trigonella foenum-graecum* leaves, given either orally or intra-peritoneally, showed hypoglycaemic effect in normoglycaemic and alloxan-induced hyperglycaemic rats but only intra-peritoneal administration of an ethanol extract (0.8 g/kg) of fenugreek leaves to diabetic rats produced a significant reduction of blood glucose concentration at 2 and 24 h only. The LD_{50} values for intra-peritoneal and oral administration of aqueous extract of fenugreek leaf in mice were 1.9 and 10 g/kg, respectively. The main organ affected after intra-peritoneal administration of the aqueous extract was the liver, while oral administration of the aqueous extract did not produce any sign of organ damage (21). The safety and efficacy of aqueous extract of *Trigonella foenum-graecum* leaves was investigated using 20 male volunteers aged 20-30 years. The extract effectively reduced blood glucose in normal subjects safely. It also reduced serum potassium level and this hypokalaemic effect merits further investigation (32). Supplementation of the diet with fenugreek leaves showed a significant effect on hyperglycaemia, hypoinsulinaemia and glycosylated haemoglobin in streptozotocin-induced diabetic rats. Fenugreek leaves improved the body weight and liver glycogen and also showed a significant effect on key carbohydrate metabolic enzymes in diabetic rats. The effect of fenugreek leaves was found to be similar to that of glibenclamide (45). Rats, made diabetic by intraperitoneal injection of streptozotocin (40 mg/kg), were fed diets supplemented with fenugreek leaves for 45 days. Fenugreek leaves lowered the lipid profile in streptozotocin-induced diabetic rats (47). Fenugreek leaf powder supplementation also significantly lowered lipid peroxidation and significantly increased the antioxidant system in streptozotocin-induced diabetic rats. The effect at a dose of 1 g/kg of body weight of fenugreek leaf powder was similar to that of glibenclamide (53).

The effects of lipid extract and the defatted fraction of fenugreek seeds were tested for their putative hypoglycaemic activity by oral administration to normal or diabetic dogs for 8 days. While the lipid extract was devoid of any activity, the fibre-rich defatted fraction lowered basal blood glucose level, plasma glucagon and somatostatin levels and reduced the orally induced hyperglycaemia. The addition of this fraction to the insulin treatment resulted in a decrease of hyperglycaemia and glycosuria in diabetic dogs. The defatted part, which in addition to fibres contains steroid saponins, was thus proved to be responsible for the anti-diabetic action of fenugreek seeds. The addition of this fraction to the food of diabetic hypercholesterolaemic dogs caused a decrease of cholesterolaemia and reduction of hyperglycaemia (3, 4). The defatted fenugreek seed yielded, on fractionation, a fibre-rich and a saponin and protein-rich sub-fraction. The effects of chronic administration of each sub-fraction on hyperglycaemia and the levels of pancreatic hormones were studied in alloxan-induced diabetic dogs. The addition of fibre-rich sub-fraction to insulin treatment resulted in a clear decrease of hyperglycaemia and glycosuria accompanied by a reduction of the high plasma glucagon and somatostatin levels in diabetic dogs. The treatment also decreased the hyperglycaemic response to the oral glucose tolerance test. The other sub-fraction was virtually devoid of the desired activity. The existence of one or more unknown active pharmacological compounds in fibre-rich sub-fraction is a possibility (5).

Oral administration of an alcoholic extract of *Trigonella foenum-graecum* seeds significantly reduced the blood sugar levels of normal as well as of alloxan-induced diabetic rats (39, 42). Oral administration of a single dose (0.5 ml) of 40-80% decoctions of fenugreek seeds to normal as well as alloxanized mice was followed by hypoglycaemia developed over a 6-h period. Reduction in blood glucose concentration was highly significant and dose-dependent. The hypoglycaemia caused by the ethanol extract (200-400 mg/kg) in alloxanized mice was also dose-dependent and comparable in effect to tolbutamide (7).

The effect of fenugreek seeds on postprandial glucose and insulin levels following the meal tolerance test (MIT) was studied in non-insulin dependent diabetics

(NIDDM). The addition of powdered fenugreek seed (15 g), soaked in water, to meals reduced the subsequent postprandial glucose levels significantly. The plasma insulin also tended to be lower in non-insulin dependent dibetics, given fenugreek (8). Oral administration of fraction G-2 of *Trigonella foenum graecum* (100mg/kg) for 15 days considerably improved the glucose tolerance in alloxan diabetic rabbits. This fraction also increased serum insulin levels of these animals. Following treatment with this fraction, total serum cholesterol and HDL-cholesterol returned back to normal levels. It was suggested that this active hypoglycaemic principle (G-2) stimulated the peripheral utilization of glucose by extra-hepatic tissues as well as at the pancreatic level (11). The effect of fenugreek seeds on blood glucose and the serum lipid profile was evaluated also in insulin-dependent (Type I) diabetic patients. Defatted fenugreek seed powder (100 g), was divided into two equal doses and incorporated into the diet, served during lunch and dinner. The fenugreek diet significantly reduced fasting blood sugar and improved the glucose tolerance test. It also reduced 24-h urinary glucose excretion. Significant reductions of serum total cholesterol, LDL and VLDL cholesterol and triglycerides were also noticed. The usefulness of fenugreek seeds in the management of diabetes was thus indicated (13). In normal rats, fenugreek seed powder inhibited the increase of blood sugar levels during oral glucose tolerance test. The seed powder also lowered the blood sugar levels of streptoztocin-induced diabetic rats (17). Oral administration of fenugreek seeds (2 and 8 g /kg) to normal and alloxan induced diabetic rats, significantly lowered the blood sugar levels of both groups of animals in a dose dependent manner (18). In a metabolic study, 10 non-insulin dependent diabetic patients were randomly given diets with or without fenugreek seed powder (25 g) for 15 days. At the end of the study, an intravenous glucose tolerance test was done, which showed that fenugreek, in the diet, significantly reduced the area under the plasma glucose curve and enhanced the metabolic clearance rate. It also increased erythrocyte insulin receptors. It was suggested that fenugreek improved the peripheral glucose utilization, which in turn, improved the glucose tolerance. The fenugreek seed exerted hypoglycaemic effect by acting at the insulin receptors at gastrointestinal level (16). The traditional recipe, "Pongal" containing raw or germinated fenugreek seeds (12.5 g) was found to lower the blood sugar levels in normal and non-insulin dependent diabetic patients as compared to Pongal without fenugreek seeds (20). Administration of sprouted fenugreek seeds (30 g/day) to non-insulin dependent diabetes mellitus patients lowered their blood sugar levels. The fenugreek also exhibited mild hypocholesterolaemic activity (22). Administration of fenugreek seed powder to patients of non-insulin dependent diabetes twice daily for 12 months significantly lowered their blood sugar levels. It was suggested that fenugreek might be effective in the treatment of diabetes (23). Administration of single dose of fenugreek (50 mg/kg) significantly attenuated the oral glucose tolerance test curve, as evidenced by decreased area under the curve. However, the fasting blood sugar levels remained unchanged. Repeated administration of the fraction G-II lowered fasting blood sugar levels of mild diabetic animals. The severely diabetic rabbits, treated for 30 days, exhibited a significant reduction of fasting blood sugar along with normalization of oral glucose tolerance (24). Fenugreek seed powder (*Methika Churna*), given to 15 patients of type-2 diabetes, at a dose of 9g/day for three months, significantly decreased their blood sugar, cholesterol and triglyaeride levels. It was suggested that fenugreek could be effectively used in controlling blood sugar or lipid levels of diabetic patients (26).

Hypoglycaemic and hypolipidaemic effect of diets supplemented with 20% *Trigonella foenum graecum* seeds was studied in streptozotocin-induced diabetic rats. The rats, not pre-treated with supplemented diets and given diets only after induction of diabetes, did not show any effect on blood sugar or lipid levels but the animals, put on fenugreek diet for five weeks prior to streptozotocin injection and maintained on the same diet for another six weeks after induction of diabetes exhibited a significant reduction in the blood sugar, free fatty acids, cholesterol and triglycerides levels (9). Increased lipid peroxidation and alterations in circulating antioxidants were observed in the diabetic rats but supplementation of fenugreek seeds in the diet of these rats lowered lipid peroxidation. The contents of glutathione and *beta*-carotene were increased and the *alpha*-tocopherol content was lowered. The levels of antioxidants in normal rats, which were fed fenugreek-supplemented diet, were higher than the control animals, which were fed commercial rat chow. The disrupted antioxidant status due to free radicals in diabetic animals was normalised by fenugreek seed supplementation in the diet (31). Administration of *T. foenum-graecum* seed (Kasoori methi) powder (10 g), 3-4 hours before glucose load to normal volunteers showed little effect on blood sugar and glucose tolerance. However, in men with sedentary habits and diabetic tendency, the seed powder of fenugreek produced reproducible hypoglycaemic effect (12).

Oral administration of both aqueous and methanol extracts (1 g/kg b.w.) of fenugreek seeds to normal mice produced hypoglycaemic effect; the effect was more pronounced in aqueous extract. The presence of hypoglycaemic activity in aqueous and methanol extracts indicates that the active compounds are polar in nature (36). The fenugreek seed powder, its methanol and aqueous extracts and also soluble dietary fibre of fenugreek showed sustained glucose reducing activity in normal and streptozotocin-induced diabetic Long Evans rats. The whole seed powder was found to be non-toxic up to a dose of 10 mg/kg. In human volunteers, the whole seed powder and soluble dietary fibre of fenugreek exhibited similar hypoglycaemic activity (14). Effect of fenugreek seeds on the fasting blood glucose level in the streptozotocin-induced diabetic rats was studied and from the results of investigation it was concluded that fenugreek decreases the fasting blood glucose level considerably by improving diabetes mellitus (48). Chronic administration of a fenugreek seed extract in rats was found to enhance food consumption and motivation to eat and also induce hyperinsulinaemia as well as hypocholesterolaemia (15). Thyroxine treatment in rats (300 μg/kg b.w./day) not only increased the levels of both the thyroid hormones (T3 and T4) but also elevated the level of serum glucose concentration and reduced the serum cholesterol level. Administration of fenugreek seed extract (220 mg/kg/day) in hyperthyroid animals decreased the serum glucose concentration as well as the serum thyroid hormones. Fenugreek seed extract was thus proved to be effective in the treatment of thyroxine-induced hyperglycaemia (44). Fenugreek seed powder was sequentially extracted with methanol and water. The seed powder, its methanol extract, and the residue left after methanol extraction showed significant hypoglycaemic effects when fed simultaneously with glucose. The water extract of the residue left after methanol extraction also showed significant hypoglycaemic activity at different prandial states. This soluble dietary fibre fraction showed no effect on the fasting blood glucose levels of non-diabetic or NIDDM model rats but showed a significant hypoglycaemic effect in NIDDM model rats when fed simultaneously with glucose. The results confirm the involvement of soluble dietary fibre fraction, having a galactomannan as it major constituent, in the hypoglycaemic effect of *T. foenum graecum* seeds (19). The chronic effect of soluble dietary fibre fraction on serum fructosamine, insulin and lipid levels, and on platelet aggregation in Type-2 diabetic rats has also been studied. Oral administration of this soluble dietary fibre of fenugreek seeds (0.5 g/kg, twice daily for 28 days) lowered the serum fructosamine level with no significant change in the insulin level as compared with the control but atherogenic lipids, cholesterol and LDL-cholesterol were found to decrease significantly with no significant effect on platelet aggregation (41). Administration of soluble dietary fibre fraction (5 g/kg b.w.) to normal, type-1 or type-2 diabetic rats significantly improved oral glucose tolerance. This fibre fraction suppressed the elevation of blood glucose after oral sucrose ingestion in both non-diabetic and type-2 diabetic rats. Daily oral administration of this fibre fraction to type-2 diabetic rats for 28 days decreased serum glucose, increased liver glycogen content and enhanced total antioxidant status. Serum insulin and insulin secretion were not affected by this fraction, which, however, increased glucose transport in 3T3-L1 adipocytes and insulin action. The findings indicated that the soluble dietary fibre fraction of *T. foenum-graecum* seeds exerts anti-diabetic effects mediated through inhibition of carbohydrate digestion and absorption, and enhancement of peripheral insulin action (59). The effect of oral administration of whole seed powder of fenugreek (5% in the diet) for 21 days on glycolytic, gluconeogenic and NADP-linked lipogenic enzymes were studied in liver and kidney tissues of alloxan-induced diabetic Wistar rats. In the diabetic liver, the activities of the glycolytic and lipogenic enzymes were significantly lower but those of gluconeogenic enzymes were higher. In the kidney tissues, however, the activities of the glycolytic and gluconeogenic enzymes were significantly higher but the activities of the lipogenic enzymes were lower. *Trigonella* seed powder treatment to diabetic rats for 21 days brought down the elevated fasting blood glucose levels to control levels and restored to control values the altered enzyme activities in both the liver and kidney. These biochemical effects exerted by *Trigonella* seeds make it a possible new therapeutic in type-1 diabetes (35). Administration of *Trigonella* seed powder to alloxan-induced diabetic rats significantly restored the altered enzyme activity to almost normal levels. Diabetes-induced structural changes in liver and kidney were also normalized following *Trigonella* seed powder (43). Histopathological abnormalities in tissues of diabetic rats were studied and the protective effect of fenugreek seed powder was evaluated. The activity of the enzyme, glutamate dehydrogenase was significantly higher while that of D-β-hydroxybutyrate dehydrogenase was significantly lower in liver and kidney of alloxan-induced diabetic rats. Histopathological studies showed liver degenerative and early nephropathic changes in diabetic rats. Ultrastructure of the diabetic liver revealed a reduction in the rough endoplasmic reticulum and swelling of mitochondria in the hepatocytes. Fenugreek treatment to the diabetic rats effectively prevented the alteration in the activities of the two enzymes and partially prevented the structural abnormalities suggesting a protective effect of fenugreek seed powder on the liver and kidney of the diabetic rats (49).

The protective effect of the aqueous extract of fenugreek seeds on the activity of calcium-dependent adenosine triphosphatase (Ca^{2+} ATPase) in liver homogenate was studied in the presence of Fe^{2+} ascorbate *in vitro*. Ca^{2+} ATPase activity in liver was protected by the aqueous extract to nearly 80% of the initial activity. The enhanced lipid peroxidation and increased susceptibility to oxidative stress associated with depletion of antioxidants in liver, kidney and pancreas of diabetic rats were normalized by a diet supplemented with fenugreek seed powder for 30 days at a dosage of 2 g/kg body weight. The findings suggest that the soluble portion of the seeds could be responsible for the antioxidant property (37). The mechanism of action of an orally active hypoglycaemic principle, isolated from water extract of seeds of *Trigonella foenum graecum,* was investigated in alloxan-induced sub-diabetic and overtly diabetic rabbits of different severities. Oral administration of the active principle (50 mg/kg b.w. for 15 days) to the sub-diabetic and mild diabetic rabbits produced significant attenuation of the glucose tolerance curve and improvement in the glucose induced insulin response, suggesting that the hypoglycaemic effect might be due to stimulation of insulin synthesis and/or secretion of insulin from the *beta* pancreatic cells of Langerhans. Prolonged administration (30 days) of the active principle to the severely diabetic rabbits significantly lowered fasting blood glucose level, but elevated the fasting serum insulin level to a much lower extent, suggesting an extra-pancreatic mode of action for the active principle. It may also be possible that the active principle increases the sensitivity of tissues to available insulin (40). The *in vivo* hypoglycaemic activity of a dialysed fenugreek seed extract was studied in alloxan-induced diabetic mice and found to be comparable to that of insulin (1.5 U/kg). The extract also improved intra-peritoneal glucose tolerance in normal mice. The mechanism by which dialysed extract attenuated hyperglycaemia was investigated *in vitro*. From the results of detailed investigation it was suggested that *in vivo* the hypoglycaemic effect of dialysed fenugreek seed extract is mediated, at least in part, by the activation of an insulin signalling pathway in adipocytes and liver cells (52). The effects of 21 days oral administration of fenugreek seed extract (1.5 g/kg b.w.) on the liver and kidney glycogen content and on some key liver enzymes of carbohydrate metabolism were studied in streptozotocin-induced diabetic rats. Administration of fenugreek extract to STZ-diabetic rats reduced blood glucose level by 58%, restored liver glycogen content and significantly decreased kidney glycogen as well as liver glucose-6-phosphatase activity. The extract was able to inhibit *alpha*-amylase activity in a dose-dependent manner *in vitro*. This inhibition was reversed by increasing substrate concentration in a pattern which complies well with the effect of competitive inhibitors. This *in vitro* inhibition was confirmed by *in vivo* suppression of starch digestion and absorption induced by fenugreek seed extract in normal rats. The findings suggest that the hypoglycaemic effect of fenugreek is mediated through insulinomimetic effect as well as by inhibition of intestinal *alpha*-amylase activity (56).

The amino acid, 4-hydroxyisoleucine was isolated in the pure form from fenugreek seeds. This amino acid was found to increase glucose-induced insulin release in the concentration range of 100 μmol/l to 1 mmol/l, through a direct effect on isolated islets of Langerhans from both rats and humans. The stimulating effect of 4-hydroxyisoleucine was strictly glucose dependent and it was ineffective at low or basal glucose concentrations. From the results of detailed investigation it was inferred that the anti-diabetic properties of fenugreek seeds are, at least in part, due to insulinotropic amino acid, 4-hydroxyisoleucine. This secretagogue may be considered as a novel drug for the treatment of NIDDM. In addition to anti-diabetic effect, the seed extract also exhibited hypocholesterolaemic activities (25, 27). The structural requirement for the insulinotropic amino acid 4-hydroxyisoleucine, derived from fenugreek seeds was studied by using synthetic amino acid and analogues. It was observed that only the isomer, (2S,3R,4S) of 4-hydroxyisoleucine acts in the micromolar range. On incubated isolated rat islets, the threshold concentration for a significant increase in insulin release was 200 μM for (2S,3R,4S) 4-hydroxyisoleucine (33). Rich in protein, fenugreek seeds contain the unique free amino acid, 4-hydroxyisoleucine, which has been characterized as one of the active ingredients for blood glucose control. This unusual amino acid also significantly decreased the plasma triglyceride levels, total cholesterol, and free fatty acids accompanied by an increase in HDL-cholesterol/Total cholesterol ratio in the dyslipidemic hamster model (57). As a part of safety evaluation of novel ingredients for use in blood glucose control, the potential genotoxicity of a fenugreek seed extract, containing a minimum of 40% 4-hydroxyisoleucine, was evaluated using the standard battery of tests (reverse mutation assay; mouse lymphoma forward mutation assay; mouse micronucleus assay). The negative assay results provide support that addition of fenugreek seed to foodstuffs formulated for people with diabetes is quite safe (50).

In diabetic rats, the decreased hepatic glyoxalase-1 activity and hyperglycaemia were restored back to almost normal levels following treatment with sodium orthovanadate and fenugreek seed powder. Combination of vanadate and fenugreek was relatively more effective (28). The significantly increased activities of glucose-6-phosphatase and fructose-1,6-bisphosphatase in diabetic liver and kidney were found to be lowered to almost control values by the use of the anti-diabetic compounds like insulin, sodium orthovanadate and fenugreek seed powder. The highest percentage of reversal to normal values was seen using the combination of vanadate and fenugreek seed powder. The lowered rate of growth of the animals as well as the increased blood sugar levels were reversed almost to the control levels by this combination therapy. The inclusion of the fenugreek seed powder overcame the toxicity of vanadium and much lower levels of vanadate were needed when it was given in combination with fenugreek seed powder. The combined effects of vanadate and fenugreek seed powder in restoring the above parameters were better than those induced by insulin administration (29). As compared to control rats, creatine kinase activities were found to decrease significantly in the tissues of experimental diabetic rats. Like insulin and vanadate, fenugreek seed powder also normalized the decreased creatine kinase activities to almost control values (30). As oxygen free radicals are considered to be responsible for the severity and complications of diabetes, the level of antioxidant enzymes catalase, superoxide dismutase and glutathione peroxidase as well as the oxidative damage were examined in the tissues of control, diabetic and treated rats. Vanadate and fenugreek administration to diabetic animals showed a reversal of the disturbed antioxidant levels and peroxidative damage. As oxidative stress plays a key role in the complications of diabetes, antioxidant property of vanadate and fenugreek seeds can be valuable in the treatment of the reversal of the complications of diabetes (38). Vanadate treatment to diabetic rats has been reported to correct the altered carbohydrate metabolism and antioxidant status. However, vanadate exerts these effects at relatively high doses and several toxic effects are produced. Investigation was, therefore, made to assess whether low doses of vanadate in combination with fenugreek seed powder can solve this problem. Alloxan-diabetic rats were treated separately with insulin, vanadate (0.6 mg/ml), fenugreek seed powder and a combined dose of vanadate (0.2 mg/ml) and fenugreek for 21 days. At the end of the experimental period, blood glucose levels and activities of pyruvate kinase, phosphoenolpyruvate carboxykinase, glutathione peroxidase, glutathione reductase, superoxide dismutase and catalase were measured in the liver and kidney. Rats treated with a combined dose of vanadate and fenugreek had glucose levels comparable to control ones. Similar results were obtained with the activities of the enzymes concerned. Lower doses of vanadate in combination with fenugreek seed powder were found to effectively counter diabetic alterations without any toxic side effects (46).

Lens, an insulin-independent tissue, was found severely affected in diabetes showing visual signs of cataract. The activity of the enzymes hexokinase, aldose reductase and sorbitol dehydrogenase was significantly increased whereas the activity of glucose-6-phosphate dehydrogenase, glutathione peroxidase and glutathione reductase decreased significantly in lenses from the third week of alloxan-induced diabetic rats. Significant increase in accumulation of metabolites, sorbitol, fructose, glucose was also found in diabetic lenses. The level of peroxidation, as measured by thiobarbituric acid reactive substances, increased whereas the levels of antioxidant reduced glutathione decreased significantly in diabetic condition. Insulin restored the levels of altered enzyme activities and metabolites almost to control levels. Sodium orthovanadate (0.6 mg/ml) and fenugreek seeds, administered separately to diabetic animals, could partially reverse the diabetic changes, metabolic and morphological, while vanadate in lowered dose in combination with fenugreek seeds was found to be most effective in restoring the altered lens metabolism and morphological appearance in diabetes. It was concluded from the observation that vanadate at lowered doses administered in combination with fenugreek seeds was most effective in controlling the altered glucose metabolism and antioxidant status in diabetic lenses (51). Not only increased blood glucose levels of diabetic rats were normalized with a lower dose of vanadium and fenugreek treatment, the sciatic nerve was also protected against the structural abnormalities found in diabetes. From the results it was suggested that lower doses of Na_3VO_4 might be used in combination with fenugreek seed as an efficient anti-diabetic agent to effectively control the long-term complications of diabetes in tissues like peripheral nerve (54). The effects of the anti-diabetic compounds (insulin, vanadate, fenugreek seed and vanadate in combination with fenugreek seed) were examined on general physiological parameters and distribution of glucose transporter (GLUT4) in skeletal muscle by immunoblotting and immunohistochemistry. Treatment of alloxan-diabetic rats with all these anti-diabetic compounds revived normoglycaemia and restored the disturbances in the distribution of GLUT4 in skeletal muscle. Fenugreek seed treatment was only partially effective in the restoration of diabetic alterations. The treatment of diabetic rats with combined doses of vanadate and fenugreek seed was most effective in the normalization of plasma glucose levels and correction of altered GLUT4 distribution (55). Treatment of diabetic rats with insulin, fenugreek seed powder, vanadate and a combined therapy of lower dose of vanadate with fenugreek seed powder revived normoglycaemia and restored the altered level of Na^+/K^+-ATPase, lipid peroxidation and membrane fluidity and also induced the redistribution of GLUT4 transporter. Fenugreek seed powder treatment alone is partially effective in restoring the above diabetes-induced alterations. Combined therapy of vanadate and fenugreek seed was most effective in normalization of altered membrane linked functions and GLUT4 distribution without any harmful side effect (58).

The beneficial hypoglycaemic effect of millets, fenugreek seeds and legumes in diabetic subjects has been amply demonstrated but the bitter taste of fenugreek seeds and coarse nature of millets have been limitations in using them in daily dietaries. However, the millets, fenugreek seeds and legumes in judicious combination, after suitable processing, were used to formulate three nutritious food products—dhokla (leavened steamed cake), uppuma (kedgeree) and laddu (sweet balls), which are popular traditional snack foods in India. Evaluation of these food products for glyaemic response in five normal and five diabetic subjects showed hypoglycaemic effects in terms of glycaemic-index. These food products may have an important role in dietary management for diabetic people (34).

A rabbit model (alloxan recovered model) has been developed for testing the hypoglycaemic activity of *Trigonella foenum graecum* and other drugs. Intravenous administration of alloxan (80 mg/kg b.w.) to rabbits showed initial increase of their fasting blood glucose levels up to 15 days but thereafter these increased levels came down to normal or near normal levels. These rabbits, called alloxan-recovered rabbits, are considered suitable for screening hypoglycaemic activity of herbal drugs. In such rabbits hypoglycaemic effect could be assessed by improvement in glucose tolerance test (10).

1. Mishkinsky JS, A Goldschmied, B Joseph, Z Ahronson, FG Sulman; Hypoglycaemic effect of *Trigonella foenum graecum* and *Lupinus termis* (Leguminosae) seeds and their major alkaloids in alloxan-diabetic and normal rats, *Arch Int Pharmacodyn Ther* **210**(1), 27-37 (1974)
2. Ghafghazi T, HS Sheriat, T Dastmalchi, RC Barnett; Antagonism of cadmium and alloxan-induced hyperglycaemia in rats by *Trigonella foenum graecum*, *Pahlavi Med J* **8**(1), 14-25 (1977)
3. Ribes G, Y Sauvaire, JC Baccou, G Valette, D Chenon, ER Trimble, MM Loubatieres-Mariani; Effects of fenugreek seeds on endocrine pancreatic secretions in dogs, *Ann Nutr Metab* **28**(1), 37-43 (1984)
4. Valette G, Y Sauvaire, JC Baccou, G Ribes; Hypocholesterolaemic effect of fenugreek seeds in dogs, *Atherosclerosis* **50**(1), 105-11 (1984)
5. Ribes G, Y Sauvaire, C Da-Costa, JC Baccou, MM Loubatieres-Mariani; Antidiabetic effects of sub-fractions from fenugreek seeds in diabetic dogs, *Proc Soc Exp Biol Med* **182**(2), 159-66 (1986)
6. Jain SC, NK Lohiya, A Kapoor; *Trigonella foenum-graecum* Linn.: a hypoglycaemic agent, *Indian J Pharm Sci* **49**(3), 113-14 (1987)
7. Ajabnoor MA, AK Tilmisany; Effect of *Trigonella foenum graceum* on blood glucose levels in normal and alloxan-diabetic mice, *J Ethnopharmacol* **22**(1), 45-49 (1988)
8. Madar Z, R Abel, S Samish, J Arad; Glucose-lowering effect of fenugreek in

non-insulin dependent diabetics, *Eur J Clin Nutr* **42**(1), 51-54 (1988)

9. Amin Riyad M, Abdul-Ghani, S Abdul-Salam, SM Suleman, Effect of Fenugreek and Lupin seeds on the development of experimental diabetes in rats, *Planta Med* **54**(4), 286-90 (1988)
10. Babu BV, R Moorti, S Pugazhenthi, KM Prabhu, PS Murthy; Alloxan recovered rabbits as animal, model for screening for hypoglycaemic activity of compounds, *Indian J Biocem Biophys* **25**(6), 714-18 (1988)
11. Murthy RR, Murthy PS, Prabhu K , Effects on blood glucose and serum insulin levels in alloxan induced diabetic rabbits by fraction G-2 (*Trigonella foenum graecum*), *Biomedicine* 10 (1)25 -29 (1990)
12. Pahwa ML, Effect of Methi intake on blood sugar in humans, *Oriental J Chem* **6**(2),124-26 (1990)
13. Sharma RD, TC Raghuram, NS Rao; Effect of fenugreek seeds on blood glucose and serum lipids in type I diabetes, *Eur J Clin Nutr* **44**(4), 301-06 (1990)
14. Nahar N, Nur-e-Alam, T Nasreen, M Mosihuzzaman, L Ali, R Begam, AKA Khan, Studies of blood glucose lowering effects of *Trigonella foenum graecum* (fenugreek) seeds, *7th Asian Symposium on Med Plants , Spices and other Nat Prod (ASOMPS*) Manila, February 2-7, (1992).
15. Petit P, Y Sauvaire, G Ponsin, M Manteghetti, A Fave, G Ribes; Effects of a fenugreek seed extract on feeding behaviour in the rat: metabolic-endocrine correlates, *Pharmacol Biochem Behav* **45**(2), 369-74 (1993)
16. Raghuraman TC, RD Sharma, B Sivakumar, BK Sahay; Effect of fenugreek seeds on intravenous glucose disposition in non insulin dependent diabetic patients, *Phytother Res* **8**(2), 82-86 (1994).
17. Ahmad M, Ismail N, Ismail Z, Pharmacognostic profile of *Trigonella* seeds and its hypoglycaemic activity. *Nat Prod Sci* **1**(1), 25-30 (1995)
18. Khosla P, DD Gupta, RK Nagpal; Effect of *Trigonella foenum graecum* (fenugreek) on blood glucose in normal and diabetic rats, *Indian J Physiol Pharmacol* **39**(2), 173-74 (1995)
19. Ali L, AK Azad Khan, Z Hassan, M Mosihuzzaman, N Nahar, T Nasreen, M Nur-e-Alam, B Rokeya; Characterization of the hypoglycaemic effects of *Trigonella foenum graecum* seed, *Planta Med* **61**(4), 358-60 (1995)
20. Neerja A , P Rajyalakshmi, Hypoglycaemic effect of processed fenugreek seeds in humans, *J Food Sci Technol* **33**(5), 427-30 (1996)
21. Abdel-Barry JA, IA Abdel-Hassan, MH Al-Hakiem; Hypoglycaemic and antihyperglycaemic effects of *Trigonella foenum-graecum* leaf in normal and alloxan-induced diabetic rats, *J Ethnopharmacol* **58**(3), 149-55 (1997)
22. Chandra V, Aruna K, Glycaemic and cholesterolaemic effect of sprouted fenugreek on diabetic subjects, *Indian J Nutr Diet* **34**(10), 246-51 (1997)

23. Renu Singh , Blood sugar lowering effect of fenugrrek in non insulin dependent diabetes, *Bull Environ Sci* **16**, 17-18 (1998)

24. Puri D , Anti-diabetic effect of a plant product, *J Int Med Sci Acad* **11**(2), 97–101 (1998)

25. Sauvaire Y, P Petit, C Broca, M Menteghetti, Y Baissac, J Fernandez-Alvarez, R Gross, M Roye, A Leconte, R Gomis, G Ribes; 4-Hydroxyisoleucine: a novel amino acid potentiator of insulin secretion, *Diabetes* **47**(2), 206-10 (1998)

26. Kuppu RK, A Srivastava, CV Krishnaswami, G Vijaykumar, M Chellamariappan, PV Asha Bai, O Buchi Babu, Hypoglycaemic and hypotriglyceridaemic effects of Methika Churna (fenugreek), *Antiseptic* **95**(3), 78-79 (1998)

27. Al-Haberi M, A Raman, Anti-diabetic and hypocholesterolaemic effects of fenugrrek, *Phytother Res* **12**(4), 233-42 (1998)

28. Jayadev Raju , D Gupta, AR Rao, NZ Baquer, Effect of anti-diabetic compounds on glyoxalase 1 activity in experimental diabetic rat liver, *Indian J Exp Biol* **37**(2), 193-95 (1999)

29. Gupta D, J Raju, NZ Baquer; Modulation of some gluconeogenic enzyme activities in diabetic rat liver and kidney: effect of anti-diabetic compounds, *Indian J Exp Biol* **37**(2), 196-99 (1999)

30. Genet S, RK Kale, NZ Baquer; Effects of vanadate, insulin and fenugreek (*Trigonella foenum graecum*) on creatine kinase levels in tissues of diabetic rat, *Indian J Exp Biol* **37**(2), 200-02 (1999)

31. Ravikumar P, CV Anuradha; Effect of fenugreek seeds on blood lipid peroxidation and antioxidants in diabetic rats, *Phytother Res* **13**(3), 197-201 (1999)

32. Abdel-Barry JA, IA Abdel-Hassan, AM Jawad, MH Al-Hakiem; Hypoglycaemic effect of aqueous extract of the leaves of *Trigonella foenum-graecum* in healthy volunteers, *East Mediterr Health J* **6**(1), 83-88 (2000)

33. Broca C, M Menteghetti, R Gross, Y Baissac, M Jacob, P Petit, Y Sauvaire, G Ribes; 4-Hydroxyisoleucine: effects of synthetic and natural analogues on insulin secretion, *Eur J Pharmacol* **390**(3), 339-45 (2000)

34. Pathak P, S Srivastava, S Grover; Development of food products based on millets, legumes and fenugreek seeds and their suitability in the diabetic diet, *Int J Food Sci Nutr* **51**(5), 409-14 (2000)

35. Raju J, D Gupta, AR Rao, PK Yadava, NZ Baquer; *Trigonella foenum graecum* (fenugreek) seed powder improves glucose homeostasis in alloxan diabetic rat tissues by reversing the altered glycolytic, gluconeogenic and lipogenic enzymes, *Mol Cell Biochem* **224**(1-2), 45-51 (2001)

36. Zia T, SN Hasnain, SK Hasan; Evaluation of the oral hypoglycaemic effect of

Trigonella foenum-graecum L. (methi) in normal mice, *J Ethnopharmacol* **75**(2-3), 191-95 (2001)

37. Anuradha CV, P Ravikumar; Restoration on tissue antioxidants by fenugreek seeds (*Trigonella foenum graecum*) in alloxan-diabetic rats, *Indian Physiol Pharmacol* **45**(4), 408-20 (2001)
38. Genet S, RK Kale, NZ Baquer; Alterations in antioxidant enzymes and oxidative damage in experimental diabetic rat tissues: effect of vanadate and fenugreek (*Trigonella foenum graecum*), *Mol Cell Biochem* **236**(1-2), 7-12 (2002)
39. Vats V, JK Grover, SS Rathi; Evaluation of anti-hyperglycaemic and hypoglycaemic effect of *Trigonella foenum graecum* Linn., *Ocimum sanctum* Linn., and *Pterocarpus marsupium* Linn. and alloxanized diabetic rats, *J Ethnopharmacol* **79**(1), 95-100 (2002)
40. Puri D, KM Prabhu, PS Murthy; Mechanism of action of a hypoglycaemic principle isolated from fenugreek seeds, *Indian J Physiol Pharmacol* **46**(4), 457-62 (2002)
41. Hannan JM, B Rokeya, O Faruque, N Nahar, M Mosihuzzaman, AK Azad-Khan, L Ali; Effect of soluble dietary fibre fraction of *Trigonella foenum graecum* on glycaemic, insulinaemic, lipidaemic and platelet aggregation status of Type 2 diabetic model rats, *J Ethnopharmacol* **88**(1), 73-77 (2003)
42. Grover JK,Vats V , Yadav SP , Anti-hyperglycaemic and hypoglycaemic effect of *Trigonella foenum graecum* (FG) and *Ocimum sanctum* (OS) in normal and diabetic rats ,*National Convention on Current Trends in Herbal Drugs and Annual Conference of Indian Society of Pharmacognosy : Herbs :The Natural Alternative*, Gandhi Nagar, Gujrat, India p. A-03, January 17-18, 2003.
43. Thakran S , NZ Baquer, Biochemical and histological changes in mitochondria of experimentally induced diabetes in rats after *Trigonella foenum graecum* therapy, 2nd *World Congress ,Biotechnological Development of Herbal Medicine*, Lucknow,UP, India, p.43, February 20-22, 2003
44. Tahiliani P, A Kar; Mitigation of thyroxine-induced hyperglycaemia by two plant extracts, *Phytother Res* **17**(3), 294-96 (2003)
45. Devi BA, N Kamalakkannan, PS Prince; Supplementation of fenugreek leaves to diabetic rats. Effect on carbohydrate metabolic enzymes in diabetic liver and kidney, *Phytother Res* **17**(10), 1231-33 (2003)
46. Mohamad S, A Taha, RN Bamezai, SF Basir, NZ Baquer; Lower doses of vanadate in combination with *Trigonella* restore altered carbohydrate metabolism and antioxidant status in alloxan-diabetic rats, *Clin Chim Acta* **342**(1-2), 105-14 (2004)
47. Annida B, P Stanely Mainzen Prince; Supplementation of fenugreek leaves lower lipid profile in streptozotocin-induced diabetic rats, *J Med Food* **7**(2), 153-56 (2004)

48. Mondal DK, BM Yousuf, LA Banu, R Ferdousi, M Khalil, KM Shamim; Effect of fenugreek seeds on the fasting blood glucose level in the streptozotocin-induced diabetic rats, *Mymensingh Med J* **13**(2), 161-64 (2004)
49. Thakran S, MR Siddiqui, NZ Baquer; *Trigonella foenum graecum* seed powder protects against histopathological abnormalities in tissues of diabetic rats, *Mol Cell Biochem* **266**(1-2), 151-59 (2004)
50. Flammang AM, MA Cifone, GL Erexson, LF Stankowski Jr., Genotoxicity testing of a fenugreek extract, *Food Chem Toxicol* **42**(11), 1769-75 (2004)
51. Preet A, BL Gupta, PK Yadava, NZ Baquer, Efficacy of lower doses of vanadium in restoring altered glucose metabolism and antioxidant status in diabetic rat lenses, *J Biosci* **30**(2), 221-30 (2005)
52. Vijayakumar MV, S Singh, RR Chhipa, MK Bhat; The hypoglycaemic activity of fenugreek seed extract is mediated through the stimulation of an insulin signalling pathway, *Br J Pharmacol* **146**(1), 41-48 (2005)
53. Annida B, P Stanely Mainzen Prince, Supplementation of fenugreek leaves reduces oxidative stress in streptozotocin-induced diabetic rats, *J Med Food* **8**(3), 382-85 (2005)
54. Preet A, BL Gupta, MR Siddiqui, PK Yadava, NZ Baquer; Restoration of ultrastructural and biochemical changes in alloxan-induced diabetic rat sciatic nerve on treatment with Na_3VO_4 and *Trigonella*—a promising anti-diabetic agent, *Mol Cell Biochem* **278**(1-2), 21-31 (2005)
55. Mohammad S, A Taha, RN Bamezai, NZ Baquer; Modulation of glucose transporter (GLUT4) by vanadate and *Trigonella* in alloxan-diabetic rats, *Life Sci* **78**(8), 820-24 (2006)
56. Gad MZ, MM El-Sawalhi, MF Ismail, ND El-Tanbouly; Biochemical study of the anti-diabetic action of the Egyptian plants Fenugreek and Balanites, *Mol Cell Biochem* **281**(1-2), 173-83 (2006)
57. Narender T, A Puri, Shweta, T Khaliq, R Saxena, G Bhatia, R Chandra; 4-Hydroxyisoleucine an unusual amino acid as anti-dyslipidemic and anti-hyperglycaemic agent, *Bioorg Med Chem Lett* **16**(2), 293-96 (2006)
58. Siddiqui MR, K Moorthy, A Taha, MF Hussain, NZ Baquer; Low doses of vanadate and *Trigonella* synergistically regulate Na^+/K^+-ATPase activity and GLUT-4 translocation in alloxan-diabetic rats, *Moll Cell Biochem* **285**(1-2), 17-27 (2006)
59. Hannan JM, L Ali, B Rokeya, J Khaleque, M Akhter, PR Flatt, YH Abdel-Wahab; Soluble dietary fibre fraction of *Trigonella foenum-graecum* (fenugreek) seed improves glucose homeostasis in animal models of type 1 and type 2 diabetes by delaying carbohydrate digestion and absorption, and enhancing insulin action, *Br J Nutr* **97**(3), 514-21 (2007)

Triticum aestivum Linn. (Poaceae) (Wheat)

Blood glucose and plasma immunoreactive insulin concentrations were measured during oral glucose tolerance test in 10 obese children. Oral glucose was given by itself or combined with 15 g unprocessed wheat bran. Wheat bran significantly reduced the blood glucose and plasma immunoreactive insulin concentrations at 30 min of the tolerance test. Thus supplementation of obese children's diet with unprocessed wheat bran was found to be advantageous (1). The postprandial glucose and hormonal responses were followed in nine non-insulin-dependent diabetics after four randomized breakfast meals containing mainly wheat products. The results indicate that baked whole-grain wheat bread is to be preferred to corresponding extruded products in non-insulin-dependent diabetes mellitus (2). *In vivo* glycaemic and insulin responses and *in vitro* starch digestibility of seven processed wheat products (shortbread biscuits, custard, quick-cooking wheat, wholemeal bread, water biscuits, puffed wheat, and puffed crisp bread) were determined. The degree of starch gelatinization in the foods was also measured. The calculated glycaemic indices ranged from 43±10 for custard to 81±9 for puffed crisp bread. Insulin responses paralleled the glycaemic responses, which correlated positively with the percentage of starch digested *in vitro*. The degree of starch gelatinization also correlated positively with the percentage starch digested *in vitro*. Differences in the glycaemic and insulin responses to wheat products may be explained in part by the extent of processing and the degree of gelatinization achieved (3). From an investigation, conducted to study the effect of different thermal processes used to produce ready-to-eat cereals from whole grain wheat, it was concluded that the glycaemic response to wheat products is affected by the processing conditions used. The more severe are the processing conditions, the more rapid is the digestion of starch (4). The effects of single and long-term administration of wheat albumin were examined on blood glucose levels and blood glucose control, respectively. From the results of detailed investigation it was concluded that in the treatment of type-2 diabetic patients, wheat albumin might be a useful functional food, which, with diet and exercise, could help to improve blood glucose control without any critical adverse effects (5).

1. Molnar D, I Dober, G Soltesz; The effect of unprocessed wheat bran on blood glucose and plasma immunoreactive insulin levels during oral glucose tolerance test in obese children, *Acta Paediatr Hung* **26**(1), 75-77 (1985)

2. Hagander B, I Bjorck, NG Asp, I Lundquist, P Nilsson-Ehle, J Schrezenmeir, B Schersten; Hormonal and metabolic responses to breakfast meals in niddm: comparison of white and whole-grain wheat bread and corresponding extruded products, *Hum Nutr Appl Nutr* **39**(2), 114-23 (1985)

3. Ross SW, JC Brand, AW Thorburn, AS Truswell; Glycaemic index of processed wheat products, *Am J Clin Nutr* **46**(4), 631-35 (1987)

4. Holm J, B Hagander, I Bjorck, AC Eliasson, I Lundquist; The effect of various thermal processes on the glycaemic response to whole grain wheat products in humans and rats, *J Nutr* **119**(11), 1631-38 (1989)
5. Kodama T, T Miyazaki, I Kitamura, Y Suzuki, Y Namba, J Sakurai, Y Torikai, S Inoue; Effects of single and long-term administration of wheat albumin on blood glucose control: randomized controlled clinical trials, *Eur J Clin Nutr* **59**(3), 384-92 (2005)

Triticum repens Linn. (Poaceae)
(Couch Grass)

Triticum repens is a very common species of grass, native to most of Europe, Asia, and northwest Africa. The hypoglycaemic effect of an aqueous extract of *T. repens* rhizomes was investigated in normal and streptozotocin-induced diabetic rats. While an oral administration of a single dose of the aqueous extract (20mg/kg) caused a significant decrease of blood glucose levels in streptozotocin-induced diabetic rats, daily oral administration of the extract for two weeks normalized the blood glucose levels of the diabetic animals. Significant reduction in blood glucose levels was also noticed in normal rats after both acute and chronic treatment. As no changes were observed in basal plasma insulin concentrations after treatment in either normal or diabetic rats, the underlying mechanism of this activity appeared to be independent of insulin secretion.

Eddouks M, M Meghrani, JB Michel; Hypoglycaemic effect of *Triticum repens* P. Beauv. in normal and diabetic rats, *J Ethnopharmacol* **102**(2), 228-32 (2005)

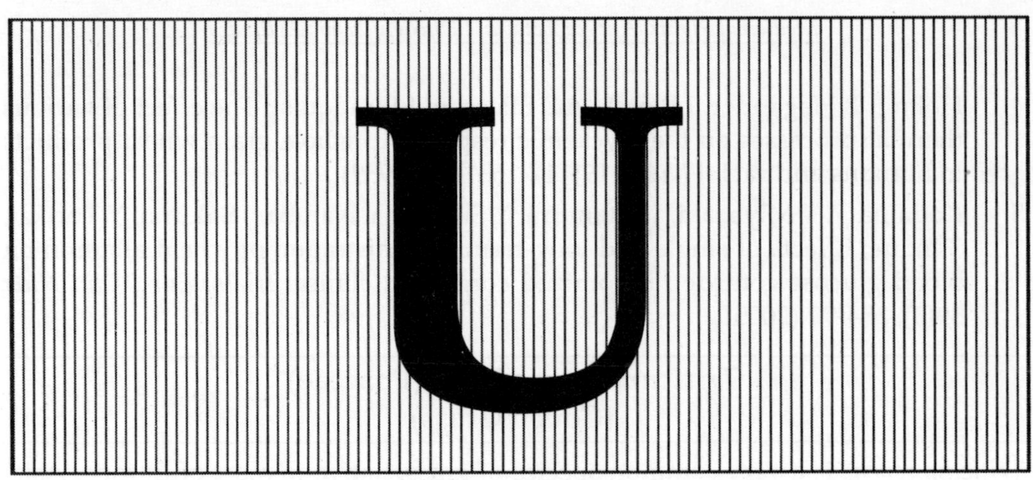

Urtica dioica Linn. (Urticaceae)
(Stinging nettle)

The stinging nettle is a flowering plant, native to Europe, Asia, northern Africa and North America. This species have spiny hairs, or stinging trichomes, the tips of which come off when touched, transforming the hair into a needle that injects a cocktail of poisons, which cause itching. The blood glucose lowering effect of stinging nettle is found in old writings such as those of Avicenna and its hypoglycaemic effect has also been verified without establishing the mechanism of its action. Bioactivity directed fractionation of the leaf extract of *U. dioica* led to the isolation of an active fraction, named F-1. The intra-peritoneal injection of active fraction was found to increase the insulin content of blood sera with a simultaneous decrease of blood sugar in normal and streptozotocin-induced diabetic rats. The results show that the blood lowering effect of the extract was due to the enhancement of insulin secretion by islets of Langerhans (1). Administration of an aqueous extract of *U. dioca* (250 mg/kg), 30 minutes before glucose loading, significantly decreased the blood sugar levels of normal rats and the effect persisted up to three hours. The extract, however, failed to elicit hypoglycaemic effect in alloxan-induced diabetic rats. The extract also decreased glucose absorption by a segment of jejunum *in situ* as compared to control rats during two hours. In an oral glucose tolerance test model, the *U. dioca* extract showed significant anti-hyperglycaemic activity (2) *Urtica diocia* exhibited potent *alpha* glycosidase inhibitory activity *in vitro*. The inhibitory effect of this drug against different source of enzyme (baker's yeast, rabbit liver and small intestine) was also evaluated (3).

1. Farzami B, D Ahmadvand, S Vardasbi, FJ Majin, Sh. Khaghani; Induction of insulin secretion by a component of *Urtica dioica* leaf extract in perifused Islets of Langerhans and its *in vivo* effects in normal and streptozotocin diabetic rats, *J Ethnopharmacol* **89**(1), 47-53 (2003)

2. Bnouham M, FZ Mehrfour, A Ziyyat, H Mekhfi, M Aziz, A Legssyer; Anti-hyperglycaemic activity of the aqueous extract of *Urtica dioica*, *Fitoterapia* **74**(7-8), 677-81 (2003)
3. Onal S, S Timur, B Ocutucu, F Zihnioglu; Inhibition of *alpha*-glucosidase by aqueous extracts of some potent anti-diabetic medicinal herbs, *Prep Biochem Biotechnol* **35**(1), 29-36 (2005)

Urtica pilulifera Linn. (Urticaceae)
(Roman Nettle)

The leaves of the plants have stinging hairs, causing irritation to the skin.

For hypoglycaemic activities see **Plant Lectins** in Appendix.

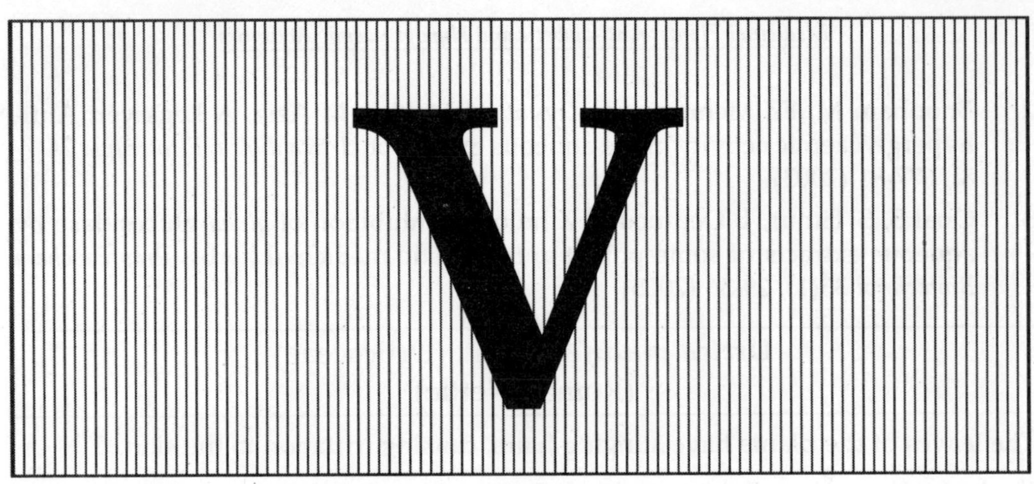

Vaccinium angustifolium Ait. (Ericaceae)
(Bilberry)

The plant is used as a natural health product and recommended for the treatment of diabetes in Canada. Ethanol extracts (12.5 μg/ml) of root, stem, leaf, and fruit were tested for anti-diabetic activity in peripheral tissues and pancreatic *beta* cells using a variety of cell-based bioassays. The results of detailed investigation demonstrated that the active principles of the plant possess insulin-like and glitazone-like properties and confer protection against glucose toxicity. Enhancement of proliferation of *beta* cells represents another potential anti-diabetic property of the plant.

Martineau LC, A Couture, D Spoor, A Benhaddon-Andaloussi, C Harris, B Meddah, C Leduc, A Burt, T Vuong, P Mai Le, M Prentki, SA Bennett, JT Arnason, PS Haddad; Anti-diabetic properties of the Canadian lowbush blueberry *Vaccinium angustifolium* Ait, *Phytomedicine* **13**(9-10), 612-23 (2006)

Vaccinium myrtillus Linn. (Ericaceae)
(Blueberry)

It is a deciduous small shrub growing on mountains and in the woods of Europe, Asia and North America. Blueberry leaf infusions are traditionally used as a folk medicine for the treatment of diabetes. Administration of a dried aqueous alcoholic extract of *V. myrtillus* leaves to streptozotocin-induced diabetic rats for 4 days significantly lowered their plasma glucose levels. A fall in plasma triglycerides was also noted.

Cignarella A, M Nastasi, ECavalli, L Puglisi; Novel lipid-lowering properties of *Vaccinium myrtillus* L. leaves, a traditional anti-diabetic treatment, in several models of rat dyslipidaemia: a comparison with ciprofibrate, *Thromb Res* **84**(5), 311-22 (1996)

Vaccinium uliginosum Linn. (Ericaceae) (Bog Bilberry)

It is native to cool temperate regions of the Northern hemisphere. It bears a dark blue-black berry 5-8 mm diameter, with a white flesh, edible and sweet when ripe in late summer. Methanol extract of *V. uliginosum* inhibited *alpha*-amylase activity of mouse plasma. It also showed depressive effect on elevation of postprandial blood glucose to some extent.

Kobayashi K, E Baba, FT Fushiya, J Batkhuu, T Dash, C Sanchir, F Yoshizaki; Screening of some Mongolian plants for influence on amylase activity in mouse plasma and gastrointestinal tube, *Biol Pharm Bull* **26**(7), 1045-48 (2003)

Vernonia amygdalina Del. (Asteraceae / Compositae)

Vernonia amygdalina is a shrub and its leaves, which have a characteristic odour and a bitter taste, are eaten as leaf vegetables. The aqueous extract *V. amygdalina* leaves produced a dose related fall in blood sugar level in rabbits. A dose of 80 mg/kg body weight produced a maximum lowering of blood sugar in fasted normal and alloxan-induced diabetic rabbits. The hypoglycaemic effects of the leaf extract were compared with those of tolbutamide. It has been suggested that the mechanism, by which the plant extract exhibits its hypoglycaemic activity, is not related to insulin secretion.

Akah PA, CL Okafor; Blood sugar lowering effect of *Vernonia amygdalina* Del. in an experimental rabbit model, *Phytotherapy Res* **6**(3), 171-73 (1992)

Vernonia colorata (Willd.) Drake (Asteraceae / Compositae)

The plant is distributed throughout Africa, particularly in Benin, Cameroon, Senegal, Togo etc. The aqueous extract of *V. colorata* leaves is used by African traditional medicine practitioners as a remedy for the treatment of diabetes. An aqueous extract of *V. colorata* (300 mg/kg, per os) induced a significant hypoglycaemic effect in normoglycaemic rats. It also reduced significantly the fasting glucose level of the hyperglycaemic rats, induced with oral administration of glucose (4 g/kg). Like glibenclamide (0.2 mg/kg, per os), the aqueous extract of *V. colorata* (300 mg/kg, per os) decreased the blood glucose in alloxan-induced diabetic rats. The aqueous extract of the leaves of *V. colorata* was thus proved to possess both hypoglycaemic and anti-diabetic effect in normoglycaemic and alloxan-induced diabetic rats (1). The acetone extract of the leaves of *V. colorata* (100 mg/kg, per os) induced a significant decrease of blood glucose in normoglycaemic rats but its hexane extract significantly increased the glycaemia in normoglycaemic rats. Like glibenclamide, acetone extract of the plant showed anti-hyperglycaemic effect in oral glucose tolerance test in alloxan-induced diabetic rats. The opposite effects elicited by hexane and acetone extracts of *V. colorata* leaves indicate the difference in their mechanisms of action (2).

1. Sy GY, RB Nongonierma, M San, A Cisse, B Faye; Anti-diabetic activity of the leaves of *Vernonia colorata* (Wilid.) Drake (Composees) in alloxan-induced diabetic rats, *Dakar Med* **49**(1), 36-39 (2004) [Article in French]

2. Sy GY, A Cisse, RB Nongonierma, M San, NA Mbodj, B Faye; Hypoglycaemic and anti-diabetic activity of acetonic extract of *Vernonia colorata* leaves in normoglycaemic and alloxan-induced diabetic rats, *J Ethnopharmacol* **98**(1-2), 171-75 (2005)

Viburnum dilatatum Thunb (Adoxaceae / Caprifoliaceae) (Gamazumi)

Viburnum dilatatum is a wild deciduous tree that bears small crimson fruits, known as gamazumi. In view of the reported radical scavenging activity of gamazumi, the anti-oxidative functions of the crude extract of gamazumi were studied in rats having diabetes induced by the administration of streptozotocin. While in rats given water, plasma levels of glucose, total cholesterol, and lipid peroxide and erythrocyte levels of thiobarbituric acid reactive substances increased with time over the experimental period of 10 weeks, these increases were inhibited in rats given the extract of gamazumi. These results demonstrated an inhibitory effect of the extract on the oxidative stress induced by diabetes and suggested that it may be useful for the prevention of diabetic complications (1). The elevation of plasma glucose level after oral administration of glucose (2 g/kg) to streptozotocin-induced diabetic rats was suppressed by the repeated administration of freeze-dried powder of *V. dilatatum* fruit juice. The action was dependent on the dose of fruit juice powder. Increase of insulin secretion was not found in rats with or without administration of fruit juice and it was expected that the fruit juice had some effects on glucose uptake. Of the five compounds identified from *V. dilatatum* fruit, cyanidin 3-sambubioside and 5-caffeoyl quinic acid showed inhibitory activity on sucrase and maltase and these were identified as active compounds for the *alpha*-glucosidase inhibitory and anti-hyperglycaemic effects of *Viburnum dilatatum* fruits (2).

1. Iwai K, A Onodera, H Matsue; Inhibitory effects of *Viburnum dilatatum* Thunb. (gamazumi) on oxidation and hyperglycaemia in rats with streptozotocin-induced diabetes, *J Agric Food Chem.* **52**(4), 1002-07 (2004)

2. Iwai K, MY Kim, A Onodera, H Matsue; *Alpha*-glucosidase inhibitory and anti-hyperglycaemic effects of polyphenols in the fruit of *Viburnum dilatatum* Thunb, *J Agric Food Chem* **54**(13), 4588-92 (2006)

Vigna angularis (Willd.) Ohwi & H Ohashi (Fabaceae) Syn: *Phaseolus angularis* (Willd.) W. F. Wight (Adzuki bean)

HP-20 column chromatography of a hot water extract, obtained by boiling adzuki beans, produced a fraction that exhibited inhibitory activity against *alpha*-

glucosidase, *alpha* -amylase, maltase, sucrase, and isomaltase. The active fraction showed potential hypoglycaemic activity in both normal mice and streptozotocin-induced diabetic rats after an oral administration of sucrose, but did not show any effect on the blood glucose concentration after glucose administration, suggesting that the active fraction suppressed the postprandial blood glucose level by inhibiting *alpha*-glucosidase and *alpha*-amylase, irrespective of the endogenous blood insulin level.

Itoh T, N Kita, Y Kurokawa, M Kobayashi, F Horio, Y Furuichi; Suppressive effect of a hot water extract of adzuki beans (*Vigna angularis*) on hyperglycaemia after sucrose loading in mice and diabetic rats, *Biosci Biotechnol Biochem.* **68**(12), 2421-26 (2004)

Vigna unguiculata (L) Walp. (Fabaceae)
(Cowpea)

The presence of insulin-like antigens has been detected in a large range of plant species and the one isolated from the developing fruits of cowpea not only showed the same electrophoretic mobility as bovine insulin but also showed the same amino acid sequence. Insulin was measured by ELISA (Enzyme-linked immunosorbent assay) using an anti-human insulin antibody and was detected both in empty pods and seed coats but not in the embryo. The highest concentrations (about 0.5 ng/µg of protein) of the protein were detected in seed coats (1, 2).

1. Silva LB, SS Santos, CR Azevedo, MA Cruz, TM Venancio, CP Cavalcante, AF Uchoa, S Astolfi Filho, AE Oliveira, KV Fernandes, J Xavier-Filho; The leaves of green plants as well as a cyanobacterium, a red alga, and fungi contain insulin-like antigens, *Braz J Med Biol Res* **35**(3), 297-303 (2002)
2. VenancioTM, AE Oliveira, LB Silva, OL Machado, KV Fernandes, J Xavier-Filho; A protein with amino acid sequence homology to bovine insulin is present in the legume *Vigna unguiculata* (cowpea), *Braz J Med Biol Res* **36**(9), 1167-73 (2003)

Vinca rosea Linn. (Apocynaceae) Syn. *Catharanthus roseus* (Madagascar periwinkle, H. Sadabahar)

It is an evergreen herbaceous plant with white to dark pink flowers. In the wild, it is an endangered plant but widely cultivated and is naturalised in subtropical and tropical areas of the world. While Ghosh and Gupta (1) reported that water extracts of leaves, stems and roots of the plant failed to exhibit any hypoglycaemic activity in normal and alloxanised rats, Chattopadhyay and co-workers (2) reported that oral administration of water-soluble fraction of the alcoholic extract of *Vinca rosea* leaves led to marked lowering of blood glucose level in normal and streptozotocin-induced diabetic rats and that the hypoglycaemic effect of the fraction was comparable with that of tolbutamide. Significant fall of blood sugar level in diabetic patients after treatment with a paste of fresh leaves of *V. rosea* (10 g daily in two divided doses) has also been reported (3). Administration of aqueous extracts of *V. rosea* flower and leaf has been found to regulate the blood sugar level in alloxan-induced diabetic male albino rats. The extracts not only produced blood glucose homeostasis but also reversed changes in carbohydrate, protein, lipid metabolisms following a single dose (150 mg/kg b.w.) of alloxan monohydrate. The metabolic and pathologic changes that took place in pancreatic islet cells, liver and kidney due to alloxan administration were also reversed. *V. rosea* was found to manifest its beneficial activity through rejuvenation, regeneration and stimulation of *beta* cell (4).

1. Ghosh RK, I Gupta; Effect of *Vinca rosea* and *Ficus racemosus* on hyperglycaemia in rats, *Indian J Animal Health* **19**(2), 145-49 (1980)
2. Chattopadhyay RR, SK Sarkar, S Ganguly, RN Banerjee, TK Basu; Hypoglycaemic and anti-hyperglycaemic effect of leaves of *Vinca rosea* Linn, *Indian J Physiol Pharmacol* **35**(3),145-51 (1991)
3. Goyal DK, SK Tiwari; Study on Sadabahar (*Vinca rosea* Linn.)in Madhumeha (Diabetes mellitus), *J Res Ayur Siddha* **20**(3-4), 93-100 (1999)
4. Ghosh S, SA Suryawanshi; Effect of *Vinca rosea* extracts in treatment of alloxan diabetes in male albino rats, *Indian J Exp Biol* **39**(8), 748-59 (2001)

Viscum album Linn. (Santalaceae/Loranthaceae) (European mistletoe)

It is a hemi-parasitic shrub, which grows on the stems of other trees. It yields yellow berry containing several seeds embedded in the very sticky, glutinous fruit pulp. Mistletoe is traditionally used for the treatment of diabetes. An aqueous extract of mistletoe (1-10 mg/ml) evoked a stepwise stimulation of insulin secretion from clonal pancreatic *beta*-cells, an effect which was abolished by diazoxide. The insulin-releasing effect of mistletoe extract was unaltered by glucose, L-alanine, 3-isobutyl-1-methylxanthine, or a depolarising concentration of potassium chloride. The findings indicated the presence of insulin-releasing natural product(s) in the plant, responsible for its reported anti-diabetic property (1). In normglycaemic and streptozotocin-induced diabetic rats, the hypoglycaemic effects of aqueous and ethanol extracts of three sub species of *Viscum album* (ssp. *album*, ssp. *austriacum*, ssp. *abietis*) were investigated. The antioxidant activity of these extracts was also studied in liver, kidney and heart tissues. All the three subspecies of *Viscum album* elicited potent anti-hyperglycaemic and antioxidant activities (2). The plant also exhibited potent *alpha* glycosidase inhibitory activity (3),

1. Gray AM, PR Flatt; Insulin-secreting activity of the traditional anti-diabetic plant *Viscum album*, (mistletoe)., *J Endocrinol* **160**(3), 409-14 (1999)
2. Orhan DD, M Aslan, N Sendogdu, F Ergun, E Yesilada; Evaluation of the hypoglycaemic effect and antioxidant activity of three *Viscum album* subspe-

cies (European mistletoe) in streptozotocin-diabetic rats, *J Ethnopharmacol* **98**(1-2), 95-102 (2005)

3. Onal S, S Timur, B Ocutucu, F Zihnioglu; Inhibition of *alpha*-glucosidase by aqueous extracts of some potent anti-diabetic medicinal herbs, *Prep Biochem Biotchnol* **35**(1), 29-36 (2005)

Vitex megapotamica (Spreng) Moldenke (Verbenaceae)

Oral administration of crude extract of *V. megapotamica* significantly reduced serum glucose levels in both normal and alloxan-induced diabetic animals. The serum glucose lowering effect was observed in normal rats at 2-3 h, after oral administration of the crude extract at a dose of 800 mg/kg. The hypoglycaemic effect of *V megapotamica* in diabetic rats was evident at 1 to 3 h after treatment with the extract (800 mg/kg). The ethyl acetate-soluble fraction (400 mg/kg) produced the maximum hypoglycaemic effect (28%,) in diabetic rats and it was more effective than n-butanol-soluble fraction.

Zanatta L, E de-Sousa, LH Cazarolli, AC Junior, MG Pizzolatti, B Szpoganicz, FR Silva; Effect of crude extract and fractions from *Vitex megapotamica* leaves on hyperglycaemia in alloxan-diabetic rats, *J Ethnopharmacol* **109**(1), 151-55 (2007)

Vitis vinifera Linn. (Vitaceae) (Common grape vine, S. Draksha, H. Angur)

Progressive insulin resistance is known to contribute to both enhanced glycosylation of proteins and nucleic acids and augmented free radical damage. In order to ameliorate these basic disorders and lessen signs and symptoms of chronic age-related disorders, ingestion of chromium and antioxidants which improve insulin sensitivity and/or lessen free radical formation are often recommended. Using 104 F344/BN rats, it was observed that prolonged supplementation of diets with a combination of agents known to sensitize insulin response and act as antioxidants (chromium polynicotinate, grape seed extract, and zinc monomethionine) can markedly lower systolic blood pressures in normotensive rats, lessen oxidative damage to fats as suggested by decreased TBARS formation, and lower HbA1c without showing signs of toxicity (1).

Bioassay-guided isolation and purification of hexane and ethyl acetate extracts of Cabernet Sauvignon grape skin yielded nine compounds, which were fully identified. The compounds were assayed for insulin production using an INS-1 cell assay. Of the isolated compounds, oleanolic acid and oleanolic aldehyde showed a dose-dependent insulin production in this assay (2).

Procyanidins are flavonoids with an oligomeric structure, and it has been shown that they can improve the pathological oxidative state in a diabetic situation. Oral administration of an extract of grape seed procyanidins to streptozotocin-induced diabetic rats elicited anti-hyperglycaemic effect, which was significantly increased when procyanidin administration was accompanied by a low dose of insulin. Grape seed procyanidins stimulated glucose uptake in L6E9 myotubes and 3T3-L1 adipocytes in a dose-dependent manner. Like insulin action, the effect of grape seed procyanidin on glucose uptake was sensitive to wortmannin, an inhibitor of phosphoinositol 3-kinase and to SB203580, an inhibitor of p38 MAPK. Procyanidins of grape also stimulated glucose transporter-4 translocation to the plasma membrane. In summary, procyanidins were found to have insulin-like effects in insulin-sensitive cells that could help to explain their anti-hyperglycaemic effect *in vivo*. These effects in combination to their antioxidant activity explain why grape seed procyanidins can improve diabetic situations (3). The effects of a grape seed procyanidin extract on the metabolic fate of glucose in adipocytes were investigated and it was found that grape seed procyanidin mimicked the anabolic effects of insulin but it stimulated glycogen synthesis less than insulin. The differences between the effects of grape seed procyanidins and the effects of insulin indicate that the former uses mechanisms complementary to those of insulin signaling pathways to bring about these effects (4). Natural grape seed proanthocyanidins are potent free radical scavengers and hence provide significant protection against oxidative stress. The possible protective role of grape seed proanthocyanidins against free radical-mediated damage in pancreatic tissues of alloxan-induced diabetic rats was studied and the results revealed that oral administration of the procyanidin (50 and 100 mg/kg b.w.) for 72 h significantly increased pancreatic glutathione levels and inhibited the increase in lipid peroxidation caused by alloxan. This was accompanied by a significant increase in serum insulin levels (5). Red wines and grape juices contain polyphenolics with antioxidant and anti-platelet properties that may be protective against oxidative stress leading to hypertension, insulin resistance, and type-2 diabetes. Diabetics given 150 ml of muscadine grape wine or de-alcoholised muscadine grape wine showed lower levels of blood glucose, insulin, and glycated haemoglobin, indicating better glycaemic control. Elevated dietary vitamin C and E levels were observed in diabetics given de-alcoholised muscadine grape wine, indicating improved antioxidant status. It was thus concluded that daily intake of 150 ml of muscadine grape wine or its de-alcoholised version with meals improved several metabolic responses among diabetics compared with diabetics given muscadine grape juice (6).

1. Preuss HG, S Montamarry, B Echard, R Scheckenbach, D Bagchi; Long-term effects of chromium, grape seed extract, and zinc on various metabolic parameters of rats, *Mol Cell Biochem* **223**(1-2), 95-102 (2001)

2. Zhang Y, B Jayaprakasam, NP Seeram, LK Olson, D DeWitt, MG Nair; Insulin secretion and cyclooxygenase enzyme inhibition by cabernet sauvignon grape skin compounds, *J Agric Food Chem* **52**(2):228-33 (2004)

3. Pinent M, M Blay, MC Blade, MJ Salvado, L Arola, A Ardevol; Grape seed-derived procyanidins have an anti-hyperglycaemic effect in streptozotocin-

induced diabetic rats and insulinomimetic activity in insulin-sensitive cell lines, *Endocrinology* **145**(11), 4985-90 (2004)

4. Pinent M, MC Blade, MJ Salvado, L Arola, A Ardevol; Metabolic fate of glucose on 3T3-L1 adipocytes treated with grape seed-derived procyanidin extract (GSPE). Comparison with the effects of insulin, *J Agric Food Chem* **53**(15), 5932-35 (2005)
5. El Alfy AT, AA Ahmed, AJ Fatani; Protective effect of red grape seeds proanthocyanidins against induction of diabetes by alloxan in rats, *Pharmacol Res* **52**(3), 264-70 (2005)
6. Banini AE, LC Boyd, JC Allen, HG Allen, DL Sauls; Muscadine grape products intake, diet and blood constituents of non-diabetic and type 2 diabetic subjects, *Nutrition* **22**(11-12), 1137-45 (2006)

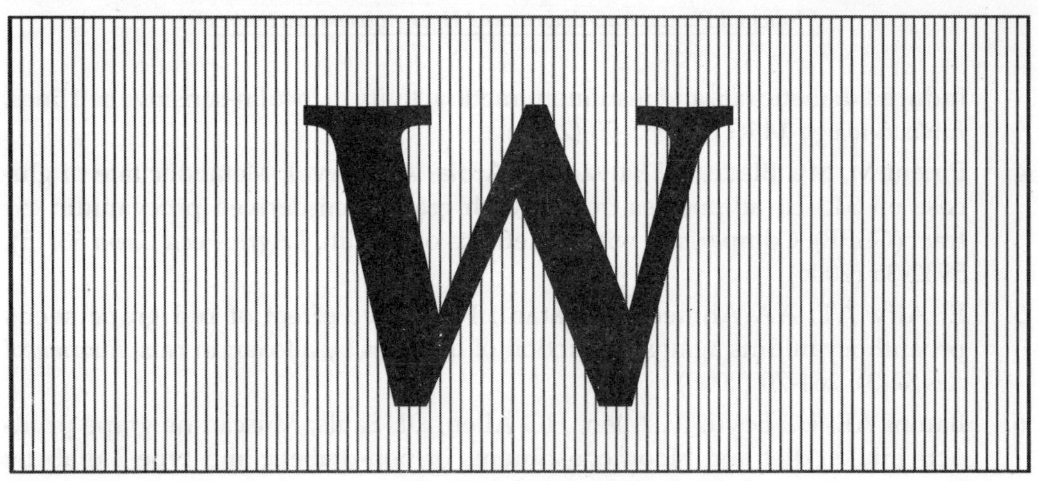

Wedelia paludosa DCC Syn. *Acmela brasiliensis*) (Asteraceae)

Wedelia paludosa is an ornamental plant, widely used in natural medicine in South Brazil. Kaurenoic acid, a bioactive diterpene present in the roots and stems of the plant, is responsible, at least in part, for the hypoglycaemic potential detected in this plant.

Bresciani LF, RA Yunes, C Burger, LE de Oliveira, KL Bof, V Cechinel-Filho; Seasonal variation of kaurenoic acid, a hypoglycaemic diterpene present in *Wedelia paludosa* (*Acmela brasiliensis*) (Asteraceae), *Z Naturforsch* [C]. **59**(3-4), 229-32 (2004)

Withania coagulans (Stocks) Dunal (Solanaceae) (Vegetable Rennet, H. Panirband)

This shrub, common in Afghanistan and East India, has the property of coagulating milk, and has been used for making cheese. It is for this reason that the plant is known as a vegetable-rennet. Administration of aqueous extract of the fruits of *Withania coagulans* significantly lowered the blood sugar, serum cholesterol, serum lipid peroxide, and hepatic lipid peroxide levels at the highest concentration of 1g/kg; p.o. in streptozotocin-induced diabetic rats. In normal rats as well, the blood sugar levels were significantly decreased following treatment with the above drug. *Withania coagulans* also exhibited free radical scavenging activity in an *in vitro* system using DPPH (1). An aqueous extract of the fruits of *W. coagulans* was found to increase the glucose utilisation by isolated rat hemi-diaphragm in comparison to control. The extract did not show any synergistic effect with insulin (2).

1. Hemalatha S, AK Wahi, PN Singh, JP Chansouria; Hypoglycaemic activity of *Withania coagulans* Dunal in streptozotocin induced diabetic rats, *J Ethnopharmacol* **93**(2-3), 261-64 (2004)
2. Hemalatha S, N Sachdeva, AK Wahi, PN Singh, JPN Chansouria; Effect of aqueous extract of fruits of *Withania coagulans* on glucose utilisation by rat hemidiaphragn, *Indian J Nat Prod* **21**(2), 20-21 (2005)

Withania somnifera Dunal (Solanaceae) (Winter cherry, S. Ashwagandha)

Withania somnifera grows as a stout shrub that reaches a height of 170cm. It is an important Indian medicinal plant that grows prolifically in India, Pakistan, Sri Lanka and Bangladesh. It is commercially cultivated in Madhya Pradesh in India. Treatment of mild NIDDM subjects with the powder of *W. somnifera* roots for 30 days significantly decreased their blood glucose levels and the effect was comparable to that of oral hypoglycaemic drugs. Significant increase in urine sodium, urine volume and significant decrease in serum cholesterol, triglycerides, LDL and VLDL cholesterol were observed indicating that root of *W. somnifera* is a potential source of hypoglycaemic, diuretic and hypocholesterolaemic agents.

Andallu B, B Radhika; Hypoglycaemic, diuretic and hypocholesterolemic effect of winter cherry (*Withania somnifera*, Dunal) root, *Indian J Exp Biol* **38**(6), 607-09 (2000)

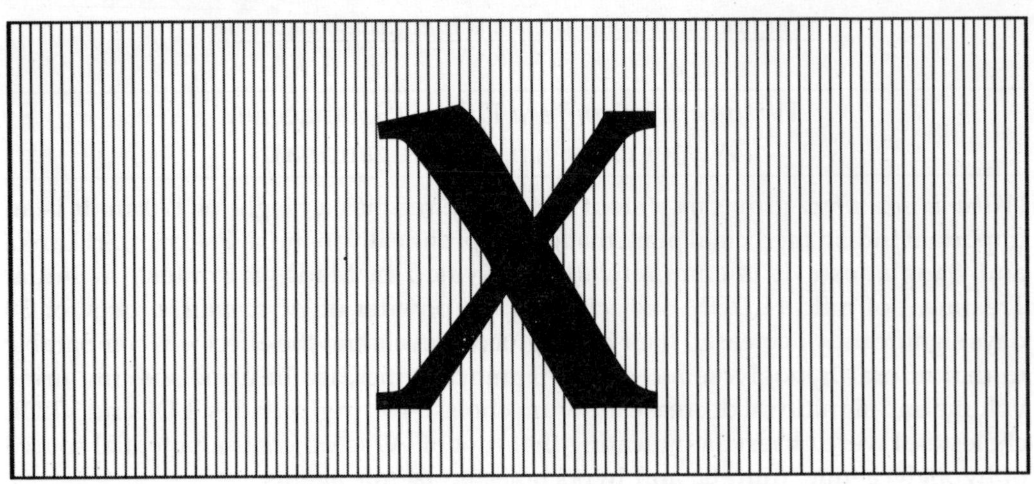

Xanthium pungens Linn. (Asteraceae / Compositae)

The wild herb of *X. pungens* was collected from Nile delta of Egypt and studied for its hypoglycaemic effect in rats. Bioassay directed fractionation of its extract led to the isolation of a polysaccharide which was found to be hypoglycaemic. The structure of the compound has been clarified.

Ammar N, S Al-Okbi, G Wassel, M Shabana, M Shabana; Hypoglycaemic activity of *Xanthium pungens,* Compositae, *J Res Edu in Indian Med* **11**(2), 19-23 (1992)

Xanthium strumarium Linn. (Asteraceae / Compositae) (H. Chotagokhru, S. Sarpakshi)

The origin of *X. strumarium* is North America. It was introduced in India and it spread like a weed. It commonly grows in wasteland and along river banks in warmer parts. A hypoglycaemic agent was isolated from *Xanthium strumarium* and it was fully characterised.

Kupiecki FP, CD Ogzewalla. FM Schell; Isolation and characterization of a hypoglycaemic agent from *Xanthium strumarium, J Pharm Sci* **63**(7), 1166-67 (1974)

Xanthocercis zambesiaca (Baker) Dumaz-le-Grand (Fabaceae / Leguminosae)

Xanthocercis zambesiaca is the single species of tree in the genus *Xanthocercis,* from the family Fabaceae. It is native to South Africa, Zambia and Zimbabwe. The blood glucose level of streptozotocin-induced diabetic rats fell after i.p. injection of the aqueous methanol extract (50 mg/kg) of the leaves and root of the plant. The nitrogen-containing sugars, fagomine, 4-O-β-D-glucopyranosylfagomine, 2,5-dideoxy-2,5-imino-D-mannitol and castanospermine reduced the blood glucose level after ip injection of 150 μmol/kg. Fagomine increased plasma insulin level in streptozotocin-induced diabetic mice and potentiated the glucose-induced insulin release from the rat isolated-perfused pancreas. Anti-hyperglycaemic effects of N-containing sugars from *Morus bombycis, Aglaonema treubii,* and *Castanospermum australe* were also studied.

Nojima H, I Kimura, FJ Chen, Y Sugihara, M Haruno, A Kato, N Asano; Anti-hyperglycaemic effects of N-containing sugars from *Xanthocercis zambesiaca, Morus bombycis, Aglaonema treubii,* and *Castanospermum australe* in streptozotocin-diabetic mice, *J Nat Prod* **61**(3), 397-400 (1998)

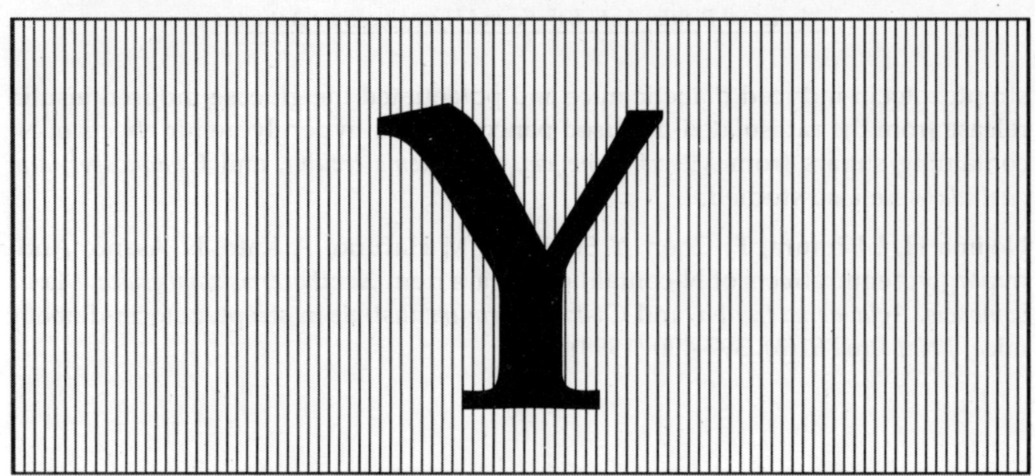

Yucca schidigera Roezl ex Ortgies (Agavaceae / Lillaceae) (Spanish Dagger)

The plant was extracted with n-butanol to yield a butanol-extractable fraction (saponin fraction) and a non-butanol fraction (non-saponin fraction). The total plant material and the non-butanol fraction were found to significantly increase serum insulin levels in the absence of any fluctuations in serum glucose levels. Both fractions displayed effects, indicating that the active constituents of the plant are present in both fractions.

Duffy CF, GF Killeen, CD Connolly, RF Power; Effects of dietary supplementation with *Yucca schidigera* Roezl ex Ortgies and its saponin and non-saponin fractions on rat metabolism, *J Agric Food Chem* **49**(7), 3408-13 (2001)

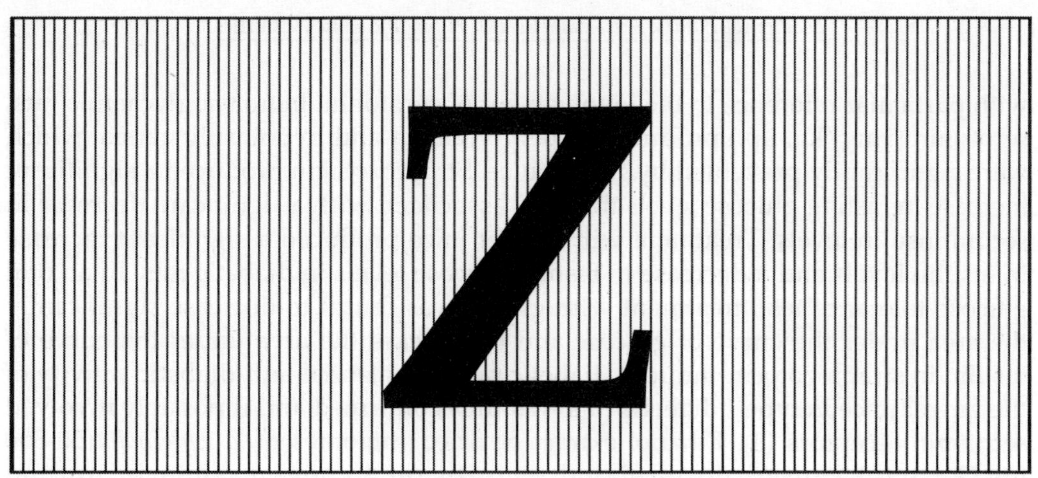

Zea mays Linn. (Poaceae)
(Maize)

The test group of diabetic patients (9 cases) on maize bran showed statistically significant reduction in the level of blood sugar, glycosylated protein, triglycerides and low-density lipoproteins. The control group (5 cases) did not show any significant change in these parameters except the reduction in blood sugar. The findings suggest that a high fibre (maize bran) diet improves the glycaemic control of diabetic patients and reduces serum lipid levels.

Gupta OP, S Bajaj, P Srivastava, AK Chaurasia; Role of maize bran on cardiovascular status, lipid profile, and glycaemia control in diabetes mellitus, *J Assoc Physicians India* **35**(5), 353-55 (1987)

Zingiber officinale Roscoe (Zingiberaceae)
(Ginger, S. Adrak)

The term ginger is generally used to describe the edible part of the plant, which is commonly used as a spice in cooking throughout the world. An ethanol extract of the rhizomes of *Zingiber officinale* was investigated for hypoglycaemic, anti-inflammatory, analgesic, antipyretic and antimicrobial activities. The extract produced blood glucose lowering in rabbits (1). Anti-hyperglycaemic and anti-hyperlipidaemic activity of dry ginger was evaluated in 20 patients each of mild non-insulin dependent diabetes and mild hypercholesterolaemia. The treated diabetic patients exhibited a significant decrease of blood and urinary sugar levels after 30 days. Similarly, a significant lowering of serum total cholesterol, triglycerides, LDL and VLDL-cholesterol along with an increase of HDL-cholesterol was observed in ginger-treated hypercholesterolaemic cases. No adverse effects were noted in these patients (2). The effect of administration of ginger juice (4 ml/kg, p.o. daily) for 6 weeks on streptozotocin-induced type-I diabetic rats was studied with particular reference to the involvement of serotonin. In normoglycaemic rats, serotonin (1mg/kg, i.p.) produced hyperglycaemia and hypoinsulinaemia, which were significantly prevented by ginger juice. Streptozotocin produced a significant increase in fasting glucose levels that was associated with a significant decrease in serum insulin levels. Treatment with ginger juice produced a significant increase in insulin levels and a decrease in fasting glucose levels in diabetic rats. In an oral glucose tolerance test, treatment with ginger was found to decrease significantly the area under the curve of glucose and to increase the area under the curve of insulin in streptozotocin-induced diabetic rats. A potential anti-diabetic activity of the ginger juice in type-I diabetic rats was thus confirmed and it possibly involved serotonin receptors (3). Ethanol extract of dried rhizomes of *Z. officinale* (50-800 mg/kg p.o.) caused dose-related, significant hypoglycaemia in normal (normoglycaemic) and streptozotocin-induced diabetic rats (4). Gingerol, the major component of ginger, is known to improve diabetes. The assay for aldose reductase inhibitors in ginger led to the isolation of five active compounds. Of these, 2-(4-hydroxy-3-methoxyphenyl)ethanol and 2-(4-hydroxy-3-methoxyphenyl)ethanoic acid were good inhibitors of recombinant human aldose reductase. These compounds significantly suppressed not only sorbitol accumulation in human erythrocytes but also lens galactitol accumulation in 30% of galactose-fed cataract rat model. A structure-activity relationship was also established (5). Daily administration of an aqueous extract of raw ginger (500 mg/kg, i.p.) for a period of 7 weeks to streptozotocin-induced diabetic rats significantly lowered their serum glucose, cholesterol and triacylglycerol levels. The treatment also resulted in a significant reduction in urine protein levels and decreased both water intake and urine output in the streptozotocin-induced diabetic rats. Thus, ginger may be of great value in managing the effects of diabetic complications in human subjects (6).

1. Mascolo N, R Jain, SC Jain, F Capasso; Ethnopharmacologic investigation of ginger (*Zingiber officinale*), *J Ethnopharmacol* **27**(1-2), 129-40 (1989)
2. Andallu B, B Radhika, Evaluation of rhizomes of *Zingiber officinale* for hypoglycaemic and hypolipidaemic activity, *Ethnobotany* **13**(1-2), 150 -154 (2001)
3. Akhani SP, SL Vishwakarma, RK Goyal; Anti-diabetic activity of *Zingiber officinale* in streptozotocin-induced type-1 diabetic rats, *J Pharm Pharmacol* **56**(1), 101-05 (2004)
4. Ojewole JA; Analgesic, antiinflammatory and hypoglycaemic effects of ethanol extract of *Zingiber officinale* (Roscoe) rhizomes (Zingiberaceae) in mice and rats, *Phytother Res* **20**(9), 764-72 (2006)
5. Kato A, Y Higuchi, H Goto, H Kizu, T Okamoto, N Asano, J Hollinshead, RJ Nash, I Adachi; Inhibitory effects of *Zingiber officinale* Roscoe derived components on aldose reductase activity *in vitro* and *in vivo*, *J Agric Food Chem* **54**(18), 6640-44 (2006)

6. Al-Amin ZM, M Thomson, KK Al-Qattan, R Peltonen-Shalaby, M Ali; Anti-diabetic and hypolipidaemic properties of ginger (*Zingiber officinale*) in streptozotocin-induced diabetic rats, *Br J Nutr* **96**(4), 660-66 (2006)

Zizyphus mauritiana Lam. (Rhamnaceae) (Indian Jujube, H. Ber)

Zizyphus mauritiana is a tropical fruit tree that is native to southern Asia (mainly India) though it is also cultivated and naturalised elsewhere in the dry tropics, notably in Africa. The effect of an aqueous extract of the leaves of *Z. mauritiana* on blood sugar levels was investigated in glucose loaded or alloxan-induced diabetic rats. In Wistar rats, administration of the extract (300 mg/kg) 90 minutes before starting the oral glucose tolerance test significantly reduced the blood sugar levels. Alloxan-induced diabetic rats also exhibited significant lowering of blood sugar levels following treatment with the extract (300 mg/kg b.w.) and the results were comparable to glibeclamide (0.2 mg/kg).

Cisse A, A Ndiaye, P Lopez-Sall, F Seck, B Faye, B Faye; Anti-diabetic activity of *Zizyphus mauritiana* Lam (Rhamnaceae)], *Dakar Med*; **45**(2), 105-07 (2000) [Article in French]

Zizyphus rugosa (Lam) (Rhamnaceae) (Wild jujube)

The flavonoid fraction of the stem bark of the plant, which yielded 3-O-rhamnosides of kaempferol, quercetin and myricetin, showed hypoglycaemic activity in experimental rabbits.

Khosa RL, VB Pandey, JP Singh; Experimental studies on *Zizyphus rugosa* (Lam) bark, *Indian Drugs* **20**(6), 241 (1983).

Zizyphus sativa Gaertn. (Rhamnaceae)

Zizyphus sativa is a small tree growing on the shores of the Mediterranean, and cultivated in Italy, Spain, and the south of France. Its fruits have a reddish-brown skin, a yellowish, sweet, acidulous pulp, and an oblong, pointed stone in the centre. Oral administration of an alcoholic extract of *Z. sativa* leaves (100-400 mg/kg) to normal rats showed a dose-dependent statistically significant lowering of blood glucose level after 2, 4 and 6 h. The effect was most pronounced at 6 h with blood glucose returning to control values at 24 h. In alloxan-induced diabetic rats, no significant effect was observed with the extract and tolbutamide.

Anand KK, B Singh, D Chand, BK Chandan, VN Gupta; Effect of *Zizyphus sativa* leaves on blood glucose levels in normal and alloxan-diabetic rats, *J Ethnopharmacol* **27**(1-2), 121-27 (1989)

Zizyphus spina-christi (L.) Desf. (Rhamnaceae)

Z. spina-christi is a tree indigenous to the south of Iran and its leaves are used in Iranian and Egyptian folk medicine. Treatment of streptozotocin-induced diabetic rats for four weeks with the butanol extract of *Z. spina-christi* leaves as well as with its principle saponin glycoside, christinin-A (3-O-[α-L-fucopyranosyl(1→2)-α-D-glucopyranosyl(1→3)-α-L-arabinopyranosyl] jujubogenin), significantly reduced serum glucose level, liver phosphorylase and glucose-6-phosphatase activities, and significantly increased serum pyruvate level and liver glycogen content. A marked improvement in glucose utilization was also observed in diabetic rats. Treatment of diabetic rats with the butanol extract for four weeks significantly increased serum insulin and pancreatic cAMP levels.

Glombitza KW, GH Mahran, YW Mirhom, KG Michel, TK Motawi; Hypoglycaemic and anti-hyperglycaemic effects of *Zizyphus spina-christi* in rats, *Planta Med* **60**(3), 244-47 (1994)

Zygophyllum cornutum Coss. (Zygophyllaceae)

Zygophyllum cornutum was identified as a new plant with hypoglycaemic properties (1). Quercetin-3'-methyl ether 3-O-β-D-glucopyranoside, the major flavonoid constituent of the plant, might be one of the active principles (2).

1. Perez C, R Paris; A new plant with hypoglycaemic properties, *Zygophyllum cornutum* Cosson, *Ann Pharm Fr* **16**(2), 86-90 (1958) [Article in French]
2. Aclinou P, K Abdessemed, G Massiot, L Le-Men-Oliver; Plants of Aures III, Structure of a flavonoid of *Zygophyllum cornutum*, *Plantes Medicinales et Phytother* **22**(4), 212-18 (1988)

Zygophyllum gaetulum Emb. & Maire (Zygophyllaceae)

The leaves of the plant are traditionally used for the treatment of diabetes in Morocco. Its ability to lower the blood glucose level was studied in 13 patients with non-insulin-dependent diabetes mellitus. A single oral dose of its aqueous extract (440 mg/kg) produced a significant hypoglycaemic effect 6 h after administration. Ingestion of the same dose twice daily resulted in a significant reduction of blood glucose level during the first week, and maintained the patient in normoglycaemia throughout the 2 week period, with no change in body weight (1).

Oral and intra-peritoneal administration of the infusion of the plant (0.7 g/kg) produced a significant hypoglycaemic effect in normal as well as in hyperglycaemic rats. The infusion increased significantly plasma insulin levels in normal rats. It is suggested that the hypoglycaemic activity of the plant may be mediated through enhancement of peripheral metabolism of glucose and an increase in insulin release (2).

The aqueous infusion of the aerial parts of *Zygophyllum gaetulum* was tested orally (1 g/kg body weight) for hypoglycaemic activity in alloxan-induced diabetic rats. The infusion was partitioned between water and butanol to yield a butanol-soluble fraction (B), and an aqueous fraction (W) which on reduction in volume gave a precipitate (WP) and supernatant (WS). Fractions (B) and (WP) caused significant reduction in blood glucose concentration, while the ingestion of (WS) produced no significant reduction in blood glucose level (3)

1. Jaouhari, J.T., Lazrek, H.B., Seddik, A., Jana, M., Hypoglycaemic response to *Zygophyllum gaetulum* extracts in patients with non-insulin-dependent diabetes mellitus, *J Ethnopharmacol* **64**(3), 211-17 (1999)
2. Skim F, HB Lazrek, A Kaaya, H el-Amri, M Jana; Pharmacological studies of two anti-diabetic plants: *Globularia alypum* and *Zygophyllum gaetulum, Therapie* **54**(6), 711-15 (1999)
3. Jaouhari, J.T., Lazrek, H.B., Jana, M., The hypoglycaemic activity of *Zygophyllum gaetulum* extracts in alloxan-induced hyperglycaemic rats, *J Ethnopharmacol* **69**(1), 17-20 (2000)

Zygophyllum geslin Coss (Zygophyllaceae)

The plant is used as a folk medicine in Algeria for the treatment of diabetes mellitus. The preliminary phytochemical screening revealed the presence of flavonoids, saponins, tannins and alkaloids. Oral administration of the aqueous extract of the plant to hyperglycaemic and alloxan-induced diabetic rats caused significant hypoglycaemic effect between 1 and 4h of the treatment.

Smati D, V Hammiche, H Nehari, B. Alamir, R. Merad; *Zygophyllum geslini* Coss: Chemical investigation, hypoglycaemic activity, *Acta Horticulturae* (332), 243-48 (1993)

APPENDIX - 1

ANTI-DIABETIC HERBAL FORMULATIONS

[In addition to reports on hypoglycaemic and anti-diabetic activities of individual plants, numerous herbal and herbo-mineral formulations have been studied for these activities and the findings published. These findings are presented here in a chronological order (based on the first publication on the topic). The trivial names of the formulations and names of the plants and minerals used are presented in bold letters.]

The blood sugar lowering effect of a composite herbo-mineral preparation, **Geriforte,** was evaluated in 10 normal and 25 uncomplicated cases of diabetes mellitus. Both normal and diabetic subjects elicited a decrease in fasting as well as post glucose-load blood sugar levels following treatment with Geriforte. However, the decrease in the blood sugar levels was relatively more marked in diabetic patients than in the normal volunteers. Administration of Geriforte (2 tablets tds) to diabetic patients for 1-6 weeks reduced their requirement of insulin. No adverse reaction was observed when Geriforte was given with insulin. It was suggested that the hypoglycaemic effect of Geriforte could be due to ***Eugenia jambolana,*** **Shilajeet, Abhrak bhasma** and **Yashad bhasma**, present in it (1). Administration of Geriforte to diabetic patients led to a significant decrease of blood sugar and serum protein levels (2). The anti-diabetic effect of Geriforte was studied in 25 patients of maturity onset diabetes mellitus. The patients exhibited a significant fall in blood sugar levels following treatment with Geriforte (3).

1. Nigam P, S Kirti, S Saxena, P Srivastava, LD Joshi; Effect of indigenous drug (Geriforte) on glucose tolerance test in normal and diabetic individuals and effect on insulin requirement, *J Diabetes Assoc India* **19**(3), 159-64 (1979)
2. Ganeriwal SK, BV Reddy, PS Baji, RM Shaikh, VS Majage, JR Kher; Effect of Geriforte on blood chemistry, *Indian Practitioner* **34**(8), 559-65 (1981)
3. Damle VB, AG Gore, Study of Geriforte in maturity onset diabetes mellitus, effect on requirement of oral hypoglycaemic agent, *Indian Practitioner* **35**(10), 495-99 (1982)

Tablets of **HAAS**, a composite drug, were tested for their anti-diabetic activity in sixty patients and significant improvements in blood and urine sugar levels were observed. No side effect was observed.

Salve SR, SJ Nalgirkar; Role of tablets of HAAS (Shiladhatu Vatti) in clinical diabetes, *J Sci Res Plants Med* **3**(1), 1-5 (1982)

A herbal formulation,-**Whangryonhaedok–Tang,** elicited potent anti-diabetic activity in mice. This compound drug also showed anti-inflammatory, antibacterial and hypocholesterolaemic effects.

Hong ND, JW Kim, HK Doo, NJ Kim; Studies on efficacy of combined preparations of crude drugs (V) Effect of Whangryonhaedok-Tang on anti-inflammatory, Ileum of mice, blood pressure, blood glucose, total cholesterol and antibacterial activity, *Korean J Pharmacogn* **13**(1), 26-32 (1982).

Hypoglycaemic activity and toxicity of **"Triphala"**, a Siddha medicine, have been studied. Oral administration of the drug (90 mg/kg) showed significant hypoglycaemic activity in fasting rabbits. The drug was found to be non-toxic (1, 2).

1. Ghosh D, R Uma, P Thejomoorthy, G Veluchamy; Hypoglycaemic and toxicity studies of Triphala: a Siddha medicine, *Acta Biochim Biophys Acad Sci Hung* **17**(1-2), p.26 (1982).
2. Ghosh D, R Uma; Hypoglycaemic and toxicity studies of Triphala, a Siddha drug, *J Res Ayur Siddha* **11** (1-4), 78-80 (1990)

A herbal mixture consisting of 50 g each of ***Enicostemma littorale, Tinospora cordifolia, Swertia chirata, Trigonella faenum-graecum, Fumaria officinalis, Gymnema sylvestre, Wrightia tinctoria*** and 15 g each of seeds of ***Syzygium cumini, Picrorrhiza kurroa, Momordica charantia, Glycyrrhiza glabra, Curcuma longa, Emblica officinalis*** and 12.5 g each of ***Cyperus rotundus, Rosa alba, Rosa damascena*** has been tried successfully on diabetic patients. However, it was not useful in juvenile diabetes, in persons prone to ketosis and at early stages of diabetes.

Mehta KC; Indian herbal drugs in the treatment of diabetes, *Curr Med Pract* **26**(10), 305-09 (1982)

Administration of the extract of **Daeshiho-Tang** significantly decreased blood sugar and cholesterol levels of diabetic rabbits. The drug also exhibited hypotensive, vasodialatory and SGOT and SGPT lowering activities.

Hong ND, IK Chang, NJ Kim, JG Shon; Studies on the efficacy of combined preparation of crude drugs (XIII): Effect of Daeshiho-tang on the blood vessels, activities of the liver enzymes, biliary secretion and anti-diabetic actions, *Korean J Pharmacogn* **14**(1), 30-38 (1983).

"Vijayasara compound", a composite drug consisting of ***Pterocarpus marsupium*** extract, ***Momordica charantia*** fruit, ***Syzygium cumini*** seed, ***Ficus glomerata*** bark extract, ***Withania somnifera*** root, **Shilajit** and **Vanga Bhasma**, showed a marked reduction in blood sugar of diabetic patients after one week of treatment with 8 tablets per day.

Ojha JK, VV Prasad, B Singh; A preliminary clinical trial of "Vijayasara compound", in cases of insulin-independent diabetes, *Nagarjun* **27**(2), 37-39 1983)

The drug **"Chandraprabhavati"** showed significant response in the management of diabetes mellitus of experimental rabbits when given at a dose of 600 mg/kg b.w.

Tripathi SN, HM Chandola, VDS Jamval; Hypoglycaemic effect of Chandraprabhavati on different experimental models of diabetes mellitus, *J Res Ayur Siddha* **4**(1-4), 99-110 (1983)

Oral administration of **Amlaki-Haridra** (prepared from ***Emblica officinalis*** and ***Curcuma longa***) produced significant reduction in blood sugar levels in diabetic patients.

Mishra SK, SK Pandey, SN Sharma, GD Singh; Effect of Amlaki-Haridra on Madhumeha, *Nagarjun* **26**(5), 105-07 (1983)

The effect of treatment of diabetic patients with the Siddha medicine, **Kadal Azhinjil** was studied on 25 diabetic patients. The medicine contains ***Salacia chinensis, Terminalia chebula, Terminalia bellerica*** and ***Phyllanthus emblica***. Out of 25 patients, four showed more than 50 %, eleven 40-50 %, and six showed less than 40% reduction in blood sugar level, after treatment for four months. The urine sugar level was reduced much earlier.

Sivaprakasam K, KK Rao, R Yasodha, G Veluchamy; Siddha remedy for diabetes mellitus, *J Res Ayur Siddha* **5**(1-4), 25-32 (1984)

Aqueous extract of a powder containing a mixture of 12 plants (***Carum roxburghianum*** (Ajmoda), ***Holarrhena antidysenterica, Aristolochia bracteata, Enicostemma littorale, Picrorrhiza kurroa, Swertia chirata, Centratherum anthelminticum, Caesalpinia bonducella, Tinospora cordifolia, Terminalia chebula, Mallotus philippensis***) and **black salt** showed significant hypoglycaemic activity in normal and alloxan-induced diabetic dogs. The extract did not exhibit any hypoglycaemic activity in normal rats but lowered the blood sugar in alloxan-induced diabetic rats.

Ainapure SS, PD Arjaria, VR.Sawant, PS. Baid, SS. Maste, AB. Varda; Hypoglycaemic activity of an indigenous preparation, *Indian J.Pharmacol* **17**(4), 238-39 (1985)

The therapeutic effect of "**Ganshao Jiangtang**" tablet consisting of radix ***Paeoniae albae*** (Chinese Peony Root) and radix ***Glycyrrhizae uralensis*** (Licorice root) was studied in 214 patients of diabetes mellitus. Of these 180 cases were treated with this tablet alone and 34 patients were treated with tablet plus Western medicines. Hypoglycaemic action was noticed in both the cases. It is suggested that in mild and moderate type of diabetic patients, this tablet can be used alone but in severe cases, it must be used with insulin. The dose is 3-4 tablets after meals but not more than 4 times a day.

Wang Z *et al*, Preliminary observation of hypoglycaemic responses in 214 diabetes mellitus patients treated with "Ganshao Jiangtang" tablet, *J Integ Trad West Med* **6**(10), 593-95 (1986).

A blood glucose lowering extract of a mixture of five plants, used by Kuwaiti diabetics, was studied for the identification of its active component(s). Only the extracts of **myrrh** (an aromatic gum resin obtained from trees and shrubs of the genus *Commiphora*) and **aloe gums** (latex from *Aloe vera*) effectively increased glucose tolerance in both normal and diabetic rats. The remaining components, gum olibanum, *Nigella sativa* seeds and gum assafoetida were without effect.

Al-Awadi FM, KA Gumaa; Studies on the activity of individual plants of an anti-diabetic plant mixture, *Acta Diabetol Latina* **24**(1), 37-41 (1987)

Xiaoke tea is a traditional herbal preparation for the treatment for diabetes mellitus in China. It is composed of Oolong tea mixed with a variety of precious Chinese medicinal herbs. An aqueous extract of Xiaoke (1 g of dried plant preparation in 64 ml of water), supplied *ad lib* in place of drinking water during the induction and development of streptozotocin diabetes in mice, reduced plasma glucose concentrations by 25 days. It did not significantly alter plasma insulin concentrations. Consumption of the Xiaoke extract by insulin-treated diabetic BB/E Wistar rats did not affect glycaemic control or body wt. When insulin treatment was reduced or discontinued, Xiaoke failed to prevent the progression of severe hyperglycaemia and weight loss. The results suggest that the slowly generated anti-hyperglycaemic effect of Xiaoke in streptozotocin diabetic mice may involve an extra-pancreatic effect on food intake, glucose production or glucose clearance.

Baily CJ, D Brown, W Smith, AJ Bone; Xiaoke, a traditional Chinese treatment for diabetes: Studies in streptozotocin diabetic mice and spontaneously diabetic BB/E rats, *Diabetes Res* **4**(1), 15-18 (1987)

A single administration of a **Vegetal complex of *Phaseolus vulgaris*** was found to reduce the level of glycaemia for 6-8 h in alloxan-induced diabetic rabbits. A similar effect was produced by chlorpropamide but the complex produced a longer hypoglycaemic effect. The vegetable complex demonstrated its sugar reducing action by extra-pancreatic means.

Khaleeva LD, LN Maloshtan, AG Sytnik; Comparative evaluation of the hypoglycaemic activity of the vegetal complex of *Phaseolus vulgaris* and chlorpropamide in experimental diabetes, *Probl Endokrinol* (Mosk) **33**(2), 69-71 (1987) [Article in Russian]

Treament with "**Nisha kathakathi Kashayam**", an Ayurvedic drug, reduced the blood sugar levels of experimentally induced fasting diabetic rabbits. A mixture of this Kashayam and **Rasnarirandadi Kashayam** is used for the treatment of diabetic hypertension. A combination of Nisha Kathakathi and "Rasnarirandadi Kashayam" significantly lowered blood cholesterol, triglycerides and free fatty acids and also reduced the possibility of development of atherosclerosis in diabetic rabbits (1). The effects of administration of a mixture (2:1, v/v) of Ayurvedic drugs "**Nisha kathakathi Kashayam**",and "**Rasnarirandadi Kashayam**" at a dose of 1 ml/kg b.w./day were studied in normal, diabetic, diabetic hypertensive and diabetic hypercholesterolemic rabbits. Administration of the individual kashayams decreased fasting blood glucose and serum cholesterol levels but the effect was more significant, when the mixture was used. Treatment with a combination of "Nisakathakathi Kashayam" and "Rasnairandadi Kashyam" reduced hypercholesterolemia, hypertriglyceridemia and hyperlipidaemia in diabetic hypertensive rabbits (2).

1. Santosh Kumari KS, KS Devi, Blood glucose and lipids in diabetic rabbits treated with indigenous medicines, *Arogya: J Health Sci* **16**(2), 138-43 (1990)
2. Santosh Kumari KS, KS Devi, Pharmacological and biochemical effects of a few indigenous drugs, *Indian J Pharmacol* **23**(3), 160-63 (1991)

The effect of **QS,** a mixture of ***Helleborus niger*** and ***Anacyclus pyrethrum*** in the proportion of 3:1, was studied clinically in patients, previously treated with diet therapy and other oral hypoglycaemic agents. Treatment with **QS** for 3-6 weeks significantly decreased plasma glucose and serum cholesterol levels. The hypoglycaemic effect was noted in patients treated with **QS** for 12 weeks. Fasting plasma glucose and postprandial plasma glucose levels of these patients were maintained at a lower level even six months after discontinuation of the drug. The dose of insulin was also reduced in patients with Insulin dependent diabetes mellitus.

Naveed W; Therapeutic evaluation of *Helleborus niger* and *Anacyclus pyrethrum* (QS) in diabetes mellitus, *J Res and Edu in Indian Med* **9**(2), 113-17 (1990)

Supplementation of 5% of diets of streptozotocin-induced diabetic rats with ***Curcuma xanthorrhiza*** improved their diabetic symptoms such as growth retardation, hyperphagia, polydipsia, elevation of glucose and triglyceride in the serum. *C. xanthorrhiza* specifically modified the amount and composition of fecal bile acids. Significance of these findings was discussed in the light of the improvement of several diabetic symptoms.

Yasni S, K Imaizumi, M Sugano; Effect of Indonesian medicinal plant *Curcuma xanthorrhiza* Roxb. on the levels of serum glucose and triglyceride, fatty acid desaturation and bile acid excretion on streptozotocin-induced diabetic rats, *Agric Biol Chem* **55**(12), 3005-10 (1991)

Vatharasavangam, a Siddha drug, was studied for its hypoglycaemic activity in rabbits. The insulin level in alloxan-induced hyperglycaemic animals increased significantly after treatment with this drug. The insulin released from the islets in hyperglycaemic rabbits decreased to low glucose stimulus but Vatharasavangam-treated rabbits showed a significant increase in the insulin released from the islet cells to the low glucose stimulus. Similarly, a significant increase of insulin secretion was observed in response to high glucose stimulus after 30 min in this drug treated rabbits, when compared to hyperglycaemic rabbits. The acid phosphatase activity of islet cells in the hyperglycaemic rabbits also increased significantly after treatment with this Siddha drug. Vatharasavangam was thus considered to act by stimulating *beta*-cells to secrete insulin to the glucose signal and improve blood glucose homeostasis.

Padmini E, CE Meenakshi, DB Motlag; Effect of a Siddha drug (Vatharasavangam) on insulin release from isolated pancreatic islets in rabbits, *Indian J Med Res* **92**, 178-82 (1990)

Administration of a Chinese traditional medicine, **Tian-shou** liquor to 43 patients of diabetes mellitus for 6 weeks, significantly lowered their blood sugar and cholesterol levels.

Liag-Lun Z; Study of Tian-shou liquor on activity of cell membrane and energy metabolism in diabetes mellitus, *Chinese J Integrated Trad Western Med* **10**(8), 455-57 (1990)

Significant improvement without any side effect was observed in 25 patients of diabetes mellitus by administration of capsules of a composite herbal drug containing ***Coccinia indica, Cuminum cyminum, Eugenia jambolana, Gymnema sylvestre, Momordica charantia, Phyllanthus niruri, Swertia chirata*** and ***Tephrosia purpurea.***

Kamick CR; A clinical trial of a composite herbal drug in the treatment of diabetes mellitus (Madhumeha), *Aryavaidyan* **5**(1), 36-46 (1991).

Asanad, an Ayurvedic drug was given to 25 diabetic patients (2 tabs tds for 8 weeks and when symptoms abated 2 tabs bd for another 4 weeks). The patients showed remarkable improvement with respect to frequency of urination, fatigue, and thirst and reduced sugar in blood and urine.

Goel N, NC Shah, Clinical evaluation of the anti-diabetic action of asanad, *Deerghayu International* **7**(1), 16-17 (1991).

A marked increase in fasting glycaemia was observed in alloxan-induced diabetes in rats. Administration of a single dose of **"Hipogalegin"** (0.45 g/kg b.w.) led to a marked decrease of glycaemia in fasted diabetic animals. The diabetic animals, not receiving "Hypogalegin", died during the first two weeks. On the other hand, treated animals continued to survive even up to 94th day after induction of diabetes.

Coprean D, R Giurgea, M Tamas, M Rosea, D Coprean, B Cuparencu; The hypoglycaemic effect of "Hipogalegin", *Rev Roum Physiol* **28**(1-2), 23-26 (1991)

The hypoglycaemic effect of ***Coccinia indica*** and **Nisamalaki** was evaluated in human maturity onset diabetes taking 18 patients of mild and moderate diabetes in the age group of 30-60 years and of both sexes. Fresh stems of *C. indica* were finely cut; shade dried, powdered and filled in capsules. The powdered drug, at the dose levels of 3-8 g/day and 4 g/day with 1 g of Nishamalaki in divided doses, was administered, respectively for mild and moderately diabetic patients for a period of 3 months. The treatment resulted in a significant decrease in fasting blood glucose levels along with a fall of urea and cholesterol levels.

Kuppurajan, K, C Seshadri, R Revathi, V Raja Gopal; Hypoglycaemic effect of *Coccinia indica* and nisamalaki in diabetes mellitus, *Indian Medicine* (Vijayawada) **3** (2-3), 6—9 (1991),

Controlled diet is recognised to be the main therapy for good metabolic control in non-insulin dependent diabetes mellitus (NIDDM). The present research focuses on the management approaches of NIDDM with the objective of studying the efficacy of herbal supplements to diet among the selected non-insulin dependent diabetics. Controlled diet includes wheat, ragi, hand-pounded rice and foods that are bitter and astringent. Herbal supplements like ***Gymnema sylvestre*** **(Sarkaral koll)**, ***Syzygium cumini*** (Jambu seeds), ***Emblica offlcinalis*** (Amla) and ***Curcuma longa*** (turmeric). given 3 times daily for a month, followed by physical and yogic excercises can cure NIDDM.

Kalpana, N, P Parvathi Easwaran, S. Uma Mageshwari; Management approaches of non insulin dependent diabetes mellitus *Indian J Nutri Dietet,* **29(9)**, 278, 1992).[

An aqueous decoction of equal parts of ***Balsamodendron myrrha, Styrax benzoin, Ferula foetida, Aloe vera,*** and ***Nigella sativa*** was found to lower the blood glucose levels significantly. The maximum effect was noted at 8-12 hours after the oral administration of the drug at a dose of 3.5 ml/kg.

Akhtar MS, MU Shah; Elemental constituents of anti-diabetic screening of a folkloric medicinal plant prescription, *Int J Toxicol, Occupational Environ Health* **2**(1), 46 (1993).

Anti-diabetic effect of a herbal formulation **D-400 (Diabecon)**, containing *Eugenia jambolana, Tinospora cordifolia, Pterocarpus marsuoium, Ficus glomerulata, Momordica charantia* and *Ocimum sanctum*, was evaluated in 20 patients of persistent postprandial hyperglycaemia. This compound effectively lowered fasting and postprandial blood sugar levels in these patients without any adverse effect (1).

Administration of **D-400** to patients of diabetes mellitus for 12 weeks significantly lowered the fasting and postprandial blood sugar levels of newly diagnosed patients and the cases already stabilized on anti-diabetic treatment. Of the diabetic patients on anti-diabetic treatment, 80% did not require oral hypoglycaemic agents and in remaining 20% cases the doses of oral hypoglycaemic drugs could be reduced. Requirement of insulin was also reduced in these patients. D-400 did not affect hepatic, renal or haemopoetic function. No side effect was noted during the trial (2).

D-400 was administered to healthy male students (3 tablets, tds) for 42 days to assess the safety and tolerability of this drug. Detailed investigations for master health check were done before starting the drug and after 15 and 45 days of treatment. At the end of the trial period, the biochemical and haematological tests did not show any abnormality and these were comparable with initial base line observations. It was concluded that D-400 was quite safe and meets minimum safety evaluation criteria (3).

Treatment with **D-400** showed significant reduction of blood sugar levels of normal rats as compared to control groups. The fall was seen at one month and remained so till 3 months. Hyperglycaemic response to adrenaline was significantly lowered following D-400 treatment. The hypoglycaemia following tolbutamide treatment was potentiated by D-400. Blood sugar remained persistently low in tolbutamide plus D-400 treated group after 3 and 4 hours. In the alloxan-induced diabetic rats, a significant lowering of blood and urinary sugar was noticed on day 20, 30 and 40 following treatment with D-400. Liver glycogen depletion was significantly inhibited in the D-400 treated group. D-400 also significantly potentiated the hypoglycaemic action of insulin in alloxan-induced diabetic rats (4).

Effect of **D-400** was evaluated in 12 newly detected cases of diabetes and 17 patients of diabetes mellitus who were already on oral hypoglycaemic agents. Treatment with D-400 (2 tablets, tds) for 6 months significantly lowered the postprandial blood sugar levels of both groups of diabetic patients (5)

The effect of **D-400** was studied on streptozotocin-induced diabetes in rats. D-400 treated group showed lower glycosylated haemoglobin (HbA1c), triglycerides and higher HDL levels. The drug blunted the hyperglycaemic response after oral administration of glucose (6). A significant reduction in blood urea nitrogen, serum creatinine, and serum uric acid levels was observed in the D-400-treated group. Considerable lowering of AUC (area under the curve) was also observed in oral glucose tolerance test. There was a rise in hepatic glycogen level close to normal after D-400 treatment. D-400 therapy significantly increased islet number and *beta* cell count in the pancreas and appeared to bring about blood sugar homoeostasis by increasing insulin secretion and repair/regeneration of endocrine pancreas in diabetic rats (7). **D-400** treatment (1 g/kg/day, p.o.) showed progressive and significant increase in liver glycogen at 2, 4 and 8 weeks, respectively. Streptozotocin-induced decrease in pancreatic islet cell, superoxide dismutase, was reversed by D-400 treatment for a period of 8 weeks. The free radical scavenging activity of D-400 may be attributed to **shilajeet**, one of its important ingredients. Streptozotocin-induced histopathological changes in pancreas and liver were also partially reversed by D-400 (8).

D-400 was investigated for its interaction with oral hypoglycaemic agents namely, tolbutamide and glibenclamide in alloxan-induced diabetic rabbits. Administration of D-400 at a dose of 1 g/kg for 15 days significantly elevated plasma tolbutamide and glibenclamide concentrations with simultaneous reduction of blood glucose. Plasma tolbutamide and glibenclamide concentrations were significantly lowered after withdrawal of D-400 treatment. Elevation of plasma concentration of tolbutamide was observed only for the first 4 h after which it declined towards normal levels and no significant difference between D-400-treated and control group was observed at the end of 8 h. (9).

The pharmacokinetic interaction of D-400 (**Diabecon**) with the commonly used drugs like rifampicin and nifedipine was studied in animal models as well as in healthy human volunteers. The results of detailed studies revealed that Diabecon (D-400) did not alter the pharmacokinetic profiles of rifampicin and nifedipine (10).

Administration of **Diabecon**, a herbo-mineral formulation to diabetic patients (2 tabs, tds) led to a significant reduction of fasting and postprandial blood sugar levels of both NIDDM and IDDM patients after 2 months of treatment. The requirement of oral hypoglycaemic agents and insulin, respectively for NIDDM and IDDM patients, was also reduced following treatment with Diabecon. Significant lowering of serum cholesterol and microalbuminuria was also noted in diabecon-treated diabetics. No side effects were observed during the trial (11).

Apart from ageing, diabetes has been considered to be one of the major risk factors of cataract, the leading cause of blindness worldwide. The high sugar levels in diabetes may cause tissue disruption by osmotic changes induced *via* aldose reductase mediated polyol pathway. Therefore, agents that can inhibit aldose reductase and prevent sorbitol accumulation may be helpful in combating sugar-induced cataract. The aldose reductase inhibitory activity of **Diabecon**, used for diabetes, was studied together with its effect against sugar-induced lens opacity in organ culture. Aqueous extract of **Diabecon** showed potential inhibitory activity against rat lens aldose reductase. It also inhibited aldose reductase activity in lens incubated with 100 mM glucose. The results of detailed investigation suggest that **Diabecon** protect the lens against sugar-induced cataract by multiple mechanisms and that *Gymnema sylvestre*, one of the constituent herbs of Diabecon, is mainly responsible for this activity (12).

1. Dubey GP, A Agrawal, A Singh; Evaluation of D-400, an indigenous herbal preparation in diabetes mellitus, *Indian J Int Med* **3**(6), 183-86 (1993)
2. Yajnik VH , Acharya HK, Vithlani MP, Yajnik NV, Efficacy and safety of D – 400, a herbal formulation in diabetic patients, *Probe* 33(4), 331-36 (1994)
3. Mohan R, BL Chauhan, SK Mitra, RD Kulkarni; Safety, efficacy and tolerability of D-400, an Ayurvedic hypoglycaemic formulation in healthy male medical students, *Probe* **33**(4), 348 –55 (1994)
4. Anturlikar SD, S Gopumadhavan, BL Chauhan, SK Mitra; Effect of D-400, a herbal formulation, on blood sugar of normal and alloxan-induced diabetic rats, *Indian J Physiol Pharmacol* **39**(2), 95-100 (1995)
5. Singh AK, BP Shaw, Evaluation of D-400, a herbomineral preparation in patients with diabetes mellitus, *The Antiseptic* **92**(7), 263-65 (1995).
6. Mitra SK, S Gopumadhavan,, TS Muralidhar, SD Anturlikar, MB Sujatha; Effect of D-400, a herbomineral preparation on lipid profile, glycated haemoglobin and glucose tolerance in streptozotocin-induced diabetes in rats, *In-*

dian J Exp Biol **33**(10), 798-800 (1995)

7. Mitra SK, S Gopumadhavan,, TS Muralidhar, SD Anturlikar, MB Sujatha; Effect of a herbomineral preparation D-400 in streptozotocin-induced diabetic rats, *J Ethnopharmacol* **54**(1), 41-46 (1996)
8. Mitra SK, S Gopumadhavan,, TS Muralidhar, SJ Seshadri; Effect of D-400, a herbomineral formulation on liver glycogen content and microscopic structure of pancreas and liver in streptozotocin-induced diabetes in rats, *Indian J Exp Biol* **34**(10), 964-67 (1996)
9. Sundaram R, MV Venkataranganna, S Gopumadhavan, SK Mitra; Interaction of a herbomineral preparation D-400, with oral hypoglycaemic drugs, *J Ethnopharmacol* **55**(1), 55-61 (1996)
10. Mitra SK, R Sundaram, MV Venkataranganna, S Gopumadhavan ; Pharmacokinetic interaction of Diabecon (D-400) with rifampicin and nifedipine, *Eur J Drug Metab Pharmacokinet* **24**(1), 79-82 (1999)
11. Malhotra AK, Effect of Diabecon in diabetic patients with microalbuminuria, *Indian Practitioner* **52**(9), 595-97 (1999).
12. Moghaddam MS, PA Kumar, GB Reddy, VS Ghole; Effect of Diabecon on sugar-induced lens opacity in organ culture: mechanism of action, *J Ethnopharmacol* **97**(2), 397-403 (2005)

A herbal preparation consisting of **Guargum** (*Cyamopsis tetragonolobus*), **Methi** (*Trigonella foenum-graecum*), **Tundika** (*Cephalandra indica*) and **Meshasringi** (*Gymnema sylvestre*) in powder form was administered to thirty control and thirty NIDDM patients twice daily before principal meals for four weeks. Oral glucose tolerance test showed improvement in both control and patient groups. Serum total and LDL cholesterol levels also fell significantly in both the groups after the trial period. No side effect of the powder was observed even after a long-term use. This powder, therefore, can be effectively used to reduce postprandial blood glucose and LDL cholesterol in NIDDM patients as a long-term measure.

Bhardwaj PK, DJ Dasgupta, BS Prashar, SS Kaushal; Control of hyperglycaemia and hyperlipidaemia by plant product, *J Assoc Physicians India* **42**(1), 33-35 (1994)

Administration of **Kyung-Ok-Ko** (300, 600 and 1200 mg/kg) to experimental animals significantly decreased their blood sugar, cholesterol and triglyceride levels in a dose dependent manner.

Whang WK, IS Oh, SH Lee, SB Choi, IH Kim; The physiological activities of Kyung-Ok-Ko (2): Effects on the hyperglycaemia, hypertension, anti-fatigue and decrease of body weight, *Korean J Pharmacogn* **25**(1), 51-58 (1994)

A combination of dried water extract of ***Pterocarpus marsupium*** stem and fresh mature leaves of **Jarul** (*Lagerstroemia speciosa*) in equal proportions improved the signs and symptoms of diabetic patients. This formulation also diminished diabetic complications.

Chaurasia A K, SD Dubey, JK Ojha, Role of Vijaysar and Jarul on insulin dependent diabetes, *Aryavaidyan* **7**(3), 147–152 (1994)

The anti-diabetic effect of a herbal product containing ***Cyamopsis tetragonoloba, Trigonella foenum-graecum, Cephalandra indica*** and ***Gymnema sylvestre*** was examined in 67 diabetic patients and 12 normal subjects. In the first phase of the study, out of 25 cases of both insulin dependent and non-insulin dependent diabetes, only 11 patients showed lowering of blood sugar levels following administration of this compound. In the second phase of the study, 42 cases of non-insulin dependent diabetes were given the test drug and all of them exhibited a decrease in the blood sugar levels. It was suggested that this compound could be used as an adjuvant in the treatment of diabetes mellitus.

Sadhukhan B, Roychowdhury, P Banerjee, S Sen, Clinical evaluation of a herbal anti-diabetic product, *J Indian Med Assoc* **92**(4), 115-17 (1994).

The hypoglycaemic effect of a herbal composite drug, **Diacont,** was evaluated in normal and alloxan-induced diabetic rats. Aqueous solution of this drug (2g/kg) significantly reduced the blood sugar levels of diabetic animals without any side effect.

Upadhya OP; Evaluation of hypoglycaemic effect of a composite herbal drug, Diacont, *Sachitra Ayurveda* **47**(6), 452-54 (1994)

The clinical efficacy of a formulation containing **Chandraprabha vati, Trivang Bhasma** and ***Pterocarpus marsupium*** was assessed in 25 patients of Madhumeha (Diabetes mellitus)

Sharma BB, NK Malviya; A clinical trial of Chandraprabha vati, Trivang bhasma and Vijaysar in Madhumeha, *Seminar on Research in Ayurveda and Siddha , CCRAS* , New Delhi, p.23, March 20 -22, 1995.

Administration of a Siddha herbo-mineral compound, **Abraka Chenduram** (200mg, bd) for 45 days to 130 patients of non-insulin dependent diabetes mellitus significantly decreased their fasting and postprandial blood sugar levels. Another Siddha compound, **Sandanpodi** (300mg, bd) also produced significant lowering of fasting and postprandial blood sugar levels of 20 diabetic patients. These compounds did not cause any adverse effect.

Ravishanker, RK Singhal; Effect of Siddha herbo-mineral and herbal drugs in the management of diabetes mellitus (Neerazhivu), *Seminar on Research in Ayurveda and Siddha, CCRAS*, New Delhi, p.19, March 20-22, 1995.

Shokatsu-cha, a Chinese traditional medicine formulation containing Dioscoreae rhizome (dried rhizome of *Dioscorea opposita*), Adenophorae radix (*Adenophora tetraphylla* root), Rehmanniae radix (root of *Rehmannia glutinosa*), Anemarrhenae rhizome (rhizome of *Anemarrhena asphodeloides*), *Salvia mittiorrhizae* radix, Epimedii folium (*Epimedium brevicornum* leaves) and Lycii fructus (fruit of *Lycium barbarum*) has been claimed to be effective in diabetes mellitus. Oral administration of Shokatsu-cha to streptozotocin-induced diabetic rats and mice for 10 days suppressed the streptozotocin-induced increase of blood sugar levels. The Shokatsu-cha extract and its ethanol-eluted fraction also inhibited the intestinal glucose absorption in diabetic rats and lowered the blood sugar levels of diabetic mice.

Sanae F, K Miyamoto, H Sanamishi, H Kizu, T Tomimori, J Sun, X Sun, Hypoglycaemic effects of Shokatsu-cha (Xia-Ke-Ca) in streptozotocin-induced diabetes mellitus, *Phytother Res* **10**(2), 127-30 (1996).

The root bark of ***Salacia prinoides*** and seeds of ***Strychnos potatorum*** were powdered and two types of tablets (each 500 mg), one containing only *Salacia prinoides* and other a 1:1 mixture of both the drugs were prepared. Forty two non-insulin dependent diabetic patients were treated with herbal drugs for 2 months. Both the herbal treatments exhibited a lowering effect on blood glucose, serum total cholesterol and triglycerides and improvement on serum HDL-cholesterol, chromium and magnesium levels significantly. In general, the single herbal tablet of *Salacia prinoictes* had a more pronounced hypoglycaemic effect than the mixed herbal tablet.

Kowsalya S, U Chandrasekhar, JB Sharmila; Development and evaluation of hypoglycaemic tablets from selected herbs, *Indian J Nutr Dietet* **33**(9), 208-15 (1996).

PRL-12, a tribal herbal preparation of Kerala, is used as a potent anti-diabetic agent. To validate its efficacy, the anti-diabetic effect of this preparation was examined in alloxan-induced diabetic rats. In PRL-12-treated rats, maximum glucose tolerance was observed at the end of 90 minutes. In diabetic rats, maximum fall in blood sugar occurred after 6 hours of administration of this drug.

Rathinam K, KS Oomen, JM Rao, Effects of herbal tribal preparation PRL 12 in reducing the blood sugar level, *Biomedicine* **17**(1), 49-52 (1997)

Oral administration of a 10% decoction of a widely used Egyptian formulation (**PSP**) containing *Aloe vera, Lupinus termis, Trigonella foenum-graecum, Commiphora mukul, Bryonia cretica* and *Rheum officinale* to alloxanised male rats (1gm/kg), gradually lowered the blood sugar levels after 2, 4 and 8 weeks. The compound also decreased the blood cholesterol, triglycerides, creatinin and AST levels.

Nada SA, SAE Bharandy, SA Negm, Evaluation of the hypoglycaemic activity of a traditional herbal preparation in male diabetic rats, *Fitoterapia* **8**(3), 240-44 (1997)

The anti-diabetic effect of **Seishin-Kanro-to,** a traditional herbal formulation containing rhizome of *Anemarrhena asphodeloides* and radix of *Rehmannia glutinosa,* was investigated in KK-Ay mice, a non-insulin dependent diabetic animal model. Seishin-Kanro-to (1700 mg/kg) significantly decreased the blood sugar levels of

KK Ay mice 7 hours after single oral administration. This formulation also lowered the blood sugar levels and improved glucose tolerance following its chronic administration for 5 weeks. It was suggested that this formulation could be used in patients of diabetes mellitus.

Miura T, M Kako, E Ishihara, H Usami-Yano, K Tanigawa, K Sudo, Y Seino; Anti-diabetic effects of Seishin-Kanro-to in KK-Ay mice, *Planta Med* **63**(4), 322 (1997).

Administration of **Amrycard**, a herbal formulation consisting of *Cinnamomum tamala, Aegle marmelos, Gymnema sylvestre, Pterocarpus marsupium, Azadirachta indica, Tinospora cordifolia,* and *Trigonella foenum-graecum,* to Insulin dependent diabetics (2caps. tds), moderate diabetics (2caps. bd) and mild diabetics (1cap, tds) for 3 weeks, produced an overall improvement in all cases (1). Administration of **Amrycard**, (2caps, tds) for 6 months to patients of diabetes mellitus, significantly lowered their fasting and postprandial blood sugar levels (2). The drug also produced significant lowering of fasting and postprandial blood sugar levels in non-insulin dependent diabetic patients (3).

1. Bhagwan Singh, Clinical trial on Amrycard capsules in the treatment of diabetes mellitus (Madhumeha), *Indian J Clin Practice* 1(9), 31-34 (1997)
2. Sarma BP, NN Barman; Diabetes mellitus and its management by herbomineral agent (Amrycard) in N.E. region of India, *Seminar on Herbs and Herbal Medicines,* Patna, p.42, January 16-19, (1999)
3. Sarma BP, NN Barman; Diabetes mellitus and its management by herbomineral agents (Amrycard) in N.E. region of India, *Proc Int Congress on Ayurveda,* Chennai, India, p.190, January 28-30, (2000)

Pancreas Tonic, a dietary supplement containing extracts of *Syzygium cumini, Gymnema sylvestre, Trigonella foenum-graecum, Azadirachta indica, Ficus racemosa* and *Tinospora cordifolia* was found to possess hypoglycaemic activity. The effect of Pancreas Tonic on serum glucose, glycosylated hemoglobin, and pancreatic islet cell regeneration of rats was studied. The diabetic group had significantly higher serum glucose and glycosylated hemoglobin levels compared with controls, but the dietary supplement-treated group showed significantly lower serum glucose and glycosylated hemoglobin levels compared with the untreated diabetic group. Histological examination of the pancreas showed a generalized reduction in size and number of islets in the diabetic group but the dietary supplement helped regeneration of islet cells. Pancreas Tonic was thus found to induce an anti-diabetic effect through regeneration of pancreatic islet cells in experimental rats. Pancreas Tonic, fed to animals with partially chemically damaged pancreas, for 12 weeks resulted in lowering of blood sugar levels and regeneration of pancreatic *beta* cells. Similar response was also observed in diabetic patients (1, 2).

1. Rao RM, FA Salem, I Gleason-Jordan; Anti-diabetic effects of a dietary supplement "Pancreas Tonic", *J Natl Med Assoc* **90**(10), 614-18 (1998)

2. M/s Botanical Indian Laboratories Pvt. Ltd., New Delhi, Pancreas tonic:-An ideal herbal food supplement for diabetes mellitus, *Antiseptic* **99**(1), 12-13 (2002).

Extracts of **P55A** (a 1:1 mixture of the barks of *Phellodendron amurense* and *Aralia elata*) have been used traditionally by Koreans to treat diabetes. Experiments were conducted to ascertain whether **P55A** could mimic insulin actions such as activation of ERK2, PI 3-kinase and glycogen synthesis in liver cells. The butanol extract of P55A was found to activate ERK2 in the cytosol and nucleus of HepG2 cells; the extent of ERK2 activation was much higher in the nucleus. It also significantly increased the level of glycogen in HepG2 cells. Association of PI 3-kinase and IRS-1 in the cytoplasm was also stimulated by the butanol extract of P55A. Active compounds of **P55A** were thus found to regulate blood glucose levels by activating ERK2 and PI 3-kinase and by stimulation of glycogen synthesis in the liver (1). Enhanced activity of the polyol pathway and oxidative damage has been implicated in the pathogenesis of diabetic cataract. **P55A**, which showed significant aldose reductase activity, caused a dramatic reduction in the high sorbitol contents observed in the lenses of diabetic rats. In addition, the greatly elevated content of thiobarbituric acid reactive substances (TBARS) and carbonylated protein in diabetic rats were reduced by P55A treatment. These results suggest that **P55A** extract exerts an antioxidant effect by reducing lipid peroxidation and protein carbonylation as well as having an inhibitory action against aldose reductase in the lenses of diabetic rats (2).

1. Kim SJ, YY Kim, Ho Ko Kwang, EK Hong, YB Han, BH Kang, H Kim; Butanol extract of 1:1 mixture of *Phellodendron* cortex and *Aralia* cortex stimulates PI 3-kinase and ERK2 with increase of glycogen levels in HepG2 cells, *Phytother Res* **12**(4), 255-60 (1998)
2. Lee Y, H Kim, HS Choi, BH Kang, YB Han, SJ Kim; Effects of water extract of 1:1 mixture of *Phellodendron* cortex and *Aralia* cortex on polyol pathway and oxidative damage in lenses of diabetic rats, *Phytother Res* **13**(7), 555-60 (1999)

The anti-diabetic activity of the Ayurvedic formulation, **Ayush-82**, a combination of **Chadraprabha vati, Trivang bhasma** and ***Pterocarpus marsupium*** and the seed powder of ***Trigonella foenum-graecum,*** was assessed in three groups of non-insulin dependent diabetic patients. All these formulations significantly reduced the fasting and postprandial blood sugar levels with marked improvement in the sign and symptoms of these patients.

Naresh Kumar, Anil Kumar, ML Sharma; Clinical evaluation of single and herbo-mineral compound drugs in the management of Madhumeha, *J Res Ayur Siddha* **20**(1-2), 1-9 (1999).

Anti-hyperglycaemic effects of a herbo-mineral compound (**Mehamrut**) containing 6 herbal ingredients [Saptarangi (*Casearia esculenta*), Gudmar (*Gymnema sylvestre*), Amla (*Emblica officinalis*), Methi (*Trigonella foenum-graecum*), Haldi (*Curcuma longa*) and Jambul beej (*Eugenia jambolana*)] and 12 minerals were evaluated in 12 cases of type-2 diabetes mellitus. Administration of Mehamrut (1-2 tabs, tds) for 6 weeks lowered the fasting and postprandial blood sugar and fructosamine levels of diabetic patients. It was suggested that this compound might be used as an adjuvant therapy in poorly controlled type-2 diabetes mellitus.

Joshi SR, J Shroff, PS Shah, S Irani, M Oswal, L Peduekar, S Keer, Katana; Effect of herbomineral preparation (**Mehamrut**) as an adjuvant in type-2 diabetes: a pilot study, *Indian Practitioner* **52**(4) 233-39 (1999).

A herbal powder, prepared from the plant drugs ***Syzygium cumini*** (Jamun), ***Gymnema sylvestre*** (Gurmar), ***Momordica charantia*** (bitter gourd), ***Solanum melongena*** (brinjal), found effective in controlling blood sugar levels in cases of diabetes mellitus. It has been patented. It was well tolerated by insulin dependent diabetes mellitus patients without any side effects.

Tomer OS, P Glomski, K Borah, Use of Jamun, A herbal powder comprising Bittergourd, Gurmar and egg-plant as anti-diabetic agents, *US.* US 5, 900, 240 (1999).

The anti-hyperglycaemic traditional Chinese prescription, **Byakko-ka-ninjin-to,** is composed of five crude drugs, ginseng, anemarrhena, licorice, gypsum and rice. The importance of Ca^{2+} as gypsum or $CaCl_2$ in the blend has been demonstrated.

Kimura I, N Nakashima, Y Sugihara, C Fu-jun, M Kimura; The anti-hyperglycaemic blend effect of traditional chinese medicine byakko-ka-ninjin-to on alloxan and diabetic KK-CA(y) mice, *Phytother Res* **13**(6), 484-88 (1999)

An Ayurvedic formulation consisting of ***Emblica officinalis, Curcuma longa, Tinospora cordifolia, Cyperus rotundus, Terminalia chebula, Syzygium cumini*** and ***Swertia chirayita*** was found to be effective in the management of diabetes mellitus.

Rajgopalan K, K Sasidharan; Evaluation of the clinical management of *Prameha roga* (Diabeties mellitus), *Aryavaidyan* **14**(1), 33-43 (2000)

The anti-hyperglycaemic activity of a herbo-mineral compound, **DM-5,** containing Sudarshan churna, Rasayana churna, Haridra churna, Suvarna makshik and Bang bhasma, was evaluated in patients of diabetes mellitus. DM-5 showed anti-diabetic effect in these patients.

Belani JM, VN Lathia; Effect of DM-5 compound in Madhumeha (Diabetes mellitus), *Proc Int Congress on Ayurveda 2000,* Chennai, TN, India, p.191, January 28-30, (2000).

Administration of a formulation containing Amrita (***Tinospora cordifolia***), Pippali (***Piper longum***) and Nimb (***Azadirachta indica***) powder (5 g, bd) for 3 months to patients of diabetes mellitus led to a significant lowering of their blood sugar.

Mehra PS, PK Madikonde, RH Singh; Amrita-Pippali-Nimb yoga in diabetes with special reference to Agni and Ojas, *Proc Int Congress on Ayurveda,-2000* , Chennai,

TN, India, p. 99-100, January 28 –30, (2000)

"**Diabetin**", an herbal formulation, possesses a sugar-reducing and anorexigenic properties. It facilitates loss of body mass and delays the manifestations of diabetic angio- and neuro-pathies. It is recommended for the treatment of a mild form of diabetes. It can be used in combination with other oral sugar-lowering drug preparations.

Bodnar PM, GP Mykhal'chyshyn, VM Reznichenko, OP Moshchych, VS Pylypchuk; Phytopreparation Diabetin in treatment of patients with insulin-independent diabetes mellitus, *Lik Sprava* (6), 94-96 (2000) [Article in Ukrainian]

"**Antidiabetis**" is a patented (**P-9801091** Zagreb, Croatia) herbal preparation and it contains the following plants: *Vaccinium myrtillus, Taraxacum officinale, Cichorium intybus, Juniperus communis, Centaurium umbellatum, Phaseolus vulgaris, Achillea millefolium, Morus nigra, Valeriana officinalis,* and *Urtica dioica* The anti-hyperglycaemic effect of ethanol extract of this preparation as well as of the residue, obtained by removal of solvent from ethanol extract at 45°C, were studied. The results of the study revealed that the residue from the ethanol extract of the herbal preparation significantly decreased the levels of glucose and fructosamine in alloxan-induced non-obese diabetic mice (1). Changes in the concentration of glutathione S-transferases and malondialdehyde were assessed in the liver of normal and non-obese diabetic mice with and without treatment with this plant extract. A 7-day treatment with P-9801091 plant extract at a dose of 20 mg/kg body weight led to a significant increase in the catalytic concentration of glutathione S-transferases in the liver of non-obese diabetic (NOD) mice and a decrease in malondialdehyde concentration, which could be explained by its anti-hyperglycaemic effect (2).

1. Petlevski R, M Hadzija, M Slijepcevic, D Juretic; Effect of 'antidiabetis' herbal preparation on serum glucose and fructosamine in NOD mice, *J Ethnopharmacol* **75**(2-3), 181-84 (2001)
2. Petlevski R, M Hadzija, M Slijepcevic, D Juretic, J Petrik, Glutathione S-transferases and malondialdehyde in the liver of NOD mice on short-term treatment with plant mixture extract P-9801091, *Phytother Res* **17**(4), 311-14 (2003)

The anti-diabetic potency of **Tincture of Panchparna**, a polyherbal formulation, was evaluated. Treatment of diabetic animals with **panchparna** tincture (1.0 ml/kg b.w.) for 30 days showed a decrease in serum glucose and serum cholesterol levels in comparison to control animals. The formulation, however, failed to show any hypoglycaemic or hypolipidaemic activity in normal animals. Hepatic glycogen levels were increased in treated diabetic animals, but there was no change in the treated control animals.

Annapurna A, DK Mahalakshmi, KM Krishna; Anti-diabetic activity of a polyherbal preparation (tincture of panchparna) in normal and diabetic rats, *Indian J Exp Biol* **39**(5), 500-02 (2001)

The effects of ***Fagopyrum tatarium*** **complex prescription (FTCP)**, a Chinese herbal formulation, were studied in type-2 diabetic rats. FTCP was close or superior to glyburide (glibenclamide) in preventing obesity, decreasing blood glucose level and improving insulin-sensitivity. FTCP could also prevent chronic complication of diabetes. No toxicity or side effect of FTCP was found.

Gao T, Q You; The study of *Fagopyrum tataricum* complex prescription on type-II diabetes rats, *Zhong Yan Cai* **24**(6), 424-26 (2001) [Article in Chinese]

In alloxan-induced diabetic animals, the anti-hyperglycaemic and hypoglycaemic effects of a herbal compound, **DWN-12** was examined. Administration of DWN-12 to alloxanised animals for 4 days significantly lowered the blood glucose, blood and tissue cholesterol, triglycerides, phospholipids and blood urea levels.

Resmi CR, F Aneez, B Sinilal, MS Latha; Anti-diabetic effect of a herbal drug in alloxan diabetic rats, *Indian Drugs* **38**(6), 319-22 (2001).

Diamed is a herbal formulation composed of the aqueous extracts of three medicinal plants (*Azadirachta indica, Cassia auriculata* and *Momordica charantia*). Oral administration of Diamed to rats with alloxan-induced experimental diabetes at different doses (0.25 g, 0.30 g or 0.35 g/kg) for 30 days resulted in a significant reduction in blood glucose, glycosylated haemoglobin, and an increase in plasma insulin and total haemoglobin. The effect was highly significant after administration of the drug at a dose of 0.35g/kg body weight. Diamed also prevented a decrease in body weight and significantly improved glucose tolerance in the diabetic animals. The effect was comparable with 600μg/kg glibenclamide.

Pari L, R Ramakrishnan, S Venkateswaran; Anti-hyperglycaemic effect of Diamed, a herbal formulation, in experimental diabetes in rats, *J Pharm Pharmacol* **53**(8), 1129-43 (2001)

Aavirai Kudineer (AK) is a herbal decoction of seven botanical drugs, cited in a Tamil Siddha medical text. The anti-diabetic efficacy of this formulation was evaluated using normal and alloxan-induced diabetic rats. Improved glucose tolerance was observed within 1 hr in **AK** -treated rats (10 ml/kg b.w.) as compared to control. A significant decrease in hyperglycaemic characteristics of alloxan diabetes was noted after 15 days of **AK** treatment. The drug also reversed the elevated levels of urea, creatinine and cholesterol and decreased protein values to near normal levels. Assay of glycogen content and main carbohydrate-metabolising enzymes, *viz.* hexokinase, glucose-6-phosphatase and fructose 1,6 diphosphatase in the liver of diabetic and **AK**-treated diabetic rats clearly ascertained the hypoglycaemic efficacy of this formulation.

Bhavapriya V, S Kalpana, S Govindasamy, T Apparanatham; Biochemical studies on hypoglycaemic effect of Aavirai kudineer: a herbal formulation in alloxan diabetic rats, *Indian J Exp Biol* **39**(9), 925-28 (2001)

The administration of an aqueous extract of **turmeric** (300 mg/kg) and **abromine** powder, the partially purified alkaloid of ***Abroma augusta,*** resulted in a significant reduction of blood glucose and increase in total haemoglobin in streptozotocin-induced diabetic rats. The drug also resulted in a decrease of free radical formation in tissues like liver, lungs, kidney and brain and also of thiobarbituric acid reactive substances (1, 2).

1. Ali Hussain HEM; Hypoglycaemic, hypolipidaemic, and antioxiant properties of a combination of *Curcuma longa* Linn. and partially purified product from *Abroma augusta* Linn. in streptozotocin-induced diabetes, *Indian J Clin Biochem* **17**(2), 33-43 (2002)
2. Ali Hussain HEM; Hypoglycaemic, hypolipidaemic, and antioxiant properties of a combination of curcumin from *Curcuma longa* Linn. and partially purified product from *Abroma augusta* Linn. in streptozotocin-induced diabetes mellitus, *Chemistry Biology Interface: Synergistic New Frontiers,* P-25-26, November 21-26, 2004, New Delhi, India

Cogent db, a polyherbal drug, was investigated for its possible anti-diabetic effect in alloxan-induced diabetic rats. Oral administration of the aqueous solution of Cogent db for 40 days exhibited a significant reduction in blood glucose, glycosylated haemoglobin and increased plasma insulin, total haemoglobin along with anti-hyperlipidemic effects in diabetic rats, the effective dose being 0.45 g/kg body weight. A significant improvement in glucose tolerance was also observed in rats treated with Cogent db. The anti-diabetic effect of Cogent db was superior to that observed with glibenclamide (1).

In order to evaluate the efficacy of Cogent db as an adjuvant in the treatment of patients with type-2 diabetes, a non-randomised, non-placebo-controlled clinical trial was carried out during a 3-month period. At the end of 3 months a significant decrease in the levels of fasting and postprandial blood glucose, cholesterol, triglycerides, glycosylated haemoglobin (HbA1c) and fasting insulin was observed in the treatment group compared to the controls. Cogent db did not alter the liver function tests, haematologic parameters, or the kidney functions (2).

The effect of Cogent db on blood glucose and plasma insulin was studied in alloxan-induced diabetic rats. The effect on the activities of hepatic glucose metabolising enzymes was also studied. The results of the investigation suggest that Cogent db controls the blood glucose level by increasing glycolysis and decreasing gluconeogenesis with a lower demand of pancreatic insulin than in untreated rats. This is possible because it regulates the activities of hepatic glucose metabolising enzymes (3).

Oral administration of Cogent db for 40 days resulted in significant reduction in blood glucose, serum and tissue (liver and kidney) lipids, whereas the level of plasma insulin and the activity of hepatic lipogenic enzymes were significantly increased in alloxan diabetic rats. Cogent db exhibits a strong anti-hyperlipidaemic effect, which could exert a beneficial action against macrovascular complications (cardiovascular disease) associated with diabetes mellitus (4).

1. Pari L, G Saravanan; Anti-diabetic effect of Cogent db, a herbal drug in alloxan-induced diabetes mellitus, *Comp Biochem Physiol* **C** *Toxicol Pharmacol* **131**(1), 19-25 (2002)
2. Shekhar KC, FI Achike, G Kaur, P Kumar, R Hashim; A preliminary evaluation of the efficacy and safety of Cogent db (an Ayurvedic drug) in the glycaemic control of patients with type 2-diabetes, *J Altern Compliment Med* **8**(4), 445-57 (2002)
3. Saravanan G, L Pari, S Venkateswaran; Effect of Cogent db, a herbal drug, on plasma insulin and hepatic enzymes of glucose metabolism in experimental diabetes, *Diabetes Obes Metab* **4**(6), 394-98 (2002)
4. Saravanan G, L Pari; Effect of Cogent db, a herbal drug, on serum and tissue lipid metabolism in experimental hyperglycaemic rats, *Diabetes Obes Metab* **5**(3), 156-62 (2003)

The effectiveness of **Inolter,** a herbal product, in achieving glycaemic control and changes in lipid profile of newly diagnosed type-2 diabetics was evaluated in a randomised, placebo-controlled double blind trial. Efficacy of Inolter was determined by observing glycaemic control by estimating glycosylated haemoglobin (HbA1c) and fasting blood sugar. Alteration of lipid profile (serum cholesterol, LDL, VLDL, HDL and triglycerides) was also studied. The results of the investigation suggest that **Inolter** is a useful adjunctive therapy to exercise and diet control in newly diagnosed type-2 diabetes mellitus.

Agrawal RP, A Sharma, AS Dua, Chandershekhar, DK Kochar, RP Kothari; A randomised placebo controlled trial of Inolter (herbal product) in the treatment of type-2 diabetes, *J Assoc Physicians India* **50**(March), 391-93 (2002)

Tangniaole Capsule decreased the blood-sugar content in normal mice and rats and heightened the level of serum insulin and the content of liver glycogen in normal rats. These capsules also lowered the blood-sugar levels and increased the liver glycogen contents in adrenalin-induced hyperglycaemic rats. The treatment with the capsules also inhibited alloxan-induced hyperglycaemia of mice and rats and improved the glucose tolerance of rats.

Wang Y, S Han, G Sun, R Wang; Experimental study on the hypoglycaemic effect of Tangniaole Capsule, *Zhong Yao Cai* **25**(6), 426-28 (2002) [Article in Chinese]

In alloxan-induced diabetic albino rats, **Karnim forte,** a herbal formulation (25-27 mg/kg) caused significant lowering of blood sugar levels.

Patil R, R Mulchandani, AT Patil; Evaluation of anti-diabetic activity of a polyherbal formulation, Karnim forte, *National Convention on Current Trends in Herbal Drugs and Annual Conference of Indian Society of Pharmacgonosy : Herbs : The Natural Alternative,* Gandhinagar, Gujarat, India , January 17-18, (2003).

Significant positive effects of an **Anti-diabetic herbal formula (ADHF)** on the prevention of progressive diet-induced type-2 diabetes were demonstrated in C57BL/6J mouse model. C57BL/6J mice developed NIDDM-like symptoms when fed solely on a diabetes induction diet containing high fat, high simple carbohydrate and low fibre for 8 weeks. In contrast, C57BL/6J mice, which had ADHF mixed into their diabetes induction diet, failed to show NIDDM-like symptoms. Blood glucose and serum insulin levels were significantly reduced in mice fed ADHF mixed diabetes induction diet compared with the diabetes positive control groups fed diabetes induction diet only. Insulin resistance and histopathological changes in pancreas and liver were also reduced in ADHF-treated mice in comparison to those, receiving diabetes induction diet (1, 2).

1. Huo Y, WD Winters, DL Yao; Prevention of diet-induced type 2 diabetes in the C57BL/6J mouse model by an anti-diabetic herbal formula, *Phytother Res* **17**(1), 48-55 (2003).
2. Winters WD, Y Huo, DL Yao; Inhibition of the progression of type 2 diabetes in the C57BL/6J mouse model by an anti-diabetes herbal formula, *Phytother Res* **17**(6), 591-98 (2003)

Guduchi (*Tinospora cordifolia*) and Chitrak (*Plumbago zeylanica*) are known to possess anti-diabetic properties. A clinical trial of **Guduchi-Chitrak yoga** (1:1) with thirty six diabetic patients of both sexes, having increased fasting blood sugar level along with polyuria, polydipsia and polyphagia, showed symptomatic improvement as well as fall in blood and urine glucose.

Trivedi VP, R Singh; Preliminary clinical evaluation of Guduchi-Chitrak yoga for its anti-diabetic activity, 2nd. *World Congress on Biotechnological Developments of Herbal Medicine"*, NBRI, Lucknow, India, p.162 February 20-22, 2003

Dianex, a polyherbal anti-diabetic formulation, was screened for its toxic effects, if any. For acute toxicity studies, Dianex was administered orally in graded doses of 0.75-10 g/kg to the mice. For sub-acute toxicity studies, different doses of Dianex (1.0, 1.5 and 2.5 g/kg) were administered orally to the rats once daily for 30 days. No mortality was observed up to 10 g/kg of Dianex in acute toxicity study. Daily administration of Dianex, at a dose as high as 2.5 g/kg, did not result in any mortality or changes in gross behaviour and body weight. No change in weight and histology of different organs or serum and liver biochemistry was also observed. However, significant increase in RBC count and haemoglobin level was observed in the treated animals at all doses. Other peripheral blood constituents were in the normal range. The dose of Dianex (0.25-0.5 g/kg) necessary to produce significant anti-diabetic activity in mouse is much lower than the doses used in the present study. Therefore, such doses were considered to be safe for daily administration without causing any serious side effect (1).

Dianex, composed of the aqueous extracts of *Gymnema sylvestre, Eugenia jambolana, Momordica charantia, Azadirachta indica, Cassia auriculata, Aegle marmelos, Withania somnifera* and *Curcuma longa,* was screened for its hypoglycaemic activity in normal and streptozotocin-induced diabetic mice. Dianex produced significant hypoglycaemic activity at 250-500 mg/kg doses in both normal and diabetic mice in acute (6 h) and long-term (6 weeks) studies. The elevated triglycerides, cholesterol, ALT, AST, urea and creatinine levels in diabetic mice were also significantly reduced at these doses. Both liver glycogen and protein levels were significantly increased in diabetic mice. Dianex increased the glucose tolerance significantly in both normal and diabetic mice at all the doses tested. The formulation decreased streptozotocin-induced injury to the tissues, at all the doses tested. It also produced significant free radical scavenging activity. Dianex may be useful in the treatment of diabetes mellitus (2). Dianex was found to be an effective adjuvant drug with either oral anti-diabetic agents or insulin that can be used in the control of blood sugars in diabetic patients. Dianex was proved to be a safe drug that does not cause any clinical, haematological or biochemical alteration in major organ systems (3).

1. Mutalik S, B Sulochona, M Chetana, N Udupa, P Uma Devi; Preliminary studies on acute and subacute toxicity of an anti-diabetic herbal preparation, Dianex, *Indian J Exp Biol* **41**(4), 316-20 (2003)
2. Mutalik S, M Chetana, B Sulochona, P Uma Devi, N Udupa; Effect of Dianex, a herbal formulation on experimentally induced diabetes mellitus, *Phytother Res* **19**(5), 409-15 (2005)
3. Sudha V, KL Bairy,U Shashikiran, A Sachidananda, B Jayaprakash, S Shalini; Efficacy and tolerability of Dianex in Type-2 diabetes mellitus: a non-randomised, open label non-comparative study, *Med J Malaysia* **60**(2),204-11 (2005)

Treatment of normal and diabetic rabbits with a combination of the **leaf juice of *Catharanthus roseus*** and **seed powder of fenugreek** caused a significant reduction of blood glucose levels. The effect was found to be dose dependent and more than the sum of the effects of individual components.

Satyanarayana S, GS Sarma, A Ramesh, K Sushruta, N Srinivas; Evaluation of herbal preparations for hypoglycaemic activity in normal and diabetic rabbits, *Pharmaceut Biol* **41**(6), 466-72 (2003)

Anti-diabetic effects of **Diastal A**, a herbal formulation containing *Emblica officinalis, Gymnema sylvestre*, and *Azadirachta indica,* were investigated in patients of diabetes mellitus. Administration of this compound led to a significant lowering of fasting blood sugar and glycosylated haemoglobin levels of diabetic patients. No adverse effects were observed during treatment. The drug was non-toxic and could be safely used for a longer period.

Upadhya L, K Tripathi; Clinical evaluation of a herbal compound in the management of diabetes mellitus, *Antiseptic Suppl. (Alternative Medicine)* **100**(9), 67-69 (2003).

Amomi Semen is a folk medicine for the treatment of diabetes in Korea. Its aqueous ethanol extract significantly stimulated glucose uptake in 3T3-L1 adipocytes at the concentration of 0.5 mg/ml. The extract significantly potentiated insulin-stimulated glucose uptake in a dose-dependent manner at a concentration range from 0.02 to 0.5 mg/ml. Based on this finding, it has been suggested that the anti-diabetic action of **Amomi** may be mediated through the stimulation of glucose uptake and potentiation of insulin action.

Kang Y, HY Kim; Glucose uptake-stimulatory activity of Amomi Semen in 3T3-L1 adipocytes, *J Ethnopharmacol* **92**(1), 103-05 (2004)

Oral administration of aqueous extracts of seed coat of ***Eugenia jambolana,*** leaves and flowers of ***Clitoria ternatea*** and ***Phyllanthus emblica*** to alloxan-induced diabetic rats for a period of 60 days caused a significant decrease in serum glucose and cholesterol levels. Increase in total white blood cells, total red blood cells, T-lymphocytes and B-lymphocytes were also observed in treated animals. The plant extracts also strengthened immune system.

Daisy P, N Priya, M Rajathi; Immunomodulatory activity of *Eugenia jambolana, Clitoria ternatea m*and *Phyllanthus emblica* on alloxan-induced diabetic rats, *J Exp Zoology* **7**(2), 269-78 (2004)

Hyponidd is a herbomineral formulation composed of the extracts of ten medicinal plants (*Momordica charantia, Melia azadirachta, Pterocarpus marsupium, Tinospora cordifolia, Gymnema sylvestre, Enicostemma littorale, Emblica officinalis, Eugenia jambolana, Cassia auriculata* and *Curcuma longa*). The possible anti-hyperglycaemic and antioxidant effect of Hyponidd was studied in diabetic rats. Oral administration of hyponidd (100 and 200 mg/kg) for 45 days, resulted in significant decrease of blood glucose levels and significant increase of hepatic glycogen and total haemoglobin levels. In an oral glucose tolerance test, significant improvement was observed in the experimental diabetic rats, treated with hyponidd. Hyponidd administration also decreased levels of glycosylated haemoglobin, plasma thiobarbituric acid reactive substances, hydroperoxides, ceruloplasmin and *alpha*-tocopherol in diabetic rats. Plasma reduced glutathione and vitamin C were significantly elevated by oral administration of hyponidd. The effect of hyponidd, at a dose of 200 mg/kg, was more effective than glibenclamide (600 μg/kg) in restoring the values to near normal. The results showed that hyponidd exhibits anti-hyperglycaemic and antioxidant activity in streptozotocin-induced diabetic rats.

Babu PS, P Stanely Mainzen Prince, Anti-hyperglycaemic and antioxidant effect of hyponidd, an ayurvedic herbomineral formulation in streptozotocin-induced diabetic rats, *J Pharm Pharmacol* **56**(11), 1435-42 (2004)

The effect of **Diasulin**, a polyherbal drug composed of ethanol extracts of ten medicinal plants, on blood glucose, plasma insulin and the activities of hepatic glucose metabolic enzymes was studied in alloxan-induced diabetic rats. Treatment with diasulin resulted in a significant reduction in blood glucose and glycosylated haemoglobin, an increase in plasma insulin and total haemoglobin and a significant improvement in glucose tolerance. Diasulin also significantly reduced the activities of glucose-6-phosphatase and fructose-1,6-bisphosphatase in the liver, whereas the level of plasma insulin and hepatic hexokinase activity was significantly increased in alloxan diabetic rats. Diasulin was thus found to control the blood glucose level by increasing glycolysis and decreasing gluconeogenesis with a lower demand of pancreatic insulin than in untreated rats. The effect of different doses of Diasulin on blood glucose, plasma insulin, lipid peroxides and tissue lipids was examined in alloxan-induced diabetic rats. In addition to a significant reduction of blood glucose and increase in plasma insulin, diasulin also resulted in a significant decrease in tissue lipids and lipid peroxide formation. The effect produced by diasulin was comparable with that of glibenclamide (1, 2).

1. Pari L, R Saravanan; Anti-diabetic effect of diasulin, a herbal drug, on blood glucose, plasma insulin and hepatic enzymes of glucose metabolism in hyperglycaemic rats, *Diabetes Obes Metab* **6**(4), 286-92 (2004)
2. Saravanan R, L Pari; Anti-hyperlipidaemic and anti-peroxidative effect of Diasulin, a polyherbal formulation in alloxan induced hyperglycaemic rats, *BMC Compliment Altern Med* **5**, 14 (2005)

The anti-diabetic and antioxidant effects of the herbal formulation, **ADD-199,** was investigated in streptozotocin-induced diabetic C(3)H mice and the results were compared with those of glibenclamide and metformin. Plasma glucose, insulin and lipids as well as liver glycogen, lipids and lipid peroxidation were measured following treatment for 8 weeks. Glibenclamide and ADD-199 increased insulin levels in diabetic mice whilst metformin had no effect. Basal plasma glucose levels in diabetic controls were reduced by ADD-199 (100 mg/kg) in less than 2 weeks compared to 4 and 6 weeks for glibenclamide and metformin. The hypoglycaemic effect of ADD-199 appeared to be associated with the alkaloidal content of the extract. The anti-hyperglycaemic and antioxidant actions of ADD-199 at a dose of 100mg/kg/day are comparable to those of the maximum daily therapeutic doses of glibenclamide (0.25 mg/kg) and metformin (50 mg/kg). The sub-chronic toxicity of the aqueous extract of **ADD-**199, prepared from *Maytenus senegalensis, Annona senegalensis, Kigelia africana* and *Lannea welwitschia,* was evaluated in albino rats. Administration of the extract (100 or 500 mg/kg b.w.) for 30 days did not affect plasma alanine aminotransferase, alkaline phosphatase and albumin or creatinine kinase levels. Similarly plasma creatinine, blood urea levels, PCV, haemoglobin, RBC, platelets, lymphocytes counts remained unaffected following treatment with the extract (**ADD-199**). ADD-199 did not affect the Zoxazolamine-induced paralysis and pentobarbitol-induced sleeping time or certain hepatic cytochrome P450 isoenzymes activities in rats. It was suggested ADD-199 on sub-chronic administration did not cause any overt organ specific toxicity (1, 2).

1. Okine LK, AK Nyarko,N Osei-Kwabena, IV Oppong, F Barnes, M Ofosuhene; The anti-diabetic activity of the herbal preparation ADD-199 in mice: a comparative study with two oral hypoglycaemic drugs, *J Ethnopharmacol* **97**(1), 31-38 (2005)
2. Nyarko AK, LK Okine, RK Wedzi, PA Addo, M Ofosuhene; Subchronic toxicity studies of the anti-diabetic herbal preparation ADD-199 in the rats: absence of organ toxicity and modulation of cytochrome P450, *J. Ethnopharmacol* 97(2), 319-25 (2005).

Oral administration of aqueous extract of ***Piper nigrum*** seeds and ***Vinca rosea*** flowers to alloxan-induced diabetic rats once a day for 4 weeks significantly lowered the blood sugar level and serum lipids. The reduced levels of antioxidant enzymes (catalase and glutathione peroxidase) in alloxanised rats were normalised by this treatment. The findings suggest that the treatment with *Piper nigrum* and *Vinca rosea* is useful not only in controlling glucose and lipid levels but also in strengthening antioxidant potential.

Kaleem M, Sheema, H Sarmad, B Bano; Protective effects of *Piper nigrum* and *Vinca rosea* in alloxan-induced diabetic rats, *Indian J Physiol Pharmacol* **49**(1), 65-71 (2005)

The anti-diabetic activity of **Glycoban,** a herbal formulation containing *Gymnema sylvestre, Eugenia jambolana, Aegle marmelos, Azadirachta indica, Momordica charantia, Ocimum sanctum, Ficus glomerata, Enicostema littorale, Tinospora cordifolia, Gossypium herbaceum* and *Strychnos nux vomica,* was studied in 45 patients of diabetes mellitus. Administration of Glycoban (2caps, each containing 610mg of drug, bd) to newly diagnosed mild cases of diabetes mellitus (NIDDM) significantly lowered their blood sugar levels without any observable side effect

Bhimani S, Clinical study of efficacy of Glycoban capsules in patients of non-insulin dependent (NIDDM) diabetes mellitus, *Antiseptic* **102**(2), 71-75 (2005).

The effect of supplementation of a powdered mixture of three traditional medicinal plants,-**bittergourd** (*Momordica charantia*), **jamun** (*Eugenia jambolana*) seeds, and **fenugreek** (*Trigonella foenum graecum*) seeds-in raw or cooked form, on blood glucose was studied in 60 non-insulin-dependent male diabetics. A significant decrease in oral hypoglycaemic drug intake was observed in treated patients. It was concluded that 2 g of a powdered mixture of traditional medicinal plants in either raw or cooked form could be successfully used for lowering blood glucose in diabetics.

Kochhar A, M Nagi; Effect of supplementation of traditional medicinal plants on blood glucose in non-insulin-dependent diabetics: a pilot study, *J Med Food* **8**(4), 545-49 (2005)

The effects of **Huang Lian Jie Du (HLJD)** decoction on vascular endothelial function in type-2 diabetic rats were investigated and its prophylactic and therapeutic significance was explored. From the results of the investigation, it was inferred that HLJD decoction possesses the ability to protect vascular endothelium from early damage in type-2 diabetic animals. The protective effects of HLJD on endothelium might be related to its ability of reducing the blood glucose, adjusting plasma lipids profiles, improving insulin resistance, antagonising inflammatory mediators and inducing endothelium-dependent vascular relaxation.

Xiao YL, FE Lu, LJ Xu, SH Leng, KF Wang; Protective effects of Huang Lian Jie Du decoction on vascular endothelial function in type-2 diabetic rats, *Zhongguo Zhong Za Zhi* **30**(22), 1767-70 (2005) [Article in Chinese]

Anti-diabetic activity of **SMK001,** a polyherbal formulation was investigated in streptozotocin-induced diabetic rats. The test compound was given orally once a day for 4 weeks starting from 21 days after streptozotocin injection. The treated diabetic rats exhibited a reduction in blood and urinary sugar levels in a dose dependent manner. SMK001, at a dose of 100 mg/kg, showed more favourable effect than glibenclamide.

Kim JD, SM Kang, BI Seo, HY Choi, HS Choi, SK Ku, Anti-diabetic activity of SMK 001 a polyherbal formulation in streptozotocin-induced diabetic rats: Therapeutic study, *Biol Pharmaceut Bull* **29**(3), 477-82 (2006) .

The effects of **Okchun-San** (OCS), a Korean herbal medicine formula, on the blood glucose levels in diabetic C57BL/KsJ db/db mice were examined. The herbal medicines were prepared from dried herbs by adding Coicis semen (OCS-C) or Oryzae semen (OCS-O). The experimental animals were divided into a control group and three sample groups; the sample groups received OCS-C (200 mg/kg), OCS-O (200 mg/kg), or acarbose (5 mg/kg) orally once a day for 12 days. On day 5 and 12, the animals of above treated groups showed lower fasting blood sugar levels than the controls. During intra-peritoneal glucose tolerance test, OCS-C group showed improved glucose sensitivity compared to the control group. These results suggest that OCS-C can be useful as an anti-diabetic therapy for Type-2 diabetic patients by lowering the blood glucose level.

Chang MS, MS Oh, DR Kim, KJ Jung, S Park, SB Choi, BS Ko, SK Park, Effects of Okchun-San, a herbal formulation on blood glucose and body weight in a model of type-2 diabetes, *J Ethnopharmacol* **103**(3), 491-95 (2006).

Chungkookjang (CKJ) is a traditional fermented unsalted soybean, used as an anti-diabetic drug. With an aim to find out the anti-diabetic candidates, present in CKJ, both cooked soybeans and CKJ were extracted with ethanol (70%) and subjected to chromatography over XAD-4 column. A comparison of the constituents of the fractions of the two columns indicated that the contents of isoflavonoid aglycones were elevated during fermentation. The fractions enriched with aglycones enhanced insulin-stimulated glucose uptake in 3T3-L1 adipocytes. This increase in glucose uptake resulted from stimulating a translocation of the glucose transporter (GLUT-4) into the plasma membrane through the phosphorylation of insulin receptor substrate (IRS-1) and Akt. The results of the investigation suggest that an increase in isoflavonoid aglycones in CKJ, in comparison to cooked soybeans, enhances glucose utilization by activating insulin signaling and stimulating PPAR-*gamma* activity in adipocytes. CKJ also contains small peptides, which improve glucose-stimulated insulin secretion in insulinoma cells. CKJ was found to be superior to cooked soybeans in anti-diabetic action (1). It was further observed that fermented soybeans mainly with *Bacillus subtilis* improved hepatic insulin sensitivity better than unfermented soybeans by enhancing hepatic insulin signaling cascade in diabetic rats (2).

1. Kwon DY, JS Jang, JE Lee, YS Kim, DH Shin, S Park; The isoflavonoid aglycone-rich fractions of Chungkookjang, fermented unsalted soybeans, enhance insulin signaling and peroxisome proliferator-activated receptor-*gamma* activity *in vitro*, *Biofactors* **26**(4), 245-58 (2006)
2. Kwon DY, SM Hong, JE Lee, SR Sung, S Park; Long-term consumption of fermented soybean-derived Chungkookjang attenuates Hepatic Insulin Resistance in 90% pancreatectomized diabetic rats, *Horm Metab Res* **39**(10),752-57 (2007)

Fermented Papaya Preparation (FPP) is a natural drug that has been commercially sold in Japan and Philippines as a nutriceutical. It was a bio-normaliser with antioxidant action, being a potent hydroxyl scavenger. The wide use of **FPP**, especially by elderly people, made the authors feel that the product possesses blood sugar level lowering activity. With an aim to scientifically verify the possibility that individuals, who are taking the nutriceutical FPP, might have a decrease of plasma sugar levels, 25 patients affected by type-2 diabetes mellitus under treatment with the oral anti-diabetic drug, glibenclamide and 25 clinically-healthy subjects were given 3 grams of FPP daily, during lunch, for two months. The results of this study confirmed that use of FPP could induce a significant decrease in plasma sugar levels in both healthy subjects and type-2 diabetic patients. This hypoglycaemic effect, associated with clinical signs, induced the diabetic patients to reduce the dosage of their anti-diabetic oral therapy. The FPP administration is, therefore, suggested as an adjuvant drug to join the oral anti-diabetic therapy in type-2 diabetes mellitus.

Danese C. D Esposito, V D'Alfonso, M Cirene, M Ambrosino, M Colotto; Plasma glucose level decreases as collateral effect of fermented papaya preparation use, *Clin Ter* **157**(3), 195-98 (2006)

Fangchinoline, the main constituent of *Stephania tetrandra,* decreased the high level of blood glucose and increased the low level of blood insulin in streptozotocin-diabetic mice at a dose of 0.3-3 mg/kg. The combined effects of **fangchinoline** with the isoflavonoid constituents (**formononetin, calycosin** and **ononin**) of *Astragalus membranaceus* on the hyperglycaemia and hypoinsulinaemia of streptozotocin-diabetic mice were investigated. Formononetin, calycosin and ononin (0.03-0.1 mg/kg) alone did not affect the blood glucose or blood insulin level of the diabetic mice but formononetin and calycosin (0.03-0.1 mg/kg) potentiated the anti-hyperglycaemic action of fangchinoline (0.3 mg/kg), but ononin did not. The combined effect of fangchinoline with formononetin and calycosin on hyperglycaemia in the diabetic mice accounted well for the therapeutic effect of the combination of *S. tetrandra* with *A. membranaceus* in **Boi-ogi-to**. The anti-hyperglycaemic action of formononetin appeared to be due to its potentiating action on insulin release.

Wenjie MA, N Masaaki, T-N Tatsuo, K Shinjiro; Combined effects of fangchinoline from *Stephania tetrandra* Radix and formononetin and calycosin from *Astragalus membranaceus* Radix on hyperglycaemia and hypoinsulinaemia in streptozotocin-diabetic mice, *Biol Pharm Bull* **30**(11), 2079-83 (2007)

APPENDIX - 2

DIETARY FIBRES IN THE MANAGEMENT OF DIABETES

[Dietary fibre is a complex mixture of plant materials that are resistant to breakdown by the human digestive system. Dietary fibres have also been commonly called "roughage". There are two major kinds of dietary fibres—water-insoluble fibres like cellulose, hemicellulose, lignin and bran and water-soluble fibres like gums, mucilages and pectins. Insoluble fibre is most frequently found in whole-grain products while soluble fibres are common in fruits, vegetables, dry beans and peas, and some cereals such as oats. Soluble fibre has been defined as the edible parts of plants that are resistant to digestion and absorption in the human small intestine with complete or partial fermentation in the large intestine. A simple example of soluble and insoluble fibres is a plum, the skin of which is insoluble fibre but its pulp contains soluble fibres.]

It has been observed that removal of fibre from food can result in faster and easier ingestion, decreased satiety, and disturbed glucose homoeostasis, which is probably due to inappropriate insulin release. These effects favour over-nutrition and, if often repeated, might lead to diabetes mellitus.

Haber GB, KW Heaton, D Murphy, LF Burroughs; Depletion and disruption of dietary fibre: Effects on satiety, plasma-glucose, and serum-insulin, *Lancet* **2**(8040), 679-82 (1977)

To define the type of dietary fibre with the greatest therapeutic potential in patients of diabetes mellitus, groups of four to six volunteers underwent 50-g glucose tolerance tests with and without the addition of either of **guar, pectin, gum tragacanth**, methylcellulose, **wheat bran**, or cholestyramine equivalent to 12 g fibre. The addition of each substance significantly reduced blood glucose concentration at one or more points during the glucose tolerance tests and generally reduced serum insulin concentrations. The greatest response was seen with guar, but this effect was abolished when non-viscous guar, obtained by hydrolysis, was used. The reduction in the mean peak rise in blood glucose concentration for each substance correlated positively with its viscosity. Viscous types of dietary fibre are, therefore, most likely to be therapeutically useful in modifying postprandial hyperglycaemia.

Jenkins DJ, TM Wolever, AR Leeds, MA Gassull, P Haisman, J Dilawari, DV Goff, GL Metz, KG Alberti; Dietary fibres, fibre analogues, and glucose tolerance: importance of viscosity, *Br Med J* **1**(6124), 1392-94 (1978)

The effects of high-carbohydrate, **high plant fibre diets** (HCF) on glucose and lipid metabolism were studied on 20 lean men receiving insulin therapy for diabetes mellitus. All men received control diets for 7 days followed by HCF diets for 16 days. The daily dose of insulin was lower for each patient on the HCF diets than on the control diet. On the HCF diets, insulin therapy could be discontinued in eleven patients. Fasting and 3-hr postprandial plasma glucose values were lower in most patients on the HCF diets than on the control diets despite lower insulin doses. The study suggests that HCF diets may be the dietary therapy of choice for certain patients with the maturity-onset type of diabetes.

Anderson JW, K Ward; High-carbohydrate, high-fibre diets for insulin-treated men with diabetes mellitus, *Am J Clin Nutr* **32**(11), 2312-21 (1979)

It is known that dietary fibre retards glucose absorption in normal and diabetic subjects but it is not clear which type of fibre would be most suitable for this purpose. In order to throw light on this point, the effect of **pectin** on postprandial blood glucose responses was compared with those of fibre from **barley** and **citrus**. The tests showed that pectin administration considerably inhibited the postprandial rise in blood glucose, while citrus fibre showed no such effect. Barley/citrus fibre (a mixture of cellulose, hemicellulose, lignin and pectin) failed to show the same inhibiting effect on postprandial rise in blood glucose as pure pectin in insulin-dependent diabetics. Thus, specific type of fibre must be considered when prescribing dietary fibre to diabetics.

Vaaler S, KF Hanssen, O Aagenaes; Effect of different kinds of fibre on postprandial blood glucose in insulin-dependent diabetics, *Acta Med Scand* **208**(5), 389-91 (1980)

Diets high in complex carbohydrate result in lower insulin requirements than the high-fibre diets conventionally used to treat diabetes. In diabetics, a diet providing 70% of energy from carbohydrate and containing 35 to 40 g of fibre per 1000 calories rapidly reduces the plasma glucose level and the requirement for insulin or sulfonylurea.

Anderson JW; High-fibre diets for diabetic and hypertriglyceridaemic patients, *Can Med Assoc J* **123**(10), 975-79 (1980)

In a randomised cross-over study with 18 NIDDM and 9 IDDM diabetics, it was revealed that a diet, high in complex carbohydrate and **leguminous fibre**, improves all aspects of diabetic control and continued use of a low carbohydrate diet no longer appears justified.

Simpson HC, RW Simpson, S Lousley, RD Carter, M Geekie, TD Hockaday, JL Mann; A high carbohydrate leguminous fibre diet improves all aspects of diabetic control, *Lancet* **1**(8210), 1-5 (1981)

The role of dietary fibre in satiety, glucose, and insulin was studied with fruit and fruit juice. Healthy volunteers ingested sugar-equivalent meals of **oranges** and **orange juice** and of **grapes** and **grape juice**. With oranges, there was a significantly smaller insulin response to fruit than to juice and less postabsorptive fall in plasma glucose. With grapes, the insulin response to the whole fruit was, paradoxically, more than that to the juice, while postabsorptive glucose values were similar. The glucose in grapes appeared to be more insulinogenic than that in oranges and apples. The plasma insulin and glucose responses to fruit appear to depend on the fibre as well as the glucose content of the fruit.

Bolton RP, KW Heaton, LF Burroughs; The role of dietary fibre in satiety, glucose, and insulin: studies with fruit and fruit juice, *Am J Clin Nutr* **34**(2), 211-17 (1981)

To assess the effect of dietary fibre on glucose tolerance, four different meals of varying fibre contents but having identical protein, fat and carbohydrate content were fed to eight healthy men (aged 22-45 years). Each meal provided 75 g of carbohydrate either as liquid glucose formula, or as **brown rice, pinto beans**, or **All Bran** (A Kellogg product). The mean plasma glucose and insulin responses were highest for the glucose formula, and least for All Bran and pinto beans. Rice produced nearly as great a rise in insulin and glucose as did the glucose formula. The higher the content of neutral detergent fibre in a meal, the lower was the magnitude of the insulin response evoked. It was concluded that dietary fibres dampened the insulin response to a high carbohydrate meal.

Potter JG, KP Coffman, RL Reid, JM Krall, MJ Albrink; Effect of test meals of varying dietary fibre content on plasma insulin and glucose response, *Am J Clin Nutr* **34**(3), 328-34 (1981)

Dietary fibres comprise a heterogeneous group of indigestible plant compounds, which can modify various digestive processes. Most importantly, the fibres possess the ability to inhibit digestion and absorption of carbohydrates, which enables better treatment of diabetics.

Hansen WE; Effect of bulk materials on the upper intestinal tract, *Klin Wochenschr* **60**(24), 1475-83 (1982) [Article in German]

Four different breakfasts were given to 21 insulin-dependent diabetic children in random order. Three diets differed in fibre content and the fourth one contained **beans** as part (38%) of the dietary fibre source. Each morning the children were asked to exercise vigorously for an hour and to rest for an hour, resulting in comparable rest and exercise periods for each child. The low-fibre diet resulted in the highest blood glucose concentrations after breakfast. Blood glucose levels of children on the high and medium-fibre diet did not differ. The bean diet produced the lowest mean blood glucose level but the children did not like this diet. It appears that the potentially major benefits from beans are limited by their impalatability. The more acceptable cereal fibre produces a smaller but important benefit on morning hyperglycaemia after breakfast.

Baumer JH, JA Drakeford, J Wadsworth, DC Savage; Effects of dietary fibre and exercise on mid-morning diabetic control—a controlled trial, *Arch Dis Child* **57**(12), (1982)

The effects of **brown rice** and **soybean dietary fibre** on the oral glucose tolerance test, plasma-insulin, glucagon, triglycerides, and cholesterol levels were studied in control and streptozotocin-induced diabetic rats. Plasma glucose level after glucose loading in diabetic rats fed soybean fibre was considerably lower than the corresponding group not receiving the fibre. Rice fibre decreased the plasma glucose of diabetic rats only at 60 min. Soybean fibre significantly lowered the glucagon and triglyceride levels in both control and diabetic rats but rice fibre had no effect on these blood parameters. The study demonstrated the potential benefit of soybean dietary fibre over rice fibre in diabetes treatment

Madar Z; Effect of brown rice and soybean dietary fibre on the control of glucose and lipid metabolism in diabetic rats, *Am J Clin Nutr* **38**(3), 388-93 (1983)

The effect of long-term high fibre diets (Weetbix, bran, baked beans, canned peas, prunes, whole wheat bread) in diabetic patients revealed a negative co-relationship between the mean plasma glucose changes and the dietary fibre,

Rosman MS, CJ Smith, WPU Jackson; The effect of long-term high-fibre diets in diabetic outpatients, *S Afr Med J* **63**(9), 310-13 (1983).

The blood glucose levels and insulin requirements in insulin-dependent diabetic patients consuming **high-bran bread** (18% dietary fibre) were compared with those consuming low bran (5% dietary fibre) or usual bread (4% dietary fibre). The insulin doses were reduced or the blood glucose concentrations were lowered in patients consuming high-bran bread.

Nygren C, G Hallmans, F Lithner; Effects of high-bran bread on blood glucose control in insulin-dependent diabetic patients, *Diabetes Metab* **10**(1), 39-43 (1984)

The effect of dietary fibre in non-insulin-dependent diabetics was studied. Once weekly over a 3-wk period, five lean, diet-controlled non-insulin-dependent diabetics ingested one of three isocaloric (337 kcal) isocarbohydrate (49 g carbohydrate) breakfasts differing primarily in dietary fibre: 3 g bran (control), 17 g bran (A), or 18 g bran and a whole apple (B). The diets of A and B were higher in protein than control; and the diet of B contained more sugar than the others because of the fruit. Compared to control, the diet A reduced plasma glucose over 180 min; but B did not. The peak blood glucose rise after B was lower than control. The diet A reduced xylose absorption suggesting a reduced rate of glucose absorption. The study suggests significant plasma glucose reductions with bran or bran and whole apple, other nutrient differences might also be related.

Parsons SR, Effects of high fibre breakfasts on glucose metabolism in non-insulin-dependent diabetics, *Am J Clin Nutr* **40**(1), 66-71 (1984)

The effectiveness and acceptability of high-carbohydrate, high-fibre diets was assessed on 14 outpatients with diabetes. Daily intake of hospital diets with 70% of energy as carbohydrate and 65 g plant fibre lowered insulin doses, serum cholesterol, and triglycerides. Home diets with 55% to 60% carbohydrate and 50 gm plant fibre daily sustained improvements throughout the observed period of up to 86 months.

Story L, JW Anderson, WJ Chen, D Karounos, B Jefferson; Adherence to high-carbohydrate, high-fibre diets: long-term studies of non-obese diabetic men, *J Am Diet Assoc* **85**(9), 1105-10 (1985)

Study showed that high-fibre intake provides well-established benefits for persons with diabetes; it lowers insulin requirements, provides better control of blood glucose, and reduces serum lipids. Foods, rich in soluble fibre, such as oat or bean products, lower cholesterol significantly for persons with hypercholesterolaemia and for healthy young subjects.

Anderson JW; Physiological and metabolic effects of dietary fibre, *Fed Proc* **44**(14), 2902-06 (1985)

Addition of purified fibre to carbohydrate test meals has been shown to flatten the glycaemic response in both normal and diabetic volunteers, reduce the insulin requirement in patients on the artificial pancreas and in the longer term reduce urinary glucose loss and improve diabetes control. The presence of fibre in a carbohydrate diet is assumed to slow down absorption and thus reduce postprandial GIP (Glucose-dependent insulinotropic polypeptide) and insulin levels and, in general, the more viscous is a purified fibre (e.g., guar and pectin) the more effective it is. In addition to fibre, many other aspects of carbohydrate foods (food form, anti-nutrients, etc.) influence the rate of digestion and it has been possible to classify starchy foods in terms of glycemic index to define the degree to which equicarbohydrate portions of different foods raise the blood glucose. Use of such data may maximize the effectiveness of high carbohydrate and high fibre diets in the management of diabetes and related disorders.

Jenkins DJ, AL Jenkins; Dietary fibre and the glycemic response, *Proc Soc Exp Biol Med* **180**(3), 422-31 (1985)

Soy fibre is a natural source of dietary fibre that consists of both cellulosic and non-cellulosic fibre materials. The effects of soy fibre on human plasma lipoprotein lipids and glucose tolerance were evaluated in patients with primary hyperlipidaemia. Results from this study suggest that supplemention of diet with soy fibre may be beneficial in dietary management of hyperlipidaemia in patients with hypercholesterolaemia and particularly in hyperlipidaemic patients with hyperinsulinaemia and impaired glucose tolerance.

Lo GS, AP Goldberg, A Lim, JJ Grundhauser, C Anderson, G Schonfeld; Soy fibre improves lipid and carbohydrate metabolism in primary hyperlipidaemic subjects, *Atherosclerosis* **62**(3), 239-48 (1986)

The hypoglycaemic activity of twenty **water-soluble mucilages** from plants of

Liliaceae, Amyrallidaceae, Dioscoreaceae, Orchidaceae, Saxifragaceae, Malvaceae, and Plantaginaceae families was evaluated. Most of the mucilages, isolated from plants of the Malvaceae family, showed considerable hypoglycaemic activity. Plantago mucilage A, the main mucilage found in the seeds of *Plantago asiatica*, also exhibited marked hypoglycaemic effect.

Tomoda M, N Shimazu, Y Oshima, M Takahashi, M Murakami, H Hikino; Hypoglycaemic activity of twenty plant mucilages and three modified products, *Planta Med* **53**(1), 8-12 (1987)

Dried beans, because of their high-fibre content and low-glycaemic index, are especially suitable for diabetic diets. Additions of sucrose up to 20% of total carbohydrate had no adverse effects on glycaemic index or insulin response of butter beans, which indicates that addition of moderate amounts of sucrose to a food of low glycaemic index may improve palatability without impairing the favourable effect on blood glucose and insulin response.

Vorster HH, E van Tonder, JP Kotze, AR Walker; Effects of graded sucrose additions on taste preference, acceptability, glycaemic index, and insulin response to butter beans, *Am J Clin Nutr* **45**(3), 575-79 (1987)

The effect of soy polysaccharide on postprandial plasma glucose levels was examined in seven obese non-insulin dependent maturity-onset diabetic patients, fed a standard meal without or with 10 g of this fibre source. Supplementation of soy polysaccharide significantly enhanced return of serum glucose levels towards fasting level but had no effect on plasma insulin levels. Soy polysaccharide appeared to lessen postprandial increases in glucagon and pancreatic polypeptide levels while it raised somatostatin levels. The changes in plasma glucagon, pancreatic polypeptide, and somatostatin levels are considered to be instrumental in the observed postprandial glucose and triglyceride effects.

Tsai AC, AI Vinik, A Lasichak, GS Lo; Effects of soy polysaccharide on postprandial plasma glucose, insulin, glucagon, pancreatic polypeptide, somatostatin, and triglyceride in obese diabetic patients, *Am J Clin Nutr* **45**(3), 596-601 (1987)

Pea fibre and sugar beet fibre were compared with wheat bran to investigate their effect on postprandial blood glucose and serum insulin responses in normal subjects. Only addition of pea fibre (15 g pure fibre) to control meal reduced the area under the incremental blood glucose curve significantly. None of the fibres significantly affected the area under the insulin-response curve, which was, however, reduced by all fibres. Pea fibre is palatable and may prove beneficial as a fibre supplement for diabetics.

Hamberg O, JJ Rumessen, E Gudmand-Hoyer; Blood glucose response to pea fibre: comparisons with sugar beet fibre and wheat bran, *Am J Clin Nutr* **50**(2), 324-28 (1989)

The soluble plant fibre psyllium significantly reduced fasting glucose and total cholesterol levels in C57BL/KsJ db/db diabetic mice relative to placebo-fed mice. Insulin levels were significantly higher in psyllium-fed animals than in placebo-fed animals. The observation indicated that psyllium might delay the progression of diabetes in the animal model. The results show that psyllium fibre can beneficially moderate glycaemic and lipid parameters in the db/db diabetes model.

Watters K, P Blaisdell; Reduction of glycemic and lipid levels in db/db diabetic mice by psyllium plant fibre, *Diabetes* **38**(12), 1528-33 (1989)

The effect of dietary fibres (natural wheat bran) in patients with decreased glucose tolerance was studied. The study revealed that dietary fibres are able to reduce release of glucagon, and exhibit their direct inhibitory effect on the level of sugar absorption from gastrointestinal tract.

Rinfel J, C Ruzsa, G Mozsik, T Javor; Hormonal changes during administration of dietary fibres in patients with decreased glucose tolerance, *Orv Hetil* **131**(4), 175-77 (1990) [Article in Hungarian]

The effect of dietary fibre from sweet lupine hull upon metabolic control was studied in 16 non-insulin dependent diabetics. Following a 2 month control period, patients received 10 g sweet lupine hull for the 3rd month and 20 g for the fourth month. During the 4th month, blood glucose decreased to control levels but no changes in body mass, HDL cholesterol, triglycerides, glycosylated Hb and non-fasting glucose and insulin levels were observed. It was concluded that a supplement of 10 to 20 g of this particular fibre did not improve metabolic control.

Diaz J, P Durruty, JC Tapia, E Carrasco, V Riesco, G Durruty, M Garcia de los Rios; The effects of a dietary fibre (white lupine bran) in the treatment of non-insulin-dependent diabetes, *Rev Med Chil* **118**(1), 24-32 (1990) [Article in Spanish]

A randomised cross-over design was used to determine the clinical usefulness of adding 16 g of beet fibre to the ordinary diet of non-insulin dependent diabetic (NIDDM) out-patients. The study included five patients treated with diet alone and eight patients treated with diet and sulphonylurea Beet fibre supplementation resulted in a 10% reduction of serum cholesterol in sulphonylurea-treated patients. No differences were found for fasting blood glucose, glycated hemoglobin, serum triglycerides or body weight. In view of the limited metabolic benefit of beet fibre treatment, it was concluded that there is little use for this type of dietary fibre in the routine treatment of patients with NIDDM.

Karlander S, I Armyr, S Efendie; Metabolic effects and clinical value of beet fibre treatment in NIDDM patients, *Diabetes Res Clin Pract* **11**(2), 65-71 (1991)

The effect of a preprandial ingestion of 7 g of soy fibres or of an equal amount of purified cellulose on serum glucose and insulin was studied on eight non-insulin-dependent (type-2) diabetic patients. The study showed no difference in insulin profiles between the two treatments. However, the glycemic profiles after soya ingestion were lower than those after cellulose ingestion. The results of the study revealed that soy fibre, rather than purified cellulose, has a favourable effect on the rise of postprandial glycemia in type-2 diabetic patients.

Librenti MC, M Cocchi, F Orsi, G Pozza, P Micossi; Effect of soya and cellulose fibres on postprandial glycemic response in type II diabetic patients, *Diabetes Care* **15**(1), 111-13 (1992)

Influences of a control diet with no vegetable fibre and a purified fibre diet (Isapgol, Plantago) were compared to results achieved with different levels of several vegetables (leaves of *Alternanthera sessilis* and *Colocasia antiquorum* and fruits of *Momordica charantia*) in eight normal and six non-insulin dependent diabetic patients. A negative correlation between the levels of fibre and blood glucose levels in terms of mean percent peak rise, AUC and percent glycemic response was observed. *Momordica charantia* was found to be more effective than the leafy vegetables.

Sreedevi, A Chhaturvedi; Effect of vegetable fibres on postprandial glycaemia, *Plant Foods Human Nutr* **44**(1), 71-78 (1993)

Three dietary fibres (**wheat bran, sugar beet** or **isapghula**) with different physicochemical properties were studied in healthy humans for their effects on small intestinal motility and postprandial hyperglycaemia. Test meals composed of glucose alone or glucose with 15 g of wheat bran, sugar beet or isapghula (psyllium) fibres were ingested to subjects and their duodeno-jejunal motor activity was evaluated electromyographically for 180 minutes. Addition of sugar beet or isapghula to the glucose meal altered duodeno-jejunal motility and inhibited stationary contractile activity but wheat bran had no activity. Blood glycaemic response to the glucose meal was reduced by sugar beet and isapghula but remained unchanged with wheat bran. From the observations it was suggested that the contractile activity induced by dietary fibre in the small intestine plays a major role in delayed glucose absorption.

Cherbut C, S Bruley des Varannes, M Schnee, M Rival, JP Galmiche, J Delort-Laval; Involvement of small intestinal motility in blood glucose response to dietary fibre in man, *Br J Nutr* **71**(5), 675-85 (1994)

A study showed that both **oat bran**, a native source of *beta*-glucan and **oat gum** (isolated *beta*-glucan), when incorporated into a meal, act similarly by lowering postprandial plasma glucose and insulin levels. A diet rich in *beta*-glucan may, therefore, be of benefit in the regulation of postprandial plasma glucose levels in subjects with Type 2 diabetes.

Braaten JT, FW Scott, PJ Wood, KD Riedel, MS Wolynetz, D Brule, MW Collins, High *beta*-glucan oat bran and oat gum reduce postprandial blood glucose and insulin in subjects with and without type 2 diabetes, *Diabet Med* **11**(3), 312-18 (1994)

Oat gum is composed mainly of the polysaccharide (1→3) (1→4)-*beta*-D-glucan, which is highly viscous in aqueous solution. The effect of viscosity on plasma glucose and insulin levels of healthy humans consuming 50 g glucose was studied. Increasing the dose of oat gum successively reduced the plasma glucose and insulin responses relative to a control without gum. The changes in plasma glucose and insulin are attributable to viscosity, and that changes occur at relatively low doses and viscosities.

Wood PJ, JT Braaten, FW Scott, KD Riedel, MS Wolynetz, MW Collins; Effect of dose and modification of viscous properties of oat gum on plasma glucose and insulin following an oral glucose load, *Br J Nutr* **72**(5), 731-43 (1994)

A study on healthy middle-aged volunteers revealed that low doses of **psyllium** and **citrus pectin** at breakfast and lunch have no effects on the postprandial plasma measurements (plasma glucose, insulin:glucose ratio, total-, LDL- and HDL-cholesterol, and triacylglycerol). Sugar-beet fibre, taken daily for 3 weeks, was found to affect both fasting and postprandial plasma metabolites favourably in these individuals.

Frape DL, AM Jones; Chronic and postprandial responses of plasma insulin, glucose and lipids in volunteers given dietary fibre supplements, *Br J Nutr* **73**(5), 733-51 (1995)

Oat bran contains an unusually high amount of a viscous polysaccharide, called *beta*-glucan. The glycaemic response with increasing amounts of *beta*-glucan present in an extruded breakfast cereal was compared with that of a continental breakfast (bread, milk, cheese, ham). A study with eight NIDDM subjects revealed a linear inverse relationship between the amount of *beta*-glucan and plasma glucose peak or area under the glucose curve. A 50% decrease in glycemic response was observed after the ingestion of 35 g carbohydrate containing approximately 5 g *beta*-glucan. Postprandial insulin increase was, however, as high as the continental breakfast irrespective of the levels of *beta*-glucan.

Tappy L, E Gugolz, P Wursch; Effects of breakfast cereals containing various amounts of *beta*-glucan fibres on plasma glucose and insulin responses in NIDDM subjects, *Diabetes Care* **19**(8), 831-34 (1996)

The low cost, high-protein and high-fibre pasta products processed exclusively from whole durum meal, and that supplemented with 12% defatted soy flour with or without methionine (0.3%) were evaluated in comparison with the regular pasta made of pure durum semolina. The products were administered to alloxan-induced diabetic hypercholesterolemic albino rats to study their effects on the levels of blood glucose and plasma lipid fractions. It was observed that administration of high-protein and high-fibre pasta samples made of whole durum meal, supplemented with defatted soy flour with or without methionine significantly reduced the elevated blood glucose as well as plasma cholesterol and plasma lipid fractions in hypercholesterolaemic diabetic rats. Considering nutritional values, protein cost as well as hypoglycaemic and hypocholesterolaemic effects, the pasta composed of whole durum meal supplemented with 12% defatted soy fibre and 0.3% methionine represented the best high-fibre; high-protein and high-quality product.

Taha SA, MM Wasif; Hypoglycaemic effect and protein nutritive quality of soy and methionine-supplemented whole durum pasta products, *Nahrung* **40**(5), 281-87 (1996)

High fibre diet has been shown to up-regulate proglucagon mRNA and secretion of glucagon-like peptide-1 and insulin compared with an elemental fibre-free diet. In order to ascertain whether physiochemical and fermentative properties of the fibre alter the expression of intestinal hormones and intestinal absorptive properties, experiments were carried out on Sprague-Dawley rats, which were fed either a 50 g/kg cellulose or rhubarb fibre diet for 14 days. Ileal proglucagon mRNA levels were found to be significantly higher in rats, fed rhubarb fibre than in those fed cellulose fibre. It was observed that replacement of cellulose fibre with rhubarb fibre in a diet up-regulated ileal proglucagon mRNA and resulted in a reduced passive permeability but did not affect glucose transport of the small intestine. This work established the importance of dietary fibre fermentability in modulating intestinal proglucagon expression and possibly glucose homeostasis.

Reimer RA, AB Thomson, RV Rajotte, TK Basu, B Ooraikul, ML McBurney; A physiological level of rhubarb fibre increases proglucagon gene expression and modulates intestinal glucose uptake in rats, *J Nutr* **127**(10), 1923-28 (1997)

Diabetic individuals can benefit from diets that are high in ***beta*-glucan**, which, as a component of oats and barley, can be incorporated into breakfast cereals and other products.

Wursch P, FX Sunyer; The role of viscous soluble fibre in the metabolic control of diabetes: A review with special emphasis on cereals rich in *beta*-glucan, *Diabetes Care* **20**(11), 1774-80 (1997)

The root mucilage of *Glossostemon bruguieri* (Moghat) showed remarkable hypoglycaemic activity, decreasing the blood glucose level in diabetic rats by 54.5% within 15 days. Moghat roots deserve further investigation as a potential medicinal and nutritive food.

Ibrahim N, W el-Eraky, S el-Gengaihi, AS Shalaby; Chemical and biological evaluation of proteins and mucilages from roots and seeds of *Glossostemon bruguieri* Desf. (Moghat), *Plant Foods Hum Nutr* **50**(1), 55-61 (1997)

The effects of sugar beet fibre in formula diet on blood glucose, serum insulin and serum hydroxyproline were studied in humans. Formula diet with sugar beet fibre reduced the postprandial blood glucose response, serum insulin response and serum hydroxyproline response compared with the same without fibre. Sugar beet fibre was shown to be capable of diminishing the glycemic responses in the relatively small amount used.

Thorsdottir I, H Andersson, S Einarsdon; Sugar beet fibre in formula diet reduces postprandial blood glucose, serum insulin and serum hydroxyproline, *Eur J Clin Nutr* **52**(2), 155-56 (1998)

The effect of neutral detergent fibre from **cocoanut kernel** (*Cocos nucifera* L) on the concentration of blood glucose, serum insulin and excretion of minerals was studied in rats. Increase in the intake of fibre resulted in significant decrease in the level of blood glucose and serum insulin. Faecal excretion of Cu, Cr, Mn, Mg, Zn and Ca was found to increase in rats fed different levels of cocoanut fibre when compared to fibre-free group. The result of the investigation suggests that inclusion of cocoanut fibre in the diet results in significant hypoglycaemic action.

Sindurani JA, T Rajamohan; Effects of different levels of coconut fibre on blood glucose, serum insulin and minerals in rats, *Indian J Physiol Pharmacol* **44**(1), 97-100 (2000)

Insoluble fibre-rich fractions, isolated from the **peel of *Citrus sinensis*** cv. *Liucheng*, were found to effectively adsorb glucose, retard glucose diffusion, and inhibit the activity of *alpha*-amylase to different extents. These properties of insoluble fibre-rich fractions of *C. sinensis* might create a concerted benefit in decreasing the rate of glucose absorption and eventually lower the concentration of postprandial serum glucose.

Chau CF, YL Huang, MH Lee; *In vitro* hypoglycaemic effects of different insoluble fibre-rich fractions prepared from the peel of *Citrus sinensis* L. cv. *Liucheng, J Agric Food Chem* **51**(22), 6623-26 (2003)

Modification of carbohydrate intake by high-fibre **rye bread** did not alter insulin sensitivity in postmenopausal, hypercholesterolaemic women. High- fibre rye bread appears to enhance insulin secretion, possibly indicating improvement of *beta* cell function.

Juntunen KS, DE Laaksonen, KS Poutanen, LK Niskanen, HM Mykkanen; High-fibre rye bread and insulin secretion and sensitivity in healthy postmenopausal women, *Am J Clin Nutr* **77**(2), 385-91 (2003)

The glycaemic and insulinemic responses to 3 different meals based on **dried peas, potatoes,** or both were compared in patients with type-2 diabetes undergoing dietary treatment. The increases in postprandial plasma glucose and insulin concentrations were delayed and significantly smaller after the pea meal than after the potato meal. The results of the investigation suggest that carbohydrates in dried peas may be largely disregarded in carbohydrate counting and that type-2 diabetic patients should probably increase their consumption of low-glycaemic, high-fibre foods at the expense of high-glycaemic, low fibre foods.

Schafer G, U Schenk, U Ritzel, G Ramadori, U Leonhardt; Comparison of the effects of dried peas with those of potatoes in mixed meals on postprandial glucose and insulin concentrations in patients with type 2 diabetes, *Am J Clin Nutr* **78**(1), 99-103 (2003)

The long-term effects of dietary fibre intake on glucose tolerance and lipid metabolism were studied in type-2 diabetic model GK rats, which were fed either a **barley** (high-dietary fibre) diet, **rice** (low-dietary fibre) diet, or **cornstarch** (very-low-dietary fibre) diet. The intake of barley diet significantly improved the area under the plasma glucose concentration time curves, lowered the fasting plasma glucose and glycosylated haemoglobin levels, and decreased plasma total cholesterol, triglycerides, and free fatty acid levels. The study demonstrated that long-term intake of barley has beneficial effects on glucose tolerance and lipid metabolism.

Li J, T Kaneko, LQ Qin, J Wang, Y Wang, A Sato; Long-term effects of high dietary fibre intake on glucose tolerance and lipid metabolism in GK rats: comparison among barley, rice, and cornstarch, *Metabolism* **52**(9), 1206-10 (2003)

The effect of the administration of 30% neutral detergent fibre diet from black gram (***Phaseolus mungo***) on the metabolism of carbohydrates was studied in rats. The experimental group showed a significant increase in liver glycogen level and a significant decrease in blood glucose. Significant increases in the activities of hexokinase, glycogen phosphorylase, fructose-1, 6-diphosphatase, glucose-6-phosphate dehydrogenase and isocitrate dehydrogenase were observed in the experimental group. The activities of phosphoglucomutase and glucose-6-phosphatase were significantly lower in rats fed the fibre diet. Blackgram fiber was thus found to exhibit significant hypoglycaemic action in experimental animals

Boby RG, S Leelamma; Blackgram fibre (*Phaseolus mungo*): mechanism of hypoglycaemic action, *Plant Foods Hum Nutr* **58**(1), 7-13 (2003)

The role of **rye fibre** in insulin and glucose metabolism was studied using endosperm rye bread, traditional rye bread, and high-fibre rye bread and refined wheat bread as control. Each bread provided 50 g available carbohydrate. Postprandial insulin, glucose-dependent insulinotropic polypeptide, and C-peptide responses to the rye breads were significantly lower than the response to the control and no significant differences in insulin and C-peptide responses to the rye breads were found. *In vitro* starch hydrolysis was slower in all rye breads than in the control. The structure of continuous matrix and starch granules differed between the rye and control breads. From the study it was inferred that structural differences between rye and wheat breads rather than the total fibre content explain the lower postprandial insulin response to rye bread than to wheat bread.

Juntunen KS, DE Laaksonen, K Autio, LK Niskanen, JJ Holst, KE Savolainen, KH Liukkonen, KS Poutanen, HM Mykkanen; Structural differences between rye and wheat breads but not total fibre content may explain the lower postprandial insulin response to rye bread, *Am J Clin Nutr* **78**(5), 957-64 (2003)

Glucomannan, the main polysaccharide of the tubers of the *Amorphophallus konjac*, has an extraordinarily high water-holding capacity and has the highest molecular weight and viscosity of any known dietary fiber. Glucomannan exhibits hypoglycaemic and hypoinsulinaemic activity, which is considered to be due to delayed gastric emptying and slowing down of glucose delivery to the intestinal mucosa.

Gonzalez Canga A, N Fernandez Martinez, AM Sahagun, JJ Gracia Vieitez, MJ Diez-Liebana, AP Calle Pardo, LJ Castro Robles, M Sierra Vega; Glucomannan: properties and therapeutic applications, *Nutr Hosp* **19**(1), 45-50 (2004) [Article in Spanish]

It is generally believed that the so-called Mediterranean diet prevents diet-related degenerative diseases. Recent studies reveal that diets, which are similar to the **Mediterranean diet** (higher amount of fibre and a higher intake of unsaturated fat together with a higher intake of fruits and vegetables), together with exercise and a low body mass index (< 25) protect one from the development of type-2 diabetes.

Biesalski HK; Diabetes preventive components in the Mediterranean diet, *Eur J Nutr* **43**(Suppl 1), 26-30 (2004)

The **high fibre cereal** was found to reduce glucose responses to the same extent in normal and hyperinsulinaemic men, but reduce insulin responses only in hyperinsulinaemic subjects.

Wolever TM, JE Campbell, D Geleva, GH Anderson; High- fibre cereal reduces postprandial insulin responses in hyperinsulinemic but not normoinsulinemic subjects, *Diabetes Care* **27**(6), 1281-85 (2004)

Beta-glucans, isolated from the African grass *Rhynchelytrum repens*, showed hypoglycaemic activity in streptozotocin-induced diabetic rats by reducing blood sugar to normal levels for a period of approximately 24 h. This performance was better than that obtained with pure *beta*-glucan from barley, which decreased blood sugar levels for about 4 h. The activity of *beta*-glucans from *R. repens* is responsible for the use of this plant extract as a hypoglycaemic drug in folk medicine.

De Paula AC, RV Sousa, RC Figueiredo-Ribeiro, MS Buckeridge; Hypoglycaemic activity of polysaccharide fractions containing beta-glucans from extracts of *Rhynchelytrum repens* (Willd.) C.E. Hubb., Poaceae, *Braz J Med Biol Res* **38**(6), 885-93 (2005)

The influence of a short-term dietary intervention with purified insoluble fibre on acute and delayed responses of glucose, insulin, glucose-dependent insulinotropic polypeptide (GIP) and glucagon-like peptide-1was investigated. From the results of the investigation it was proved that consumption of highly purified insoluble dietary fibres accelerated the acute GIP and insulin response.

Weickert MO, M Mohlig, C Koebnick, JJ Holst, P Namsolleck, M Ristow, M Osterhoff, H Rochlitz, N Rudovich, J Spranger, AF Pfeiffer; Impact of cereal fibre on glucose-regulating factors, *Dibetologia* **48**(11), 2343-53 (2005)

Epidemiological observations suggest that intake of cereal fibre is linked to reduced risk of type-2 diabetes. Based on recent findings, the authors hypothesized that intake of purified insoluble oat fibre may improve whole-body insulin sensitivity and this was subjected to test in a randomized, controlled, single-blind, cross-over study with 17 overweight or obese subjects with normal glucose metabolism. The study showed that increased insoluble dietary fibre intake for 3 days significantly improved whole-body insulin sensitivity.

Weickert MO, M Mohlig, C Schofl, AM Arafat, B Otto, H Viehoff, C Koebnick, A Kohl, J Spranger, AF Pfeiffer; Cereal fiber improves whole-body insulin sensitivity in overweight and obese women, *Diabetes Care* **29**(4), 775-80 (2006)

Investigation showed that products prepared from barley flour enriched with *beta*-glucan exhibit favourable responses on glucose metabolism, and particularly on insulinemic responses.

Casiraghi MC, M Garsetti, G Testolin, F Brighenti; Post-prandial responses to cereal products enriched with barley *beta*-glucan, *J Am Coll Nutr* **25**(4), 313-20 (2006)

APPENDIX - 3

FRUITS AND FRUIT PRODUCTS AND THEIR EFFECTS ON BLOOD GLUCOSE RESPONSES

The increase in blood glucose in insulin-dependent diabetics after different fruit meals (apple, banana and orange) was investigated. The effects of fruit loads were compared with those of an equal amount of glucose dissolved in water. The postprandial blood glucose responses to pure glucose, apple and banana were almost identical, but the response after orange was somewhat weaker. It was, therefore, inferred that fructose, present in these fruits, represents an important source of rapidly absorbable carbohydrate and, therefore, fruits should be used only in mixed meals.

Vaaler S, R Wiseth, O Aagenaes; Increase in blood glucose in insulin-dependent diabetics after intake of various fruits, *Acta Med Scand* **212**(5), 281-83 (1982)

The effect of dietetic fruit products (pectin nectar, apricot nectar, apple and strawberry jam), sweetened by sorbitol, on the blood sugar and insulin levels was studied in insulin-dependent diabetic patients and the results were compared with those sweetened by sugar. The study was conducted by using "Biostator", an artificial endocrine pancreas, which was able to supply appropriate amounts of insulin to the patients depending on the degree of glycaemia produced by the products. It was observed that though the blood sugar levels were slightly increased with the dietetic products, the peaks of the blood sugar curves were lower and less insulin was supplied automatically by the biostator during the loading with these products in comparison to the products, sweetened by sugar.

Todorova S, N Veleva, I Arnaudov, T Taneva, D Andreev; Effect of dietetic fruit products prepared with sorbitol and pectin on the blood sugar and insulin levels in diabetic patients, *Vutr Boles* **21**(5), 88-96 (1982) [Article in Bulgarian]

Postprandial hyperglycaemia was studied after ingestion of peeled and non-peeled fruits (pears) in type-2 diabetics. No significant differences were noted in terms of mean blood glucose, serum insulin and serum triglyceride levels between fruits with or without peels. Peeled and non-peeled fruits appear to produce the same hyperglycaemia in type-2 diabetics, in spite of the high fibre content of the peel.

Katsilambros N, P Philippides, J Boletis, K Mavroudis, D Frangaki, M Marangos, GK Daikos; Postprandial hyperglycemia after ingestion of peeled and non-peeled fruits in type-2 diabetics, *J Endocrinol Invest* **8**(3), 189-91 (1985)

The serum insulin and plasma glucose responses to milk and fruit products were studied in non-insulin-dependent type-2 diabetic patients. The responses following the ingestion of foods containing sucrose, glucose, fructose or lactose in portions that contained 50 g of carbohydrate were compared with those obtained following the ingestion of pure fructose, sucrose, glucose + fructose and lactose. The results showed that the glucose response was essentially the same whether the carbohydrate was given as a pure substance, or in the form of a naturally occurring food. Thus the plasma glucose response to ingestion of fruits and milk products can be predicted from the constituent carbohydrate present. However, this was not true with serum insulin response.

Gannon MC, FQ Nuttall, PA Krezowski, CJ Billington, S Parker; The serum insulin and plasma glucose responses to milk and fruit products in type 2 (non-insulin-dependent) diabetic patients, *Diabetologia* **29**(11), 784-91 (1986)

Postprandial glucose and insulin responses to various tropical fruits (pineapple, mango, banana, durian and rambutan) of equivalent carbohydrate content were determined in non-insulin-dependent diabetic subjects. The results showed that the glucose-response curves to mango and banana were significantly less than those to rambutan, durian and pineapple. The insulin response curve and insulin area after ingestion of durian was statistically greater than that seen after ingestion of other fruits.

Roongpisuthipong C, S Banphotkasem, S Komindr, V Tanphaichitr; Postprandial glucose and insulin responses to various tropical fruits of equivalent carbohydrate content in non-insulin-dependent diabetes mellitus, *Diabetes Res Clin Pract* **14**(2), 123-31 (1991)

Glycaemic responses to orange and apple were compared with that of white bread in non-insulin-dependent diabetic subjects and it was found that the fruits had lower glycaemic indices in comparison to white bread. The low glycaemic response to orange and apple might be ascribed to the high content of fructose which is rapidly cleared and metabolised by the liver, without elevating the blood glucose.

Gregersen S, O Rasmussen, S Larsen, K Hermansen; Glycaemic and insulinaemic responses to orange and apple compared with white bread in non-insulin-dependent diabetic subjects, *Eur J Clin Nutr* **46**(4), 301-03 (1992)

In order to study the effect of ripening of banana on the postprandial blood glucose and insulin responses, three meals, consisting of 120 g under-ripe banana, 120 g over-ripe banana or 40 g white bread were fed to ten non-insulin dependent type-2 diabetic patients on separate days. The mean postprandial blood glucose response area to white bread was found to be significantly higher than under-ripe and over-ripe banana. Glycaemic indices of the under-ripe and over-ripe bananas also differed. The mean insulin response areas to the three meals were similar. The low glycaemic response of under-ripe bananas in comparison to over-ripe bananas may be ascribed to the high content of starch, which is hydrolysed only slowly by *alpha*-amylase in humans (1). Ercan and co-workers, however, demonstrated that glucose, insulin, C-peptide, and glucagon area responses varied little with ripeness of the bananas (2).

1. Hermansen K, O Rasmussen, S Gregersen, S Larsen; Influence of ripeness of banana on the blood glucose and insulin response in type 2 diabetic subjects, *Diabet Med* **9**(8), 739-43 (1992)
2. Ercan N, FQ Nuttall, MC Gannon, JT Lane, LA Burmeister, SA Westphal; Plasma glucose and insulin responses to bananas of varying ripeness in persons with noninsulin-dependent diabetes mellitus, *J Am Coll Nutr* **12**(6), 703-09 (1993)

The glycaemic indices (GI), peak incremental indices (PI) and time of peak increment (TPI) of eight different fruits were determined. Glycaemic indices of these fruits were positively correlated with total free glucose and negatively with fructose, both free and total (free + that as part of sucrose), present in the fruits. No important differences in glycaemic responses to common fruits were observed in type 2 diabetic patients,

Lunetta M, M Di Mauro, S Crimi, L Mughini; No important differences in glycaemic responses to common fruits in type 2 diabetic patients, *Diabet Med* **12**(8), 674-68 (1995)

Effects of oral administration of concentrated juice of plum (ekisu) on lipid and glucose tolerance were assessed in insulin-resistant obese Wistar fatty rats. It was found to decrease blood glucose and plasma triglyceride concentrations compared with controls. Treatment with plum for 2 weeks reduced areas under the curve (AUCs) for glucose and insulin during a glucose tolerance test. In db/db mice, plum decreased these AUCs, and also blood glucose during an insulin tolerance test. Results suggest that plum probably increases insulin sensitivity in these rats *via* adiponectin-related mechanisms.

Utsunomiya H, T Yamakawa, J Kamei, K Kadonosono, S Tanaka; Anti-hyperglycaemic effects of plum in a rat model of obesity and type 2 diabetes, Wistar fatty rat, *Biomed Res* **26**(5), 193-200 (2005)

APPENDIX - 4

HYPOGLYCAEMIC GLYCANS

[Glycans are relatively complex carbohydrates having a general formula of $C_n(H_2O)_{n-1}$ where n is usually a large number between 200 and 2500. Glycans can be homo or hetero-polymers of monosaccharide residues, and can be linear or branched. Glycans usually consist solely of O-glycosidic linkages of monosaccharides. A heteroglycan is composed of more than one monomer type. Glucans (or *beta*-glucans), which are polysaccharides of D-glucose monomers linked by glycosidic bonds, have been discussed under dietary fibres, as these are found in the bran of cereal grains.]

Hikino and co-workers isolated numerous glycans from a variety of plants and studied their hypoglycaemic activity. These glycans include aconitans A, B, C and D, from *Aconitum carmichaeli* (6), anemarans A, B, C and D from *Anemarrhena asphodeloides* (3), arborans A and B from *Aloe arborescens* var. *natalensis* leaves (16), atractans A, B and C from *Atractylodes japonica* (4), coixans A, B and C from *Coix lachryma-jobi* var. *ma-yuen* seeds (14), dioscorans A, B, C, D, E and F from *Dioscorea japonica* (15) ephedrans A, B, C, D and E from *Ephedra distachya* (7), eleutherans A, B, C, D, E, F, and G from *Eleutherococcus senticosus* (13), lithospermans A, B and C from *Lithospermum erythrorhizon* (5), oryzarans A, B, C, and D from *Oryza sativa* roots (17), oryzabrans A, B, C and D from *Oryza sativa* bran (20), panaxans A, B, C, D, E, F, G, H, I, J, K, L, M, N, O, P, Q, R, S, T and U from *Panax ginseng* (1, 9, 10, 12, 18), quinquefolans A, B, and C from *Panax quinquefolium* (19), saccharans A, B, C, D, E, and F from *Saccharum officinarum* (8), and trichosans A, B, C, D, and E from *Trichosanthes kirilowii* (22).

Most of these glycans, isolated by bioactivity-guided fractionation of aqueous or aqueous methanol extracts of the plant materials, showed significant hypoglycaemic activity in normal and alloxan-induced hyperglycaemic mice. Structural information about panaxan A and panaxan B were also secured (2, 11). The mechanisms of hypoglycaemic activity of aconitan A, a glycan from *Aconitum carmichaeli* roots, were studied (21).

Hypoglycaemic actions of some heteroglycans of *Ganoderma lucidum* fruit bodies were also studied (23).

MVS-I, the major neutral polysaccharide obtained from the seeds of *Malva verticillata*, is mainly composed of *beta*-1,3-linked D-glucan and of *alpha*-1,5-linked L-arabino-*beta*-3,6-branched D-galactan. MVS-1 showed remarkable hypoglycaemic activity (24).

3. Konno C, K Sugiyama, M Kano, M Takahashi, H Hikino; Isolation and hypoglycaemic activity of panaxans A, B, C, D and E, glycans of *Panax ginseng* roots, *Planta Med* **50**(5), 434-36 (1984)

4. Tomoda M, K Shimada, C Konno, K Sugiyama, H Hikino; Partial structure of panaxan A, a hypoglycaemic glycan of *Panax ginseng* roots, *Planta Med* **50**(5), 436-38 (1984)

5. Takahashi M, C Konno; H Hikino; Isolation and hypoglycaemic activity of anemarans A, B, C and D, glycans of *Anemarrhena asphodeloides* rhizomes, *Planta Med* (2), 100-02 (1985)

6. Konno C, Y Suzuki, K Oishi, E Munakata, H Hikino; Isolation and hypoglycemic activity of atractans A, B and C, glycans of *Atractylodes japonica* rhizomes, *Planta Med* (2), 102-03 (1985)

7. Konno C, T Mizuno, H Hikino; Isolation and hypoglycaemic activity of lithospermans A, B and C, glycans of *Lithospermum erythrorhizon* roots, *Planta Med* (2), 157-58 (1985)

8. Konno C, M Murayama, K Sugiyama, M Arai, M Murakami, M Takahashi, H Hikino; Isolation and hypoglycaemic activity of aconitans A, B, C and D, glycans of *Aconitum carmichaeli* roots, *Planta Med* (2), 160-61 (1985)

9. Konno C, T Mizuno, H Hikino; Isolation and hypoglycaemic activity of ephedrans A, B, C, D and E, glycans of *Ephedra distachya* herbs, *Planta Med* (2), 162-63 (1985)

10. Takahashi M, C Konno, H Hikino; Isolation and hypoglycaemic activity of saccharans A, B, C, D, E, and F, glycans of *Saccharum officinarum* stalks, *Planta Med* (3), 258-60 (1985)

11. Hikino H, Y Oshima, Y Suzuki, C Konno; Isolation and hypoglycaemic activity of Panaxans F, G, and H, glycans of *Panax ginseng* roots, *Shoyakugaku Zasshi* **39**(4), 331-33 (1985)

12. Konno C, M Murakami, Y Oshima, H Hikino; Isolation and hypoglycemic activity of panaxans Q, R, S, T and U, glycans of *Panax ginseng* roots, *J Ethnopharmacol* **14**(1), 69-74 (1985)

13. Tomoda M , K Shimado, C Konno, H Hikino; Structure of panaxan B, a hypoglycaemic glycan of *Panax ginseng* roots, *Phytochemistry* 24(10), 2431-33 (1985)

14. Oshima Y, C Konno, H Hikino; Isolation and hypoglycaemic activity of panaxans I, J, K and L, glycans of *Panax ginseng* roots, *J Ethnopharmacol* **14**(2-3), 255-59 (1985)

15. Hikino H, M Takahashi, K Otake, C Konno; Isolation and hypoglycaemic activity of eleutherans A, B, C, D, E, F, and G: glycans of *Eleutherococcus senticosus* roots, *J Nat Prod* **49**(2), 293-97 (1986)

16. Konno C, H Hikino; Isolation and hypoglycaemic activity of coixans A, B and C, glycans of *Coix lachryma*-jobi var. *ma-yuen* seeds, *Planta Med* Feb(1), 64-65 (1986)

17. Hikino H, C Konno, M Takahashi, M Murakami, Y Kato, M Karikura, T Hayashi; Isolation and hypoglycaemic activity of dioscoransA, B, C, D, E and F; glycans of *Dioscorea japonica* rhizophora, *Planta Med* No. 3, 168-71 (1986)

18. Hikino H, M Takahashi, M Murakami, C Konno, Y Mirin, M Karikura; Isolation and hypoglycaemic activity of arborans A and B, glycans of *Aloe arborescens* var. *natalensis* leaves, *Int J Crude Drug Res* **24**(4), 183-186 (1986)

19. Hikino H, M Murakami, Y Oshima, C Konno; Isolation and hypoglycaemic activity of oryzarans A, B, C, and D: glycans of *Oryza sativa* roots, *Planta Med* (6), 490-92 (1986)

20. Konno C, H Hikino, Isolation and hypoglycemic activity of panaxans M , N , O and P glycans of *Panax ginseng* roots, *Int J Crude Drug Res* **25**(1), 53-56 (1987)

21. Oshima Y, K Sato, H Hikino; Isolation and hypoglycaemic activity of quinquefolans A, B, and C, glycans of *Panax quinquefolium* roots, J Nat Prod **50**(2), 188-90 (1987)

22. Hikino H, M Takahashi, Y Oshima, C Konno; Isolation and hypoglycaemic activity of oryzabrans A, B, C and D, glycans of *Oryza sativa* bran, *Planta Med* **54**(1), 1-3 (1988)

23. Hikino H, M Kobayashi, Y Suzuki, C Konno; Mechanisms of hypoglycaemic activity of aconitan A, a glycan from *Aconitum carmichaeli* roots, *J Ethnopharmacol* **25**(3), 295-304 (1989)

24. Hikino H, M Yoshizawa, Y Suzuki, Y Oshima, C Konno; Isolation and hypoglycaemic activity of trichosans A, B, C, D, and E: glycans of *Trichosanthes kirilowii* roots, *Planta Med* **55**(4), 349-50 (1989)

25. Hikino H, T Mizuno; Hypoglycaemic actions of some heteroglycans of *Ganoderma lucidum* fruit bodies, *Planta Med* **55**(4), 385 (1989)

26. Tomoda M, N Shimizu, R Gonda, M Kanari, H Yamada, H Hikino; Anti-complementary and hypoglycaemic activities of the glycans from the seeds of *Malva verticillata*, *Planta Med* **56**(2), 168-70 (1990)

APPENDIX - 5

HYPOGLYCAEMIC PLANT LECTINS

[Lectins are sugar-binding proteins which are highly specific for their sugar moieties. They typically play a role in biological recognition phenomena involving cells and proteins. Lectins are glycoproteins that are known for their ability to clump (agglutinate) erythrocytes *in vitro*. The terms phytohaemagglutinins, phytagglutinins, and lectins are used interchangeably. Lectin-containing plants are common in the most types of beans, including soybeans. Lectins' interaction with certain carbohydrates is very specific. Lectins may bind with free sugar or with sugar residues of polysaccharides, glycoproteins, or glycolipids. Different lectins have different levels of toxicity, though not all lectins are toxic.]

Wheat germ agglutinin produces several alterations in the ability of fat cells to bind and respond to insulin. It markedly stimulates glucose oxidation but causes only a modest stimulation of glucose transport. At a concentration of 0.25-20 µg/ml, this lectin increased the binding of insulin by adipocytes, apparently by increasing the binding affinity of the insulin receptor. At lower concentrations (0.25-2.5 µg/ml), the elevation in binding was accompanied by an increase in the sensitivity of the adipocytes to insulin stimulation of glucose transport. At higher concentrations, this lectin appeared to act at another site(s) to inhibit the activation of the transport system by insulin (1). Treatment of rat adipocytes with wheat germ agglutinin was found to markedly enhance insulin binding by increasing the affinity of the insulin receptor. The increase in receptor affinity produced by wheat germ agglutinin treatment was not caused by the formation of receptor clusters. Instead, it appears that a simple interaction between the plant lectin and the receptor is sufficient to induce the changes in the insulin binding properties of adipocytes (2).

1. Livingston JN, BJ Purvis; Effects of wheat germ agglutinin on insulin binding and insulin sensitivity of fat cells, *Am J Physiol* **238**(3), E267-75 (1980)
2. Livingston JN, BJ Purvis; The effects of wheat germ agglutinin on the adipocyte insulin receptor, *Biochim Biophys Acta* **678**(2), 194-201 (1981)

The plant lectin concanavalin A shows a striking resemblance with a portion of insulin in peptide sequence as well as in three-dimensional conformational homology. This amino acid sequence has been demonstrated to be essential for the bioactivity of insulin. The insulinomimetic activity of concanavalin A and its structural and conformational resemblance with insulin offer insight into the mechanism of insulin action (1). Insulin directly inhibits protein phosphorylation in isolated rat liver nuclear envelopes. Concanavalin A and agents that mimic insulin also directly regulate nuclear functions (2).

1. Franzusoff AJ; Insulinomimetic homology of concanavalin A, *Med Hypotheses* **10**(3), 223-28 (1983)

2. Purrello F, DB Burnham, ID Goldfine; Insulin receptor antiserum and plant lectins mimic the direct effects of insulin on nuclear envelope phosphorylation, *Science* **221**(4609), 462-64 (1983)

Rats fed a diet containing kidney bean (*Phaseolus vulgaris*) showed a decline in the level of circulating insulin and caused an increase in the level of mRNAs for the insulin receptor and GLUT-4 in the gastrocnemius muscle. Since the kidney bean-fed rats are euglycaemic the results suggest that insulin receptor and GLUT-4 mRNA levels are regulated in response to circulating insulin concentrations rather than glucose. In the soleus muscle of rats fed the diet containing kidney bean; however a decline was observed in the level of GLUT-4 mRNA. It has been proposed that a component of kidney beans, most likely the lectin phytohaemagglutinin, has systemic effects which lead to changes in expression of the insulin receptor and GLUT-4 genes and to the sensitivity of muscle to insulin (1).

The effects of inclusion of raw kidney bean (*Phaseolus vulgaris*) in a high-quality control diet were tested in nutritional trials on the growth and metabolism of obese Zucker (fafa) rats and their lean littermates. The growth of both obese and lean rats on bean diets was retarded by the daily bean intake in a dose-dependent manner and the weight reduction of these rats could be accounted for exclusively by reduced lipid content. Plasma insulin levels were significantly depressed in the obese Zucker rats on bean diets but the pancreas was not significantly enlarged nor its insulin content changed in 10 d trials. The results suggest the use the bean lectin as a dietary adjunct or therapeutic agent to stimulate gut function and ameliorate obesity (2).

1. Knott RM, G Grant, S Bardocz, A Pusztai, AF de Carvalho, JE Hesketh; Alterations in the level of insulin receptor and GLUT-4 mRNA in skeletal muscle from rats fed a kidney bean (*Phaseolus vulgaris*) diet, *Int J Biochem* **24**(6), 897-902 (1992)
2. Pusztai A, G Grant, WC Buchan, S Bardocz, AF de Carvalho, SW Ewen; Lipid accumulation in obese Zucker rats is reduced by inclusion of raw kidney bean (*Phaseolus vulgaris*) in the diet, *Br J Nutr* **79**(2), 213-21 (1998)

Intra-peritoneal administration of lectin (100 mg/kg), isolated from *Urtica pilulifera* seeds, to streptozotocin-induced diabetic rats for 30 days significantly reduced their blood sugar levels. The changes in food and water intake, body weight and histological changes in normal and treated diabetic rats were also evaluated. The observations were compared with that of Glipizide, an oral anti-diabetic agent.

Kavalali G, H Tuncel, S Goksel, HH Hatemi; Hypoglycaemic activity of *Urtica pilulifera* in streptozotocin-diabetic rats, *J Ethnopharmacol* **84**(2-3), 241-45 (2003)

Tomato lectin phosphatidylethanolamine conjugate was synthesized and the compound was incorporated into the conventional liposomes of insulin. The blood glucose levels of the normal and diabetic mice were reduced by modified liposomes. Tomato lectin-modified liposomes were found to promote the oral absorption of insulin due to the specific-site combination on GI cell membrane.

Zhang N, QN Ping, WF Xu; The enhancing effect of tomato lectin modified liposomes of insulin on oral absorption in mice, *Yao Xue Xue Bao* **39**(5), 380-84 (2004) [Article in Chinese]

APPENDIX - 6

HYPOGLYCAEMIC PLANTS TRADITIONALLY USED IN DIFFERENT PARTS OF THE WORLD

[Tradtional medicines of a country largely depend on the plants grown in that region and, therefore, plants endemic to a certain region are generally used in that country. The plants used in different countries for the treatment of diabetes are reported in this section. Many of these plants have, however, been included in the main section of the book.]

AFRICA

Oral hypoglycaemic plants in West Africa have been grouped by Bever according to their main active components. Plants having constituents same or similar to those with known hypoglycaemic activity but reported from plants growing elsewhere in the world have also been grouped. However, the action of many of the constituents of African plants is still to be confirmed pharmacologically.

Bever BO; Oral hypoglycaemic plants in West Africa, *J Ethnopharmacol* **2**(2), 119-27 (1980)

The effects of two vegetable flours, prepared from the African plants *Detarium senegalense* and *Cissus rotundifolia*, on postprandial blood glucose and insulin concentrations in human subjects, were investigated. These flours contained significant amounts of non-starch polysaccharides (NSP) and *D. senegalense* was particularly rich in water-soluble NSP. Compared with the controls, *Detarium* and *Cissus* meals elicited significant reductions in plasma glucose levels at most postprandial time points. Significant reductions in plasma insulin levels at various postprandial time points were also seen after *Detarium* and *Cissus* breads. The main water-soluble non-starch polysaccharide fraction of *Detarium*, identified as a high-molecular-weight xyloglucan, is likely to be a primary factor in determining the physiological activity of *Detarium* flour.

Onyechi UA, PA Judd, PR Ellis; African plant foods rich in non-starch polysaccharides reduce postprandial blood glucose and insulin concentrations in healthy human subjects, *Br J Nutr* **80**(5), 419-28 (1998)

BANGLADESH

Rhizomes of *Costus speciosus*, tubers of *Nephrolepsis tuberosa*, and bulbs of *Stephania hernandifolia* are used by the local people and traditional healers in the Eastern Himalayan belt. The effects of these crude drugs on serum glucose levels were studied in non-diabetic and diabetic rat models at different prandial states. Administration of freeze-dried juices of *C. speciosus* and *N. tuberosa* simultaneously with glucose in non-diabetic rats showed no significant effect in the fasting or postprandial state. However, when fed 30 min before the glucose load both *C. speciosus* and *N. tuberosa* showed hypoglycaemic effect. Unlike these two drugs, *S. hernandifolia* increased the serum glucose levels of non-diabetic rats in all the series of experiments. In NIDDM model rats, *N. tuberosa* juice opposed the rise in serum glucose level when fed 30 min before the glucose load. In IDDM model rats, none of these three freeze-dried juices showed any effect in the fasting state.

Mosihuzzaman M, N Nahar, L Ali, B Rokeya, AK Khan, M Nur-E-Alam, RP Nandi; Hypoglycaemic effects of three plants from eastern Himalayan belt, *Diabetes Res* **26**(3), 127-38 (1994)

The plants *Pterospermum acerifolium* , *Eupatorium odoratum, Cassia tamala, Curcuma zedoria* and *Cassia sophera* from Bangladesh have been screened for their hypoglycaemic activity.

Rokeya B; Plant materials as a source of potential anti-diabetic agents in Diabetes mellitus Epidemic: combat the challenge, "Proceedings of the 4th International seminar on Asian Network of Research on Anti-diabetic plants (ANRAP), Kolkata, India, January 16-18, 2004

BRAZIL

An ethnopharmocological survey, conducted in Port Alegre, Brazil, revealed that majority of people use "jambolao", botanically identified as *Syzygium cumini,* for the treatment of diabetes. For this purpose, they use dry leaves of *S. cumini* (2.5 g/l) in the form of tea.

Coimbera Teixeira C, Danni Fuchi F, Blotta RM, A Pereira Da Costa, D Guedes Mussnich, G Gral Ranquetat; Plants employed in the treatment of diabetes mellitus: Results of an ethnopharmacological survey in Porto Alegra, Brazil,, *Fitoterapia* **63**(4), 320-22 (1992)

Intra-gastric administration of the extracts of Brazilian medicinal plants (*Epidendrum monsenii, Marrubium vulgare, Rubus imperialis* and *Wedelia paludosa*) significantly lowered the blood glucose level of diabetic rats. It has been suggested that these plants can be used as adjuvant agents in the treatment of diabetes mellitus.

Novaes AP, C Rossi, C Poffo, E Pretti Junior, AE Oliveira, V Schlemper, R Niero, V Cechinel-Filho, C Burger; Preliminary evaluation of the hypoglycaemic effect of some Brazilian medicinal plants, *Therapie* **56**(4), 427-30 (2001)

A single oral administration of Brazilian propolis (a resinous mixture, that honey bees collect from tree buds and other botanical sources to construct their hives) extract demonstrated a potent anti-hyperglycaemic effect in Sprague-Dawley rats. 3,4,5-Tri-caffeoylquinic acid that shows a strong maltase-specific inhibition, was recognized to be a prominent candidate of the extract that exerts the effect.

Matsui T, S Ebuchi, T Fujise, KJ Abesundara, S Doi, H Yamada, K Matsumoto;

Strong anti-hyperglycaemic effects of water-soluble fraction of Brazilian propolis and its bioactive constituent, 3,4,5-tri-O-caffeoylquinic acid, *Biol Pharm Bull* **27**(11), 1797-803 (2004)

Trace elements in eight hypoglycaemiant plants (*Trigonella foenum graecum, Panax ginseng, Pfaffia paniculata, Myrcia speciosa, Zea mays, Harpagophytum procumbens, Syzygium jambolona*, and *Bauhinia forficata*) were dertermined by synchrotron radiation total reflection X-ray fluorescence spectrometry. The elements P, K, Ca, Ti, Mn, Fe, Cu, Zn, Rb, and Sr were detected in all these medicinal plants.

Zucchi OL, S Moreira, EF de Jesus, HS Neto, MJ Salvador;, Characterization of hypoglycaemic plants by total reflection X-ray fluorescence spectrometry, *Biol Trace Elem Res* **103**(3), 277-90 (2005)

Crude acetone extracts of Brazilian seaweeds, *Spatoglossum schroederi* and *Caulerpa racemosa* were found to inhibit *alpha*-amylase activity.

Teixeira VL, FD Rocha, PJ Houghton, MA Kaplan, RC Pereira; *Alpha*-amylase inhibitors from Brazilian seaweeds and their hypoglycemic potential, *Fitoterapia* **78**(1), 35-36 (2007)

BULGARIA

The antioxidant activity of extracts from 23 Bulgarian medicinal plants was studied. The polyphenol contents of these plants were measured and compared with those of mate (*Ilex paraguariensis*), black tea (*Camellia sinensis*), honey bush (*Cyclopia* spp.), and rooibos (*Aspalathus linearis*), all of which are of foreign origin and used as herbal tea. The antioxidant activity was measured by the ABTS cation radical discoloration assay, and the total polyphenol content was assayed according to the Folin-Ciocalteu method. Five Bulgarian plant extracts, which exhibited antioxidant activity higher than that of mate are *Alchemilla vulgaris, Sambucus ebulus, Mentha spicata, Fragaria vesca* and *Crataegus monogyna.* The antioxidant activity of more than half of the herbal extracts of Bulgarian medicinal plants was higher than or comparable to the reference foreign plants.

Kiselova Y, D Ivanova, T Chervenkov, D Gerova, B Galunska, T Yankova; Correlation between the *in vitro* antioxidant activity and polyphenol content of aqueous extracts from Bulgarian herbs, *Phytother Res* **20**(11), 961-65 (2006)

CHILE

The hypoglycaemic activity of four plants, (*Bauhinia candicans, Galega officinalis, Morus alba*, and *Rubus ulmifolius*), that are used for the treatment of diabetes in Chilean popular medicine, was evaluated in alloxan and streptozotocin-induced hyperglycaemic rats. In normal rats, 20% dried leaf infusion of the drugs did not modify significantly the glycaemia in the period studied, but in diabetic rats, different results were observed, depending on the drug used. *B. candicans* presented a greater decrease of glycaemia in alloxan diabetic rats and *R. ulmifolius* showed a similar activity in both alloxan and streptozotocin diabetic rats. Petroleum ether extract elicited a marked hypoglycaemic effect in streptozotocin-induced model.

Lemus I, R Garcia, E Delvillar, G Knop; Hypoglycaemic activity of four plants used in Chilean popular medicine, *Phytother Res* **13**(2), 91-94 (1999)

CHINA

The effects of yinchenhao decoction on the blood glucose level were studied in a variety of animal models. The decoction inhibited hyperglycaemia of alloxan-induced mice, significantly reduced the level of fasting blood glucose in normal mice, alloxan-induced diabetic mice and rats. It also improved impaired glucose tolerance in dexamethasone-induced insulin-resistant rats. The results suggested that hypoglycaemic action of yinchenhao decoction was comparable to that of metformin and gliclazide.

Pan J, C Han, H Liu, J Du, A Li; Effects of yinchenhao decoction on normal animals and animal models of diabetes mellitus, *Zhong Yao Cai* **24** (2), 128-31 (2001) [Article in Chinese]

Touchi, a traditional Chinese food, is derived by fermentation of soybean. A water-soluble extract of Touchi was found to exert a strong inhibitory activity against rat intestinal *alpha*-glucosidase. The effect of administration of sucrose (2 g/kg) with or without Touchi extract (100 and 500 mg/kg) was studied in normal rats. Postprandial increases in blood glucose levels at 30 and 60 min after the administration of Touchi extract were significantly depressed compared with controls. In human subjects, Touchi extract decreased the glycaemic response dose dependently after sucrose loading and it elicited a significant anti-glycaemic effect at a minimum effective dose of 0.3 g. Touchi extract was found to exhibit *alpha*-glucosidase inhibitory activity, and it might have potential use in the management of patients with non-insulin-dependent diabetes mellitus.

Fujita H, T Yamagami, K Ohshima; Fermented soybean-derived water-soluble Touchi extract inhibits *alpha*-glucosidase and is anti-glycaemic in rats and humans after single oral treatments, *J Nutr* **131**(4), 1211-13 (2001)

Chinese herbal drugs are known to be a major source of medicines for the prevention and treatment of diseases including diabetes mellitus. Over 200 species of plants, including many common plants, are known to exhibit hypoglycaemic properties. The drugs and formulations that have been approved by the Chinese health regulatory agency for commercial use in China were reviewed. Pharmacological and clinical evaluations indicated that these drugs had a mild, but significant, blood glucose lowering effect and long-term use of these agents were considered to be advantageous over chemical drugs in alleviating some of the chronic diseases and complications caused by diabetes. It was further observed that the use of these herbal drugs in conjunction with conventional chemical drugs permitted lowering of doses and frequency of administration of the chemical drugs.

Jia W, W Gao, L Tang; Anti-diabetic herbal drugs officially approved in China, *Phytother Res* **17**(10), 1127-34 (2003)

The compositions and pharmacological effects of eight anti-diabetic herbal drugs that have been approved by health regulatory agency for commercial use in China were reviewed. The hypoglycaemic effect of these products was found to be due to their ability to (i) restore the functions of pancreatic tissues, (ii) increase in insulin output, (iii) inhibit the intestinal absorption of glucose and (iv) facilitate insulin-dependent processes.

Jia W, WY Gao, PG Xiao; Anti-diabetic drugs of plant origin used in China: compositions, pharmacology, and hypoglycaemic mechanisms, *Zhongguo Zhong Yao Za Zhi* **28**(2), 108-13 (2003)

EGYPT

Hypoglycaemic activity of desert plants, collected from different Egyptian localities, was studied. Of the 31 plants that were collected only *Lycium shawii, Salvia aegyptiaca, Pergularia tomentosa, Convolvulus althaeoides, Haloxylon salicornicum, Ephedra alata, Scrophularia deserti,* and *Crotalaria aegyptiaca* showed persistent hypoglycaemic effects. The plants that exhibited transient hypoglycaemic effects 1 h after administration were *Silena succulenta, Lygos raetam, Convolvulus lanatus,* and *Pulicaria incise* and the plants that exhibited this activity 3h after administration were *Ochradenus baccatus* and *Zygophyllum album*. The plants *Thymus capitatus, Launaea nudicaulis, Conyza dioscorides, Nitraria retusa,* and *Limonium tubiflorum* also demonstrated hypoglycaemic activity. The plants that were tested on alloxanised diabetic rats and were found to be superior to Daonil were *Matthiola livida, Salvia aegyptiaca, Astragalus species,* and *Arthrocnemum glaucum*.

Shabana MM, YW Mirhom,AA Genenah, EA Aboutabl, HA Amer; Study into wild Egyptian plants of potential medicinal activity. Ninth communication: hypoglycaemic activity of some selected plants in normal fasting and alloxanised rats, *Arch Exp Veterinarmed* **44**(3), 389-94 (1990)

EUROPE

Of the twelve plants, used for the traditional treatment of diabetes mellitus in northern Europe, *Ilex guayusa,* commonly known as "guayusa", was proved to have potentially useful anti-diabetic agents. The plant retarded the development of hyperglycaemia in streptozotocin-induced diabetes and reduced the hyperphagia, polydipsia, body weight loss, and glycated haemoglobin.

Swanston-Flatt SK, C Day, PR Flatt, BJ Gould, CJ Bailey; Glycaemic effects of traditional European plant treatments for diabetes. Studies in normal and streptozotocin diabetic mice, *Diabetes Res* **10**(2), 69-73 (1989)

INDIA

Folklore uses of 26 anti-diabetic plant species growing in Rayalseema region of Andhra Pradesh have been reported. The method of preparation and dose of administration of crude drugs by tribal and non-tribal herbalists are recorded. The known chemical constituents of the plants have also been reported.

Nagaraju N, KN Rao; Folk medicine for diabetes from Royalseema of Andhra Pradesh, *Ancient Sci Life* **9**(1), 31-35 (1989).

Ocimum sanctum, Aegle marmelos, Azadirachta indica and *Murraya koenigii* decreased the blood sugar of streptozotocin diabetic rabbits. The different solvent extracts of *Aegle marmelos* showed different rate of hypoglycaemic action.

Santhoskumari KS, KS Devi; Hypoglycaemic effect of a few medicinal plants, *Ancient Sci Life* **9**(4), 221-23 (1990)

Out of six plants (*Acacia auriculiformis, Acalypha ciliata, Clematis grata, Deeringia amaranthoides, Engelhardtia colebrookiana, Randia uliginosa*), collected from Garhwal region , extracts of *Acacia auriculiformis* legumes and *Acalypha ciliata* roots exhibited hypoglycaemic activity.

Uniyal SK, S Bahuguna, OP Sati; Biological screening of extracts of some medicinal plants from Garhwal, *Herba Hungarica* **29**(1-2), 37-41 (1990)

Sixty four plants, claimed to possess anti-diabetic activity in folk traditional therapy, have been identified and listed along with form of intake and dosage.

El-Gammal SY; Folk-traditional anti-diabetic herbs, *Bull Indian Inst History Med* **21**(1), 87-90 (1991)

The phytochemical investigation of some herbal drugs, claimed to possess anti-hypertensive and anti-hyperglycaemic activity by the mobile street vendors in Delhi, was carried out and the results discussed.

Sinha RK; Antihypertensive and anti-hyperglycaemic herbal drugs prescribed by mobile street vendors of herbs, *Probe* **12**(2), 135-39 (1993).

Varying degree of hypoglycaemic activity was detected in a large number of herbs examined at the laboratory level or clinically. However, encouraging results were observed with the hypoglycaemic plant drugs, ***Swertia chirayita*** and ***Trichosanthes dioica.***

Muckerjee SK , Scope and use of indigenous herbal drugs in 'Madhumeha', in Indian scenario, *International Seminar On Free Radicals Mediated Diseases and Ayurveda* , Faculty of Ayurveda, IMS, BHU, Varanasi, September 2-4, (A–11) (1996)

Numerous plants are used traditionally for the treatment of diabetes and out of these 45 plants were reviewed by the authors. Again of these plants *Allium cepa, Allium sativum, Aloe vera, Cajanus cajan, Coccinia indica, Caesalpinia bonducella, Ficus bengalenesis, Gymnema sylvestre, Momordica charantia, Ocimum sanctum, Pterocarpus marsupium, Swertia chirayita, Syzigium cumini, Tinospora cordifolia* and *Trigonella foenum graecum* were tested and found to show varying degree of hypoglycaemic and anti-hyperglycemic activity.

Grover JK, S Yadav, V Vats; Medicinal plants of India with anti-diabetic potential, *J Ethnopharmacol* **81**(1), 81-100 (2002)

Terminalia chebula, Terminalia belerica, Emblica officinalis and a combination of all these drugs in equal proportion, known as "Triphala", are used extensively in Indian system of medicine. These were found to inhibit lipid peroxide formation and to scavenge hydroxyl and superoxide radicals *in vitro*. The concentrations of plant extracts that inhibited 50% of lipid peroxidation and scavenged hydroxyl and superoxide radicals varied from drug to drug but were within a small range. Oral administration of methanol extracts (100 mg/kg b.w.) of the drugs reduced the blood sugar level in normal and in alloxan (120 mg/kg) diabetic rats significantly within 4 h. Continued, daily administration of the drug produced a sustained effect.

Sabu MC, R Kuttan; Anti-diabetic activity of medicinal plants and its relationship with their antioxidant property, *J Ethnopharmacol* **81**(2), 155-60 (2002)

The efficacy of four drugs (*Momordica charantia, Eugenia jambolana, Tinospora cordifolia* and *Mucuna pruriens)* was assessed in the prevention of murine alloxan dibetic cataract. Administration of lyophilized aqueous extracts of *Momordica charantia* and *Eugenia jambolana* (200 mg/kg p.o.) every day for four months prevented the development of cataract but the protective effect was less significant with *T. cordifolia* and *M. pruriens*.

Rathi SS, JK Grover, V Vikrant, NR Biswas; Prevention of experimental diabetic cataract by Indian Ayurvedic plant extracts, *Phytother Res* **16**(8), 774-77 (2002)

Thirty known or less known hypoglycaemic plants, selected from folklore uses, and from Ayurvedic, Unani and Siddah system of Medicine, were thoroughly investigated for their anti-diabetic activity. In these experiments, vacuum dried 95% ethanol extracts of different plants (250 mg/kg) were administered to alloxan induced diabetic rats once, twice or thrice daily for 2 weeks to bring down the fasting blood sugar level to near normal level. Comparative evaluation of hypoglycaemic activity revealed significant blood lowering activity in decreasing order in 24 samples which is as following. *Coccinia indica, Tragia oleifera, Eugenia jambolana, Tinospora cordifolia, Swertia chirayita, Momordica charantia, Ficus glomerata, Ficus benghalensis, Vinca rosea, Premna integrifolia, Mucuna pruriens, Terminalia belerica, Sesbenia aegyptiaca, Azadirachta indica, Dendrocalamus hamiltonii, Zingiber officinale, Aegle marmelos, Cinnamomum tamala, Trichosanthes cucumerina* and *Ocimum sanctum.*

Kar A, BK Choudhury, NG Bandyopadhyay; Comparative evaluation of hypoglycaemic activity of some Indian medicinal plants in alloxan diabetic rats, *J Ethnopharmacol* **84**(1), 105-08 (2003)

In order to unravel the mechanism of hypoglycaemic activity, effects of ten different plant extracts were evaluated in male mice. It was observed that while the extracts of *Inula racemosa, Boerhaavia diffusa* and *Ocimum sanctum* decreased the serum concentration of both cortisol and glucose, the extracts of *Aegle marmelos, Azadirachta indica* and *Gymnema sylvestre* exhibited hypoglycaemic activity without altering the serum cortisol concentration. As *I. racemosa, B. diffusa* and *O. sanctum* exhibited anti-peroxidative, hypoglycaemic and cortisol lowering activities, it is suggested that these three plant extracts may potentially regulate corticosteroid induced diabetes mellitus.

Gholap S, A Kar; Hypoglycaemic effects of some plant extracts are possibly mediated through inhibition in corticosteroid concentration, *Pharmazie* **59**(11), 876-78 (2004)

Herbal medicine is the dominant system of medicine practised by the local tribes of Sikkim and Darjeeling for the treatment of diabetes. A study showed that 37 species of plants belonging to 28 families are used as anti-diabetic agents in the folk medicinal practices in this region and 81% of these plants are hitherto unreported as hypoglycaemic agents.

Chhetri DR, P Parajuli, GC Subba; Anti-diabetic plants used by Sikkim and Darjeeling Himalayan tribes, India, *J Ethnopharmacol* **99**(2), 199-202 (2005)

Certain inorganic trace elements such as vanadium, zinc, chromium, copper, iron, potassium, sodium, and nickel are known to play an important role in the maintenance of normoglycaemia. The presence of some of these elements in *Murraya koenigii, Mentha piperita, Ocimum sanctum,* and *Aegle marmelos* justifies their use in diabetes and related metabolic disorder.

Narendhirakannan, RT; S Subramanian, M Kandaswamy, Mineral content of some medicinal plants used in the treatment of diabetes mellitus, *Biol Trace Elem Res* **103**(2), 109-15 (2005)

INDONESIA

Administration of Indonesian medicinal plants; *Curcuma xanthorrhiza, Zingiber aromaticum, Parkia speciosa* and *Pithecellobium jiringa* (5% of diet) to steptozotocin-induced diabetic rats improved the diabetic symptoms and triglycerides in the serum of the animals

Yasni S, K Imaizumi, M Sugano; Effects of an Indonesian medicinal plant *Curcuma xanthorrhiza* Roxb., on the levels of serum glucose and triglycerides, fatty acid desaturation, and bile acid excretion in streptozotocin-induced diabetic rats, *Agric Biol Chem* **55**(12), 3005-10 (1991).

JORDAN

A study, made between December 2003 and August 2004, revealed that about 31% of diabetic patients in Jordan use herbal products. The herbs commonly used by the diabetic patients were found to be *Trigonella foenum-graecum* (22.9%), *Lupinus albus* (14.6%), *Allium sativum* (11.5%), *Allium cepa* (5.2%), *Nigella sativa* (7.3%), *Zea mays* (6.3%), *Urtica dioica* (8.3%), *Eucalyptus globulus* (9.4%), *Olea europea* (3.1%), *Cumminum cyminum* (9.4%), *Coriandrum sativum* (10.4%), *Salvia officinalis* (3.1%), and *Tilia cordata* (1%).

Otoom SA, SA Al-Safi, ZK Kerem, A Alkofahi; The use of medicinal herbs by diabetic Jordanian patients, *J Herb Pharmacother* **6**(2), :31-41 (2006)

KOREA

In Korean folk medicine the underground parts of *Rosa rugosa* are used for treating diabetes.

Park JC, H Ito, T Yoshida, ^{1}H NMR assignment of HIV protease inhibitor procynadin B-3 isolated from *Rosa rugusa* , *Nat Prod Sci* **9**(2), 49 -51 (2003)

The effects of traditional anti-diabetic herbs on the progress of diabetes were studied in db/db mice, a typical non-insulin-dependent model. The results indicated that mulberry leaf water extract, Korean red ginseng, banaba leaf water extract, and the combination of above herbs effectively reduced blood glucose, insulin, triglyceride, and percent HbA1c. Increased expressions of liver PPAR-*alpha* mRNA and adipose tissue PPAR-*gamma* mRNA were observed in animals, fed diets supplemented with test herbs. The efficacy was highest in animals that were fed the combination diet.

Park MY, KS Lee, MK Sung; Effects of dietary mulberry, Korean red ginseng, and banaba on glucose homeostasis in relation to PPAR-*alpha*, PPAR-*gamma*, and LPL mRNA expressions, *Life Sci* **77**(26), 3344-54 (2005)

KUWAIT

The efficacy of a hypoglycaemic plant extract, in common use by Kuwaiti diabetic individuals, was evaluated using both normal and streptozotocin-induced diabetic rats. A significant decrease in blood glucose concentration was demonstrated on glucose tolerance tests, as compared to untreated animals.

Al-Awadi FM, MA Khattar, KA Gumaa; On the mechanism of the hypoglycaemic effect of a plant extract, *Diabetologia* **28**(7), 432-34 (1985)

LEBANON

The inhibitory activity against digestive enzymes related to diabetes and angiotensin converting enzyme (ACE) of extracts of nine plant species collected in Lebanon was studied. Of the different extracts of these nine plants, only methanol extracts of *Marrubium radiatum* and *Salvia acetabulosa* exhibited significant activity against *alpha*-amylase and *alpha*-glucosidase. The extracts also showed a strong inhibitory activity against ACE justifying the traditional use of these plants.

Loizzo MR, AM Saab, R Tundis, F Menichini, M Bonesi, V Piccalo, GA Statti, B de-Cindio, PJ Houghton, F Menichini; *In vitro* inhibitory activities of plants used in Lebanon traditional medicine against angiotensin converting enzyme (ACE) and digestive enzymes related to diabetes, *J Ethnopharmacol* **119**(1), 109-16 (2008)

MALAYSIA

The blood glucose lowering effects of some local herbs of Malaysia, (*Phyllanthus niruri, Zingiber zerumbet, Eurycoma longifolia* and *Andrographis paniculata*) were studied in normoglycaemic and streptozotocin-induced hyperglycaemic rats. Significant reduction in blood glucose level was observed when hyperglycaemic rats were treated with an aqueous extract of *Andrographis paniculata* (50 mg/kg b.w.). This effect was enhanced when freeze-dried material was used. Administration of aqueous extract *Eurycoma longifolia* showed positive results in hyperglycaemic rats at a dose of 150 mg/kg body weight. No significant reduction in blood glucose level was observed in hyperglycaemic rats treated with the other two drugs.

Husen R, AH Pihie, M Nallappan; Screening for anti-hyperglycaemic activity in several local herbs of Malaysia, *J Ethnopharmacol* **95**(2-3), 205-08 (2004)

Extracts of six selected Malaysian plants (*Anacardium occidentale, Averrhoa bilimbi, Lagerstroemia speciosa, Parkia speciosa, Phyllanthus amarus* and *Pithecellobium jiringa*) with a reputation of usefulness in treating diabetes were examined for *alpha*-amylase inhibition using an *in vitro* model. Of these plants, hexane extract of *Phyllanthus amarus* showed *alpha*-amylase inhibitory properties. Dotriacontanyl docosanoate, triacontanol and a mixture of oleanolic acid and ursolic acid were isolated from this extract. All compounds were tested in the *alpha*-amylase inhibition assay and the results revealed that the oleanolic acid and ursolic acid (2:1) mixture was a potent *alpha*-amylase inhibitor.

Ali H, PJ Houghton, A Soymyanath; *Alpha*-Amylase inhibitory activity of some Malaysian plants used to treat diabetes; with particular reference to *Phyllanthus amarus*, *J Ethnopharmacol* **107**(3), 449-55 (2006)

MAURITIUS

Of the seven indigenous medicinal plants of Mauritius (*Coix lacryma-jobi, Aegle marmelos, Artocarpus heterophyllus, Vangueria madagascariensis, Azadirachta indica, Eriobotrya japonica,* and *Syzigium cumini*) that were studied for their possible effects on starch breakdown by *alpha*-amylase, only *Artocarpus heterophyllus* significantly inhibited *alpha*-amylase activity *in vitro*. Results of the investigation indicated that aqueous extract of the leaves of the plant might act as a 'starch blocker' and thereby reduce post-prandial glucose peaks.

Kotowaroo MI, MF Mahomoodally, A Gurib-Fakim, AH Subratty; Screening of traditional anti-diabetic medicinal plants of Mauritius for possible *alpha*-amylase inhibitory effects *in vitro*, *Phytother Res* **20**(3),228-31 (2006)

MEXICO

A number of plants that are traditionally used in Mexico against diabetes were collected and their extracts were tested on CD1 strain mice with alloxan-induced diabetes. The plants that showed significant anti-diabetic activity are *Tecoma stans* (whole plant), *Salpianthus arenarius* (flowers), *Bidens pilosa* (whole plant or flowers), *Cecropia obtusifolia* (stems & leaves), *Psittacanthus calyculatus* (leaves, stems, flowers), *Turnera diffusa* (whole plant) and *Coutarea latiflora* (whole plant).

Perez RM, A Ocegueda, JL Munoz, JG Avila, WW Morrow; A study of the hypoglycaemic effect of some Mexican plants, *J Ethnopharmacol* **12**(3), 253-62 (1984)

The hypoglycemic effect of 12 plants, most used in Mexico for controlling diabetes mellitus, was studied in 27 rabbits submitted weekly to glucose tolerance tests after gastric administration of water, tolbutamide or a preparation of the plant. Tolbutamide and studied plants (except *Aloe barbadensis*) decreased significantly the area under glucose tolerance curve, in relation with the water control. The strongest effect was shown by *Psacalium peltatum* (27.9%), followed by *Curcubita ficifolia* (26.4%), *Lepechinia caulescens* (26.0%), *Opuntia streptacantha* (21.4%), *Solanum verbascifolim* (21.1%), *Teucrium cubense* (19.4%), *Cecropia obtusifolia* (18.9%), *Phaseolus vulgaris* (18.5%), *Tecoma stans* (17.5%), *Eriobotrya japonica* (17.2%), *Salpianthus macrodonthus* (15.0%), tolbutamide (14.3%), and *Aloe barbadensis* (1.4%).

Roman-Ramos R, H Flores-Saenz, G Partida-Hernandez, A Lara-Lemus, F Alarcon-Aguilar; Experimental study of the hypoglycaemic effect of some anti-diabetic plants, *Arch Invest Med* (Mex) **22**(1), 87-93 (1991)

The hypoglycaemic effects of 12 "anti-diabetic" plants, used in Mexico, were studied using 27 healthy rabbits with gastric administration of water, tolbutamide or a decoction of the "antidiabetic" plant before the induction of temporary hyperglycaemia by subcutaneous injection of 50% dextrose solution (4 ml/kg b.w.) at the beginning of the experiment and after 60 min. Blood glucose level was determined every 60 min for a period of 5 h. Tolbutamide and eight of the studied plants decreased significantly the hyperglycaemia as compared with control test (water). The strongest effect was produced by *Guaiacum coulteri*, followed by *Marrubium vulgare, Crataegus pubescens, Cynodon dactylon, Calea zacatechichi, Buddleia americana, Bauhinia divaricata* and *Coix lachryma*.

Roman-Ramos R, F Alarcon-Aguilar, A Lara-Lemus, JL Flores-Saenz; Hypoglycaemic effect of plants used in Mexico as anti-diabetics, *Arch Med Res* **23**(1), 59-64 (1992)

The hypoglycaemic activity of some plants, used empirically by the Mexican population as anti-diabetics, was studied. Traditional preparations of *Cucurbita ficifolia, Guaiacum coulteri, Lepechinia caulescens,* and *Psacalium peltatum* showed hypoglycaemic effect similar to tolbutamide in healthy and mild diabetic rabbits but failed to show any effect in severely diabetic rabbits.

Roman-Ramos R, A Lara-Lemus, F Alarcon-Aguilar, JL Flores-Saenz; Hypoglycaemic activity of some anti-diabetic plants, *Arch Med Res* **23**(3), 105-09 (1992)

The anti-hyperglycaemic effect of 12 edible plants was studied on 27 healthy rabbits, submitted weekly to subcutaneous glucose tolerance tests after gastric administration of water, tolbutamide or a traditional preparation of the plants. Like tolbutamide, traditional preparations of the plants (*Cucurbita ficifolia, Phaseolus vulgaris, Opuntia streptacantha, Spinacea oleracea, Cucumis sativus* and *Cuminum cyminum*) decreased significantly the area under the glucose tolerance curve and the hyperglycaemic peak. *Brassica oleracea var. botrytis, Allium cepa* and *Allium sativum* only decreased the hyperglycaemic peak.

Roman-Ramos R, JL Flores-Saenz, F Alarcon-Aguilar; Anti-hyperglycemic effect of some edible plants, *J Ethnopharmacol* **48**(1), 25-32 (1995)

The effects of three Mexican medicinal plants of the plant family, Asteraceae, (*Psacalium decompositum, Psacalium peltatum* and *Acourtia thurberi*) on blood glucose levels were investigated in fasting mice and temporally hyperglycaemic rabbits. The decoction of *P. decompositum* roots reduced the blood glucose level of normal mice after intra-peritoneal administration and significantly lowered the hyperglycaemic peak in rabbits with temporal hyperglycaemia. Plant decoctions of *P. peltatum* and *A. thurberi* showed only minor effects.

Alarcon-Aguilar FJ, R Roman-Ramos, M Jimenez-Estrada, R Reyes-Chilpa, B Gonzalez-Paredes,JL Flores-Saenz; Effects of three Mexican medicinal plants (Asteraceae) on blood glucose levels in healthy mice and rabbits, *J Ethnopharmacol* **55**(3), 171-77 (1997)

Of the 28 medicinal plants, used for the treatment of diabetes mellitus, traditional preparations of only eight of these plants were found to significantly decrease the hyperglycaemic peak and/or the area under the glucose tolerance curve, when administered intra-gastrically to temporarily hyperglycaemic rabbits. These plants were: *Guazuma ulmifolia, Tournefortia hirsutissima, Lepechinia caulescens, Rhizophora mangle, Musa sapientum, Trigonella foenum graceum, Turnera diffusa*, and *Euphorbia prostrata*.

Alarcon-Aguilar FJ, R Roman-Ramos, S Perez-Gutierez, A Aguilar-Contreras, CC Contreras-Weber, JL Flores-Saenz; Study of the anti-hyperglycaemic effect of plants used as anti-diabetics, *J Ethnopharmacol* **61**(2), 101-10 (1998)

The hypoglycaemic effects of the extracts of *Bouvardia terniflora, Brickellia veronicaefolia* and *Parmentiera edulis*, used in traditional medicine for the treatment of diabetes, were confirmed by a systematic study. Intra-peritoneal administration (300 mg/kg) of chloroform extracts of *P. edulis* and *B. terniflora* and hexane extract of *B. veronicaefolia* to alloxan-induced diabetic mice decreased the blood glucose levels.

Perez-Gutierez RM, C Perez-Gonzalez, MA Zavala-Sanchez, S Perez-Gutierez; Hypoglycaemic activity of *Bouvardia terniflora, Brickellia veronicaefolia,* and *Parmentiera edulis, Salud Publica Mex* **40**(4), 354-58 (1998) [Article in Spanish]

The hypoglycaemic activities of aqueous alcoholic extracts of *Bidens pilosa, Salvia officinalis, Psacalium peltatum,* and *Turnera diffusa* were investigated in healthy and alloxan-diabetic mice.. The extract of *S. officinalis* significantly reduced the blood glucose level of fasting normal mice 2 and 4h after intra-peritoneal administration. The extracts of *P. peltatum* and *B. pilosa* also significantly diminished glycaemia in healthy mice at 2h. The extract of *T. diffusa,* however, did not show any hypoglycaemic activity.

Alarcon-Aguilar FJ, R Roman-Ramos, JL Flores-Saenz, F Aguirre-Garcia; Investigation on the hypoglycaemic effects of extracts of four Mexican medicinal plants in normal and alloxan-diabetic mice, *Phytother Res* **16**(4), 383-86 (2002)

Mexican plants with hypoglycaemic effect, commonly used in the treatment of diabetes, have been reviewed. Out of a total of 306 species, that have records of a popular use in the treatment of diabetes, seven have been discussed in greater detail. These are: *Cecropia obtusifolia* Bertol. (Cecropiaceae), *Equisetum myriochaetum* Schlecht & Cham (Equisetaceae), *Acosmium panamense* (Benth.) Yacolev (Fabaceae), *Cucurbita ficifolia* Bouche (Cucurbitaceae), *Agarista mexicana* (Hemsl.) Judd. (Ericaeae), *Brickellia veronicaefolia* (Kunth) A. Gray (Asteraceae), and *Parmentiera aculeata* (Kunth) Seem. (Bignoniaceae).

Andrade-Cetto A, M Heinrich; Mexican plants with hypoglycaemic effect used in the treatment of diabetes, *J Ethnopharmacol* **99**(3), 325-48 (2005)

Type-2 diabetes is an increasing health problem in Mexico, as in many other countries, and the use of medicinal plants to treat this disease is widespread. The authors proposed a mathematical tool for analysing ethnopharmacological field data, with the ultimate aim to select species with most prominent impact on a community to treat a single disease. Using this tool, it was demonstrated that *Malmea depressa* (Baill.) R.E. Fr. and *Cecropia peltata* L. are culturally most salient hypoglycaemic plants in Yucatec Mayan community

Andrade-Cetto A, J Becerra-Jimenez, E Martinez-Zurita, P Ortega-Larrocea, M Heinrich; Disease-Consensus Index as a tool of selecting potential hypoglycaemic plants in Chikindzonot, Yucatan, Mexico, *J Ethnopharmacol* **107**(2), 199-204 (2006)

MONGOLIA

A preliminary investigation on the acute effect of two Mongolian medicinal plant extracts (*Dryopteris* species, Aspidiaceae) was made using oral glucose tolerance in rats. A single administration of these plant extracts was found to improve glucose utilization and insulin resistance in diabetic rats.

Khookhor O, Q Bolin, Y Oshida, Y Sato; Effect of Mongolian plants on *in vivo* insulin action in diabetic rats, *Diabetes Res Clin Pract* **75**(2), 135-40 (2007)

MOROCCO AND QUEBEC

A vastly growing and renewed interest in complementary and alternative medicines are being witnessed in the western world. An ethnopharmacological survey of the anti-diabetic plants, most frequently recommended by herbalists, naturopaths, and other traditional practitioners, was made both in Morocco, where traditional medicine is common and also in Quebec, where the use of medicinal plants is still marginal. *Trigonella foenum graecum* (fenugreek) was among the top ten most recommended anti-diabetic plants in both surveys, appearing first in Morocco and second in Québec. *Vaccinium spp.* (blueberry) received first place in Quebec. Several of the other top ten most common anti-diabetic plants in Québec are *Taraxacum officinale, Gymnema sylvestre, Glycyrrhiza glabra, Syzygium cumini, Opuntia streptacantha,* and *Panax ginseng/P. quinquefolium*. In contrast, the most commonly recommended anti-diabetic plants of Morocco are *Lupinus albus, Globularia alypum, Nigella sativa, Artemisia herba alba, Origanum compactum* and *Vitis vinifera* (red vine).

Haddad Pierre S, Depot M, Settaf, A, Cherrah Y; Use of Anti-diabetic Plants in Morocco and Québec, *Diabetes Care* **24**, :608-609 (2001)

NEPAL

Allium wallichi and *Dimeria dianthus* have been screened for their hypoglycaemic activity.

Rokeya B; Plant materials as a source of potential anti-diabetic agents in Diabetes mellitus Epidemic: combat the challenge, "Proceedings of the 4th International seminar on Asian Network of Research on Anti-diabetic plants (ANRAP), Kolkata, India, January 16-18, 2004

PAKISTAN

Dried ethanol extracts of medicinal plants collected from Islamabad and the Murree region were tested for their insulin secretagogue activity *in vitro*. The extracts were tested at various concentrations for insulin release from INS-1 cells in the presence of 5.5 mM glucose. Glibenclamide was used as a control. The different concentrations at which the plant extracts showed insulin secretagogue activity are as follows: *Artemisia roxburghiana, Salvia coccinia* and *Monstera deliciosa* showed insulin secretagogue activity at 1 µg/ml,, *Abies pindrow, Centaurea iberica* and *Euphorbia helioscopia* at 10 µg/ml, *Bauhinia variegata* and *Bergenia himalaicia* at 20 µg/ml, and *Taraxacum officinale* and *Viburnum foetens* at 40 µg/ml. These medicinal plants of Islamabad and the Murree region of Pakistan may be potential natural resources for anti-diabetic compounds.

Hussain Z, A Waheed, RA Qureshi, DK Burdi, EJ Verspohl, N Khan, M Hasan; The effect of medicinal plants of Islamabad and Murree region of Pakistan on insulin secretion from INS-1 cells, *Phytother Res* 18(1), 73-77 (2004)

Pakistan is rich in medicinally important plants. Of these plants, *Gymnema sylvestre*, *Momordica charantia* and *Eugenia jumbolana* were found to possess hypoglycemic activity of varying degree.

Khan B, MS Arayne, S Naz, N Mukhtar; Hypogylcaemic activity of aqueous extract of some indigenous plants, *Pak J Pharm Sci* **18**(1), 62-64 (2005)

PERU

Polymnia sonchifolia (common name: Yacón) is cultivated in Peru's Andean Cloud Forests for its tubers that are used as diabetic food. Yacón tubers store carbohydrates in the form of inulin, a polymer of sucrose that the human body cannot metabolise. It is, therefore, acceptable as a sweet low-calorie food for diabetics.

Zardini E; Ethnobotanical notes on Yacon (*Polymnia sonchifolia;* Asteraceae), *Economic Botany* **45**(1), 72-85 (1991)

PHILIPPINES

The validity of ethnobotanical use of a number of medicinal plants as anti-diabetic agents was tested using the oral glucose tolerance test. Of the plants (*Artemisia vulgaris, Eucalyptus tereticornis, Imperata cylindrica, Nopalea cochinellifera, Solanum nigrum, Syzygium cumini,* and *Vitex negundo*) tested, only the bark of *Syzygium cumini* and the leaves of *Vitex negundo* and *Eucalyptus tereticornis* exhibited anti-hyperglycemic activities when fed simultaneously with glucose. *Vitex negundo* exhibited greater anti-hyperglycaemic activity than *Eucalyptus tereticornis.*

Villasenor IM, MR Lamadrid;, Comparative anti-hyperglycaemic potentials of medicinal plants, *J Ethnopharmacol* **104**(1-2), 129-31 (2006)

SAUDI ARABIA

Anti-diabetic efficacy of 12 plants, used in the traditional medicine of Saudi Arabia, was tested in experimental mice. Three of these plants (*Teucrium oliverianum, Hamada salicornia* and *Allium cepa*) were found to possess significant hypoglycaemic activity. *Artemisia abyssinica, Azadirachta indica* and *Loranthus curviflorus* showed moderate activity. Five plants (*Rhazya stricta, Momordica charantia, Aloe vera, Allium sativum* and *Coriandrum sativum*) also showed significant activity. *Moringa oleifera* increased the blood glucose level of diabetic mice.

Moosa JS; A study on the crude anti-diabetic drugs, used in Arabian folk medicine, *Int J Crude Drug Res* **23**(3), 137-45 (1985)

SOVIET RUSSIA

Plants, used in folklore and traditional medicine of USSR for the treatment of diabetes (95 species), have been listed. The parts and organs of some of these popular plants and their preparations have also been described.

Kit SM, LM Budnevskaya, VS Kit; The plants used in cases of sugar diabetes, *Rastit Resur* **22**(3), 405-16 (1986) [Article in Russian]

Hypoglycaemic activity of arfazetin, a Soviet anti-diabetic species of medicinal plants, was studied in 32 patients with diabetes mellitus, types-1 and -2. In patients with type-1 diabetes mellitus, the drug was given in combination with a diet and an adequate dose of insulin and in patients with diabetes mellitus, type-2, an infusion of the drug was given in addition to a diet and hypoglycaemic drugs. In patients with type-2 diabetes, it was possible to decrease or even give up a daily dose of hypoglycemic drugs. The optimum daily dose of arfazetin was 1 glass of infusion, prepared from 5 g of dried plant, to be taken 30 min before meal.

Korotkova VD, AA Perelygina, TE Trumpe, SIa Sokolov, AM Lobanova; Arfazetin in the treatment of diabetes mellitus, *Probl Endokrinol* (Mosk) **34**(4), 25-28 (1988) [Article in Russian]

Administration of peony roots preparations provides the stable prophylactic effect against the development of experimental alloxan diabetes. This preparation and its complex with aspirin conserve the normal hemostatic system and the insulin status in diabetic animals.

Ul'ianov AM, IuA Tarasov, LA Liapina, VE Pastorova, MS Uspenskaia; Effect of a peony root preparation on the status of the insulin and hemostatic system in animals during development of alloxan diabetes, *Vopr Med Khim* **44**(3), 256-61 (1998) [Article in Russian]

SRI LANKA

The aqueous extracts of root bark of *Aegle marmelos* and *Salacia reticulata* and fruit juice of *Momordica charantia* showed significant hypoglycaemic activity in rats. The highest oral hypoglycaemic activity and maximum improvement of the oral glucose tolerance were associated with *Momordica charantia.*

Karunanayake ER, J Welihinda, SR Sirimanne, G Sinna dorai; Oral hypoglycaemic activity of some medicinal plants of Sri Lanka, *J Ethnopharmacol* **11**(2), 223-31 (1984).

Aqueous extracts of *Osbeckia octandra, Artocarpus heterophyllus* and *Bambusa vulgaris* significantly lowered the fasting blood glucose level and markedly improved glucose tolerance in Sprague-Dawley rats. Maximum hypoglycaemic activity was observed at +3 hr with *O. octandra* and *B. vulgaris*. The hypoglycaemic activity of the extracts was comparable with that of tolbutamide.

Fernando MR, MI Thabrew, EH Karunanayake; Hypoglycaemic activity of some medicinal plants in Sri-Lanka, *Gen Pharmacol* **21**(5), 779-82 (1990)

TAIWAN

The plants that are widely used in Taiwan to treat diabetes mellitus were screened for their putative effectiveness. Only six out of the ten plants exhibited blood glucose lowering activity through an insulin-independent mechanism.

Hsu FL, JT Cheng; Investigation in rats of the antihyperglycaemic effect of plant extracts used in Taiwan for the treatment of diabetes mellitus, *Phytother Res* **6**(2), 108-11 (1992)

From a survey of crude drugs in Taiwan market, the list of anti-diabetic crude drugs has been updated.

Lin CC, Crude drugs used for the treatment of diabetes mellitus in Taiwan, *Am J Chin Med* **20**(3-4), 1269-79 (1992)

TANZANIA

Cassia auriculata, Ricinus communis and *Securinega virosa* were identified as anti-diabetic plants on the basis of the information furnished by traditional healers of Kilosa district of Tanzania. These plants were proved to have hypoglycaemic activity.

Moshi MJ, ZH Mbwambo; Experience of Tanzanian traditional healers in the management of non-insulin dependent diabetes mellitus, *Pharmaceut Biol* **40**(7), 552-60 (2002)

USA (SOUTH TEXAS)

Of the 61 different plant medicines, used by patients with non-insulin dependent diabetes mellitus in South Texas, *Opuntia streptocantha* (prickly pear cactus), *Cnidoscolus chayamansa* (chaya), *Eriobotrya japonica* (loquat) and *Aloe vera* (savila) are most common. Some of these plants have been reported to have hypoglycaemic activity.

Noel PH, JA Pugh,AC Larme, G Marsh; The use of Traditional plant medicines for non-insulin dependent diabetes mellitus in South Texas, *Phytother Res* **11**(7), 512-17 (1997)

WEST INDIES

Aqueous extracts of *Bixa orellana, Capsicum frutescens,* and *Catharanthus roseus* showed significant hypoglycaemic activity in dogs. *Mikania micrantha, Anacardium occidentale, Momordica balsomnia, M. charantia, Cassia alata, Cocos nucifera,* and *Symphytum officinale* also showed significant but not sustained hypoglycaemic activity.

Morrison EY, M West; A preliminary study of the effects of some West Indian medicinal plants on blood sugar levels in the dog, *West Indian Med J* **31**(4), 194-97 (1982).

A survey of patients attending 17 government health centres in the island of Trinidad revealed that herbal medicines are taken regularly by many patients with diabetes.

The effectiveness of some of these plants, most frequently used by diabetics, has been established. Further, it was revealed that patients' culture, educational background, type of symptoms, and formal medical treatment may also influence the selection and use of these herbal medicines..

Mahabir D, MC Gulliford; Use of medicinal plants for diabetes in Trinidad and Tobago, *Rev Panam Salud Publica* **1**(3), 174-79 (1997)

APPENDIX - 7

PHYTOCHEMICALS WITH ANTI-DIABETIC POTENTIAL

[The term phytochemical is usually used to refer to compounds found in plants that are not normally involved in primary metabolic processes such as photosynthesis and cell respiration of plants. The biological activities elicited by a plant are primarily due to the presence of these chemical constituent(s) in the plant. While it has not always been possible to identify the active chemical(s), responsible for the desired activity shown by a plant, it has been successfully demonstrated in many cases. A particular phytochemical is not generally a monopoly of a single plant species and may be obtained from more than one plant, albeit in different combinations and in different yields. Many of these compounds may also be easily synthesized or prepared by easy chemical transformation of other phytochemicals. The structures of the phytochemicals, isolated from different plants and reported to have anti-diabetic activities, are shown in this Chapter. Only the structures of the phytochemicals, reported by their trivial names, have been shown and arranged in alphabetical order. The plant source of these phytochemicals and the references regarding their anti-diabetic or related activity are also shown. In case of some complex saponins and glycosides, the structures of the non-sugar parts (aglycones) have generally been shown and the site(s) of attachment of the sugar moiety. Some of the structures, particularly of the ginsenosides, have been copied directly from *Online Database for Chemicals from Around the World* **Chem Blink**]

Structure	Plant source and Reference
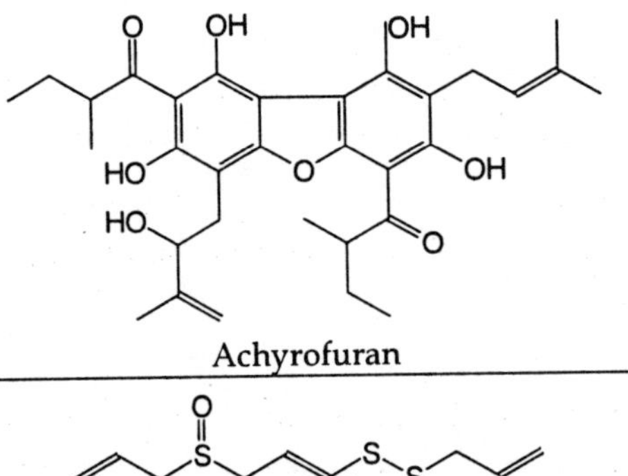 O OH OH HO O OH HO O Achyrofuran	*Achyrocline satureioides* Carney *et al, J Nat Prod* **65**(2), 203-05 (2002)
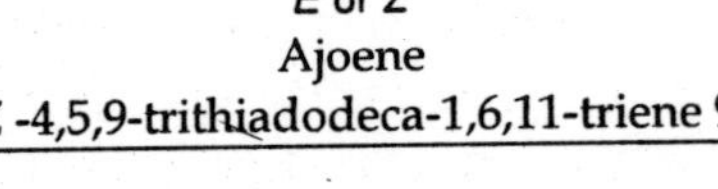 O S S S *E* or *Z* Ajoene (E and Z -4,5,9-trithiadodeca-1,6,11-triene 9-oxide)	*Allium sativum* Hattori *et al., J Nutr Sci Vitaminol* **51**(5), 382-84 (2005)

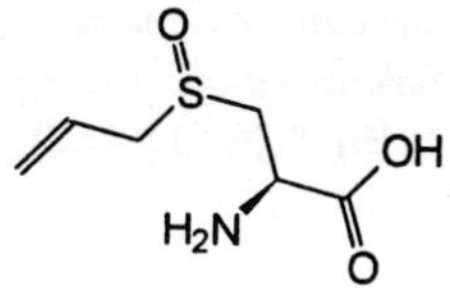 O, S, OH, H_2N, O Alliin	*Allium sativum* (Garlic) Chung LY; *J Med Food* **9**(2), 205-13 (2006)
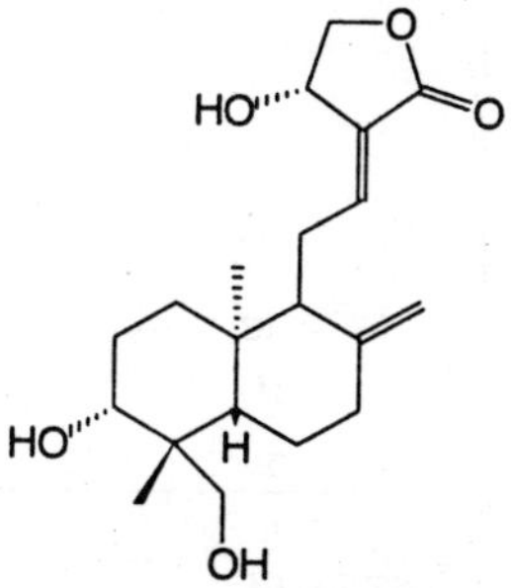 O, HO, O, HO, H, OH Andrographolide	*Andrographis paniculata* Yu *et al.*, *Planta Med* **69**(12), 1075-79 (2003)
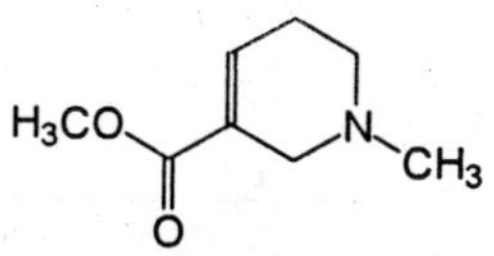 H_3CO, N, CH_3, O Arecoline	*Areca catechu* Chempakam B, *Indian J Exp Biol* **31**(5), 474-75 (1993)
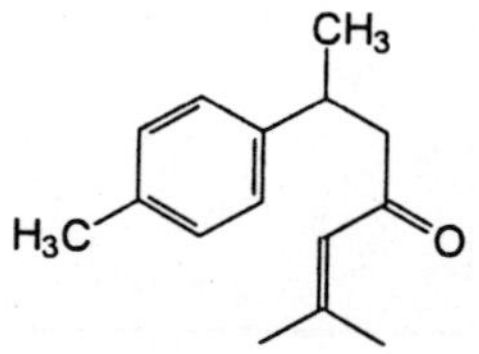 CH_3, H_3C, O Ar-Turmerone	*Curcuma longa* Kuroda *et al.*, *Biol Pharm Bull* **28**(5), 937-39 (2005)

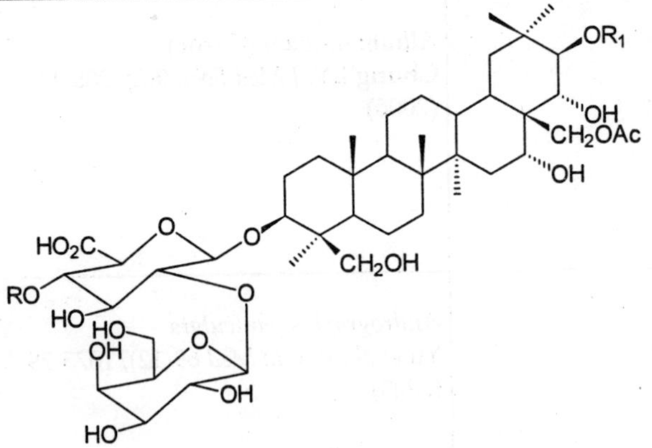 Assamicin I: R = α-Rhamnopyranosyl R_1 = Angeloyl Assamicin II: R = α-Rhamnopyranosyl R_1 = 3,4-di-O-Angeloyl-6-deoxy-β-glucopyranosyl	*Aesculus assamica* Sakurai *et al., Bioorg Med Chem Lett* **12**(5), 807-10 (2002).
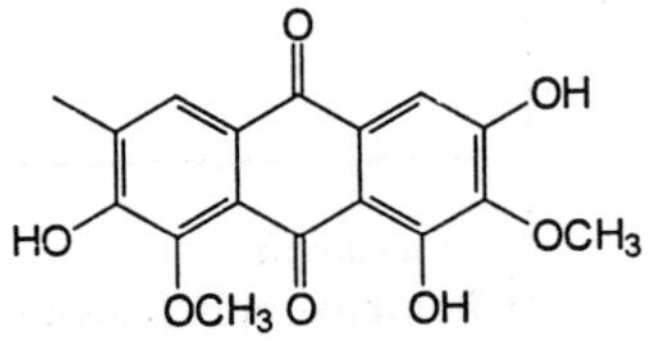 Aurantio-obtusin	*Cassia tora* Jang *et al., Biol Pharm Bull* **30**(11), 2207-10 (2007)
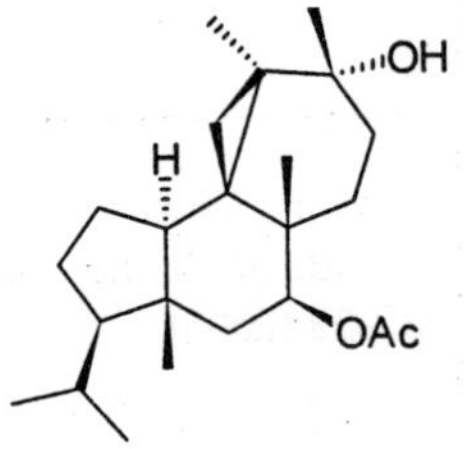 Azorellanol	*Azorella compacta* Fuentes *et al., Phytother Res* **19**(8), 713-16 (2005)
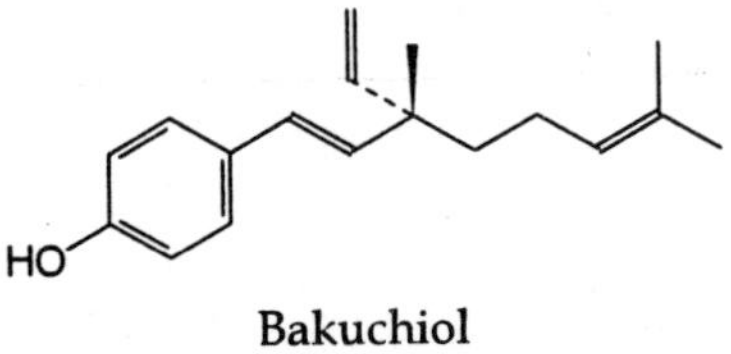 Bakuchiol 4-(3-Ethenyl-3,7-dimethyl-1,6-octadienyl)phenol	*Otholobium pubescens* Krenisky *et al., Biol Pharm Bull* **22**(10), 1137-40 (1999) *Psoralea corylifolia* Kim *et al., Planta Med* **71**(1), 87-89 (2005)

Structure	Source / Reference
HO, HO, OH, H, H, CO_2H Bassic acid	*Bumelia sartorum* Naik *et al., J Ethnopharmacol* **33**(1-2), 37-44 (1991)
H_3CO, O, OH, OH, O, OH Bellidifolin 1,5,8-Trihydroxy-3-methoxy-xanthen-9-one	*Swertia japonica* Basnet *et al., Planta Med* **60**(6), 507-11 (1994), **61**(5), 402-05 (1995)
O, O, N^+, OCH_3, OCH_3 Berberine	*Coptis chinensis* Chen *et al, Acta Pharma Sin* **21**(6), 401-06 (1986), *Berberis vulgaris,* Zhang *et al., Chin Med J* (Engl) **121**(21), 2124-28 (2008),
OH, H, O, H, HO, H Betulinic acid chemBlink	*Cassia fistula,* Vaishnava *et al., Fitoterapia* **64**(1), 95 (1993), *Morus alba* Singab *et al., J Ethnopharmacol* **100**(3), 333-38 (2005)

Borassoside A Borassoside B: R =H, R_1 = CH_2OH Borassoside C: R = CH_2OH, R_1 = H Borassoside D, E, F (differ in sugar units)	*Borassus flabellifer* Yoshikawa *et al., Chem Pharm Bull* (Tokyo) **55**(2), 308-16 (2007)
Boussingoside A1	*Boussingaultia baselloides* Espada *et al., Canad J Chem* **68**(11), 2039-44 (1990)
Brazilin	*Caesalpinia* species Kim *et al., Planta Med* **61**(4), 297-301 (1995); Won *et al., Planta Med.* **70**(8), 740-44 (2004).

Compound	Source and reference
Cacalol	*Psacalium decompositum* Inman *et al.*, *J Nat Prod* **62**(8), 1088-92 (1999)
5-Caffeoyl quinic acid (Neochlorogenic acid)	*Viburnum dilatatum* Iwai *et al.*, *J Agric Food Chem* **54**(13), 4588-92 (2006)
Calycosin	*Astragalus membranaceus* Shen *et al.*, *J Nutr* **136**(4), 899-905 (2006) Wenjie *et al.*, *Biol Pharm Bull* **30**(11), 2079-83 (2007)
Cannabisin G	*Berberis vulgaris* Zhang *et al.*, *Chin Med J* (Engl) **121**(21), 2124-28 (2008)
Capsaicin	*Capsicum frutescens* Babu & Srinivasan; *Mol Cell Biochem* **175**(1-2), 49-57 (1997) Tolan *et al.*, *Phytother Res* **15**(5), 391-94 (2001)., *Phytother Res* **18**(1), 95-96 (2004)

Compound	Source and references
Cassiaside	*Cassia tora* Lee *et al*, *Arch Farm Res* **29**(7), 587-90 (2006)
Castanospermine (1,6,7,8-Tetrahydroxyoctahydroindolizine)	*Castanospermum australe*, Saul *et al*., *Arch Biochem Biophys* **221**(2), 593-97 (1983), *Proc Nat Acad Sci*, USA, **82**(1), 93-97 (1985) *Xanthocercis zambesiaca* Nojima *et al*., *J Nat Prod* **61**(3), 397-400 (1998)
Centaureidin	*Jasonia montana* Al-Howiriny *et al*., *Nat Prod Res* **19**(3), 253-65 (2005).
Chamaemeloside Apigenin 7-[6'-(3-Hydroxy-3-methylglutaryl)glucoside]	*Chamaemelum nobile* Konig *et al*., *Planta Med* **64**(7), 612-14 (1998)
Chiro-inositol	*Fagopyrum esculentum* Kawa *et al*., *J Agric Food Chem* **51**(25), 7287-91 (2003) *Mucuna pruriens* Donati *et al*., *Phytother Res* **19**(12), 1057-60 (2005)

 Chlorogenic acid	*Cecropia obtusifolia* Andrade-Cetto *et al.*, *J Ethnopharmacol* **78**(2-3), 145-49 (2001) *Cecropia peltata* Nicasio *et al.*, *Phytother Res* **19**(8), 661-64 (2005),
Christinin A (3-O-[α-L-fucopyranosyl(1→2)-β-D-glucopyranosyl(1→3)-α-L-arabinopyranosyl] jujubogenin) **Jujubogenin**	*Zizyphus spina-christi* Glombitza *et al.*, *Planta Med* **60**(3), 244-47 (1994)
 chryso-obtusin-2-O-β-D-glucoside	*Cassia tora* Jang *et al.*, *Biol Pharm Bull* **30**(11), 2207-10 (2007)
 Chrysophanol 1,8-Dihydroxy-3-methylanthraquinone	*Rheum undulatum* Choi *et al.*, *Arch Pharm Res* **28**(9), 1027-30 (2005)

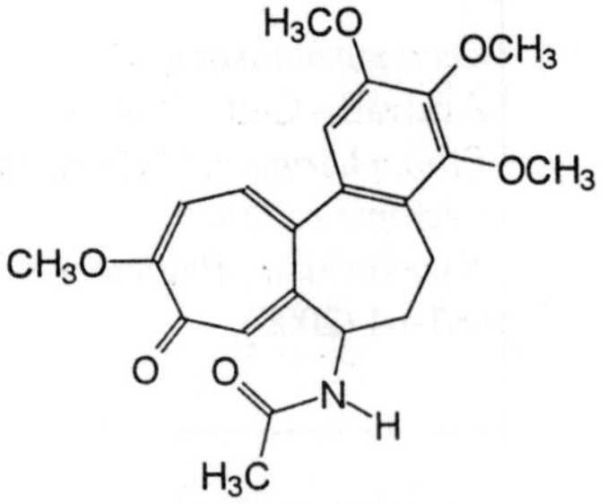 H_3CO, OCH_3, OCH_3, CH_3O, O, O, N, H, H_3C Colchicine	*Colchicum luteum* Chaudry *et al.*, *Fitoterapia* **64**(6), 510-15 (1993)
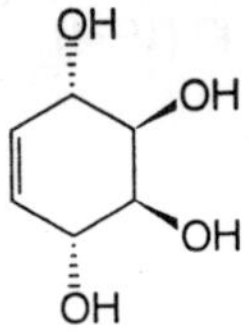 OH, OH, OH, OH Conduritol A	*Gymnema sylvestre* Miyatake *et al.*, *Biosci Biotechnol Biochem* **58**(4), 756-57 (1994)
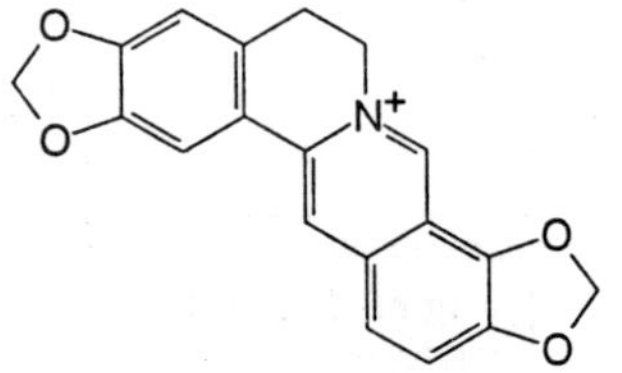 O, O, N^+, O, O Coptisine	*Coptis chinensis* Chen and Xie; *Acta Pharma Sin* **21**(6), 401-06 (1986)
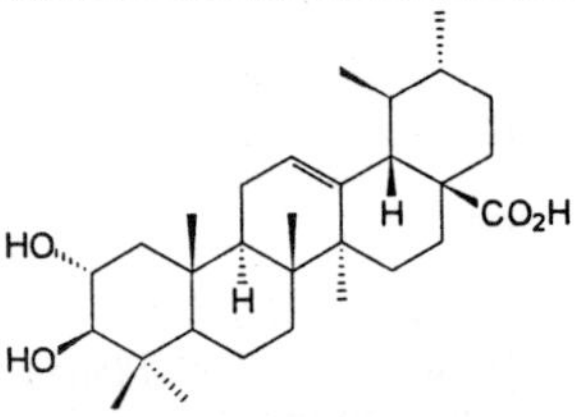 H, CO_2H, HO, H, HO Corosolic acid (2α-Hydroxy ursolic acid.)	*Lagerstroemia speciosa* Miura *et al.*, *Biol Pharmaceut Bull* **27** (7), 1104-05 (2004); **29**(3), 585-87 (2006)
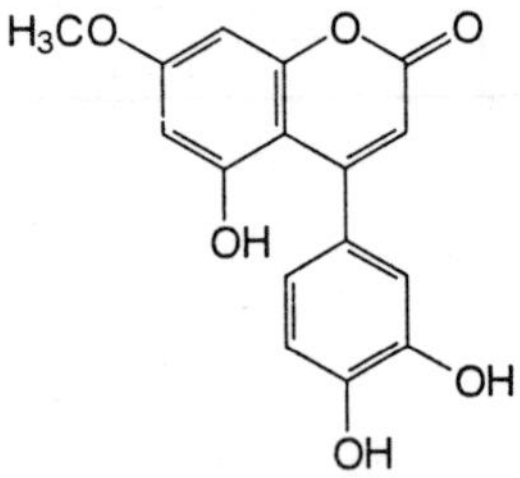 H_3CO, O, O, OH, OH, OH Coutareagenin (5-Hydroxy-7-methoxy-4-(3,4-dihyroxyphenyl)-2H-benzo-1-pyran-2-one)	*Hintonia latiflora* Korec *et al.*, *Arzneimittel-Forschung* javascript:AL_get(this, 'jour', 'Arzneimittelforschung.'); **50**(2), 122-28 (2000)

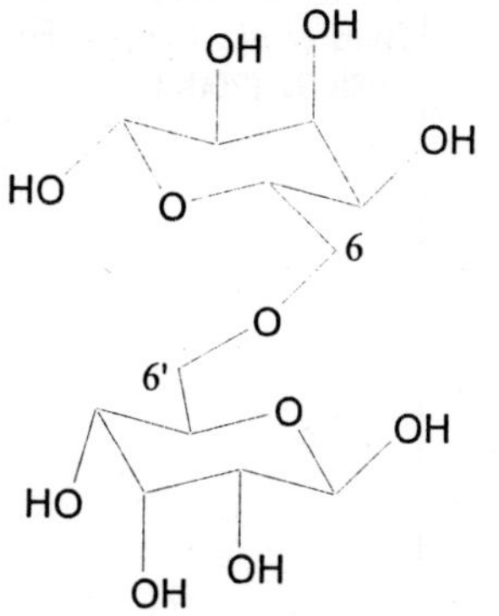 Coyolosa	*Acrocomia mexicana* Perez *et al.*, *Pharm Acta Helv* **72**(2), 105-11 (1997)
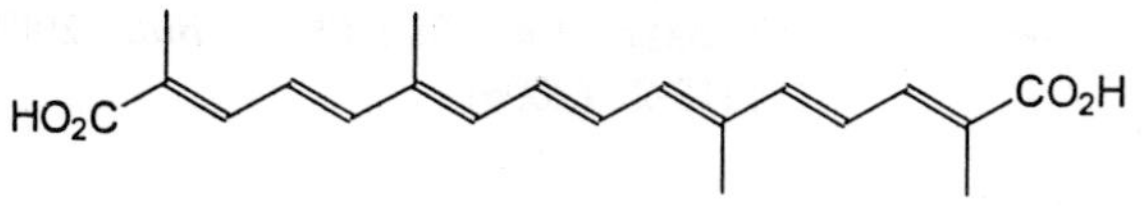 Crocetin	*Gardenia jaminoides* Xi *et al.*, *Planta Med* **71**(10), 917-22 (2005)
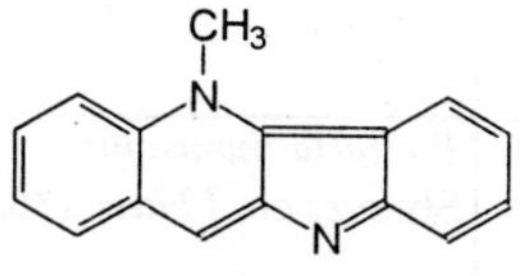 Cryptolepine	*Cryptolepis sanguinolenta* Bierer *et al.*, *J Med Chem* 41(6), 894-901 (1998), **41**(15), 2754-64 (1998); *Diabet Med* **15**(5), 367-74 (1998),
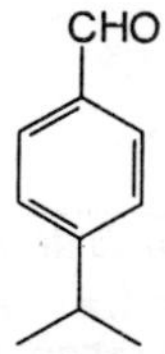 Cuminaldehyde	*Cuminum cyminum* Kalia *et al.*, *J Sci Pharm* **6**(2), 45-47 (1995); Lee *et al.*, *J Agric Food Chem* **53**(7), 2446-50 (2005)
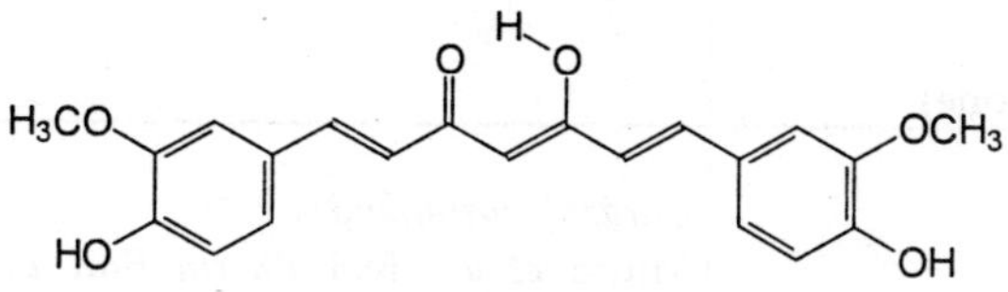 Curcumin Tetrahydrocurcumin	*Curcuma longa* Narayannasamy *et al.*, *J Herbs, Spices, Med Plants* **10**(1), 75-84 (2002), Arun *et al.*, *Plant Foods Hum Nutr* **57**(1), 141-50 (2002), Suryanarayana *et al.*, *Invest Ophthalmol Vis Sci* **46**(6), 2092-99 (2005) Pari *et al.*, *Plant Foods Hum Nutr* **62**(1), 25-29 (2007)

Compound	Source / Reference
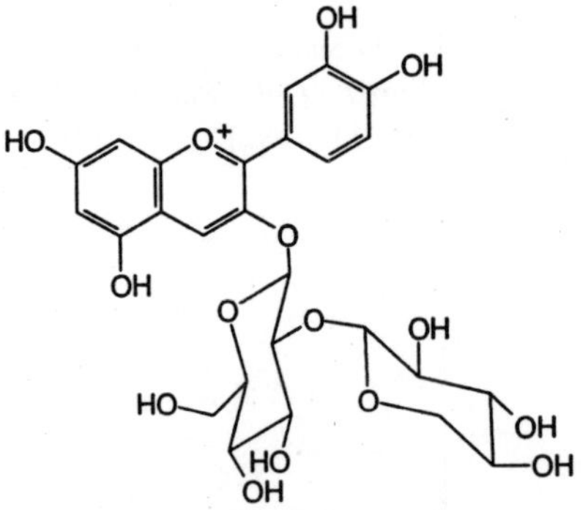 Cyanidin 3-sambubioside	*Viburnum dilatatum* Iwai *et al., J Agric Food Chem* **54**(13), 4588-92 (2006)
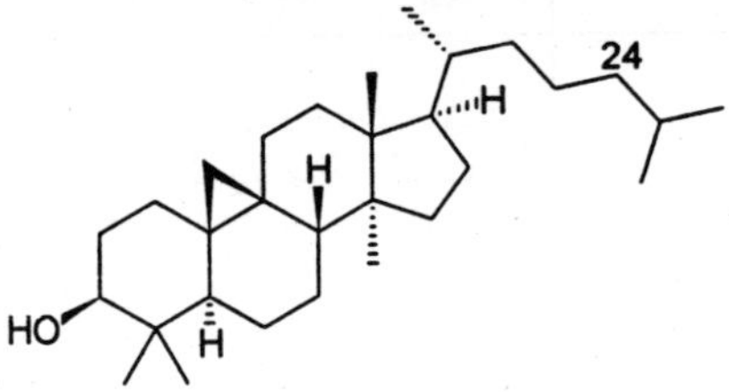 Cycloartanol 24-Methylene-cycloartanol	*Aloe barbadensis* Tanaka *et al., Biol Pharm Bull* **29**(7), 1418-22 (2006)
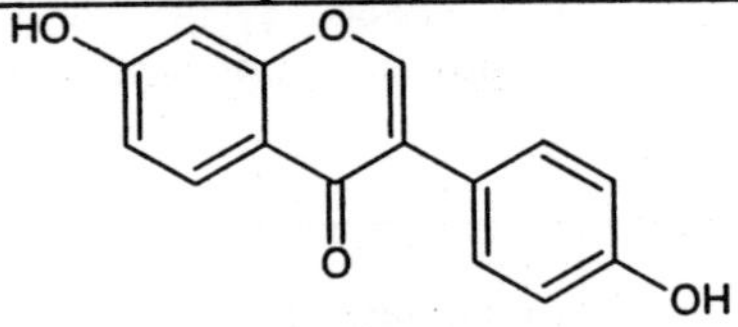 Daidzein (4',7-Dihydroxyisoflavone)	*Pueraria thomsonii* Shen *et al., J Nutr* **136,** 899-905 (2006)
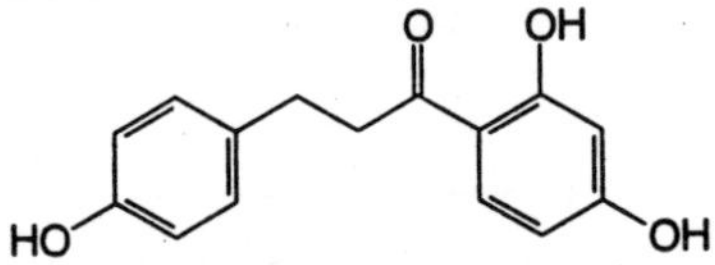 Davidigenin (4,2',4'-Trihydroxydihydrochalcone)	*Artemisia dracunculus* Logendra *et al., Phytochemistry* **67**(14), 1539-46 (2006)
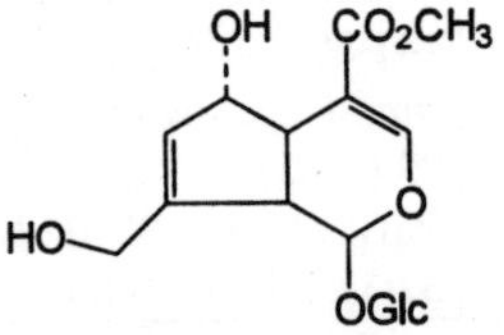 Deacetylasperulosidic acid methyl ester	*Gardenia jasminoides* Miura *et al., Biol Pharm Bull* **19**(1), 160-61 (1996).

Compound	Source and reference
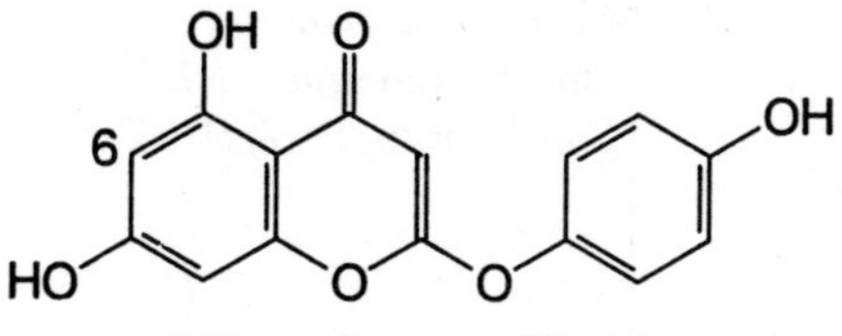 6-Demethoxycapillarisin	*Artemisia dracunculus* Logendra *et al., Phytochemistry* **67**(14), 1539-46 (2006)
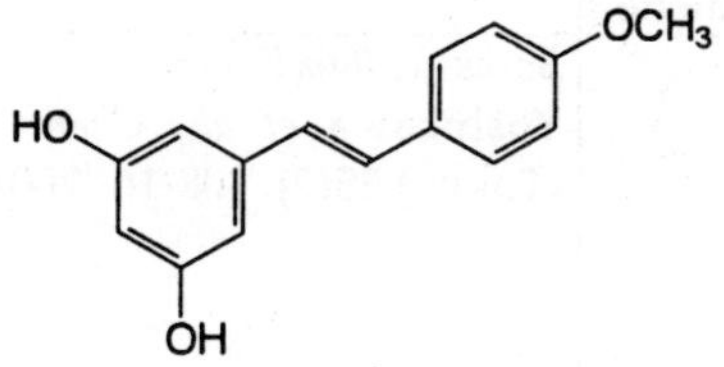 Desoxyrhapontigenin	*Rheum undulatum* Choi *et al., Arch Pharm Res* **28**(9), 1027-30 (2005)
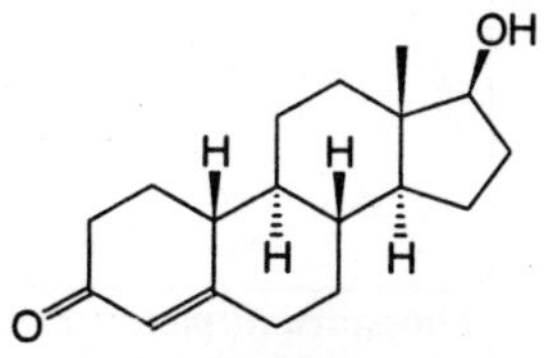 Diandrol	*Salacia diandra* Kumara *et al., IUPAC International Conference on Biodiversity and Natural Products Chemistry and Medical Applications,* New Delhi, OP-13, Jan.26-31, 2004
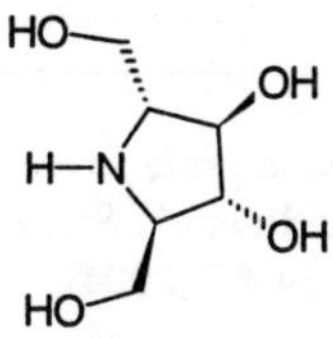 2,5-Dideoxy-2,5-imino-D-mannitol	*Xanthocercis zambesiaca* Nojima *et al., J Nat Prod* **61**(3), 397-400 (1998)
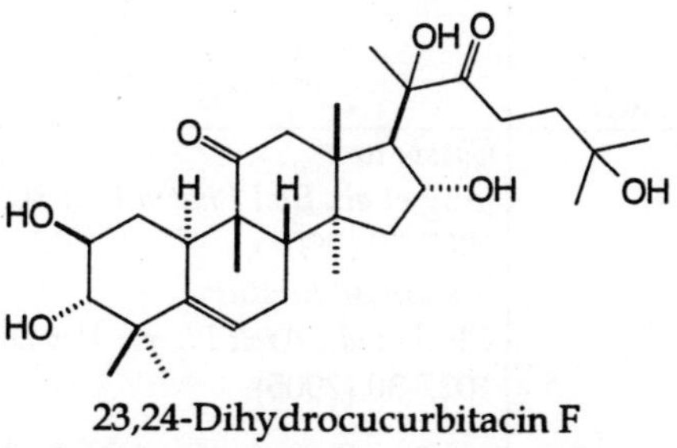 23,24-Dihydrocucurbitacin F 3-O-β D-glucopyranosyl-23,24-dihydrocucurbitacin F	*Hintonia standleyana* Guerrero-Analco *et al., Planta Med* **71**(12), 1099-105 (2005).

18, 20, 23, 25, 19, OH, O, HO 5β,19-Epoxy-3 β,25-dihydroxycucurbita-6,23(*E*)-diene	*Momordica charantia* Harinantenaina *etal., Chem Pharm Bull* (Tokyo) **54**(7),:1017-21 (2006)
OH, HO, O, H, H, H, H, H Dioscin Chem Blink	*Borassus flabellifer* Yoshikawa *et al., Chem Pharm Bull* (Tokyo) **55**(2), 308-16 (2007)
CO_2H, OH, CH_3, H_3C, N Dioscoretine	*Dioscorea dumetorum* Iwu *et al., Planta Med* **56**(1), 119-20 (1990), **56**(3), 264-67 (1990)
HO, O, OH Ellagic acid 2-(2,3,6-trihydroxy-4-carboxyphenyl) ellagic acid	*Caesalpinia ferrea* Ueda *et al., Biol Pharm Bull* **27**(10), 1584-87 (2004).
OH, O, H_3C Emodin	*Cassia tora* Jang *et al., Biol Pharm Bull* **30**(11), 2207-10 (2007), *Rheum undulatum* Choi *et al., Arch Pharm Res* **28**(9), 1027-30 (2005)

$H_3CO-C(=O)$ … Enhydrin	*Smallanthus sonchifolius* Schon *et al., Phytochem Anal* **16**(3), 161-65 (2005)
OH H N CH_3 CH_3 Ephedrine	*Ephedra sinica* Xiu *et al., Am J Chin Med* **29**(3-4), 493-500 (2001).
HO OH OH OR OH Epicatechin (R = H) Epicatechin gallate (R = galloyl)	*Pterocarpus marsupium* Chakravarthy *et al., Indian Drug* **18**(5), 184-85 (1981) Sheehan *et al., J Nat Prod* **46**(2), 232-34 (1983) Bone *et al., Biosci Rep* **5**(3), 215 21 *(1985);* Ahmad *et al., Acta Diabetol Lat* **26** (4), 291-300 (1989), Zaid *et al., J Clin Biochem* **17**(2), 27-32 (2002) *Camellia sinensis* Anderson *et al., J Agric Food Chem* **50**(24), 7182-86 (2002), Koyama *et al., Planta Med* **70**(11), 1100-02 (2004)
OH OH HO OH OH OH OH OH Epigallocatechin 3-gallate	*Camelia sinensis* Anderson and Polansky; *J Agric Food Chem* **50**(24), 7182-86 (2002), Koyama *et al., Planta Med* 70(11), 1100-02 (2004);

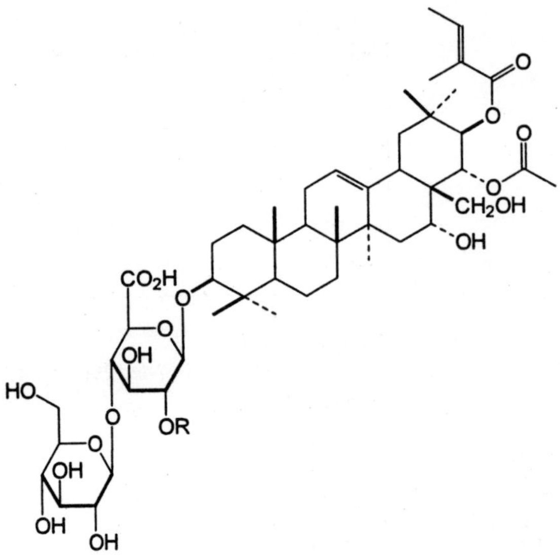 Escin 1a: R = D-Glucopyranoxyl Escin IIa: R = D-Xylopyranoxyl 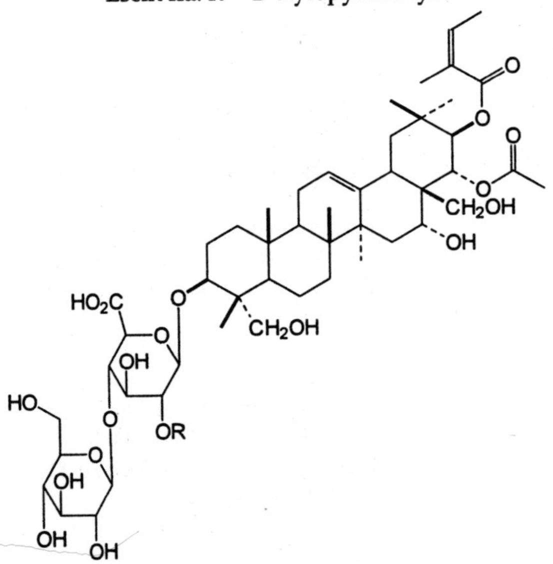 Escin Ib: R = D-Glucopyranoxyl Escin IIb: D-Xylopyranoxyl	*Aesculus hippocastanum* Yoshikawa *et al., Chem Pharm Bull* (Tokyo) **42**(6), 1357-59 (1994)., *Chem Pharm Bull* (Tokyo) **44**(8), 1454-64 (1996) *Aesculus hippocastanum* Yoshikawa *et al., Chem Pharm Bull* (Tokyo) **42**(6), 1357-59 (1994)., *Chem Pharm Bull* (Tokyo) **44**(8), 1454-64 (1996).

OH, OH, N, H, OH Fagomine 4-O-β-D-glucopyranosylfagomine	*Xanthocercis zambesiaca* Nojima *et al., J Nat Prod* **61**(3), 397-400 (1998)
OCH$_3$, H$_3$CO, H$_3$C, N, H, OH, O, N, CH$_3$, H, O, OCH$_3$ Fangchinoline	*Stephania tetrandra* Tsutsumi *et al., Biol Pharm Bull* **26**(3), 313-17 (2003) Wenjie *et al., Biol Pharm Bull* **30**(11), 2079-83 (2007)
Foetidin (A 1:1 mixture of glucosides of β-sitosterol and 5,25stigmastadiene-3β–ol)	*Momordica foetida* Marquis *et al., Planta Med* **31**(4), 367-74 (1977)
HO, O, O, OCH$_3$ Formononetin	*Astragalus membranaceus* Shen *et al., J Nutr* **136**(4), 899-905 (2006) Wenjie *et al., Biol Pharm Bull* **30**(11), 2079-83 (2007)
H$_3$CO, H$_3$CO, O, O, OH Fraxidin (8-Hydroxy-6,7-dimethoxycoumarin)	*Teramnus labialis* Fort *et al., Phytomedicine* **6**(6), 465-67 (2000)
OH, H, O, H, HO, H, H, H, HO Furost-5-ene-3β,22, 26-triol Saponins, built on furost-5-ene-3β,22, 26-triol	*Balanites aegyptiaca* Kamel *et al., Chem Pharm Bull* (Tokyo) **39**(5), 1229-33 (1991).

Structure	Source / Reference
HN, H, N, H_2N Galegine	*Galega officinalis* Patricic and Kalodera; *Acta Pharm Jugosl* **32**(3), 219-23 (1982) Pundarikakshudu *et al., Fitoterapia* **65**(5), 423-26 (1994)
OH, HO, O, OH, O, OH, HO, R, OH, OH, O Garcinia biflavonoid GB-1 (R = H) Garcinia biflavonoid GB2: (R = OH)	*Garcinia kola* Iwu *et al., J Pharm Pahrmacol* **42** (4), 290-92 (1990)
O, OH, HO, OCH_3 Gingerol	*Zingiber officinale* Kato *et al., J Agric Food Chem* **54**(18), 6640-44 (2006)
HO, OH, HO, O, O, O, OH, OH, HO, OH, O, OH, H, H, OH, OH, HO, O, HO, O, H, H, H, H, O, O, HO, OH, OH Ginsenoside-Rb_1	*Panax quinquefolius* Xie *et al., Pharmacol Res.* **42** (2), 113-17 (2004)

Ginsenoside-Rb_2	*Panax ginseng* Yokozawa *et al., Chem Pharm Bull* (Tokyo) **33**(2), 869-72 (1985), *J Pharm Pharmacol* **48**(7), 763-67 (1996)
Ginsenoside Rc	*Panax quinquefolius* Sievenpiper *et al., Eur Clin Nutr* **57**(2), 243-48 (2003) Xie *et al., Pharmacol Res* **45**(2), 113-17 (2004)
Ginsenoside Rd	*Panax quinquefolius* Xie JT *et al., Pharmacol Res* **45**(2), 113-17 (2004)

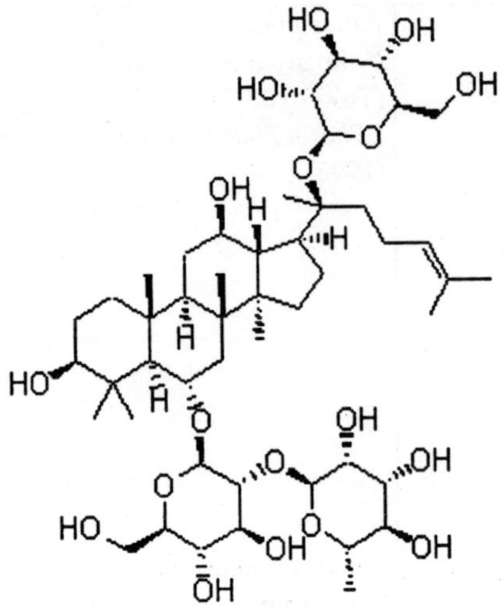 Ginsenoside Re	*Panax ginseng* Attele *et al.*, *Diabetes* **51**(6), 1851-58 (2002)
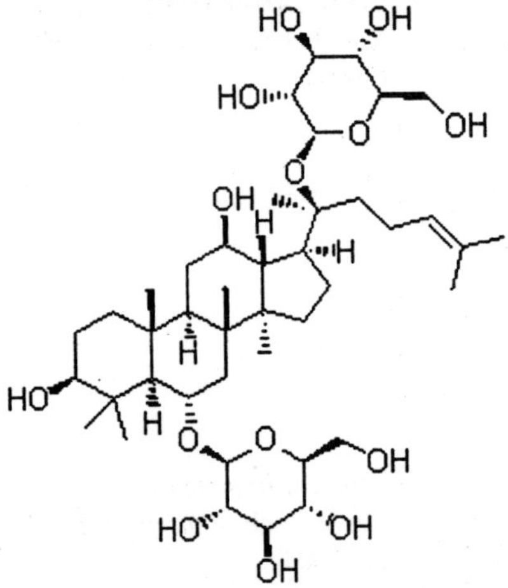 Ginsenoside Rg-1 (Sanchinoside C-1) **Courtesy: *Online Database of Chemicals* Chem Blink**	*Panax notoginseng* Jiang *et al.*, *Yao Xue Xue Bao* **17**(3), 222-25 (1982); Gong *et al.*, *Acta Pharmaceutica Sinica* **26** (2), 81-85 (1991)
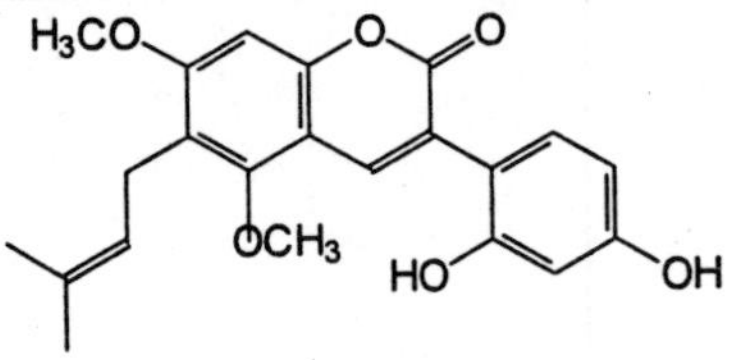 Glycyrin	*Glycyrrhiza uralensis* Kiroda *et al.*, *Bioorg Med Chem Lett* **13**(24), 4267-72 (2003).

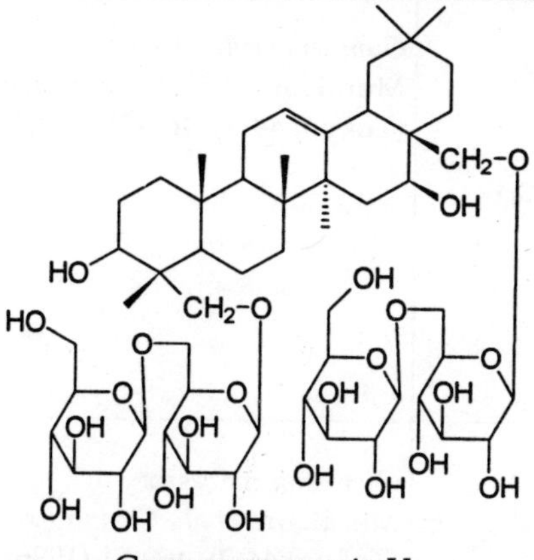 Gymnemasaponin V	*Gymnema sylvestre* Sugihara *et al., J Asian Nat Prod Res* **2**(4), 321-27 (2000)
Gymnemasin A: 3- O-[β-D glucopyranosyl(1→3)- β-D-glucuronopyranosyl]- 22 O-tigloyl-gymnemanol, **Gymnemasin B:** 3-O-[β-D-glucopyranosyl (1 →3)- β-D glucuronopyranosyl]-gymnemanol **Gymnemasin C:** 3-O- β-D-glucuronopyranosyl- 22-O-tigloyl-gymnemanol **Gymnemasin D:** 3-O- β-D-glucuronopyranosyl-gymnemanol, 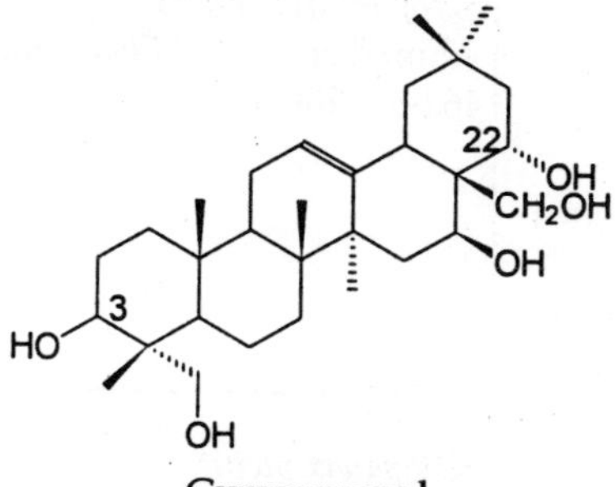 Gymnemanol	*Gymnema sylvestre* Mahato *et al., Int Seminar Trad Med,* Calcutta November 7-9, p. 128 (1992).
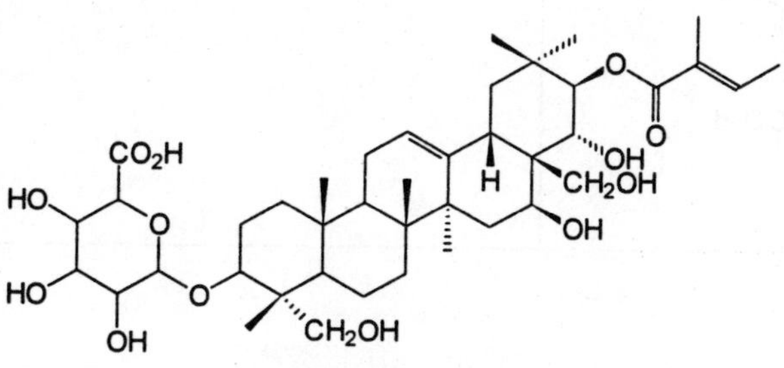 Gymnemic acid IV	*Gymnema sylvestre* Sugihara *et al., J Asian Nat Prod Res* **2**(4), 321-27 (2000).

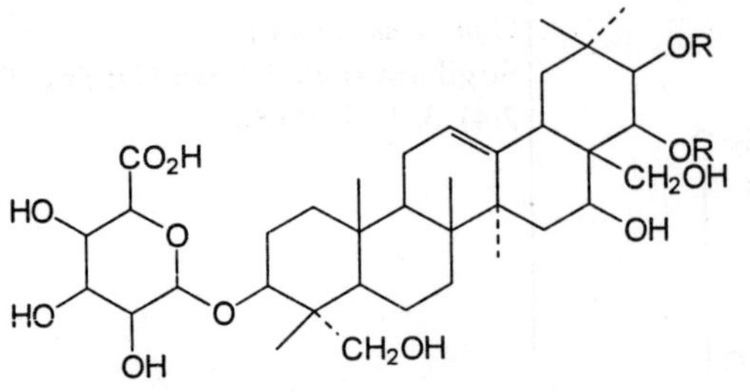 Gymnemic acid V (R= Tigloyl group)	*Gymnema sylvestre* Murakami *et al., Chem Pharm Bull* (Tokyo) **44**(2), 469-71 (1996).
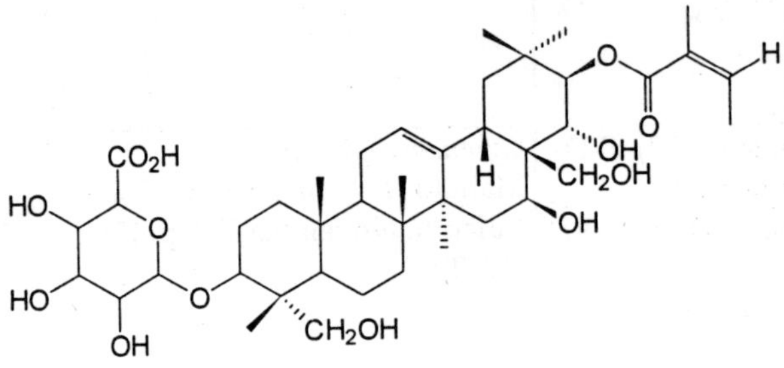 **Gymnemoside B**	*Gymnema sylvestre* Murakami *et al., Chem Pharm Bull* (Tokyo) **44**(2), 469-71 (1996)
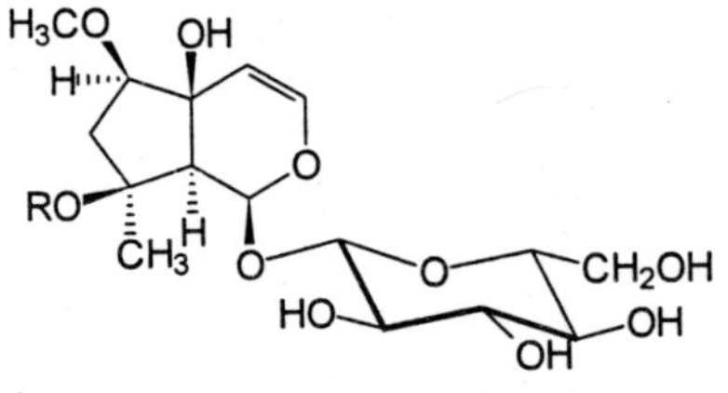 Harpagoside-B (R = Cinnamoyl)	*Scrophularia deserti* Ahmed *et al., Biol Pharm Bull* **26**(4), 462-67 (2003)
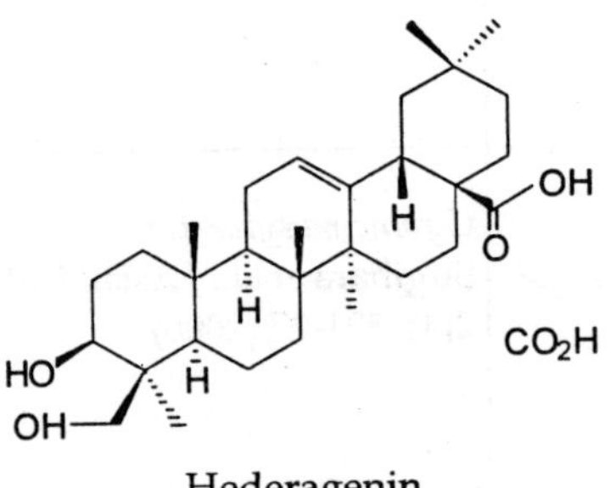 Hederagenin	*Kalopanax pictus* Park *et al., Arch Pharm Res* **21**(1), 24-29 (1998).

Compound	Source / Reference
HO OH HO H₃C O O HO O HO OH O O OH OCH OH O Hesperidin	*Schizonepeta tenuifolia* Kim *et al., Arch Pharmacal Res* **19**(6), 441-46 (1996)
OH O HO OH O Humulone	*Humulus lupulus* Aigo Nutritive Chemicals Ltd., *Japan Kakai Tokkyo Koho* JP 59, 59, 623, (Cl. A61. K35/78) 4 pp. (1984)
OH O OCH₃ HO O O CH₂OH OH O Hydnocarpin	*Hydnocarpus wightiana* Reddy *et al., Phytother Res* **19**(4), 277-81 (2005).
OH H HO OH HO O OH Hydroxybrazilin	*Hematoxylon campechianum* Moon *et al., Yakhak Hoeji* **38**(1), 97-101 (1994)

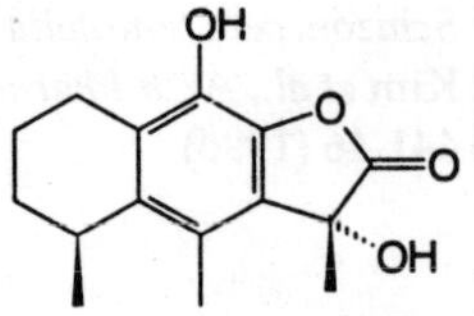 3-Hydroxycacalolide	*Psacalium decompositum* Inman *et al., J Nat Prod* **62**(8), 1088-92 (1999)
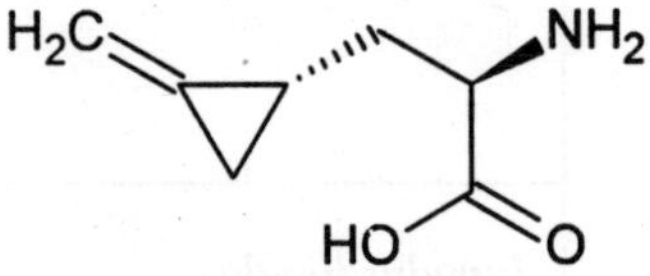 Hypoglycin A	*Blighia sapida* Sherratt *et al., Trends Pharmacol Sci* 7(5), 186-91 (1986) Foungbe *et al., Ann Pharm Fr* **44**(6), 509-15 (1986)
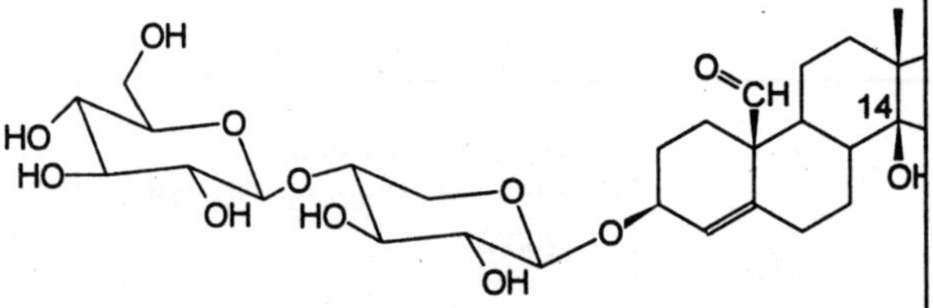 Hyrcanoside (4-O-β-D-glucopyranosyl-β-D-xylopyranosyl-card-4-en-19-al-olide) 14-Methoxy-hyrcanoside	*Securigera securidaca* Ali *et al., Pharmazie* **53**(10), 710-15 (1998)
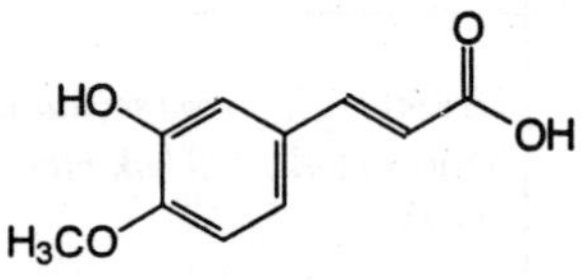 Isoferulic acid	*Cimicifuga dahurica* Liu *et al., Planta Med* **65**(8), 712-14 (1999).

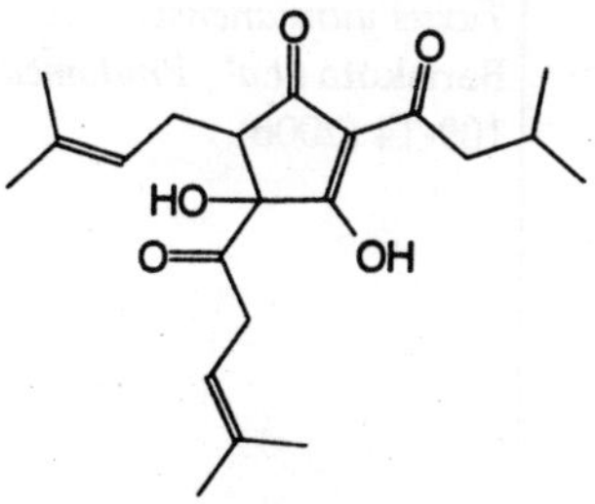 Isohumulone	*Humulus lupulus* **Yajima** *et al., J Biol Chem* **279**(32), 33456-62 (2004)
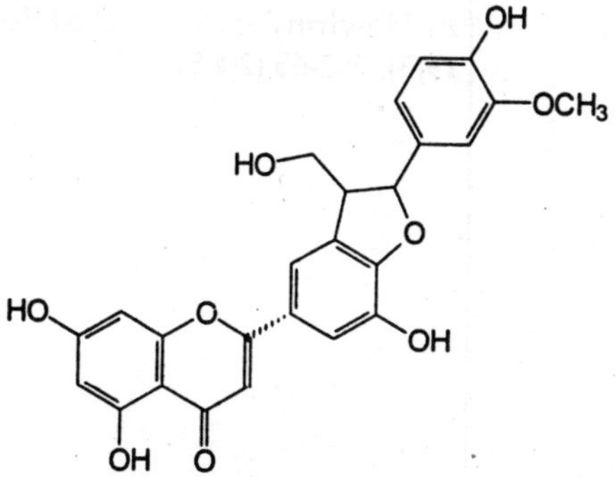 Isohydnocarpin	*Hydnocarpus wightiana* **Reddy** *et al., Phytother Res* **19**(4), 277-81 (2005).
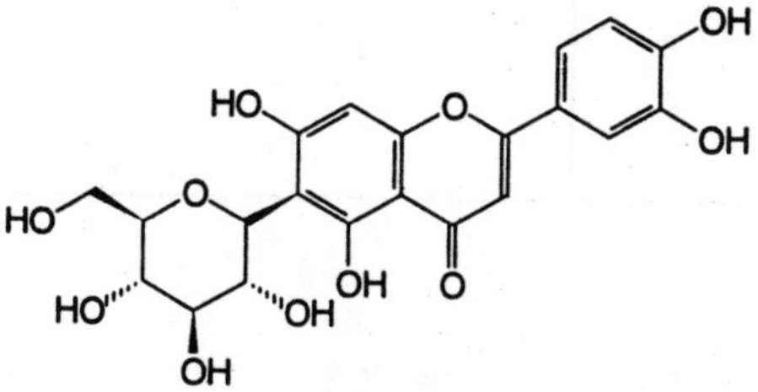 Isoorientin	*Cecropia obtusifolia* **Andrade-Cetto** *et al., J Ethnopharmacol* **78**(2-3), 145-49 (2001); *Gentiana olivieri* **Sezik** *et al., Life Sci* **76**(11), 1223-38 (2005).
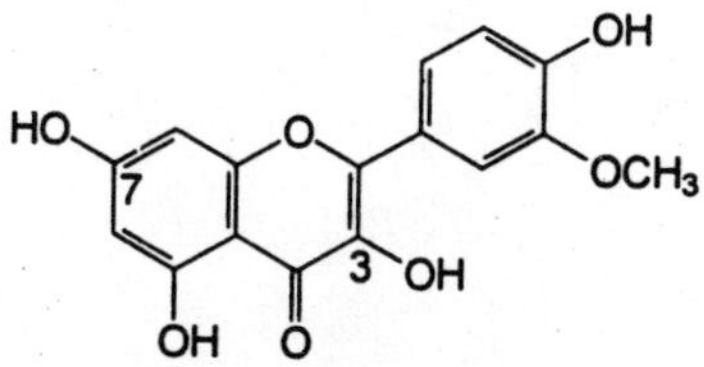 Isorhamnetin Isorhamnetin 3,7-di-O-β-D-glucopyranoside	*Brassica juncea* **Yokozawa** *et al., J Agric Food Chem* **50**(19), 5490-95 (2002)

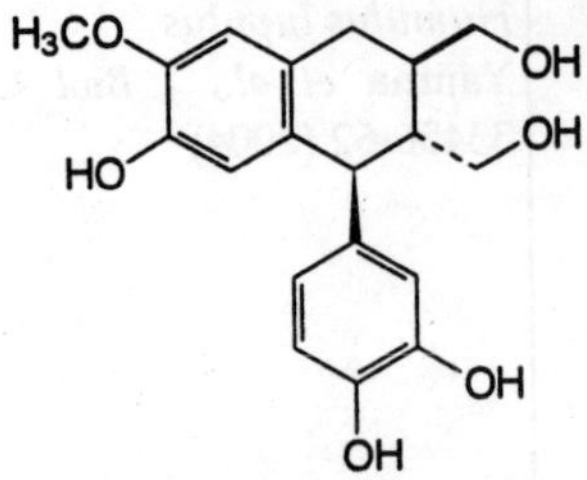 Isotaxiresinol	*Taxus yunnanensis* **Banskota *et al.*, *Phytomedicine* 13(1-2), 109-14 (2006)**
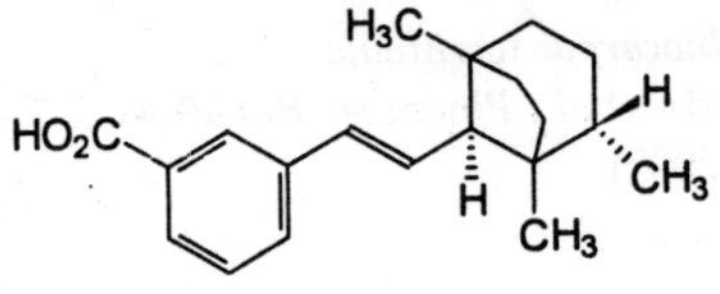 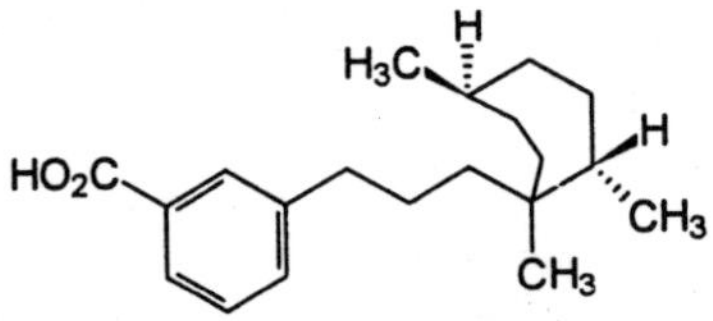 Jasonin A Jasonin B 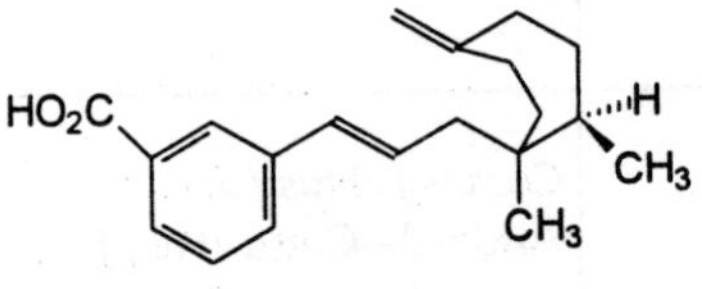 Jasonin C	*Jasonia montana* **Al-Howiriny *et al.*, *Nat Prod Res* 19(3), 253-65 (2005).**

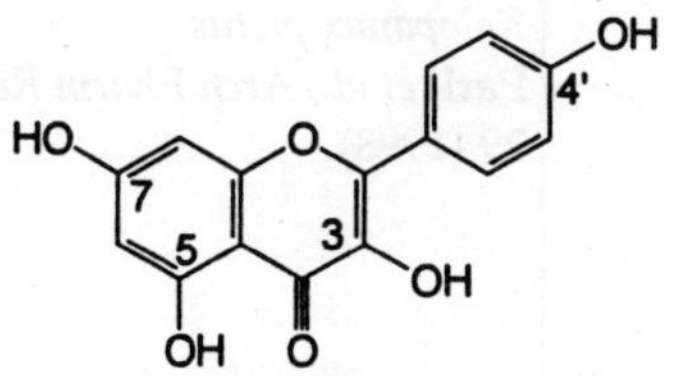 Kaempferol Kaempferol glucosides Kaempferol 3-O-β-D-glucopyranoside (Astragalin) Kaempferitrin (kaempferol-3,7-O-α-dirhamnoside) Kaempferol 3-O- α-(2''galloyl) rhamnoside	*Bridelia ferruginea* Iwu *et al., Fitoterapia* **54**(6), 243-48 (1983). *Equisetum myriochaetum,* Andrade-Cetto *et al., J Ethnopharmacol* **72**(1-2), 129-33 (2000), *Morus insignis* Basnet *et al., Chem Pharm Bull* (Tokyo) **41**(7), 1238-43 (1993) *Eucommia ulmoides* Kim *et al., J Ethnopharmacol* **93**(2-3), 227-30 (2004). *Bauhinia forficata* De-Sousa et *al., J Nat Prod* **67**(5), 829-32 (2004) Jorge *et al., Chem Biol Interact* **149**(2-3), 89-96 (2004) *Bauhinia megalandra* Estrada *et al., Phytother Res* **19**(10), 859-63 (2005)
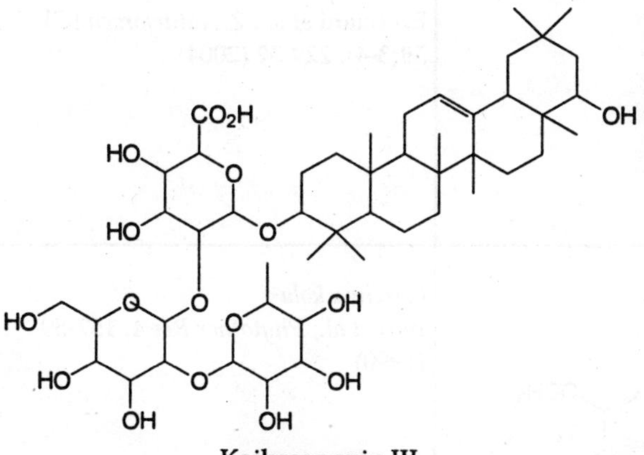 Kaikasaponin III	*Pueraria thunbergiana* Lee *et al., Arch Pharmacal Res* **23**(5), 461-66 (2000), Choi *et al., J Med Food* **7**(1), 31-37 (2004)

Kalopanaxsaponin A (3-O-[L-rhamnopyranosyl-(1→2)-α-L-arabinopyranosyl]-hederagenin)	*Kalopanax pictus* Park *et al.*, *Arch Pharm Res* **21**(1), 24-29 (1998).
Kaurenoic acid	*Wedelia paludosa* Bresciani *et al.*, *Z Naturforsch* [C]. **59**(3-4), 229-32 (2004)
Kola flavanone	*Garcinia kola* Iwu *et al.*, *Phytother Res* **4**, 157-59 (1990)

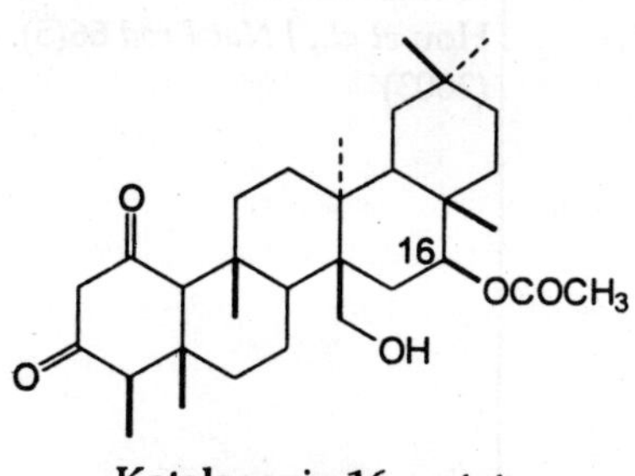 Kotalagenin 16-acetate	*Salacia oblonga* Matsuda *et al.*, *Chem Pharm Bull* (Tokyo) **47**(12), 1725-29 (1999)
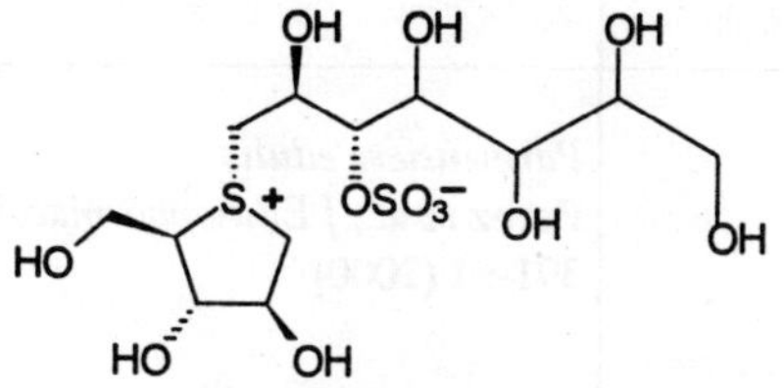 Kotalanol	*Salacia oblonga* Matsuda *et al.*, *Chem Pharm Bull* (Tokyo) **47**(12), 1725-29 (1999) *Salacia reticulata* Yoshikawa *et al.*, *Chem Pharm Bull* (Tokyo) **46**(8), 1339-40 (1998)
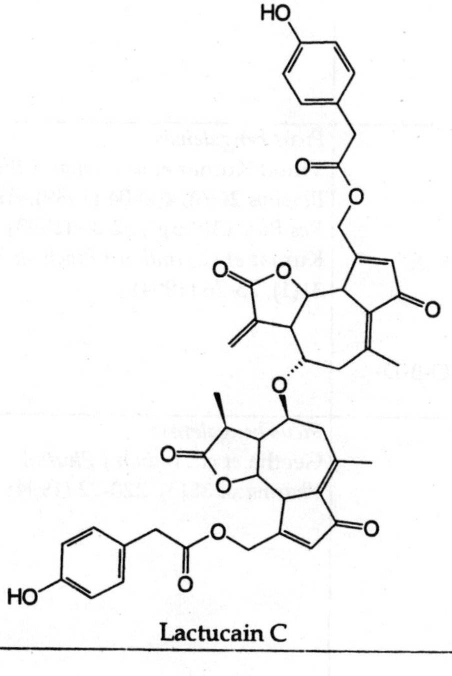 Lactucain C	*Lactuca indica* Hou *et al.*, *J Nat Prod* **66**(5), 625-29 (2003)

Compound	Source / Reference
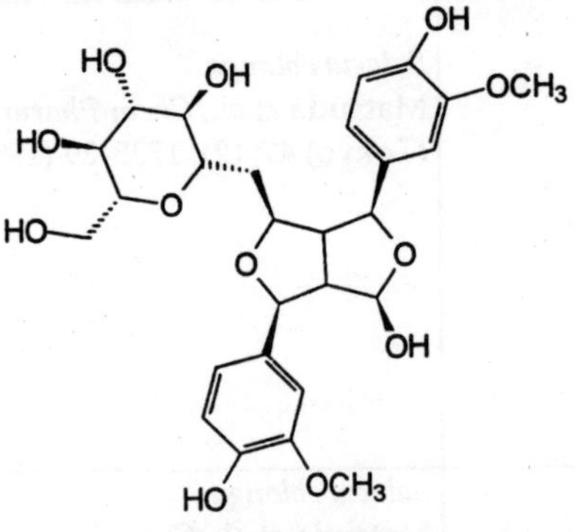 Lactucaside	*Lactuca indica* Hou *et al., J Nat Prod* **66**(5), 625-29 (2003)
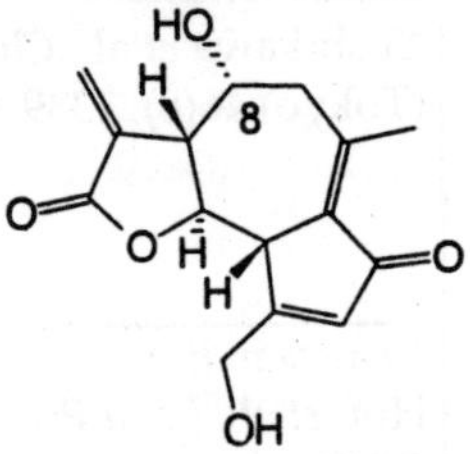 Lactucin Lactucin-8-O-methylacrylate	*Parmentiera edulis* Perez *et al., J Ethnopharmacol* **71**(3), 391-94 (2000)
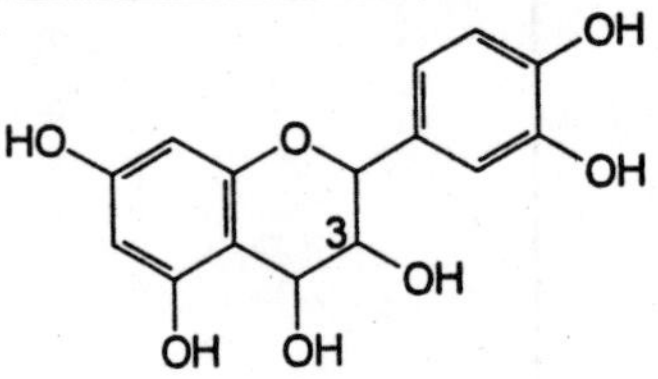 Leucocyanidin Dimethoxy derivative of leucocyanidin 3-O-β-D-galactosyl cellobioside	*Ficus bengalensis* Vinod Kumar *et al., Indian J Biochem Biophys* **26**(6), 400-04 (1989), *Amala Res Bull* **13**(Aug), 32-36 (1993) Kumar *et al., Indian J Biochem Biophys* **31**(1), 73-76 (1994)
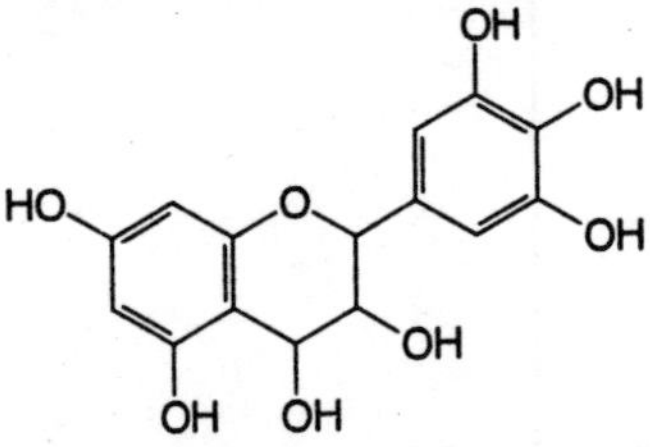 Leucodelphinidin A leucodelphinidin derivative	*Ficus bengalensis* Geetha *et al., Indian J Physiol Pharmacol* **38**(3), 220-22 (1994)

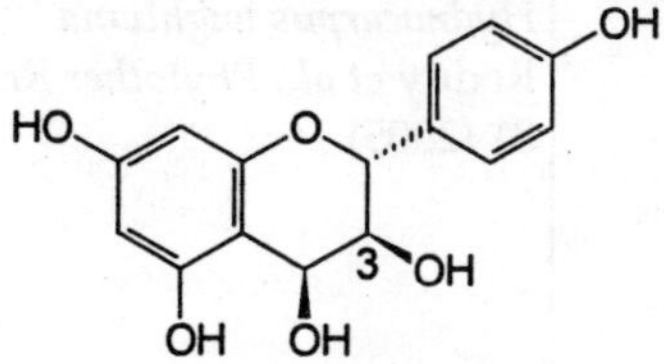 Leucopelargonidin Leucopelargonidin -3-O-□-L-rhamnoside	*Ficus bengalensis* Cherian *et al., Indian J Biochem Biophys* **29**(4), 380-82 (1992), *Indian J Exp Biol* **31**(1), 26-29 (1993), *Indian J Exp Biol* **33**(8), 608-11 (1995) Augusti *et al., Indian J Med Res* **99**(2), 82-86 (1994)
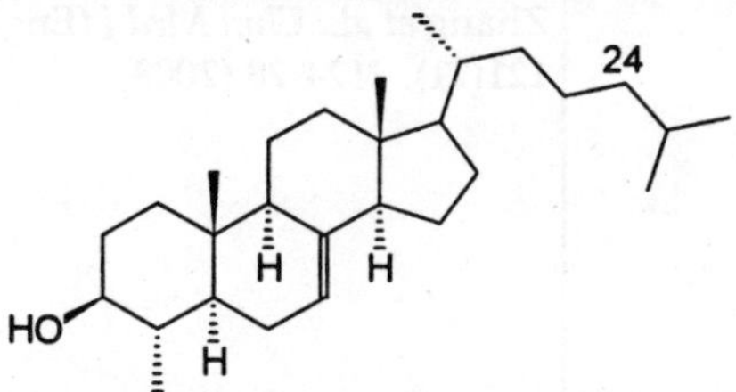 Lophenol 24-methyl-lophenol, 24-ethyl-lophenol	*Aloe barbadensis* (*Aloe vera*) Tanaka *et al., Biol Pharm Bull* **29**(7), 1418-22 (2006)
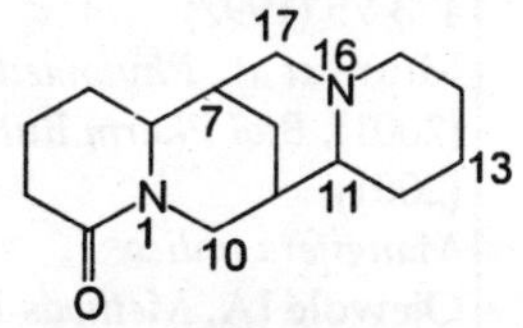 Lupanine 13-□ Hydroxy lupanine 17-Oxo-lupanine	*Genista tenera* Martins *et al., Phytochem Anal* **16**(4), 264-66 (2005) *Lupinus* species Garcia Lopez *et al., Eur J Pharmacol* **504**(1-2), 139-42 (2004).
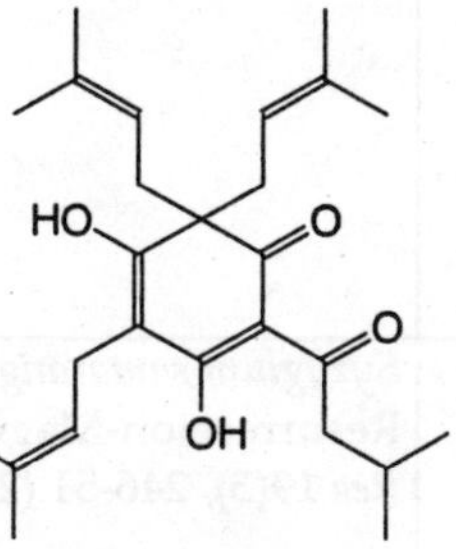 Lupulone	*Humulus lupulus* Aigo Nutritive Chemicals Ltd., *Japan Kakai Tokkyo Koho* JP 59, 59, 623, (Cl. A61. K35/78) 4 pp. 1984

Compound	Source and reference
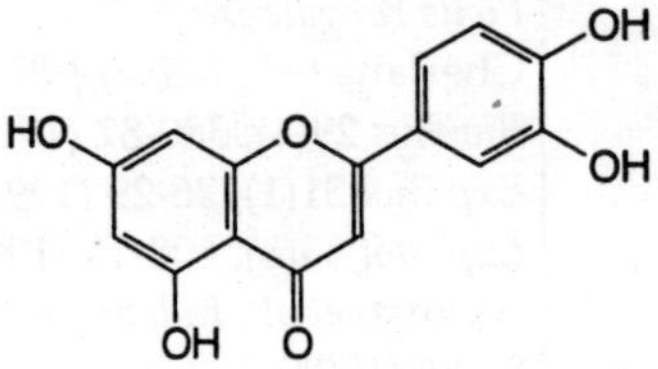 Luteolin	*Hydnocarpus wightiana* Reddy *et al., Phytother Res* **19**(4), 277-81 (2005)
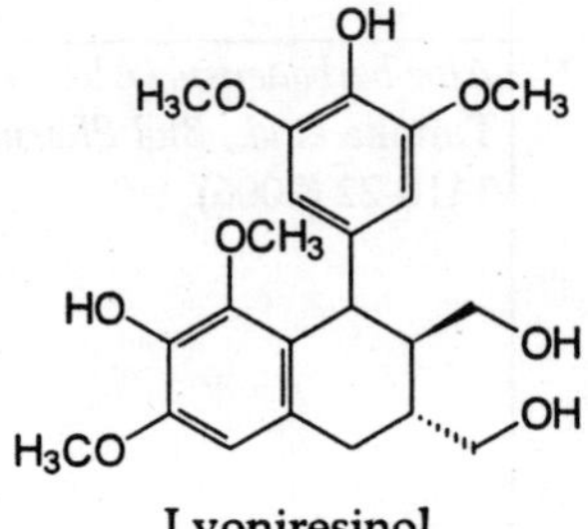 Lyoniresinol	*Berberis vulgaris* Zhang *et al., Chin Med J* (Engl) **121**(21), 2124-28 (2008)
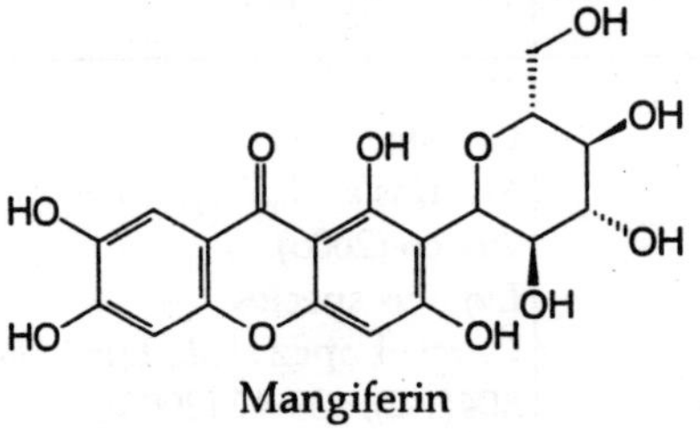 Mangiferin	*Anemarrhena asphodeloides* Hong *et al., Yao Xue Xue Bao* **32**(6), 473-75 (1997) Miura *et al., Phytomedicine* **8**(2), 85-87 (2001), *Biol Pharm Bull* **24**(9), 1009-11 (2001) *Mangifera indica* Ojewole JA; *Methods Find Exp Clin Pharmacol* **27**(8). 547-54 (2005)
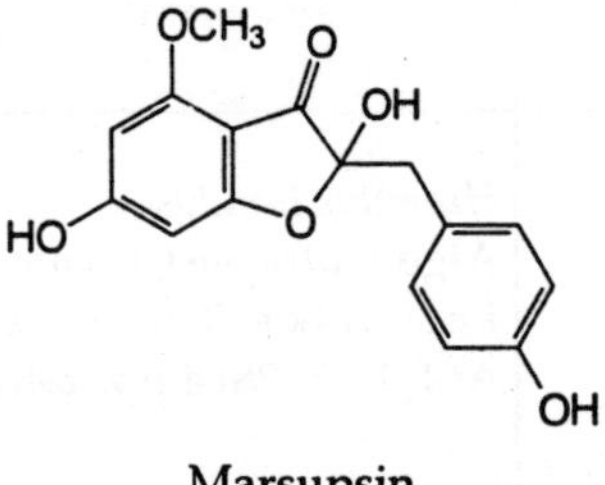 Marsupsin	*Pterocarpus marsupium* Manickam *et al., J Nat Prod* **60**(6), 609-10 (1997)
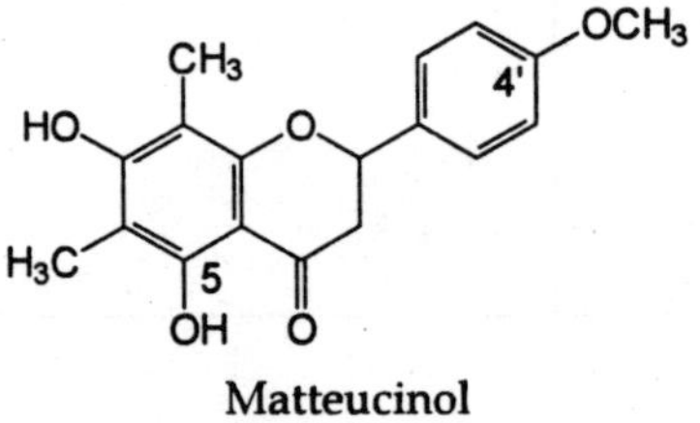 Matteucinol 5-O-Methyl-4'-desmethoxymatteucinol	*Syzygium samarangense* Resurreccion-Magno *et al., Phytother Res* **19**(3), 246-51 (2005)

HO HO HO₂C HO O O O OH OH O H H CO₂H Momordin 1c	*Kochia scoparia* Yoshikawa *et al.*, *Chem Pharm Bull* (Tokyo), **45**(8), 1300-05 (1997)
HO HO O OH Moracin M Moracin M-3-O-β-D-glucopyranoside	*Morus insignis* Basnet *et al.*, *Chem Pharm Bull* (Tokyo) **41**(7), 1238-43 (1993).
HO OH HO O OH OH O Morin	*Ficus bengalensis* Nagwa *et al.*, *Arch Pharm Res* **11**(2), 166-68 (1988)
HO O OH OH HO O OH HO OH Mulberrofuran U	*Morus insignis* Basnet *et al.*, *Chem Pharm Bull* (Tokyo) **41**(7), 1238-43 (1993).

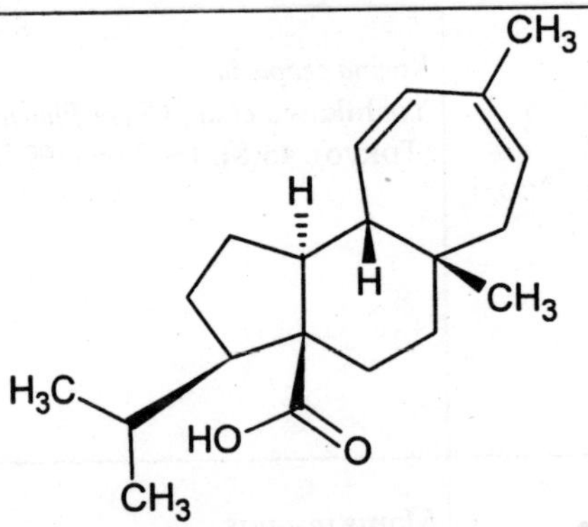 Mulin-11,13-dien-20-oic acid	*Azorella compacta* Fuentes *et al., Phytother Res* **19**(8), 713-16 (2005).
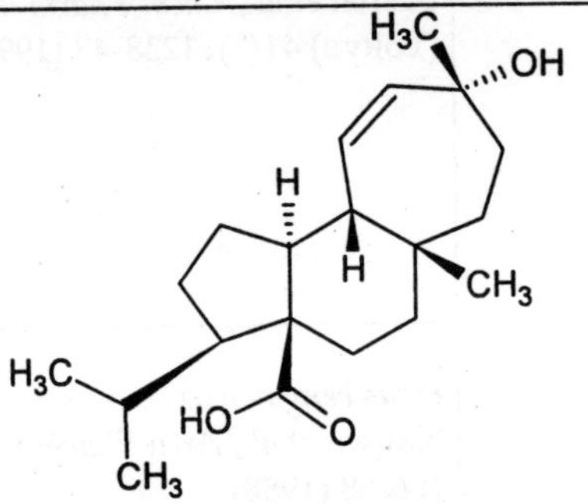 Mulinolic acid	*Azorella compacta* Fuentes *et al., Phytother Res* **19**(8), 713-16 (2005).
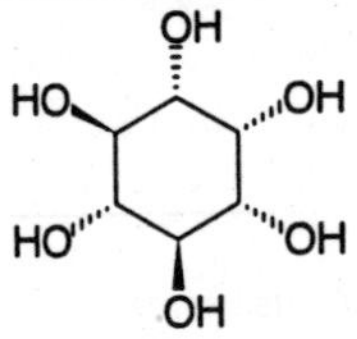 *Myo*-inositol	*Peucedanum japonicum* Lee *et al., Arch Pharm Res* **27**(12), 1207-10 (2004)
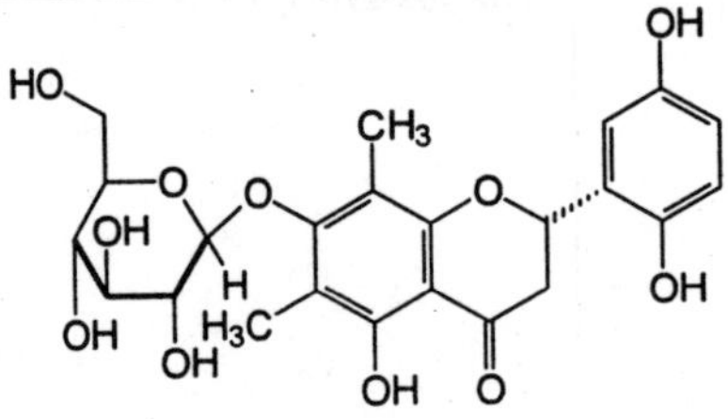 Myrciacitrin I	*Myrcia multiflora* Yoshikawa *et al., Chem Pharm Bull* (Tokyo) **46**(1), 113-19 (1998)

Compound	Source and reference
Myrciaphenone B	*Myrcia multiflora* Yoshikawa *et al.*, *Chem Pharm Bull* (Tokyo) **46**(1), 113-19 (1998)
Myricetin 4'-O-Methyl-5'-O-acetylmyricetin-3-O-gluco(2→1) rhamnoside,	*Abelmoschus moschatus* Liu *et al.*, *Planta Med* **71**(7), 617-21 (2005) *Zizyphus rugosa* Khosa *et al.*, *Indian Drugs* **20**(6), 241 (1983) *Pisonia morindifolia* Manogaran & Sulochana, *National Symposium on Emerging Trends in Indian Medicinal Plants*, Lucknow, p.27 (4-O/2), October 10-12, 2003
Naringenin Prunin (naringenin 7-O-β-D-glucoside)	*Prunus davidiana* Choi *et al.*, *Planta Med* **57**(3), 208-11(1991)
Neomangiferin (7-O-β-D-glucopyranosyl-mangiferin)	*Anemarrhena asphodeloides* Miura *et al.*, *Biol Pharm Bull* **24**(9), 1009-11 (2001)
N-Methylcytisine	*Genista tenera* Martins *et al.*, *Phytochem Anal* **16**(4), 264-66 (2005)., *Lygos raetam* Abdel Halim *et al.*, *Acta Pharm Hung* **67**(6), 241-47 (1997).

Nordihydroguaiaretic acid (Masoprocol)	*Larrea tridentata* Luo *et al., Eur J Pharmacol* **346**(1), 77-79 (1998)
Obtusifolin	*Cassia tora* Jang *et al., Biol Pharm Bull* **30**(11), 2207-10 (2007)
Oleanolic acid Oleanolic acid and ursolic acid (1:1) Oleanolic acid and oleanolic aldehyde Oleanolic acid 28-O-β-D-glucopyranoside Oleanolic acid 3-O-[β-D-xylopyranosyl (1→2)]-[β-D-glucopyranosyl (1→3)]-α-L-arabinopyranoside (Elatoside E) Oleanolic acid oligoglycosides (Betavulgarosides II, III, and IV) Oleanolic acid 3-O-glucuronide	*Aralia elata* Kim *et al., Korean J Pharmacogn* **24**(3), 219-22 (1993) *Tridax procumbens* Shaiq Ai *et al., Phytochemistry* **60**(3), 295-99 (2002) *Olea europaea* Somova *et al., J Ethnopharmacol* **84**(2-3), 299-305 (2003) *Vitis vinifera* Zhang *et al., J Agric Food Chem* **52**(2):228-33 (2004) *Aralia elata* Yoshikawa *et al., Chem Pharm Bull* (Tokyo) **42**(6), 1354-56 (1994), **43**(11), 1878-82 (1995),.**44**(10), 1923-27 (1996) *Beta vulgaris* Yoshikawa *et al., Chem Pharm Bull* (Tokyo) **44**(6), 1212-17 (1996) *Kochia scoparia* Matsuda *et al., Chem Pharm Bull* **46**(9), 1399-1403 (1998)
Oleuropeoside	*Olea europaea* Gonzalez *et al., Planta Med* **58**(6), 513-15 (1992)

Compound	Source
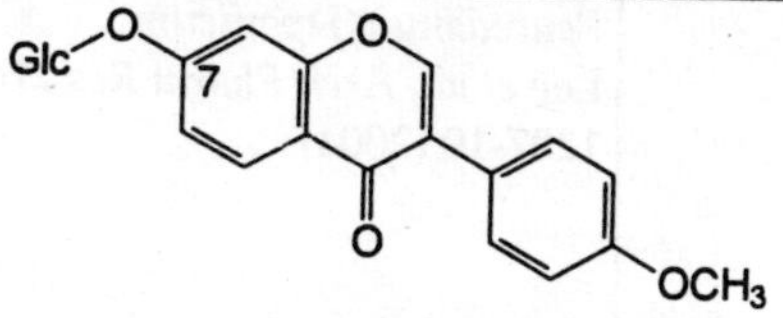 Ononin (Formononetin-7-O-β-D-glucopyranoside)	*Astragalus membranaceus* Wenjie *et al., Biol Pharm Bull* **30**(11), 2079-83 (2007)
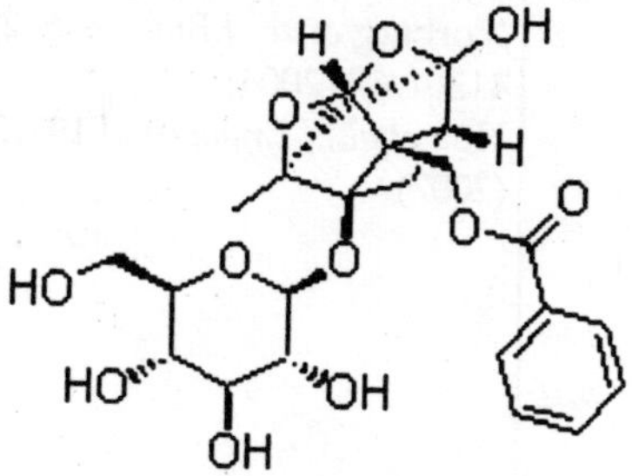 Paeoniflorin 8-Debenzoylpaeoniflorin Chem Blink	*Paeonia lactiflora* Hsu *et al., Planta Med* **63**(4), 323-25 (1997)
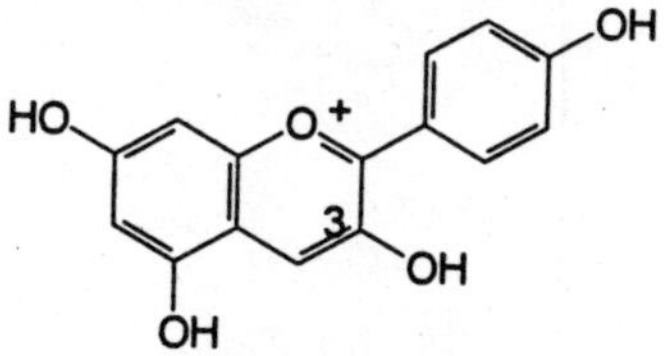 Pelargonidin Dimethoxy derivative of perlargonidin 3-O-α-L rhamnoside	*Ficus bengalensis* Cherian S *et al., Indian J Biochem Biophys* **29**(4), 380-82 (1992)
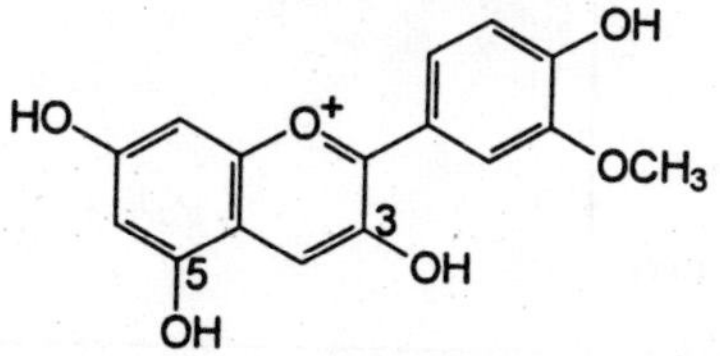 Peonidin Peonidin {3-O-[2-O-(6-O-*E*-feruloyl-β-D-glucopyranosyl)-6-O-*E*-caffeoyl-β-D-glucopyranoside]-5-O-β-D-glucopyranoside}	*Ipomoea batatas* cv. Ayamurasaki Matsui *et al., J Agric Food Chem* **50**(25), 7244-48 (2002)

Compound	Source / Reference
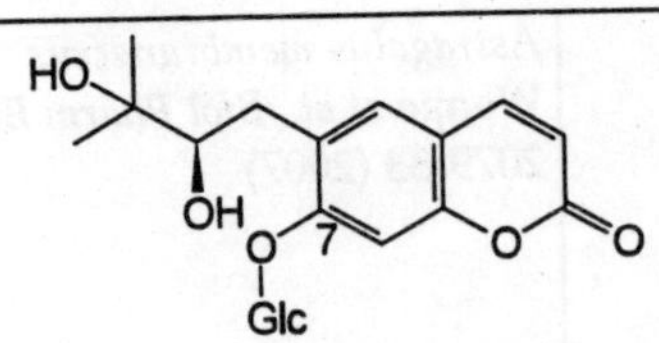 Peucedanol-7-O-β-D-glucopyranoside	*Peucedanum japonicum* Lee *et al., Arch Pharm Res* **27**(12), 1207-10 (2004)
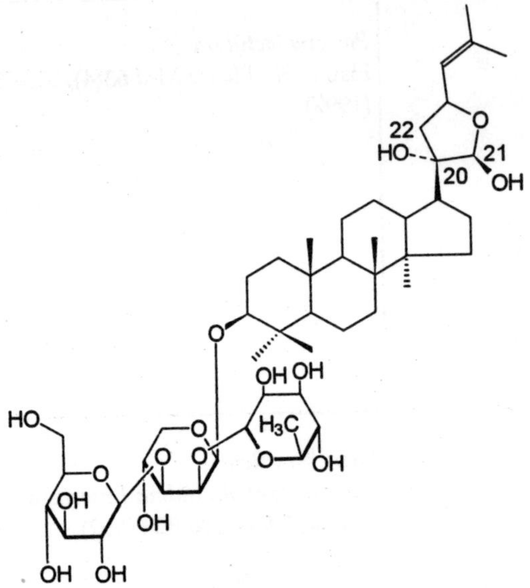 Phanoside	*Gynostemma pentaphyllum* Norberg *et al., J Biol Chem* **279**(40), 41361-67 (2004). Hoa *et al., J Endocrinol* **192**(2), 389-94 (2007)
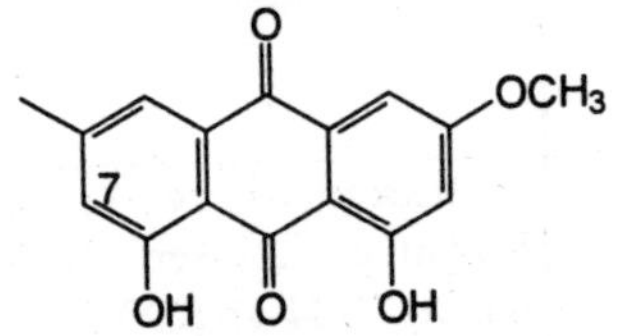 Physcion (1,8-Dihydroxy-3-methoxy-6-methyl-anthraquinone;) 7-Methylphyscion	*Cassia fistula* Vaishnava *et al., Fitoterapia* **64**(1), 95 (1993)
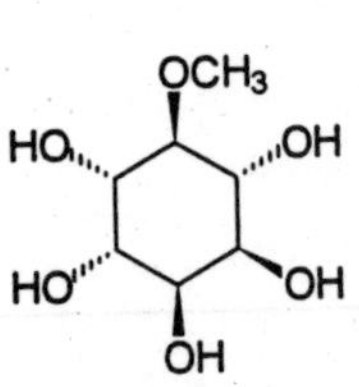 (+)-Pinitol	*Bougainvillea spectabilis* Narayanan *et al., Curr Sci* **56**(3), 139-41 (1987); Bates *et al., Br J Pharmacol* **130**(8), 1944-48 (2000) *Glycine max* Kim *et al., Eur J Clin Nutr* **59**(3), 456-58 (2005), Kang *et al., J Med Food* **9**(2), 182-86 (2006)

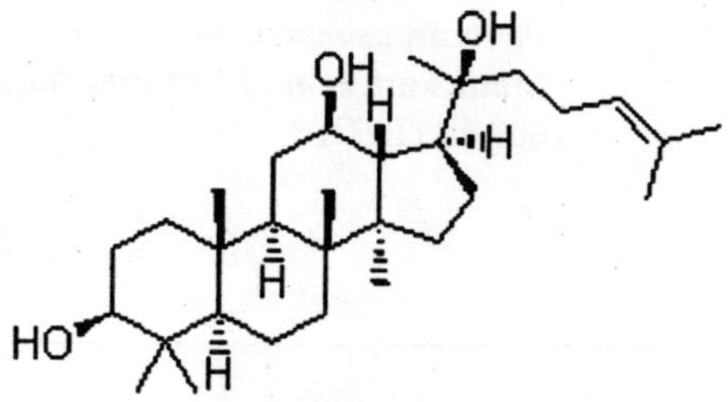 Protopanaxadiol 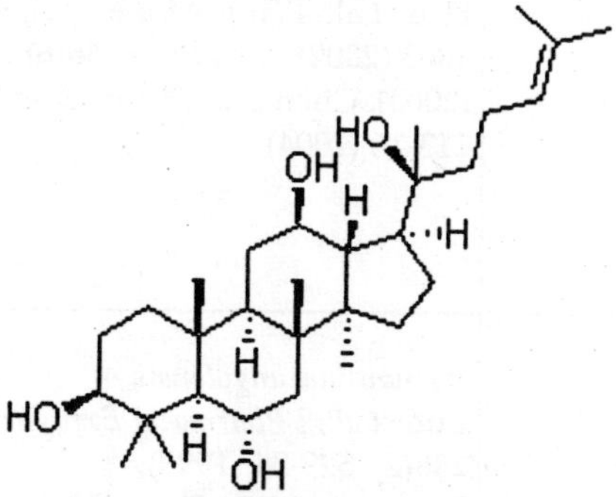 Protopanaxatriol Chem Blink	*Panax quinquefolius* **Sievenpiper** *et al., J Am Coll Nutr* **22**(6), 524-32 (2003), **23**(3), 248-58 (2004)
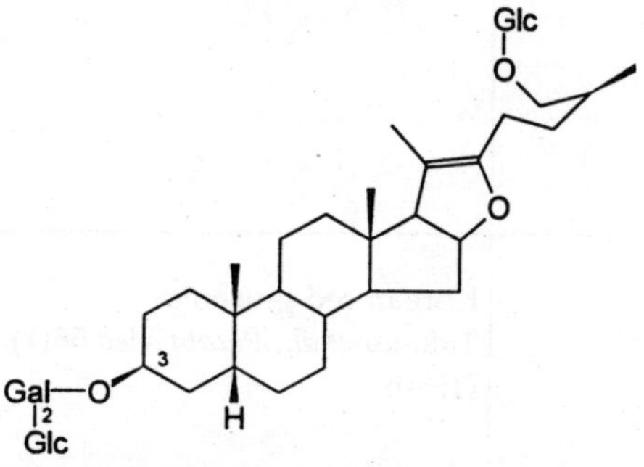 Pseudoprototimosaponin AIII	*Anemarrhena asphodeloides* **Nakashima** *et al., J Nat Prod* **56**(3), 345-50 (1993)
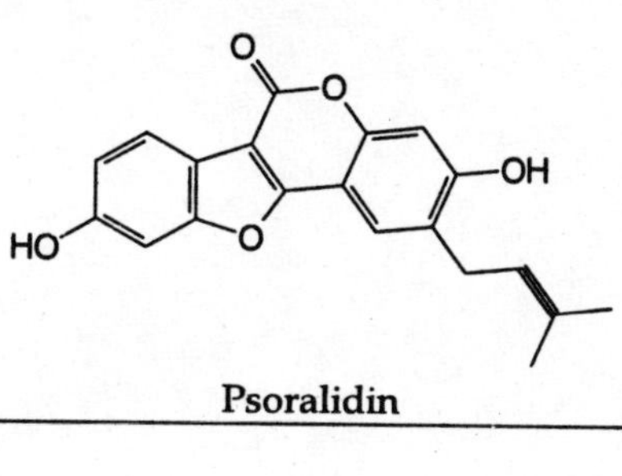 Psoralidin	*Psoralea corylifolia* *Kim et al., Planta Med* **71**(1), 87-89 (2005)

Compound	Source and reference
Pterostilbene	*Pterocarpus marsupium* Manickam *et al., J Nat Prod* **60**(6), 609-10 (1997)
Puerarin	*Pueraria lobata* Hsu *et* al., *Planta Med* **68**(11), 999-1003 (2002), *J Nat Prod* **66**(6), 788-92 (2003), Chen *et al.,Planta Med* **70**(2), 113-16 (2004)
Pycnanthuquinone A: R=α-OH Pycnanthuquinone B: R=β-OH	*Pycnanthus angolensis* Luo *et al., J Pharmacol Exp Ther* **288**(2), 529-34 (1999), Fort *et al., J Org Chem* **65**(20), 6534-39 (2000)
Pyro-glutamic acid	Korean red ginseng Takaku *et al., Planta Med* **56**(1), 27-30 (1990)

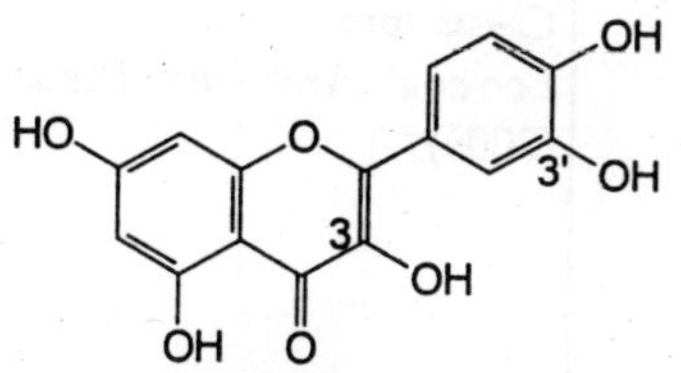 Quercetin Quercetin 3-rhamnoside (Quercitrin) Quercetin 3-O- α-(2"galloyl) rhamnoside Quercetin-3-neohesperidoside Quercetin 3-O-α-L-arabinopyranosyl-(1→2)-β-D-glucopyranoside, Quercetin-3-O- β -glucopyranoside (isoquercitrin) Quercetin-3′-methyl ether 3-O-β-D-glucopyranoside	*Ficus bengalensis* Nagwa *et al., Arch Pharm Res* **11**(2), 166-68 (1988) *Zizyphus rugosa* Khosa *et al., Indian Drugs* **20**(6), 241 (1983) *Amomum xanthioides* Kim Y-M *et al., The FASEB J* **21**, 845.4 (2007) *Bauhinia megalandra* Estrada et al., *Phytother Res* **19**(10), 859-63 (2005). *Bridelia ferruginea* Addae-Mensah *et al., Fitoterapia* **60**(4), 359-62 (1989) *Eucommia ulmoides* Kim *et al., J Ethnopharmacol* **93**(2-3), 227-30 (2004) *Morus insignis* Basnet *et al., Chem Pharm Bull* (Tokyo) **41**(7), 1238-43 (1993); *Phyllanthus sellowianus* Hnatyszyn *et al., Phytomedicine* **9**(6), 556-59 (2002) *Zygophyllum cornutum* Aclinou *et al., Plantes Medicinales et Phytother* **22**(4), 212-18 (1988)
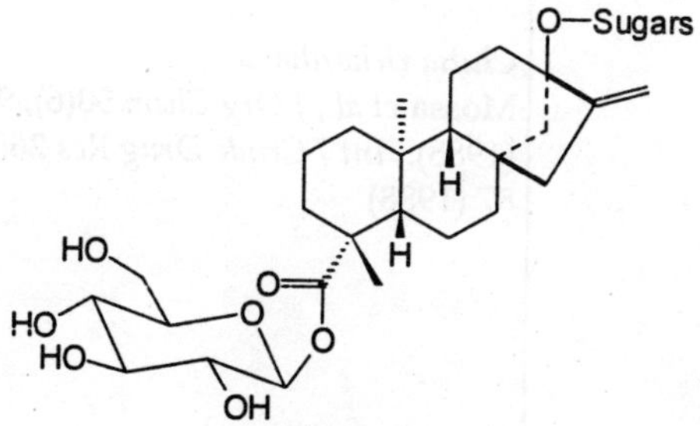 Rebaudioside A	*Stevia rebaudiana* Abudula *et al., Metabolism* **53**(10), 1378-81 (2004)
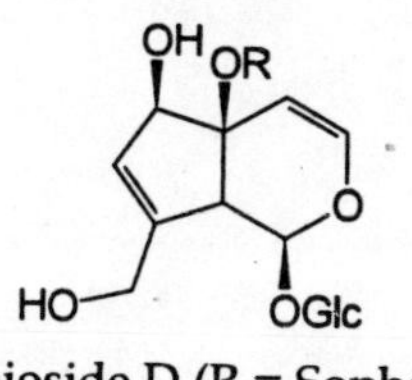 Rehmannioside D (R = Sophoroside)	*Rehmannia glutinosa* var. *hueichingensis* Oshio *et al., Phytochemistry* **21**(1), 133-38 (1982)

OH OH O 6 H_3CO O CH_3 Rubrofusarin Rubrofusarin-6-O-β-D-gentiobioside	*Cassia tora* Lee *et al*, *Arch Farm Res* **29**(7), 587-90 (2006)
OH HO O OH OR OH O Rutin (R = Rutinose) (Quercetin-3-rutinoside)	*Bridelia ferruginea* Onunkwo *et al.*, *Phytother Res* **10**(5), 418-20 (1996) *Phyllanthus sellowianus* Hnatyszyn *et al.*, *Phytomedicine* **9**(6), 556-59 (2002)
OH OH S+ OSO_3^- HO HO OH Salacinol	*Salacia chinensis* Yoshikawa *et al.*, *Yakugaku Zasshi* **123**(10), 871-80 (2003) *Salacia oblonga* Matsuda *et al.*, *Chem Pharm Bull* (Tokyo) **47**(12), 1725-29 (1999) *Salacia reticulate* Yoshikawa *et al.*, *Bioorg Med Chem* **10**(5), 1547-54 (2002)
O H O O O O O O Saudin	*Clutia richardiana* Mossa *et al.*, *J Org Chem* **50**(6), 916-18 (1985)., *Int J Crude Drug Res* **26**(2), 81-87 (1988)

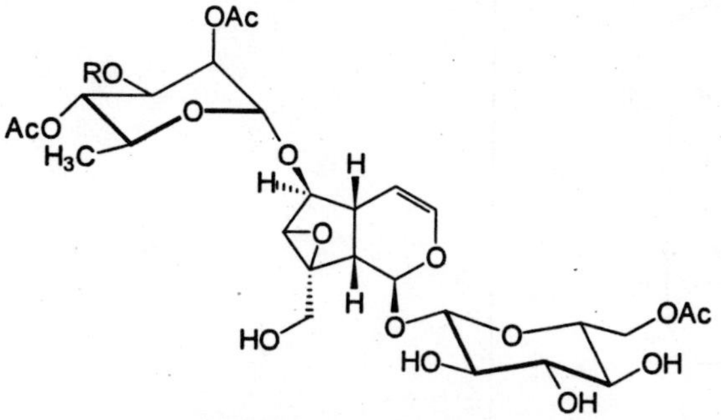 Scropolioside-D2 (R = cinnamoyl)	*Scrophularia deserti* Ahmed *et al., Biol Pharm Bull* **26**(4), 462-67 (2003)
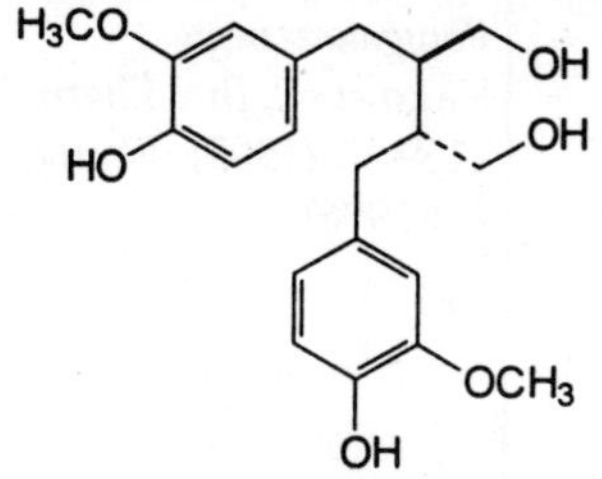 Secoisolariciresinol	*Taxus yunnanensis* Banskota *et al., Phytomedicine* **13**(1-2), 109-14 (2006)
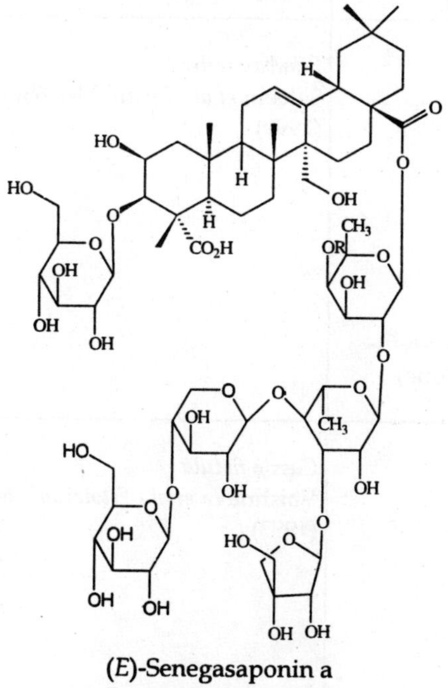 (*E*)-Senegasaponin a R = *trans*-cinnamoyl	*Polygala senega* L. var. *latifolia* Yoshikawa *et al., Chem Pharm Bull* (Tokyo) **43**(12), 2115-22 (1995)

HO, HO, O, H, H, H, OH, CH$_3$, OR, O, OH, CO$_2$H, OH, OH, OH, O, O, O, O, OH, CH$_3$, HO, OH, OH, OH, O, OH, OH, OH (*E*)-Senegasaponin b R = *trans*-cinnamoyl Senegin II (R =3,4-Dimethoxy-*trans*-cinnamoyl)	*Polygala senega* Kako *et al., Biol Pharm Bull* **18**(8), 1159-61 (1995), *Planta Med* **62**(5), 440-43 (1996)
OH, OH, HO, O, Glc, OH, OH, OH, O Shamimin (2-(2,4,5-trihydroxyphenyl)-3,5,7-trihydroxy-6-C-glucopyranosyloxy-4H-1-benzopyran-4-one)	*Bombax ceiba* Saleem *et al., Planta Med* **65**(4), 331-34 (1999).
H, H, H, H, HO β-Sitosterol	*Cassia fistula* Vaishnava *et al., Fitoterapia* **64**(1), 95 (1993).

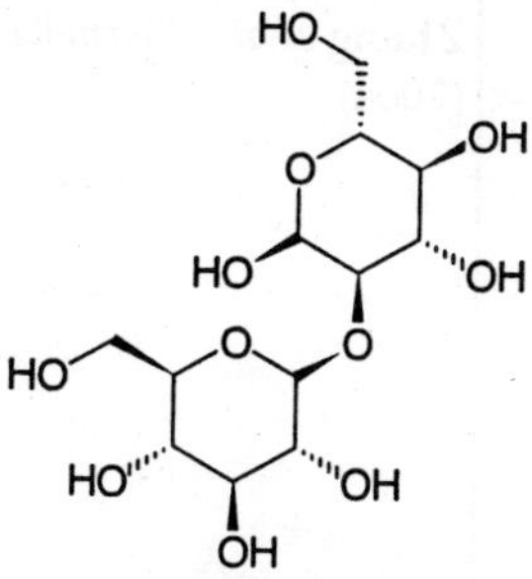 HO, OH, O, HO, OH, HO, O, O, HO, OH, OH Sophorose 6-O-caffeoylsophorose	*Ipomoea batatas* Matsui *et al., Biosci Biotechnol Biochem* **68**(11), 2239-46 (2004)
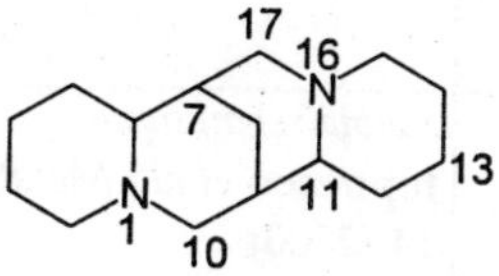 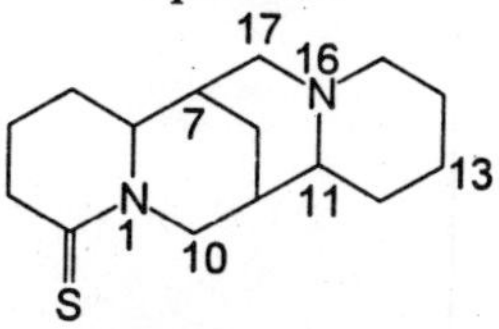 17, 16, N, 7, 13, N, 11, 1, 10 Sparteine 17, 16, N, 7, 13, N, 11, 1, 10, S 2-Thionosparteine	*Lupinus* species Garcia Lopez *et al. Eur J Pharmacol* **504**(1-2), 139-42 (2004).
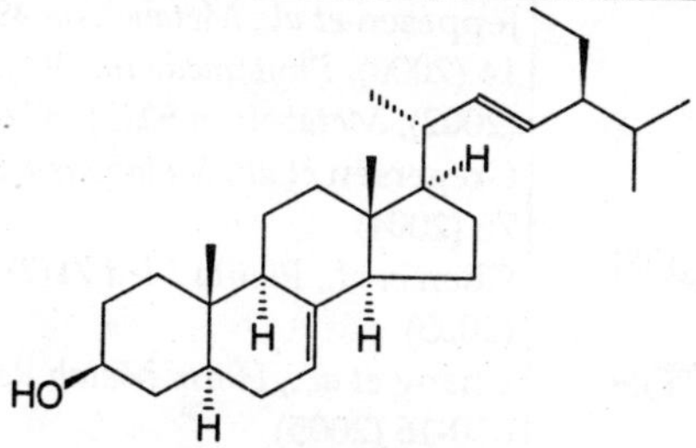 H, H, H, HO, H α-Spinasterol 3β,5α,22(*E*)-Stigmasta-7,22-dien-3-ol	*Phytolacca americana* Jeong *et al., Planta Med* **70**(8), 736-39 (2004)
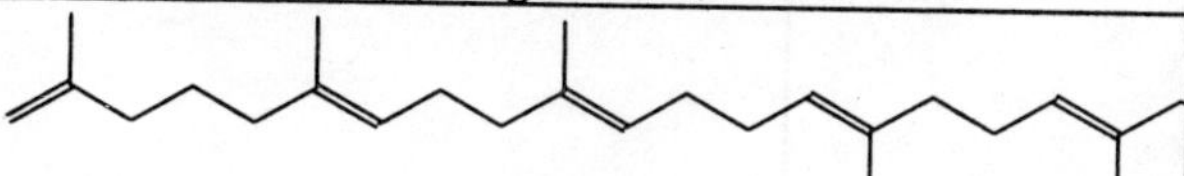 Squalene	*Amaranthus caudatus* Comforti *et al., Biol Pharm Bull* **28**(6), 1098-102 (2005)

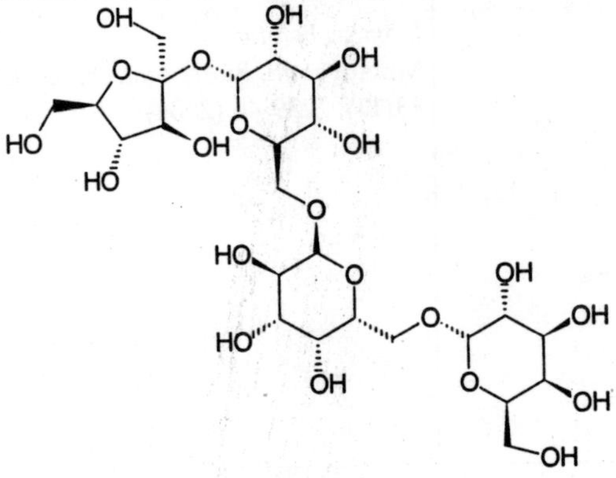 Stachyose	*Rehmannia glutinosa* Zhang *et al.*, *Pharmazie* **59**(7), 552-56 (2004)
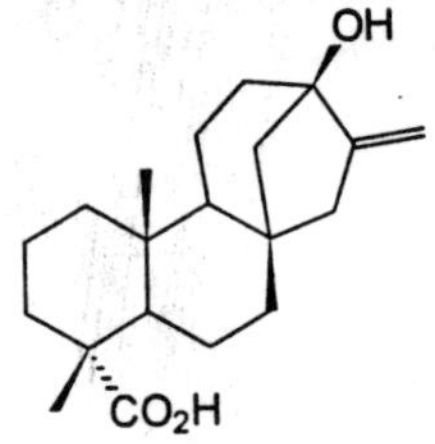 Steviol	*Stevia rebaudiana* Jeppesen *et al.*, *Metabolism* **49**(2), 208-14 (2000)
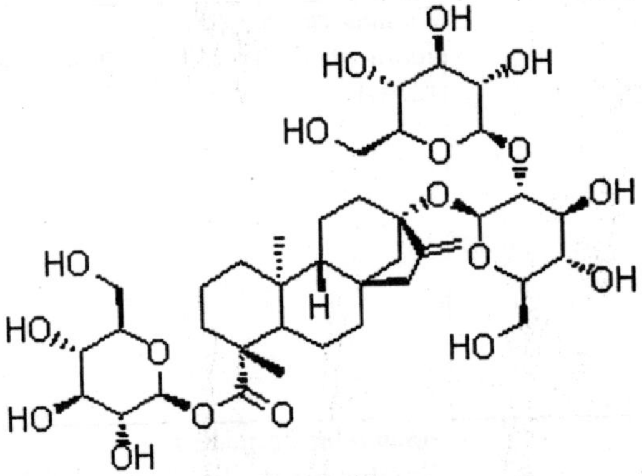 *** Stevioside Chem Blink	*Stevia rebaudiana* Jeppesen *et al.*, *Metabolism* **49**(2), 208-14 (2000), *Phytomedicine* **9**(1), 9-14 (2002), *Metabolism* **52**(3), 372-8 (2003) Gregersen *et al.*, *Metabolism* **53**(1), 73-76 (2004) Chen *et al.*, *Planta Med* **71**(2), 108-13 (2005) Chang *et al .*, *Horm Metab Res* **37**(10), 610-16 (2005) Ferreira *et al.*, *Planta Med* **72**(8), 691-96 (2006)

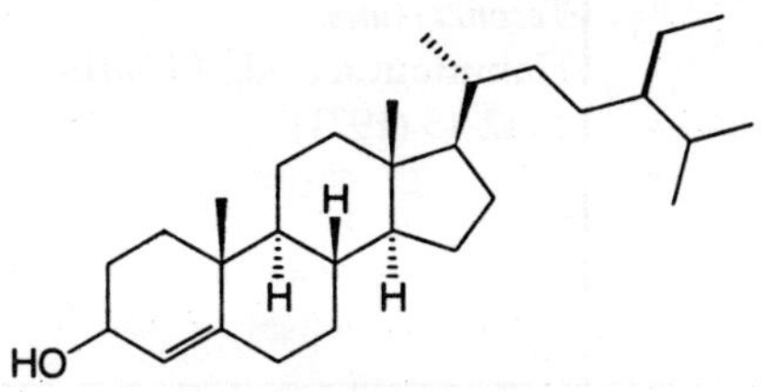 HO H H H Stigmast-4-en-3-ol Stigmast-4-en-3-one	*Anacardium occidentale* Alexander-Lindo *et al., Phytother Res* **18**(5), 403-07 (2004). *Parkia speciosa* Jamaluddin *et al., Food Chem* **54**(1), 9-13 (1995).
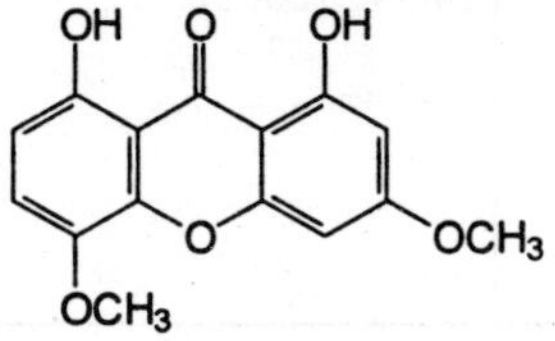 OH O OH O OCH_3 OCH_3 Swerchirin (1,8-dihydroxy-3,5-dimethoxyxanthone)	*Swertia chirayita* Bajpai *et al., Planta Med* **57**(2), 102-04 (1991) Saxena *et al., Indian J Exp Biol* **31**(2), 178-81 (1993), *Indian J Exp Biol* **34**(4), 351-55 (1996)
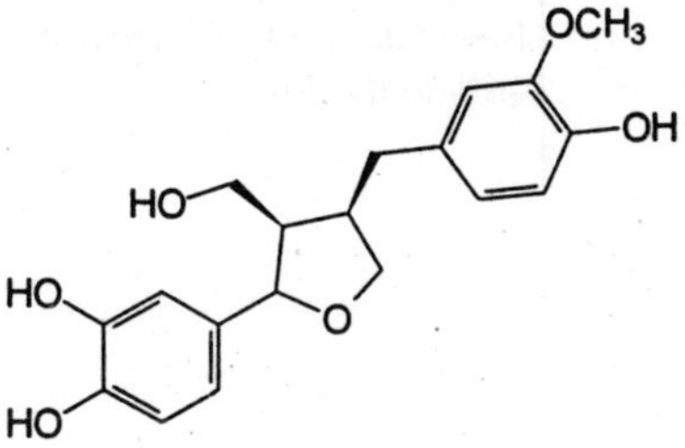 OCH_3 OH HO HO O HO Taxiresinol	*Taxus yunnanensis* Banskota *et al., Phytomedicine* **13**(1-2), 109-14 (2006)
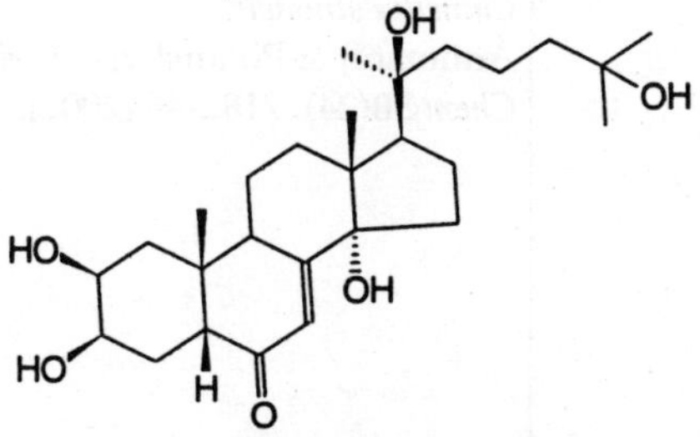 OH OH HO OH HO H O Taxisterone (22-Deoxy-20-hydroxyecdysone)	*Taxus cuspidata* Nakano *et al., Phytochemistry* **21**(11), 2749-51 (1982)

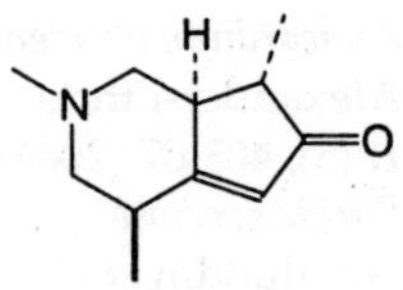 Tecomine	*Tecoma stans* Hammouda *et al., J Pharm Sci* **60**(8), 1142-45 (1971)
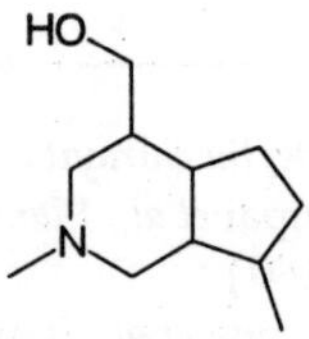 Tecostanine	*Tecoma stans* Costantino *et al., Pharmazie* **58**(2), 140-42 (2003)
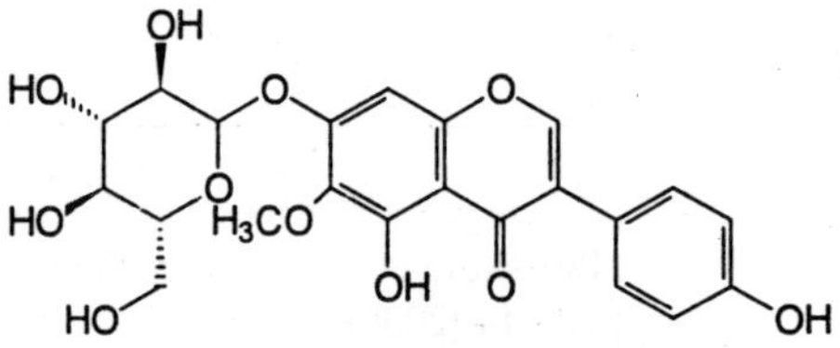 Tectoridin 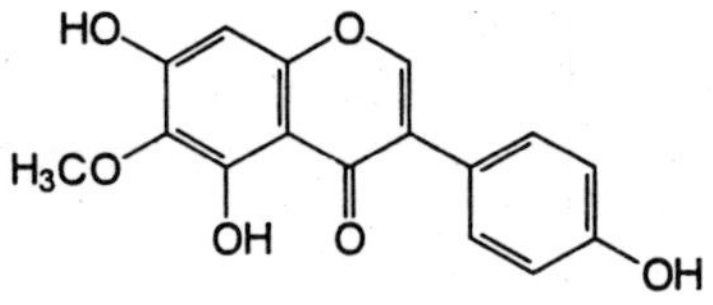Tectorigenin	*Belamcanda chinensis* Jung *et al., Arch Pharmacal Res* **25**(3), 306-12 (2002) *Pueraria thunbergiana* Lee *et al., Arch Pharmacal Res* **23**(5), 461-66 (2000)
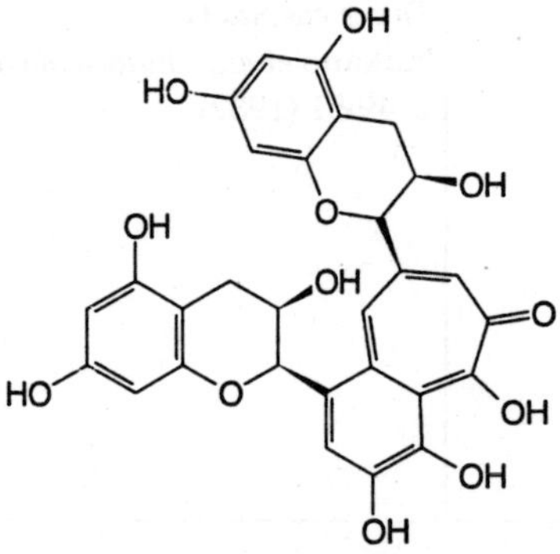 Theaflavin	*Camellia sinensis* Anderson & Polansky; *J Agric Food Chem* **50**(24), 7182-86 (2002).

Thymoquinone (2-isopropyl-5-methyl-1, 4-benzoquinone)	*Nigella sativa* El-Dakhakhny *et al., Planta Med* **68**(5), 465-66 (2002)
Toralactone-9-O- β -D-gentiobioside	*Cassia tora* Lee *et al, Arch Farm Res* **29**(7), 587-90 (2006)
Tormentic acid	*Poterium ancistroides* Villar *et al., Planta Med* (**1**), 43-45 (1986); Ivorra *et al., Planta Med* **54**(4), 282-86 (1988)
trans-Dehydrocrotonin	*Croton cajucara* Farias *et al., Planta Med* **63**(6), 558-60 (1997) Silva *et al., Diabetes Obes Metab* **3**(6), 452-56 (2001).

3,4,5-Tri-caffeoylquinic acid	Brazilian propolis Matsui *et al., Biol Pharm Bull* **27**(11), 1797-803 (2004)
3 β,7 β,25-Trihydroxycucurbita-5,23(*E*)-dien-19-al	*Momordica charantia* Harinantenaina *et al., Chem Pharm Bull* (Tokyo) **54**(7),:1017-21 (2006)
(-)-Uniflorine A Uniflorine B	*Eugenia uniflora* Matsumura *et al.,Pharmaceut Biol* **34** (4), 302-07 (2000).
12-Ursene	*Agarista mexicana* Perez *et al., Phytother Res* **16**(1), 55-58 (2002)

HO H H H CO_2H Ursolic acid	*Cornus mas* Jayaprakasam *et al.*, *J Agric Food Chem* **54**(1), 243-48 (2006). *Morus insignis* Basnet *et al.*, *Chem Pharm Bull* (Tokyo) **41**(7), 1238-43 (1993) *Olea europaea*, subspecies *Africana* Somova *et al.*, *J Ethnopharmacol* **84**(2-3), 299-305 (2003)
HO H H O O O H Vulgarin	*Artemisia cannariensis* Peran *et al.*, *Rev Iber Endocrinol* **23**(134), 171-78 (1976) [Article in Spanish]
OH HO OH OCH_3 O Xanthohumol	*Humulus lupulus* Nozawa *et al.*, *Biochem Biophys Res Commun* **336**(3), 754-61 (2005)